Clinical Diagnosis and Management of Dystonia

Clinical Diagnosis and Management of Dystonia

Edited by

THOMAS T WARNER PhD FRCP

Department of Clinical Neurosciences
Institute of Neurology, University College London
and Royal Free Hospital
National Hospital for Neurology and Neurosurgery
London, UK

SUSAN B BRESSMAN MD

Department of Neurology
Beth Israel Medical Center and
Albert Einstein College of Medicine
New York, NY, USA

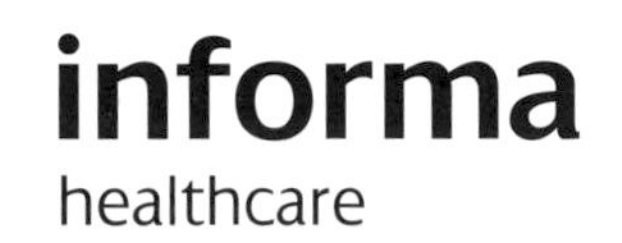

First published in the United Kingdom in 2007 by Informa Healthcare, Telephone House, 69-77 Paul Street, London EC2A 4LQ. Informa Healthcare is a trading division of Informa UK Ltd. Registered Office: 37/41 Mortimer Street, London W1T 3JH. Registered in England and Wales number 1072954.

Tel: +44(0)20 7017 5000
Fax: +44(0)20 7017 6699
Website: www.informahealthcare.com

A CIP record for this book is available from the British Library.

Library of Congress Cataloging-in-Publication Data

Data available on application

ISBN-10: 1 84184 317 2
ISBN-13: 978 1 84184 317 9

Distributed in North and South America by
Taylor & Francis
6000 Broken Sound Parkway, NW, (Suite 300)
Boca Raton, FL 33487, USA

Within Continental USA
Tel: 1 (800) 272 7737; Fax: 1 (800) 374 3401
Outside Continental USA
Tel: (561) 994 0555; Fax: (561) 361 6018
Email: orders@crcpress.com

Distributed in the rest of the world by
Thomson Publishing Services
Cheriton House
North Way
Andover, Hampshire SP10 5BE, UK
Tel: +44 (0)1264 332424
Email: tps.tandfsalesorder@thomson.com

Composition by Exeter Premedia Services Pvt. Ltd., Chennai, India
Printed and bound in India by Replika Press Pvt Ltd

Contents

Contributors

Fereshte Adib Saberi MD
Department of Neurology
Klinicum Nord
Hamburg
Germany

Alberto Albanese MD
Fondazione IRCCS Istituto Neurologico Carlo Besta
Università Cattolica del Sacro Cuore
Milan
Italy

Kotura Asanuma MD
Center for Neurosciences
Feinstein Institute for Medical Research
North Shore – Long Island Jewish Health System
Manhassett, NY
USA

Friedrich Asmus MD
Hertie-Institute for Clinical Brain Research
Department of Neurodegenerative Diseases
University of Tübingen
Tübingen
Germany

Anna Rita Bentivoglio MD
Istituto di Neurologia
Università Cattolica del Sacro Cuore
Rome
Italy

Kailash P Bhatia MD DM MRCP
Sobell Department of Motor Neuroscience and Movement Disorders
Institute of Neurology
University College London
London
UK

Jean-Pierre Bleton PT
Physiotherapy Unit
Neurology Department
Raymond Garcin Center
Sainte-Anne Hospital
Paris
France

Yvette M Bordeon MD PhD
Department of Neurology
David Geffen School of Medicine at UCLA
Reed Neurological Research Institute
Los Angeles, CA
USA

Susan B Bressman MD
Department of Neurology
Beth Israel Medical Center and
Albert Einstein College of Medicine
New York, NY
USA

Stefan J Cano PhD
Neurological Outcome Measures Unit
Institute of Neurology
University College London
London
UK

Maren Carbon MD
Center for Neurosciences
Feinstein Institute for Medical Research
North Shore – Long Island Jewish Health System
Manhassett, NY
USA

Anabel R Chade MD
Centro Neurologico Hospital Frances
Buenos Aires
Argentina

Martin Cloutier MD FRCPC
Hopital Charles-Lemoyne
Service de Neurologie
Greenfield Park, QC
Canada

Cynthia L Comella MD
Department of Neurological Sciences
Rush University Medical Center
Chicago, IL
USA

Dirk Dressler MD
Department of Neurology
Rostock University
Rostock
Germany

Mark J Edwards
Sobell Department of Motor Neuroscience and Movement Disorders
Institute of Neurology
University College London
London
UK

David Eidelberg MD
Center for Neurosciences
Feinstein Institute for Medical Research
North Shore – Long Island Jewish Health System
Department of Neurology
North Shore University Hospital
Manhasset, NY
New York University School of Medicine
New York, NY
USA

Antonio E Elia
Fondazione IRCCS Istituto Neurologico Carlo Besta
Università Cattolica del Sacro Cuore
Milan
Italy

Steven J Frucht MD
Columbia University Medical Center
Department of Neurology
The Neurological Institute
New York, NY
USA

Thomas Gasser MD
Hertie-Institute for Clinical Brain Research
Department of Neurodegenerative Diseases
University of Tübingen
Tübingen
Germany

Howard L Geyer MD PhD
Department of Neurology
Albert Einstein College of Medicine
Montefiore Medical Center
Bronx, New York, NY
USA

Paul Greene MD
Associate Professor of Clinical Neurology
Dystonia Clinical Research Center
Neurological Institute
Columbia-Presbyterian Medical Center
New York, NY
USA

Mark Hallett MD
Human Motor Control Section
National Institute of Neurological Disorders and Stroke
Bethesda, MD
USA

Joseph Jankovic MD
Parkinson's Disease Center
and Movement Disorders Clinic
Baylor College of Medicine Department of Neurology
Houston, TX
USA

Christoph Kamm MD
Hertie-Institute for Clinical Brain Research
Department of Neurodegenerative Diseases
University of Tübingen
Tübingen
Germany

Su Kanchana MD PhD
Division of Neurology,
Department of Neuroscience
Lehigh Valley Hospital and Health Network
Allentown, PA
USA

Meike Kasten MD
Klinik für Psychiatrie and Psychotherapie
Lübeck
Germany

Marianne King
Dystonia Nurse Specialist
PNRU
Sharoe Green Hospital
Fulwood, Preston
UK

Joachim K Krauss MD
Professor and Chairman
Department of Neurosurgery
Medical University Hannover, MHH
Hannover
Germany

Anthony E Lang MD FRCPC
University Health Network
Toronto Western Hospital
Department of Medicine
Division of Neurology
University of Toronto
Toronto, Ontario
Canada

Thomas J Loher MD
Department of Neurology
University of Berne
Salem Spital
Berne
Switzerland

Christy L Ludlow PhD
Laryngeal and Speech Section
National Institute of
Neurological Disorders and Stroke
Bethesda, MD
USA

Jörg Müller MD
Department of Neurology
Medical University Innsbruck
Innsbruck
Austria

Laurie J Ozelius PhD
Albert Einstein College of Medicine
Department of Genetics and Genomic Sciences
Mount Sinai School of Medicine
New York, NY
USA

Werner Poewe MD
Department of Neurology
Medical University Innsbruck
Innsbruck
Austria

Tamara Pringsheim MD
University Health Network
Toronto Western Hospital
Department of Medicine
Division of Neurology
University of Toronto
Toronto, Ontario
Canada

Caroline M Tanner MD PhD
Director, Clinical Research
The Parkinson's Institute
Sunnyvale, CA
USA

Ronald Tintner
Parkinson's Disease Center and Movement
Disorders Clinic
Department of Neurology
Baylor College of Medicine
Houston, TX
USA

Enza Maria Valente
Institute C.S.S. Mendel
Rome
Italy

Thomas T Warner PhD FRCP
Department of Neurosciences
Institute of Neurology
Royal Free Hospital
National Hospital for Neurology and Neurosurgery
University College London
London
UK

Preface

It is almost 100 years since the first clinical descriptions were made of cases of dystonia. In the ensuing century, the study of this protean movement disorder has undergone a turbulent evolution, with dramatic shifts in the views regarding its causation and phenomenology. Having been considered for a considerable period of time as a psychological or psychiatric disorder, the dystonias are now recognized to be, in the majority of cases, an organic neurological disorder.

The time, therefore, is fitting to take stock of our knowledge of the various conditions that we now recognize as dystonias. This is the primary aim of this volume. We have drawn together a series of monographs from world leaders in the field of dystonia. We hope that this book will lead the reader through the phenomenology and etiology of dystonia, to then describe specific forms. The final chapters summarise various medical and surgical treatment strategies for dystonia, including paramedical input, and the book concludes on how we can measure dystonia and its effects on quality of life.

By nature, a collection of chapters by numerous authors will contain some repetition, but we hope this has been kept to a minimum and, where it exists, is important for the issues being discussed.

We are very grateful for all the authors who contributed during the prolonged gestation of this book, and for the support they have given. The same applies to the families of the editors and publishers! Finally, both editors have benefited from working with two supreme clinical neurologists, whose contribution to the study of dystonia has been immense: the late David Marsden in London and Stanley Fahn in New York. Their energy and clinical skills in dissecting out the clinical and anatomical basis of dystonia has been inspirational.

We hope that this book will further encourage young neurologists and neuroscientists to focus their energies in the area of dystonia to take forward our understanding of this movement disorder in the next 100 years.

Tom Warner
Susan Bressman

1

Diagnosis of dystonia

Howard L Geyer and Susan B Bressman

INTRODUCTION

Dystonia is a movement disorder characterized by patterned, directional, and sustained muscle contractions that produce abnormal, often twisting, postures or repetitive movements. Dystonia can result from a wide variety of causes, and clinicians must endeavor to elucidate its etiology in every patient in order to tailor optimal counseling and therapy for each individual. Although our understanding of the basic pathophysiologic mechanisms that give rise to this condition remains incomplete, thanks to advances in fields as disparate as neuroimaging and molecular genetics, modern diagnostic testing permits a specific diagnosis to be applied in many patients with dystonia. This chapter will present one diagnostic approach to patients with dystonia.

IDENTIFYING DYSTONIA

An important first step in diagnosing dystonia is recognizing abnormal movements as dystonic. Dystonic contractions tend to exhibit consistent directionality, and are patterned, repeatedly involving the same muscle groups; this latter feature differentiates dystonia from disorders such as chorea in which it is often impossible to predict which muscles will move next. The movements typically cause twisting of body parts, as connoted by the term torsion dystonia; in body parts that do not permit twisting, such as the jaw, there is consistent directionality (e.g. jaw opening or closing). Movements are usually more sustained (i.e. of longer duration) than other hyperkinesias, such as myoclonus. Although dystonia may result in jerking movements that mimic tremor, dystonic 'tremor' exhibits a directional preponderance (i.e. relatively forceful jerks in one direction alternate with slower movements in the opposite direction) which distinguishes it from the sinusoidal oscillations of true tremor. Unlike tics, dystonia is not preceded by an urge to perform the movement, nor is it associated with relief once the movement is executed. During dystonic movements, agonist and antagonist muscles contract simultaneously.[1]

Typically, dystonia is aggravated by voluntary movement, and in action dystonia, the dystonic movements are present only with voluntary movement. When dystonia is elicited exclusively by particular actions, it is called task-specific dystonia; examples include writer's cramp, which affects the arm and hand muscles involved in writing, and the embouchure dystonia of the orobuccal muscles observed in woodwind and brass musicians. Activation of dystonic movements by actions in remote parts of the body is called overflow; examples include leg dystonia while writing and axial dystonia induced by talking. More rarely, voluntary activity actually suppresses the dystonia; such paradoxical dystonia is more common in dystonia involving facial and oromandibular muscles. For example, talking or chewing may suppress eye closure in blepharospasm or jaw opening in oromandibular dystonia. Many patients discover a tactile or proprioceptive sensory trick (geste antagonistc) that minimizes the dystonia; for instance, a patient with head tilt due to cervical dystonia may lightly touch the chin to keep the head straight. Like many movement disorders, dystonia is worsened by fatigue and emotional stress, and the movements usually abate with relaxation or sleep.

A number of conditions that can produce abnormal postures resembling dystonia should be considered in the differential diagnosis. Causes of such pseudodystonia include disorders of the central and peripheral nervous systems as well as non-neurologic conditions. Tonic seizures can produce sustained twisting movements, and should be considered when symptoms are paroxysmal. Head tilt can result from vestibulopathy, trochlear nerve palsy, or a mass lesion in the posterior fossa or retropharyngeal space. Head tilt may also develop in patients (typically young boys) with hiatal hernia and gastroesophageal reflux (Sandifer syndrome). Apraxia of eyelid opening or ptosis of any etiology can be mistaken for blepharospasm. Stiff-person syndrome causes sustained contraction of axial and proximal limb muscles, and may be etiologically related to Satayoshi syndrome, a childhood disorder with painful muscle contractions, malabsorption, and alopecia.[2,3] Neuromuscular causes of sustained muscle contraction include neuromyotonia (Isaac syndrome), myotonic disorders, and rarely inflammatory myopathies. Carpopedal spasms can result from tetany due to hypocalcemia, hypomagnesemia, or alkalosis. Orthopedic and rheumatologic processes affecting bones, ligaments, or joints can also result in abnormal postures.

CLASSIFICATION OF DYSTONIA

Classifying a patient's dystonia along each of several dimensions aids greatly in prognosis and guides the diagnostic work-up and selection of therapy (Table 1.1). These dimensions include anatomic distribution of involved body areas, age at onset, and etiology of the dystonia.

Table 1.1 Classification of dystonia

Distribution

Focal:
- e.g. cervical dystonia, blepharospasm, spasmodic dysphonia, oromandibular dystonia, brachial dystonia

Segmental:
- e.g. Meige syndrome, craniocervical dystonia, bibrachial dystonia

Multifocal

Hemidystonia

Generalized

Age of onset

Early-onset (= 26 years) dystonia

Late-onset (<26 years) dystonia

Etiology

Primary (idiopathic) dystonia

Secondary dystonia:
- Associated with inherited neurologic conditions:
  - Dystonia-plus syndromes
  - Degenerative diseases
- Symptomatic of an exogenous/environmental cause
- Associated with Parkinson's disease and other parkinsonian disorders
- Dystonic phenomenology in another movement disorder
- Psychogenic dystonia

Anatomic distribution

In focal dystonia, the abnormal movements involve a single body region, whereas segmental dystonia affects two or more contiguous body parts. When dystonia is multifocal, two or more non-contiguous body areas are involved. Hemidystonia affects one side of the body. Generalized dystonia involves the legs (or one leg and the trunk) plus at least one other area of the body.

Cervical dystonia is the most common type of focal dystonia. Various abnormal head positions can occur, including torticollis (horizontal rotation), laterocollis (lateral tilting), anterocollis (flexion), and retrocollis (extension), depending on the particular combination of neck muscles involved. For example, torticollis may result from dystonic contraction of the ipsilateral splenius capitis and contralateral sternocleidomastoid muscles. Although pain is not a common finding in most forms of dystonia, approximately 75% of patients with cervical dystonia experience neck pain.[4] Like dystonia elsewhere, contractions vary in their duration, so that neck movements may be relatively tonic or more clonic. Clonic repetitive jerking of the head may resemble tremor, but unlike true tremor usually exhibits a directional preponderance. One maneuver that may help identify a directional preponderance is to observe the resultant position when the patient is asked to 'relax and let the head (or other involved body region) go in the direction it wants'. Another method is to ask the patient to slowly move the head in various directions and then observe for a 'null point' or a direction in which the jerking is quieted; alternatively, one may also seek to identify a direction in which the jerking is more forceful.

Less prevalent than cervical dystonia are focal dystonias involving cranial muscles. Spasmodic dysphonia is dystonia of the vocal cords; abnormal adduction, which causes a strained, strangled voice, is more common than abduction, in which the voice sounds whispering and breathy. Patients with blepharospasm have abnormal contraction of the orbicularis oculi; mild cases are characterized by increased rate and flurries of blinking, whereas in more severe cases forceful eye closure may interfere with vision. In oromandibular dystonia, there is abnormal activity in lower facial, tongue, jaw, and pharyngeal muscles that can interfere with speaking or swallowing. Brachial dystonia is a form of focal dystonia that may be primarily, or exclusively, present with writing (writer's cramp); it is probably more common than usually recognized.

Segmental dystonia can involve the cranial muscles, as in the combination of blepharospasm and oromandibular dystonia, sometimes called Meige syndrome. In craniocervical dystonia, another type of segmental dystonia, the cranial musculature is involved together with neck muscles. Writer's cramp spreads from the dominant to the contralateral arm in 15% of patients, at which point it is considered segmental (bibrachial) dystonia. Hemidystonia is not typical of primary dystonia; it almost invariably implies that the dystonia is secondary to another cause, most commonly stroke, trauma, or perinatal injury.[5] Dystonia may be generalized at onset or may begin as focal or segmental dystonia and subsequently spread to become generalized.

The anatomic distribution of dystonia carries some prognostic value: complete remissions may occur in patients with cervical dystonia,[6,7] but remissions occur very rarely in generalized dystonia and are usually partial.[8]

Age at onset

The age at onset of primary dystonia is bimodally distributed, with modes at 9 years (early onset) and 45 years (late onset) and a nadir at 27 years.[9] Age at onset is closely related to anatomic distribution. Early-onset dystonia usually starts in a leg or arm, and less commonly starts in the neck, vocal cords, or other cranial muscles. Late-onset primary dystonia commonly affects the neck or cranial muscles and is less likely to begin in a limb; onset in the leg is especially unlikely. Additionally, age at onset is also an important consideration in prognosis: most early-onset patients beginning with leg or arm dystonia progress to involve more than one limb and about 50% eventually generalize, whereas late-onset primary dystonia tends to remain focal or segmental.[10–12] Generalized dystonia beginning in adulthood is far more likely to be secondary (or psychogenic) than to be primary dystonia.

Etiology

Although it is not possible to identify the cause of dystonia in every patient, every effort should be made to do so, in order to individualize more specific therapy and counseling. One etiologic classification system identifies two broad categories: primary, or idiopathic, dystonia; and secondary, or symptomatic, dystonia (see Table 1.1).[13]

Primary dystonia

In primary dystonia, dystonia is the only neurologic abnormality present, except for the occasional occurrence of tremor (resembling essential tremor) or, especially in DYT1 dystonia (see below), occasional myoclonic jerks involving dystonic muscles. Findings such as parkinsonism, ataxia, ocular motor abnormalities, weakness, spasticity, seizures, or dementia suggest that dystonia is secondary. In primary dystonia there are no structural brain abnormalities and no inborn errors of metabolism identifiable with conventional investigations. The majority of primary dystonias are focal or segmental in distribution, with onset in adulthood. Approximately 10% of patients with primary dystonia have generalized dystonia, usually starting in childhood or adolescence.[14]

For many types of primary dystonia a genetic etiology is known or suspected, although a family history of dystonia cannot always be elicited.[15,16] Four primary dystonia loci have been mapped, and for one locus (*DYT1*) the gene product has been identified. (Table 1.2 lists loci for genetic forms of primary and some secondary dystonias.[17–34]) About 90% of generalized primary dystonia in Ashkenazi Jews and up to 50% of generalized primary dystonia in other populations is due to deletion of a GAG triplet from the *DYT1* gene located at chromosome 9q34.[17] This mutation results in loss of a glutamic acid residue from the translated protein torsinA, a member of the AAA+ family of proteins (chaperone-like ATPases associated with the assembly, operation, and disassembly of protein complexes).[18,35] DYT1 dystonia is inherited in autosomal dominant fashion with reduced penetrance of 30%. Because all affected patients possess the same mutation, screening for this form of dystonia is relatively easy and is now commercially available.[36] DYT1 dystonia has a mean age at onset of 12.5 years but the range is broad (3–64 years); in 94% of cases, symptoms begin in a limb.[10] In about two-thirds of patients there is progression to generalized or multifocal dystonia, while in the remainder dystonia remains focal or segmental, usually as writer's cramp or bibrachial dystonia.[17] Progression usually occurs within 5 years of onset, but can occur later.[37]

The other familial primary dystonias whose genes have been mapped are less common. These include DYT6 (dystonia with variable expression in Mennonite/Amish families),[24] DYT7 (focal dystonia in a northwestern German family),[25] and DYT13 (craniocervicobrachial dystonia in an Italian family),[31,32] all of which are inherited in autosomal dominant fashion with reduced penetrance. Genetic testing for these dystonias is not currently commercially available.

Table 1.2 Classification of genetic dystonias

Disease	Dystonia type	Pattern of inheritance	Chromosome region	Gene locus	Protein	Reference(s)
Oppenheim's torsion dystonia	PTD	Autosomal dominant	9q34	*DYT1*	TorsinA	17,18
Early-onset (unconfirmed)	PTD	Autosomal recessive	Not mapped	*DYT2*	Not identified	19
Lubag (X-linked dystonia-parkinsonism)	Heredo-degenerative dystonia	X-linked recessive	Xq13.1	*DYT3*	Multiple transcript system	20
Whispering dystonia (one family only)	PTD	Autosomal dominant	Not mapped	*DYT4*	Not identified	21
Dopa-responsive dystonia	Dystonia-plus	Autosomal dominant	14q22.1	*DYT5*	GTP cyclohydrolase I	22,23
Craniocervical dystonia (Mennonite/Amish)	PTD	Autosomal dominant	8p21-q22	*DYT6*	Not identified	24
Familial torticollis	PTD	Autosomal dominant	18p	*DYT7*	Not identified	25
Paroxysmal dystonic choreoathetosis (non-kinesigenic) (Mount–Rebak)	Paroxysmal dystonia	Autosomal dominant	2q33-q35	*DYT8*	Myofibrillogenesis regulator 1	26
Paroxysmal dyskinesias with spasticity	Paroxysmal dystonia	Autosomal dominant	1p21	*DYT9*	Not identified	27
Paroxysmal kinesigenic dyskinesia	Paroxysmal dystonia	Autosomal dominant	16p11.2-q12.1	*DYT10*	Not identified	28
Myoclonus-dystonia	Dystonia-plus	Autosomal dominant	7q21-q23	*DYT11*	ε-sarcoglycan	29
Rapid-onset dystonia-parkinsonism	Dystonia-plus	Autosomal dominant	19q13	*DYT12*	Na^+/K^+-ATPase $\alpha 3$	30
Cranicervicobrachial	PTD	Autosomal dominant	1p36	*DYT13*	Not identified	31, 32
Dopa-responsive dystonia	Dystonia-plus	Autosomal dominant	14q13	*DYT14*	Not identified	33
Myoclonus-dystonia	Dystonia-plus	Autosomal dominant	18p11	*DYT15*	Not identified	34

PTD = primary torsion dystonia.

Secondary dystonia

When dystonia is secondary to a hereditary neurologic disorder or an exogenous insult, neurologic abnormalities in addition to dystonia are likely to be present. An important exception is dystonia resulting from dopamine receptor-blocking agents (acute dystonic reaction and tardive dystonia), which usually consists of dystonia only. Some clues suggesting that a patient's dystonia is secondary rather than primary are listed in Table 1.3. Secondary dystonias can be further classified (see Table 1.1).

Dystonia-plus syndromes One subcategory of secondary dystonia comprises the dystonia-plus syndromes. These are inherited conditions in which dystonia is accompanied by other neurological abnormalities, but (like in the primary dystonias) there is no evidence of brain degeneration. Dystonia-plus syndromes include dopa-responsive dystonia, myoclonus-dystonia, and rapid-onset dystonia-parkinsonism.

A highly treatable condition, dopa-responsive dystonia (DRD) must always be considered in the differential diagnosis of dystonia. It typically presents in early or mid-childhood with gait dysfunction, and girls are affected more commonly than boys. Classically, symptoms worsen over the course of the day and improve with sleep.[22] Parkinsonism (including rigidity, bradykinesia, stooped posture, and loss of postural reflexes) may develop, making juvenile parkinsonism an important consideration in the differential diagnosis.[38] Because increased tone and hyperreflexia are often present and ankle clonus may be found (although Babinski signs are uncommon), DRD may be misdiagnosed as cerebral palsy.[39] DRD can present in adulthood as focal dystonia[40–42] or parkinsonism.[43,44]

Classic cases of DRD are caused by heterozygous mutations in the GTP-cyclohydrolase I (*GCH1*) gene located at chromosome 14q22.1-q22.2 (classified as DYT5).[23] Inheritance of DRD is autosomal dominant, with reduced penetrance that apparently is sex-influenced (higher in girls).[45] The mutations severely impair the activity of GCH1, the enzyme which catalyzes the rate-limiting step in the synthesis of tetrahydrobiopterin (BH_4); BH_4 is a necessary cofactor for tyrosine hydroxylase, the enzyme which catalyzes the conversion of tyrosine to levodopa in the rate-limiting step of dopamine biosynthesis.[23] Over 100 mutations have been identified and de novo mutations appear to be common, making genetic testing complex and expensive.[42,45]

Whereas most DRD is due to heterozygous *GCH1* mutations, rarer DRD variants result from homozygous or compound heterozygous mutations in the *GCH1* gene[46] or in genes encoding tyrosine hydroxylase[47–49] or other enzymes involved in pterin metabolism.[50] Patients with these defects are often more severely affected, and their dystonia may be less salient than features due to deficiency of nonepinephrine and serotonin, including hypotonia, hypokinesia, oculogyric crises, ptosis, miosis, seizures, and drooling.

Myoclonus-dystonia is a rare dystonia-plus syndrome with prominent myoclonic jerks, usually affecting the arms, neck, and trunk more than the legs. The dystonia, which is usually mild, most commonly manifests as writer's cramp or torticollis. Symptoms typically begin in

Table 1.3 Clues suggesting that dystonia is secondary

- History of exogenous insult or exposure (e.g. drug exposure, head trauma, encephalitis, perinatal hypoxia)
- Dystonia at rest (rather than with action) at onset
- Atypical site for age at onset (e.g. leg onset in an adult, cranial onset in a child)
- Early onset of speech abnormality
- Hemidystonia
- Presence of abnormalities other than dystonia on neurologic examination or general medical examination:
  - e.g. parkinsonism, ataxia, dementia, seizures, myoclonus, visual loss, optic atrophy/other ophthalmoscopic abnormalities, ocular motor abnormalities, deafness, dysarthria, dysphagia, weakness, hypotonia, muscle atrophy, neuropathy, hyperreflexia, dysautonomia, Kayser–Fleischer ring, hepatosplenomegaly, characteristic rash or odor, evidence of malabsorption
- Non-physiologic findings suggesting a psychogenic basis (e.g. false weakness, false sensory loss, inconsistent or incongruous movements)
- Abnormality on brain imaging
- Abnormality in laboratory evaluation

childhood or early adolescence. Many patients, especially those with a positive family history, have a mutation in the ε-sarcoglycan gene (*SGCE*) on chromosome 7q21 (classified as DYT11).[29] Myoclonus-dystonia due to *SGCE* mutation is inherited in autosomal dominant fashion but there is imprinting (i.e. penetrance is reduced and is dependent on the parent transmitting the gene mutation); most patients inherit the mutation from the father. The symptoms characteristically respond to alcohol.[51,52]

In rapid-onset dystonia-parkinsonism, another rare dystonia-plus syndrome, dystonia and parkinsonism often begin suddenly during adolescence or early adulthood and progress over hours to weeks, after which the symptoms usually stabilize. Inheritance is autosomal dominant. The responsible gene, which maps to chromosome 19q13 (classified as DYT12), was recently identified; it codes for Na^+/K^+-ATPase α3, a catalytic subunit of the sodium–potassium pump.[30]

Degenerative neurologic disorders Inherited causes of dystonia include numerous conditions in which there is histopathologic evidence of brain degeneration; many of these are autosomal recessive disorders resulting from inborn errors of metabolism, but dystonia is also associated with various autosomal dominant, X-linked, and mitochondrially inherited disorders (Table 1.4). Neuroimaging is frequently abnormal in these heredodegenerative conditions. Dystonia is thought to result from disrupted basal ganglia function and/or impaired dopamine synthesis. In many of these disorders, other abnormalities may be more prominent than the dystonia; these may include mental retardation, seizures, optic atrophy, gaze paresis ataxia, and neuropathy. Since some of these conditions can respond to specific interventions (e.g. anti-copper therapy for Wilson's disease) or dietary restriction or supplementation, a specific diagnosis should always be sought.

Wilson's disease is a degenerative disorder with autosomal recessive inheritance that can produce secondary dystonia; as a treatable condition, it should be considered in the differential diagnosis. It results from mutations in the *ATP7B* gene on chromosome 13q14.3-q21.1 which produce a defect in copper metabolism, leading to the insidious development of neurologic, psychiatric, and/or hepatic dysfunction. Because over 200 different mutations have been reported, genetic testing is of limited feasibility. When onset is in childhood, Wilson's disease usually presents with hepatic dysfunction, but in adult-onset disease, neurologic presentation is most typical.[53] Dystonia can be generalized, segmental, or multifocal,[54] but cranial involvement is characteristic; Wilson described the typical 'sardonic' smile in his original 1912 monograph.[55] Other common neurologic abnormalities include tremor (classically 'wing-beating'),

Table 1.4 Etiologies of secondary dystonia

Dystonia-plus syndromes
Dopa-responsive dystonia
Myoclonus-dystonia
Rapid-onset dystonia-parkinsonism

Hereditary conditions associated with neurodegeneration
Autosomal dominant:
- Huntington's disease
- Machado–Joseph disease (SCA3)
- Other SCA subtypes (SCA2, SCA6, SCA17)
- Familial basal ganglia calcification (Fahr's disease)
- Dentatorubral-pallidoluysian atrophy
- Neuroferritinopathy
- Frontotemporal dementia
- Neuronal intranuclear inclusion disease (inheritance not well-established)

Autosomal recessive:
- Juvenile Parkinson's disease (*parkin*)
- Wilson's disease
- Aceruloplasminemia
- Pantothenate kinase-associated neurodegeneration (formerly Hallervorden–Spatz syndrome)
- Neuroacanthocytosis
- Ataxia with vitamin E deficiency
- Ataxia-telangiectasia
- Ataxia with oculomotor apraxia
- Sulfite oxidase (molybdenum cofactor) deficiency
- Triosephosphate isomerase deficiency
- Guanidinoacetate methyltransferase deficiency
- Infantile bilateral striatal necrosis
- Cockayne's disease
- Lysosomal storage disorders:
  - GM1 gangliosidosis
  - GM2 gangliosidosis (hexosaminidase A deficiency)
  - Niemann–Pick type C (juvenile dystonia lipidosis)
  - Metachromatic leukodystrophy
  - Krabbe's disease
  - Neuronal ceroid lipofuscinosis
- Amino and organic acid disorders:
  - Glutaric acidemia type I
  - Homocystinuria
  - Propionic acidemia
  - Methylmalonic aciduria
  - Fumarase deficiency
  - Hartnup disease

(*Continued*)

Table 1.4 (Continued)

X-linked recessive:
- Lubag (X-linked dystonia-parkinsonism)
- Lesch–Nyhan syndrome
- Deafness–dystonia–optic atrophy syndrome (Mohr–Tranebjaerg syndrome)
- Pelizaeus–Merzbacher disease
- Rett's syndrome

Mitochondrial:
- Leber's hereditary optic neuropathy
- Mitochondrial encephalomyopathy with lactic acidosis and stroke-like episodes (MELAS)
- Myoclonic epilepsy with ragged-red fibers (MERRF)
- Leigh's syndrome (subacute necrotizing encephalomyelopathy)

Acquired/exogenous causes

Toxins:
- Medications:
  - Dopamine receptor-blocking agents
  - Antiepileptic agents
  - Levodopa
  - Dopamine agonists
  - Calcium channel blockers (cinnarizine, flunarizine)
- Carbon monoxide
- Carbon disulfide
- Cyanide
- Manganese
- Methanol
- Wasp sting

Perinatal cerebral injuries:
- Cerebral palsy
- Kernicterus

Vascular lesions:
- Stroke
- Arteriovenous malformation
- Antiphospholipid syndrome

Infection:
- Encephalitis
- Subacute sclerosing panencephalitis
- Human immunodeficiency syndrome/acquired immunodeficiency syndrome (HIV/AIDS)
- Abscess

Brain tumors

Paraneoplastic syndrome

(*Continued*)

Table 1.4 (Continued)

Demyelination:
- Multiple sclerosis
- Pontine myelinolysis

Trauma:
- Head trauma
- Cervical cord injury
- Peripheral injury (including complex regional pain syndrome)

Structural:
- Atlanto-axial subluxation
- Klippel–Feil syndrome
- Syringomyelia
- Arnold–Chiari malformation

Parkinson's disease and other parkinsonisms associated with dystonia

Parkinson's disease
Progressive supranuclear palsy
Corticobasal ganglionic degeneration
Multiple system atrophy

Other movement disorders exhibiting dystonic phenomenology

Tic disorders
Familial paroxysmal kinesigenic dyskinesias
Familial paroxysmal non-kinesigenic dyskinesias
Episodic ataxia syndromes

dysarthria, dysphagia, drooling, ataxia, and dementia. In addition to brain and liver (cirrhosis, acute hepatitis) involvement, numerous systemic findings may occur, including renal, endocrine, and cardiac abnormalities.[56–59] In addition to Kayser–Fleischer rings (see below), which do not produce symptoms, ophthalmologic findings may include sunflower cataracts. As treatment can alleviate symptoms and prevent progression, especially if instituted early, the diagnosis of Wilson's disease should be considered in all patients with onset of dystonia prior to 50 years of age.

Another important hereditary condition causing dystonia is juvenile parkinsonism due to mutations in the *parkin* gene. In this autosomal recessive condition, parkinsonism usually begins before the age of 40 years and is associated with dystonia at onset, hyperreflexia, slow progression, and dyskinesias occurring early in the course of levodopa treatment.[60] The dystonia often predominates in the lower limbs, but the hands, neck, and trunk may also be involved. Symptoms typically respond to levodopa treatment at low-to-moderate doses. Genetic testing is commercially available.[61]

Many other hereditary metabolic and neurodegenerative conditions are associated with dystonia; some are listed in Table 1.4.

Other causes of secondary dystonia A variety of acquired insults can cause secondary dystonia in previously unaffected individuals (see Table 1.4). Many cases are iatrogenic, resulting from medications that block dopamine receptors; antipsychotic and antiemetic agents are the most common offenders. Other causes, including vascular, infectious, neoplastic, and traumatic etiologies, less frequently result in dystonia.

Dystonia can occur in association with other movement disorders. It frequently accompanies Parkinson's disease, often occurring as painful foot dystonia when levodopa levels are low, but it may affect other body areas as well. The camptocormia (forward flexion of the thoracolumbar spine) that occurs in patients with Parkinson's disease may be a dystonic phenomenon.[62,63] Parkinson's-plus syndromes are even more strongly associated with dystonia than is idiopathic Parkinson's disease. In one study, 59% of patients with corticobasal degeneration had dystonia, mostly involving the arms.[64] In another series, dystonia was present in 46% of patients with progressive supranuclear palsy, most commonly manifesting as limb dystonia or blepharospasm.[65,66] Whereas the prevalence of dystonia in multiple system atrophy has been reported to be as high as 46% (mostly anterocollis and unilateral limb dystonia),[67] other authors have found frequencies closer to 12%.[68]

Spinocerebellar ataxia, especially type 3 (SCA3), can be associated with dystonia. A recent series found the prevalence of dystonia to be 10% of 80 patients with SCA3,[69] while another series reported dystonia in 23% of 61 patients.[70] Also known as Machado–Joseph disease, SCA3 is the most common hereditary ataxia with autosomal dominant inheritance in the United States, constituting 21% of 149 families with dominantly inherited ataxia in one series.[71] It results from expansion of CAG repeats in the *ATXN3* gene on chromosome 14q24.3-q31, and the likelihood of dystonia is correlated with increasing repeat length.[70] Presentation is often in the third or fourth decade and begins with speech and gait dysfunction, typically followed by ophthalmoparesis, dysarthria, dysphagia, and ataxia. Other characteristic features include bulging eyes, perioral fasciculations, and peripheral neuropathy. Dystonia is highly variable in presentation[72,73] and may even respond to levodopa therapy.[74,75] Dystonia also may occur in SCA17,[76] but is uncommon in other forms of spinocerebellar ataxia.

Patients with other movement disorders can also exhibit movements that resemble dystonia but are not generally categorized as dystonia. For example, tics can be dystonic in appearance when they are slow and sustained. Similarly, paroxysmal and episodic disorders can produce dyskinetic postures resembling dystonia.[77]

Toxic causes of dystonia are most commonly iatrogenic, induced by medications prescribed for psychosis, gastrointestinal complaints, or other indications. Manganese intoxication may result in a dystonic-parkinsonian syndrome,[78] and severe exposure can lead to dystonic posturing of the limbs and trunk, as well as focal dystonia such as blepharospasm, grimacing, torticollis, and oculogyric crisis.[79,80] Other toxins associated with dystonia include carbon monoxide,[81] cyanide,[82,83] carbon disulfide,[84] and methanol.[85,86] Dystonia has been reported following a wasp sting.[87]

Dystonia can result from acquired brain lesions such as tumors, infections (e.g. abscess, encephalitis), strokes, vascular malformations, trauma, and demyelination. Structural lesions producing dystonia are most commonly located in basal ganglia and thalamus (and, for blepharospasm, in rostral brainstem).[88,89] Lesions of the parietal lobe have also been reported.[90,91] In a series of 25 patients with cervical dystonia secondary to lesions of the central nervous system, cerebellum and brainstem were the areas most commonly involved, followed by basal ganglia and cervical spinal cord.[92] Perinatal insults such as asphyxia or kernicterus may be associated with the development of dystonia, onset of which may be delayed by years.[93,94] Dystonia may develop following peripheral trauma, and may be particularly likely when complex regional pain syndrome is present, but whether peripheral injury truly plays a causal role in producing dystonia remains controversial.[95–100]

Sometimes classified as a subtype of secondary dystonia, psychogenic dystonia deserves particular mention. In one unpublished series, psychogenic dystonia was the third most common cause of secondary dystonia (after tardive dystonia and birth injury), accounting for 14% of classifiable secondary dystonias.[101] A psychogenic origin of dystonia should be suspected when manifestations vary over time, remit upon distraction or when socially convenient, or are inconsistent with normal physiologic patterns.

DIAGNOSTIC EVALUATION

The diagnosis of dystonia, like that of all neurologic disorders, relies most firmly upon a thorough history and a complete physical and neurologic examination; these usually permit presumptive classification of the dystonia as primary or secondary, which in turn guides the subsequent evaluation.

Primary dystonia

If the history and examination demonstrate no neurologic abnormalities other than dystonia, there is no history suggesting an acquired insult (including drug exposure), and there are no features suggesting a secondary cause (see Table 1.3), a primary dystonia can be postulated. However, the possibility of DRD should always be considered and, when appropriate, excluded (see below).

In patients with onset of primary dystonia prior to 26 years of age, DYT1 testing is a reasonable initial investigation, as this test correctly identifies 100% of clinically ascertained carriers.[17] We also consider DYT1 testing in patients with later onset who have an affected relative with an early age at onset. If the GAG deletion is detected, DYT1 dystonia is confirmed and no further diagnostic work-up is necessary.

If the GAG deletion is not present, a primary dystonia is still possible; unfortunately, at this time, genetic testing for primary dystonias other than DYT1 is not commercially available. It is likely that additional gene tests will become available in the future. The website http://www.geneclinics.org is a useful resource for up-to-date information about genetic testing.

When DYT1 testing is negative (or is not indicated due to onset at age 26 or later), subsequent investigation emphasizes the exclusion of secondary etiologies (including dystonia-plus syndromes) with greater certainty. In most cases a trial of levodopa to exclude DRD is warranted (see below). Magnetic resonance imaging (MRI) of the brain should be performed to exclude structural lesions as well as signal abnormalities suggestive of a metabolic disorder.

Secondary dystonia

The work-up for secondary dystonia may proceed if the evaluation for a suspected primary dystonia is negative, or may be launched ab initio when clinical features suggest a secondary cause for the dystonia.

Although the differential diagnosis of secondary dystonia (see Table 1.4) appears daunting, it can often be narrowed considerably on the basis of age at onset, family history, and presence of other features such as developmental delay, ataxia, or spasticity. Consultation with geneticists and specialists in metabolic disorders is often invaluable. When dystonia follows an exogenous insult with an appropriate temporal interval, further work-up may not be necessary.

MRI of the brain is critical in assessing secondary dystonia. Imaging may reveal a structural lesion (e.g. stroke, arteriovenous malformation, tumor, or abscess) in a brain region associated with dystonia. Caudate atrophy should prompt consideration of Huntington's disease or neuroacanthocytosis. In Wilson's disease there may be abnormalities involving the putamen, thalamus, and brainstem, including the 'face-of-the-giant-panda' sign, comprising hyperintensity in the midbrain tegmentum sparing the red nucleus, preserved signal intensity in the lateral substantia nigra pars reticulata, and hypointensity of the superior colliculus.[102,103] Pantothenate kinase-associated neurodegeneration (PKAN, formerly Hallervorden–Spatz syndrome[104]) is classically associated with the 'eye-of-the-tiger' sign: i.e. pallidal hypointensity with relative hyperintensity in the anteromedial globus pallidus on T2-weighted MRI.[105,106] Basal ganglia calcification may signify Fahr's disease. Diffuse signal abnormality in the white matter raises the possibility of a leukodystrophy. Other metabolic conditions with characteristic MRI patterns include neuroferritinopathy, glutaric aciduria, and methylmalonic aciduria. Positron emission tomography is not currently in widespread use in the evaluation of dystonia but may assume a more important role as its utility is further elucidated.[107,108] In addition to brain imaging, MRI of the cervical spine may be helpful in assessing patients with cervical or brachial dystonia, as it may disclose a lesion such as a tumor, syrinx, or demyelinating plaque.[109–111]

Along with neuroimaging, the investigation of secondary dystonia also includes ruling out treatable conditions that can cause dystonia, chiefly DRD and Wilson's disease. Methods currently available for the clinical diagnosis of DRD include empiric treatment with levodopa; measurement of tetrahydrobiopterin, neopterin, and dopamine metabolites in cerebrospinal fluid (CSF); phenylalanine loading; and measurement of BH_4 levels and GCH1 activity in fibroblasts or lymphocytes. Chronic oral levodopa replacement at a low dose usually results in a return to normal or near-normal motor function that is sustained over time.[22] We offer a therapeutic trial of levodopa to patients with onset of dystonia in childhood or adolescence, as well as to adult-onset patients with any features suggesting DRD (e.g. parkinsonism, diurnal variation, hyperreflexia). We begin with half a tablet of carbidopa/levodopa 25/100 daily, slowly increasing the dose over several weeks. While a daily dose of 600 mg of levodopa is occasionally required, most patients with DRD will respond to a dose of 300 mg/day or less. Because other forms of dystonia may demonstrate some response to levodopa,[112,113] improvement with empiric treatment is not specific for DRD; however, it is very sensitive, and if a patient responds to levodopa, treatment should usually be continued.

Another tool for diagnosing DRD is lumbar puncture for measurement of neopterin and biopterin levels in CSF; reduced levels of neopterin appear to be specific for DRD due to GCH1 deficiency.[114] A less invasive test involves demonstration of elevated phenylalanine levels, decreased tyrosine levels, and elevated phenylalanine/tyrosine ratios in serum following oral phenylalanine loading. This test detects GCH1 deficiency because biopterin is a necessary cofactor for phenylalanine hydroxylase, which catalyzes the hydroxylation of phenylalanine to tyrosine in the liver, and because DRD patients have normal baseline levels of phenylalanine and tyrosine.[115] The sensitivity and specificity of this test are still being clarified.[116] Reduced activity of GCH1 and decreased neopterin and biopterin levels have been demonstrated in lymphoblasts and cultured skin fibroblasts; these findings may prove useful for diagnosis, and prenatal diagnosis may even be possible if these techniques can be applied to amniocytes.[117,118]

Genetic testing for DRD is available through a few commercial laboratories (listed at www.geneclinics.org). Single-strand conformation polymorphism/sequence analysis of all six exons of the gene reveals a mutation in about 50–60% of clinically diagnosed cases,[119–121] but this methodology may miss large heterozygous deletions and multiplications.[122] A recent study in which sequence analysis was supplemented with quantitative duplex polymerase chain reaction identified mutations in the *GCH1* gene in 87% of DRD patients identified with rigorous inclusion criteria,[123] but such high sensitivity has not been replicated. A negative result, especially when only sequence analysis is performed, does not exclude the diagnosis of DRD. As always, it is essential that patients and families meet with an experienced genetic counselor before and after testing so that they understand the implications of a positive or negative result.

Another treatable cause of dystonia, Wilson's disease should be considered in patients whose dystonia begins prior to age 50 years. Treatment options include dietary modification, chelating agents, and agents that reduce copper absorption from the gastrointestinal tract.[124] As described above, MRI of the brain may suggest the diagnosis. Serum ceruloplasmin is a reasonable initial screening test for Wilson's disease, but is not sufficiently sensitive (85% in one study[125]) or specific.[126] Slit-lamp examination for Kayser–Fleischer rings (due to deposition of copper in Descemet's membrane) is nearly (but not quite[127,128]) 100% sensitive in patients with neurologic Wilson's disease. As urinary copper may be elevated, measurement of 24-hour urinary copper is sometimes helpful. Liver biopsy is probably the most sensitive diagnostic modality; in one study in which hepatic copper content was measured in 15 patients with neurologic Wilson's disease, the concentration was greater than 250 μg/g in 14 patients and greater than 50 μg/g in all patients.[125] Genetic testing, including mutation analysis of the *ATP7B* gene and sequence analysis/mutation scanning of select exons, is available on a limited basis, but the sensitivity of this testing depends on the patient's ethnicity and the particular mutations sought and exons examined. In practice, we rely on slit-lamp examination, 24-hour urinary copper, and serum ceruloplasmin level to screen for Wilson's disease; if these are normal and clinical suspicion is high (due to concomitant hepatic dysfunction, psychiatric or cognitive abnormalities, or suggestive family history), we may consider liver biopsy.

When neuroimaging is normal and there is no evidence for DRD or Wilson's disease, additional laboratory investigations may be helpful. Routine blood tests such as complete blood count, electrolytes, glucose, calcium, magnesium, coagulation profile, and kidney, liver, and thyroid function are usually supplemented by erythrocyte sedimentation rate, antinuclear antibody screen, and syphilis screen. More specialized testing may be indicated as well, as dictated by the clinical presentation. Features such as chorea, orolingual dystonia, seizures, and abnormal behavior and cognition might suggest the diagnosis of neuroacanthocytosis; serum creatine phosphokinase (CPK) should be measured and a peripheral blood smear performed to assess for acanthocytes. Adult-onset chorea may reflect neuroferritinopathy, and serum ferritin may be helpful in making this diagnosis. Ataxia due to vitamin E deficiency can be diagnosed by demonstrating low serum levels of this vitamin. Ataxia-telangiectasia should be suspected when ataxia accompanies recurrent infections and conjunctival telangiectasias, and may be confirmed by low serum levels of immunoglobulins and elevated α-fetoprotein. A history of thrombotic events or fetal loss may bespeak the antiphospholipid syndrome, and should prompt testing for anticardiolipin antibodies and related studies. Quantitative analysis of amino acids in serum and urine and of organic acids in urine is useful in assessing for amino acidopathies and organic acidopathies. Measurement of lysosomal enzymes in leukocytes may disclose a lysosomal storage disease. Testing for the human immunodeficiency virus is indicated when appropriate. Genetic testing is available for some of the hereditary conditions causing dystonia (e.g. Huntington's disease, juvenile parkinsonism due to the *parkin* mutation, and some spinocerebellar ataxias), and undoubtedly mutational analysis for more conditions will be offered in the future. Lactate and pyruvate can be measured in blood and CSF when a mitochondrial disorder is considered. Pterins and neurotransmitter metabolites can also be assayed in CSF.

In some cases, electrophysiologic testing modalities such as nerve conduction studies/electromyography, evoked potentials, and electroencephalography can provide useful information, but these rarely lead to a specific diagnosis. Occasionally, definitive diagnosis may require tissue biopsy. As mentioned above, liver biopsy for measurement of hepatic copper may be needed to confirm the diagnosis of Wilson's disease. Bone marrow of patients with Niemann–Pick disease type C usually contains foam cells and sea-blue histiocytes. Fibroblasts obtained by skin biopsy can be used for lysosomal enzyme screening in suspected storage diseases, as well as for filipin staining and low-density lipoprotein-induced cholesterol esterification in Niemann–Pick type C.[129] Muscle biopsy can be useful; abnormalities consistent with mitochondrial myopathy (such as ragged red fibers) suggest a mitochondrial disorder. Brain biopsy may reveal intraneuronal inclusions[130] but is not a common component of the diagnostic evaluation of dystonia.

APPLYING THE DIAGNOSIS

The ultimate goal of a precise diagnosis of dystonia is the optimization of treatment for each patient. At the current time, most patients with dystonia are treated with symptomatic therapies such as oral medications, chemodenervation with botulinum toxin, and surgical procedures that are not highly specific for the particular cause of the individual's dystonia. Nevertheless, timely assignment of a specific diagnosis allows better genetic counseling, more reliable estimation of prognosis, and design of more meaningful clinical trials. As our understanding of these complex and challenging disorders grows, individualized therapies directed at specific dystonia syndromes will undoubtedly emerge.

REFERENCES

1. Yanagisawa N, Goto A. Dystonia musculorum deformans: analysis with electromyography. J Neurol Sci 1972; 13: 39–65.
2. Satoyoshi E. A syndrome of progressive muscle spasm, alopecia, and diarrhea. Neurology 1978; 28: 458–71.
3. Drost G, Verrips A, Hooijkaas H, Zwarts M. Glutamic acid decarboxylase antibodies in Satoyoshi syndrome. Ann Neurol 2004; 55: 450–1.
4. Chan J, Brin MF, Fahn S. Idiopathic cervical dystonia: clinical characteristics. Mov Disord 1991; 6: 119–26.
5. Chuang C, Fahn S, Frucht SJ. The natural history and treatment of acquired hemidystonia: report of 33 cases and review of the literature. J Neurol Neurosurg Psychiatry 2002; 72: 59–67.
6. Jayne D, Lees AJ, Stern GM. Remission in spasmodic torticollis. J Neurol Neurosurg Psychiatry 1984; 47: 1236–7.
7. Friedman A, Fahn S. Spontaneous remissions in spasmodic torticollis. Neurology 1986; 36: 398–400.
8. Eldridge R, Ince SE, Chernow B, Milstien S, Lake CR. Dystonia in 61-year-old identical twins: observations over 45 years. Ann Neurol 1984; 16: 356–8.
9. Bressman SB, de Leon D, Brin MF et al. Idiopathic torsion dystonia among Ashkenazi Jews: evidence for autosomal dominant inheritance. Ann Neurol 1989; 26: 612–20.
10. Bressman SB, de Leon D, Kramer PL et al. Dystonia in Ashkenazi Jews: clinical characterization of a founder mutation. Ann Neurol 1994; 36: 771–7.
11. Greene P, Kang UJ, Fahn S. Spread of symptoms in idiopathic torsion dystonia. Mov Disord 1995; 10: 143–52.
12. O'Riordan S, Raymond D, Lynch T et al. Age at onset as a factor in determining the phenotype of primary torsion dystonia. Neurology 2004; 63: 1423–6.
13. Bressman SB. Dystonia genotypes, phenotypes, and classification. Adv Neurol 2004; 94: 101–7.
14. Nutt JG, Muenter MD, Aronson A, Kurland LT, Melton LJ. Epidemiology of focal and generalized dystonia in Rochester, Minnesota. Mov Disord 1988; 3: 188–94.
15. Defazio G, Livrea P, Guanti G, Lepore V, Ferrari E. Genetic contribution to idiopathic adult-onset blepharospasm and cranial-cervical dystonia. Eur Neurol 1993; 33: 345–50.
16. Stojanovic M, Cvetkovic D, Kostic VS. A genetic study of idiopathic focal dystonias. J Neurol 1995; 242: 508–11.
17. Bressman SB, Sabatti C, Raymond D et al. The DYT1 phenotype and guidelines for diagnostic testing. Neurology 2000; 54: 1746–52.
18. Ozelius LJ, Hewett JW, Page C et al. The early-onset torsion dystonia gene (DYT1) encodes an ATP-binding protein. Nat Genet 1997; 17: 40–8.
19. Khan NL, Wood NW, Bhatia KP. Autosomal recessive, DYT2-like primary torsion dystonia: a new family. Neurology 2003; 61: 1801–3.
20. Nolte D, Niemann S, Muller U. Specific sequence changes in multiple transcript system DYT3 are associated with X-linked dystonia parkinsonism. Proc Natl Acad Sci USA 2003; 100: 10347–52.
21. Parker N. Hereditary whispering dystonia. J Neurol Neurosurg Psychiatry 1985; 48: 218–24.
22. Segawa M, Hosaka A, Miyagawa F, Nomura Y, Imai H. Hereditary progressive dystonia with marked diurnal fluctuation. Adv Neurol 1976; 14: 215–33.
23. Ichinose H, Ohye T, Takahashi E et al. Hereditary progressive dystonia with marked diurnal fluctuations caused by mutations in the GTP cyclohydrolase I gene. Nat Genet 1994; 8: 236–42.
24. Almasy L, Bressman SB, Raymond D et al. Idiopathic torsion dystonia linked to chromosome 8 in two Mennonite families. Ann Neurol 1997; 42: 670–3.
25. Leube B, Rudnicki D, Ratzlaff T et al. Idiopathic torsion dystonia: assignment of a gene to chromosome 18p in a German family with adult onset, autosomal dominant inheritance and purely focal distribution. Hum Mol Genet 1996; 5: 1673–7.
26. Rainier S, Thomas D, Tokarz D et al. Myofibrillogenesis regulator 1 gene mutations cause paroxysmal dystonia choreoathetosis. Arch Neurol 2004; 61: 1025–9.
27. Auburger G, Ratzlaff T, Lunkes A et al. A gene for autosomal dominant paroxysmal choreoathetosis/spasticity (CSE) maps to the vicinity of a potassium channel gene cluster on chromosome 1p, probably within 2 cM between D1S443 and D1S197. Genomics 1996; 31: 90–4.
28. Tomita H, Nagamitsu S, Wakui K et al. Paroxysmal kinesigenic choreoathetosis locus maps to chromosome 16p11.2-q12.1. Am J Hum Genet 1999; 65: 1688–97.
29. Zimprich A, Grabowski M, Asmus F et al. Mutations in the gene encoding epsilon-sarcoglycan cause myoclonus-dystonia syndrome. Nat Genet 2001; 29: 66–9.

30. de Carvalho Aguiar P, Sweadner KJ, Penniston JT et al. Mutations in the Na^+/K^+-ATPase alpha3 gene ATP1A3 are associated with rapid-onset dystonia parkinsonism. Neuron 2004; 43: 169–75.
31. Bentivoglio AR, Ialongo T, Contarino MF, Valente EM, Albanese A. Phenotypic characterization of DYT13 primary torsion dystonia. Mov Disord 2004; 19: 200–6.
32. Valente EM, Bentivoglio AR, Cassetta E et al. DYT13, a novel primary torsion dystonia locus, maps to chromosome 1p36.13–36.32 in an Italian family with cranial-cervical or upper limb onset. Ann Neurol 2001; 49: 362–6.
33. Grötzsch H, Pizzolato GP, Ghika J et al. Neuropathology of a case of dopa-responsive dystonia associated with a new genetic locus, DYT14. Neurology 2002; 58: 1839–42.
34. Grimes DA, Han F, Lang AE et al. A novel locus for inherited myoclonus-dystonia on 18p11. Neurology 2002; 59: 1183–6.
35. Goodchild RE, Dauer WT. The AAA+ protein torsinA interacts with a conserved domain present in LAP1 and a novel ER protein. J Cell Biol 2005; 168: 855–62.
36. Klein C, Friedman J, Bressman S et al. Genetic testing for early-onset torsion dystonia (DYT1): introduction of a simple screening method, experiences from testing of a large patient cohort, and ethical aspects. Genet Test 1999; 3: 323–8.
37. Edwards M, Wood N, Bhatia K. Unusual phenotypes in DYT1 dystonia: a report of five cases and a review of the literature. Mov Disord 2003; 18: 706–11.
38. Segawa M, Nomura Y, Nishiyama N. Autosomal dominant guanosine triphosphate cyclohydrolase I deficiency (Segawa disease). Ann Neurol 2003; 54 (Suppl 6): S32-S45.
39. Nygaard TG, Waran SP, Levine RA, Naini AB, Chutorian AM. Dopa-responsive dystonia simulating cerebral palsy. Pediatr Neurol 1994; 11: 236–40.
40. Deonna T, Roulet E, Ghika J, Zesiger P. Dopa-responsive childhood dystonia: a forme fruste with writer's cramp, triggered by exercise. Dev Med Child Neurol 1997; 39: 49–53.
41. Steinberger D, Topka H, Fischer D, Muller U. GCH1 mutation in a patient with adult-onset oromandibular dystonia. Neurology 1999; 52: 877–9.
42. Tassin J, Durr A, Bonnet AM et al. Levodopa-responsive dystonia. GTP cyclohydrolase I or parkin mutations? Brain 2000; 123: 1112–21.
43. Nygaard TG, Takahashi H, Heiman GA et al. Long-term treatment response and fluorodopa positron emission tomographic scanning of parkinsonism in a family with dopa-responsive dystonia. Ann Neurol 1992; 32: 603–8.
44. Harwood G, Hierons R, Fletcher NA, Marsden CD. Lessons from a remarkable family with dopa-responsive dystonia. J Neurol Neurosurg Psychiatry 1994; 57: 460–3.
45. Furukawa Y, Lang AE, Trugman JM et al. Gender-related penetrance and de novo GTP-cyclohydrolase I gene mutations in dopa-responsive dystonia. Neurology 1998; 50: 1015–20.
46. Jarman PR, Bandmann O, Marsden CD, Wood NW. GTP-cyclohydrolase I mutations in patients with dystonia responsive to anticholinergic drugs. J Neurol Neurosurg Psychiatry 1997; 63: 304–8.
47. Knappskog PM, Flatmark T, Mallet J, Ludecke B, Bartholome K. Recessively inherited L-dopa-responsive dystonia caused by a point mutation (Q381K) in the tyrosine hydroxylase gene. Hum Mol Genet 1995; 4: 1209–12.
48. Lüdecke B, Dworniczak B, Bartholome K. A point mutation in the tyrosine hydroxylase gene associated with Segawa's syndrome. Hum Genet 1995; 95: 123–5.
49. van den Heuvel LP, Luiten B, Smeitink JA et al. A common point mutation in the tyrosine hydroxylase gene in autosomal recessive L-dopa-responsive dystonia in the Dutch population. Hum Genet 1998; 102: 644–6.
50. Hanihara T, Inoue K, Kawanishi C et al. 6-Pyruvoyl-tetrahydropterin synthase deficiency with generalized dystonia and diurnal fluctuation of symptoms: a clinical and molecular study. Mov Disord 1997; 12: 408–11.
51. Kyllerman M, Forsgren L, Sanner G et al. Alcohol-responsive myoclonic dystonia in a large family: dominant inheritance and phenotypic variation. Mov Disord 1990; 5: 270–9.
52. Saunders-Pullman R, Shriberg J, Heiman G et al. Myoclonus dystonia: possible association with obsessive-compulsive disorder and alcohol dependence. Neurology 2002; 58: 242–5.
53. El-Youssef M. Wilson disease. Mayo Clin Proc 2003; 78: 1126–36.
54. Svetel M, Kozic D, Stefanova E et al. Dystonia in Wilson's disease. Mov Disord 2001; 16: 719–23.
55. Wilson SAK. Progressive lenticular degeneration: a familial nervous disease associated with cirrhosis of the liver. Brain 1912; 34: 295–509.
56. Brewer GJ, Yuzbasiyan-Gurkan V. Wilson disease. Medicine (Baltimore) 1992; 71: 139–64.
57. Frydman M, Kauschansky A, Bonne-Tamir B, Nassar F, Homburg R. Assessment of the hypothalamic–pituitary–testicular function in male patients with Wilson's disease. J Androl 1991; 12: 180–4.
58. Kuan P. Cardiac Wilson's disease. Chest 1987; 91: 579–83.
59. Meenakshi-Sundaram S, Sinha S, Rao M et al. Cardiac involvement in Wilson's disease – an electrocardiographic observation. J Assoc Physicians India 2004; 52: 294–6.
60. Khan NL, Graham E, Critchley P et al. Parkin disease: a phenotypic study of a large case series. Brain 2003; 126: 1279–92.
61. Brice A, Dürr A, Lücking C. (Updated November 6, 2006.) Parkin type of juvenile Parkinson disease. In: GeneReviews at GeneTests: Medical Genetics Information Resource (database online). Copyright, University of Washington, Seattle, 1997–2007. Available at http://www.genetests.org. Accessed January 22, 2007.
62. Slawek J, Derejko M, Lass P. Camptocormia as a form of dystonia in Parkinson's disease. Eur J Neurol 2003; 10: 107–8.
63. Azher SN, Jankovic, J. Camptocormia: pathogenesis, classification, and response to therapy. Neurology 2005; 65: 355–9.
64. Vanek Z, Jankovic J. Dystonia in corticobasal degeneration. Mov Disord 2001; 16: 252–7.
65. Rafal RD, Friedman JH. Limb dystonia in progressive supranuclear palsy. Neurology 1987; 37: 1546–9.
66. Barclay CL, Lang AE. Dystonia in progressive supranuclear palsy. J Neurol Neurosurg Psychiatry 1997; 62: 352–6.
67. Boesch SM, Wenning GK, Ransmayr G, Poewe W. Dystonia in multiple system atrophy. J Neurol Neurosurg Psychiatry 2002; 72: 300–3.
68. Wenning GK, Tison F, Ben Shlomo Y, Daniel SE, Quinn NP. Multiple system atrophy: a review of 203 pathologically proven cases. Mov Disord 1997; 12: 133–47.
69. Schöls L, Peters S, Szymanski S et al. Extrapyramidal motor signs in degenerative ataxias. Arch Neurol 2000; 57: 1495–500.
70. Jardim L, Pereira M, Silveira I et al. Neurologic findings in Machado–Joseph disease. Arch Neurol 2001; 58: 899–904.
71. Ranum LP, Lundgren JK, Schut LJ et al. Spinocerebellar ataxia type 1 and Machado–Joseph disease: incidence of CAG expansions among adult-onset ataxia patients from 311 families with dominant, recessive, or sporadic ataxia. Am J Hum Genet 1994; 57: 603–8.
72. Cardoso F, de Oliveira JT, Puccioni-Sohler M et al. Eyelid dystonia in Machado–Joseph disease. Mov Disord 2000; 15: 1028–30.
73. Munchau A, Dressler D, Bhatia KP, Vogel P, Zuhlke C. Machado–Joseph disease presenting as severe generalised dystonia in a German patient. J Neurol 1999; 246: 840–2.

74. Nandagopal R, Moorthy SG. Dramatic levodopa responsiveness of dystonia in a sporadic case of spinocerebellar ataxia type 3. Postgrad Med J 2004; 80: 363–5.
75. Wilder-Smith E, Tan EK, Law HY et al. Spinocerebellar ataxia type 3 presenting as an L-DOPA responsive dystonia phenotype in a Chinese family. J Neurol Sci 2003; 213: 25–8.
76. Hagenah JM, Zuhlke C, Hellenbroich Y, Heide W, Klein C. Focal dystonia as a presenting sign of spinocerebellar ataxia 17. Mov Disord 2004; 19: 217–20.
77. Fahn S. Clinical variants of idiopathic torsion dystonia. J Neurol Neurosurg Psychiatry 1989; Suppl: 96–100.
78. Calne DB, Chu NS, Huang CC, Lu CS, Olanow W. Manganism and idiopathic parkinsonism: similarities and differences. Neurology 1994; 44: 1583–6.
79. Cook DG, Fahn S, Brait KA. Chronic manganese intoxication. Arch Neurol 1974; 30: 59–64.
80. Cersosimo MG, Koller WC. The diagnosis of manganese-induced parkinsonism. Neurotoxicology 2006; 27: 340–6.
81. Choi IS, Cheon HY. Delayed movement disorders after carbon monoxide poisoning. Eur Neurol 1999; 42: 141–4.
82. Grandas F, Artieda J, Obeso JA. Clinical and CT scan findings in a case of cyanide intoxication. Mov Disord 1989; 4: 188–93.
83. Borgohain R, Singh AK, Radhakrishna H, Rao VC, Mohandas S. Delayed onset generalised dystonia after cyanide poisoning. Clin Neurol Neurosurg 1995; 97: 213–15.
84. Krauss JK, Mohadjer M, Wakhloo AK, Mundinger F. Dystonia and akinesia due to pallidoputaminal lesions after disulfiram intoxication. Mov Disord 1991; 6: 166–70.
85. LeWitt PA, Martin SD. Dystonia and hypokinesis with putaminal necrosis after methanol intoxication. Clin Neuropharmacol 1988; 11: 161–7.
86. Quartarone A, Girlanda P, Vita G et al. Oromandibular dystonia in a patient with bilateral putaminal necrosis after methanol poisoning: an electrophysiological study. Eur Neurol 2000; 44: 127–8.
87. Benito-Conejero S, Lopez-Dominguez JM, Martinez-Marcos F et al. Acute dystonia following a wasp sting. Rev Neurol 2005; 41: 62–3.
88. Kostic VS, Stojanovic-Svetel M, Kacar A. Symptomatic dystonias associated with structural brain lesions: report of 16 cases. Can J Neurol Sci 1996; 23: 53–6.
89. Lee MS, Rinne JO, Ceballos-Baumann A, Thompson PD, Marsden CD. Dystonia after head trauma. Neurology 1994; 44: 1374–8.
90. Burguera JA, Bataller L, Valero C. Action hand dystonia after cortical parietal infarction. Mov Disord 2001; 16: 1183–5.
91. Khan AA, Sussman JD. Focal dystonia after removal of a parietal meningioma. Mov Disord 2004; 19: 714–16.
92. LeDoux MS, Brady KA. Secondary cervical dystonia associated with structural lesions of the central nervous system. Mov Disord 2003; 18: 60–9.
93. Saint Hilaire MH, Burke RE, Bressman SB, Brin MF, Fahn S. Delayed-onset dystonia due to perinatal or early childhood asphyxia. Neurology 1991; 41: 216–22.
94. Scott BL, Jankovic J. Delayed-onset progressive movement disorders after static brain lesions. Neurology 1996; 46: 68–74.
95. Jankovic J, Van der Linden C. Dystonia and tremor induced by peripheral trauma: predisposing factors. J Neurol Neurosurg Psychiatry 1988; 51: 1512–19.
96. Sankhla C, Lai EC, Jankovic J. Peripherally induced oromandibular dystonia. J Neurol Neurosurg Psychiatry 1998; 65: 722–8.
97. Frucht S, Fahn S, Ford B. Focal task-specific dystonia induced by peripheral trauma. Mov Disord 2000; 15: 348–50.
98. Nobrega JC, Campos CR, Limongi JC, Teixeira MJ, Lin TY. Movement disorders induced by peripheral trauma. Arq Neuropsiquiatr 2002; 60: 17–20.
99. Jankovic J. Can peripheral trauma induce dystonia and other movement disorders? Yes! Mov Disord 2001; 16: 7–12.
100. Weiner WJ. Can peripheral trauma induce dystonia? No! Mov Disord 2001; 16: 13–22.
101. Fahn S. Dystonia: phenomenology, classification, etiology, genetics and pathophysiology. In: Fahn S, Jankovic J, Hallett M, Jenner P, eds. 16th Annual Course: A Comprehensive Review of Movement Disorders for the Clinical Practitioner, Vol. 3. New York: Columbia University, 2006: 1–85.
102. Hitoshi S, Iwata M, Yoshikawa K. Mid-brain pathology of Wilson's disease: MRI analysis of three cases. J Neurol Neurosurg Psychiatry 1991; 54: 624–6.
103. Jacobs DA, Markowitz CE, Liebeskind DS, Galetta SL. The "double panda sign" in Wilson's disease. Neurology 2003; 61: 969.
104. Shevell M. Hallervorden and history. N Engl J Med 2003; 348: 3–4.
105. Sethi KD, Adams RJ, Loring DW, El Gammal T. Hallervorden–Spatz syndrome: clinical and magnetic resonance imaging correlations. Ann Neurol 1988; 24: 692–4.
106. Hayflick SJ, Westaway SK, Levinson B et al. Genetic, clinical, and radiographic delineation of Hallervorden–Spatz syndrome. N Engl J Med 2003; 348: 33–40.
107. Carbon M, Su S, Dhawan V et al. Regional metabolism in primary torsion dystonia: effects of penetrance and genotype. Neurology 2004; 62: 1384–90.
108. Asanuma K, Ma Y, Okulski J et al. Decreased striatal D2 receptor binding in non-manifesting carriers of the DYT1 dystonia mutation. Neurology 2005; 64: 347–9.
109. Cammarota A, Gershanik, OS, Garcia S, Lera G. Cervical dystonia due to spinal cord ependymoma: involvement of cervical cord segments in the pathogenesis of dystonia. Mov Disord 1995; 10: 500–3.
110. LeDoux MS, Brady KA. Secondary cervical dystonia associated with structural lesions of the central nervous system. Mov Disord 2003; 18: 60–9.
111. Uncini A, Di Muzio A, Thomas A, Lugaresi A, Gambi D. Hand dystonia secondary to cervical demyelinating lesion. Acta Neurol Scand 1994; 90: 51–5.
112. Hunt AL, Giladi N, Bressman S, Fahn S. L-dopa treatment in idiopathic torsion dystonia. Neurology 1991; 41(Suppl 1): 293.
113. Fletcher NA, Thompson PD, Scadding JW, Marsden CD. Successful treatment of childhood-onset symptomatic dystonia with levodopa. J Neurol Neurosurg Psychiatry 1993; 56: 865–7.
114. Furukawa Y, Mizuno Y, Narabayashi H. Early-onset parkinsonism with dystonia. Clinical and biochemical differences from hereditary progressive dystonia or DOPA-responsive dystonia. Adv Neurol 1996; 69: 327–37.
115. Hyland K, Fryburg JS, Wilson WG et al. Oral phenylalanine loading in dopa-responsive dystonia: a possible diagnostic test. Neurology 1997; 48: 1290–7.
116. Saunders-Pullman R, Blau N, Hyland K et al. Phenylalanine loading as a diagnostic test for DRD: interpreting the utility of the test. Mol Genet Metab 2004; 83: 207–12.
117. Bezin L, Nygaard TG, Neville JD, Shen H, Levine RA. Reduced lymphoblast neopterin detects GTP cyclohydrolase dysfunction in dopa-responsive dystonia. Neurology 1998; 50: 1021–7.
118. Bonafé L, Thöny B, Leimbacher W, Kierat L, Blau N. Diagnosis of dopa-responsive dystonia and other tetrahydrobiopterin disorders by the study of biopterin metabolism in fibroblasts. Clin Chem 2001; 47: 477–85.
119. Bandmann O, Valente EM, Holmans P et al. Dopa-responsive dystonia: a clinical and molecular genetic study. Ann Neurol 1998; 44: 649–56.
120. Steinberger D, Korinthenberg R, Topka H et al. Dopa-responsive dystonia: mutation analysis of GCH1 and analysis of therapeutic doses of L-dopa. Neurology 2000; 55: 1735–7.

121. Furukawa Y. Update on dopa-responsive dystonia: locus heterogeneity and biochemical features. Adv Neurol 2004; 94: 127–38.
122. Furukawa Y, Guttman M, Sparagana SP et al. Dopa-responsive dystonia due to a large deletion in the GTP cyclohydrolase I gene. Ann Neurol 2000; 47: 517–20.
123. Hagenah J, Saunders-Pullman R, Hedrich K et al. High mutation rate in dopa-responsive dystonia: detection with comprehensive GCHI screening. Neurology 2005; 64: 908–11.
124. Brewer GJ, Askari F, Lorincz MT et al. Treatment of Wilson disease with ammonium tetrathiomolybdate: IV. Comparison of tetrathiomolybdate and trientine in a double-blind study of treatment of the neurologic presentation of Wilson disease. Arch Neurol 2006; 63: 521–7.
125. Steindl P, Ferenci P, Dienes JP et al. Wilson's disease in patients presenting with liver disease: a diagnostic challenge. Gastroenterology 1997; 113: 212–18.
126. Walshe JM. Diagnostic significance of reduced serum caeruloplasmin concentration in neurological disease. Mov Disord 2005; 20: 1658–61.
127. Ross ME, Jacobson IM, Dienstag JL, Martin JB. Late-onset Wilson's disease with neurological involvement in the absence of Kayser–Fleischer rings. Ann Neurol 1985; 17: 411–13.
128. Demirkiran M, Jankovic J, Lewis RA, Cox DW. Neurologic presentation of Wilson disease without Kayser–Fleischer rings. Neurology 1996; 46: 1040–3.
129. Vanier MT, Rodriguez-Lafrasse C, Rousson R et al. Type C Niemann–Pick disease: spectrum of phenotypic variation in disruption of intracellular LDL-derived cholesterol processing. Biochim Biophys Acta 1991; 1096: 328–37.
130. Yerby MS, Shaw CM, Watson JM. Progressive dementia and epilepsy in a young adult: unusual intraneuronal inclusions. Neurology 1986; 36: 68–71.

2

Epidemiology of dystonia

Meike Kasten, Anabel R Chade, and Caroline M Tanner

INTRODUCTION

Epidemiology is the investigation of the distribution and determinants of a disease or condition in a population. Dystonia is the third most common movement disorder, yet little is known regarding its population distribution and causes. Barriers to good studies include its relative rarity, the lack of disease registries such as exist for cancer, and the widespread belief that a substantial proportion of cases may not seek medical attention or are misdiagnosed. Deficiencies in epidemiologic knowledge limit progress in identifying treatments, prevention, or cures for this disabling disorder. In this chapter, we provide an overview of the epidemiology of dystonia, beginning with a short review of epidemiologic concepts as they apply to dystonia. Subsequent sections review what is known regarding the frequency and distribution of dystonia and its determinants. Because much remains to be done in this area, we conclude by identifying important directions for future work.

Although dystonic syndromes can be classified in many ways (see Chapter 1), the traditional grouping into two broad categories, based on etiology, of primary and secondary dystonia is followed in this chapter.[1] Primary dystonia (also called primary torsion dystonia, PTD) is distinguished from most secondary dystonias by the absence of signs and symptoms other than dystonia or dystonic tremor. Dystonia may also be characterized by age of onset (early vs late onset), site of symptoms (focal, segmental, generalized), or specific cause.

EPIDEMIOLOGIC CONCEPTS IMPORTANT TO THE STUDY OF DYSTONIA

A complete consideration of the principles of neuroepidemiology is beyond the scope of this chapter, but may be found in several textbooks.[2–4] A brief discussion of some key aspects is presented here.

Published estimates of the frequency of dystonia suggest that dystonia is a rare disease. Whether this is a correct assessment has been questioned by some, and the final answer will require further research investigations. The uncertainty stems from several characteristics of dystonia that make epidemiologic investigations particularly challenging. First, the term dystonia covers a clinically and etiologically heterogeneous set of disorders. All of the epidemiologic studies of the distribution of dystonia to date have focused on primary dystonia. Even within this category, clinical features range from generalized disease to focal disorders involving only a few muscles, such as spasmodic dysphonia or writer's cramp. The secondary dystonias include many rare neurologic disorders, but also include more common conditions, such as dystonia due to drugs (neuroleptics and therapies for parkinsonism) and dystonia as part of more extensive neurologic injuries, such as cerebral palsy, stroke, and traumatic brain injury. A few clinical series suggest that these forms may be common, but the full impact remains an unknown, though likely significant, source of disability.

A further difficulty in studying dystonia is that the clinical features of the syndrome may be unfamiliar to many practitioners. Because primary dystonia frequently manifests clinical signs only when specific motor tasks are repetitively performed, mild cases or early cases of dystonia are commonly misdiagnosed. In the secondary dystonias, the unique dystonic phenomenology may not be recognized or may not be recorded in a format that can be easily retrieved. The threshold for recognition of dystonia as a problem appropriate for medical attention may vary as well. While those with severe, generalized disease are likely to seek medical attention, many persons with mild or moderate features of disease may not do so, or may not persist in seeking attention if the dystonia is not recognized by the first practitioner. To determine the extent to which dystonia is missed, the 'gold-standard' approach would be direct evaluation of a population by expert diagnosticians, including the appropriate provocative tests to identify task-specific syndromes. The costs and practical difficulties of such an effort have, so far, rendered this approach impossible. More efficient approaches, beginning with a questionnaire screening for symptoms of dystonia, followed by expert exam in those endorsing symptoms, have been successful in identifying undiagnosed cases. For example, a postal survey in northern England found 10% of respondents to advertisements describing dystonic syndromes were previously undiagnosed.[5] Similarly, in an Italian survey of adults aged ≥50 years, 4/6 cases of dystonia had not previously been diagnosed.[6]

EPIDEMIOLOGY OF PRIMARY DYSTONIAS

Incidence and prevalence have been estimated for primary dystonia in small studies – other measures of disease in populations, such as mortality, are not available. For primary dystonia, precision of both incidence and prevalence estimates is problematic because of the small number of cases identified in published, community-based studies.

Incidence

Incidence estimates are theoretically a better representation of disease distribution, as those with shortened survival are more likely to be included. Only two studies[7,8] have estimated overall annual incidence of primary dystonia, and the results differ considerably. Korczyn et al[7] estimated incidence in Israeli Jews based on 1969–1975 hospital discharge data verified by examination. The crude annual incidence in Jews of European descent was estimated at $0.42/10^6$ based on seven cases, and of Afro-Asian descent at $0.11/10^6$, based on a single case. Whether this figure represents all PTD or only generalized PTD is not clearly stated. Nutt et al[8] estimated PTD incidence in Rochester, Minnesota, based on records linkage with review of medical records for the period 1950–1982. Crude annual incidence of generalized PTD was $2/10^6$ person-years (p-y) (based on three cases), of torticollis was $11/10^6$ p-y (based on 11 cases), of blepharospasm was $4.6/10^6$ p-y (based on seven cases), of oromandibular dystonia was $3.3/10^6$ p-y (based on five cases), of both writer's cramp and spasmodic dysphonia was $2.7/10^6$ p-y (based on four cases each). Thus, the total knowledge of the incidence of PTD is based only on a total of 41 cases from two populations observed between 1950 and 1982. There is, at a minimum, a five-fold difference in the estimates of generalized dystonia between these two studies. Neither study presented age- or gender-specific incidence, and only one of the total cases was non-white. In a separate report, the incidence of torticollis in Finland was $1/10^6$, but no methodologic information was provided in this abstract.[9]

Prevalence

The prevalence of primary dystonia is reported in a number of different studies,[5–8,10–26] at 30–7320 cases per million for late-onset and 2–50 cases per million for early-onset dystonia. Estimates of prevalence for generalized dystonia ranged from $0.3/10^6$ in a German service-based study[14] (based on four cases) to $50/10^6$ in a Chinese community-based, door-to-door study[10] (based on three cases) and are further described in Table 2.1. For focal and segmental dystonia, estimated prevalence ranged from $30/10^6$ based on three cases identified in a door-to-door study in China[10] to $2250/10^6$ based on six cases identified in a population sample of older adults in Italy.[6] The variation in reported prevalence seen from study to study can be at least partially explained by differences in case ascertainment methods and the fact that all the reported rates are crude rates. Adjusted rates for primary dystonia are not available, and crude rates always result in larger variance because adjustment for influencing factors such as differences in mean age, gender distribution, or risk-factor profile in the study population is not possible.

Only five studies estimating the prevalence of PTD have been conducted in enumerated populations.[8,10,12,15,24] Precision in these studies is poor, as only 74 cases were identified over all four studies. Service-based studies that included patients from tertiary care or treatment centers (botulinum toxin clinics)[11,13,14,16–20,22] reported overall prevalences of 61–117/million for focal dystonia[11,13,14,16,20] and 3–50/million for generalized dystonia.[14,19] Service-based approaches do not account for differences in access to care or treatment response for dystonia subtypes. This is important, as some subtypes are harder to recognize than others, mild cases may not seek medical attention, and misdiagnosed cases may not be referred to the center. Error in estimating prevalence and bias in subgroup comparisons is likely using a service-based approach.

Age, gender, and ethnicity

The number of cases observed in enumerated populations is too small to be able to describe distribution. Therefore, we must rely on clinical series, recognizing that many differences in access to care associated with these factors could influence these observations.

Age The age at onset of primary dystonia appears to be bimodal based on clinical series, with modes at 9 years

Table 2.1 Prevalence of generalized PTD[a]

Location of study	Number of cases	Estimated prevalence/million
Germany (Castelon-Konkiewitz, 2002)[14]	4	0.3
UK (Duffey et al, 1998)[5]	37	1.4
Iceland (Asgeirsson et al, 2006)[24]	1	3.0
Japan (Sugawara et al, 2006)[25]	8	6.8
Israel (Korczyn et al, 1980)[7]	35	9.6
USA (Nutt et al, 1988)[8]	3	34
China (Li et al, 1985)[10]	3	50

[a]Results not adjusted for differences in underlying populations.
PTD = primary torsion dystonia.

(early onset) and 45 years (late onset), divided by a nadir at 27 years.[27] The age at onset appears to correlate with the subtype of dystonia (Table 2.2). Focal dystonia and dystonia with cranial symptoms are associated with older age of onset; however, incidence studies are lacking, and these observations may reflect an influence of disease duration. Table 2.2 also summarizes age and gender data from the two largest dystonia investigations: a record-linkage study in the United Kingdom[5] and a service-based study (ESDE) in Europe.[13]

Age at onset may be especially relevant in familial disease. Patients attending a botulinum toxin clinic with a family history of primary focal dystonia reported a younger age at onset (39 ± 18 years) than those without a family history (47 ± 14 years) ($p < 0.01$).[23] This pattern could reflect greater awareness and, thus, earlier recognition of dystonia in those with affected relatives, or the true genetic influence on age of onset.

Gender Most of the available prevalence studies provide male:female ratios or gender-specific prevalence rates; one large study indicates a female preponderance for focal dystonia.[13] Writer's cramp, however, seemed to be more common in men in this evaluation. The prevalence of focal dystonia in women is higher than expected, and it is not clear this is a true finding. However, female preponderance of focal dystonia might be explained by a number of factors: (1) women may be more aware of symptoms than men; (2) genetic factors may make women more susceptible; or (3) women may have more exposure to environmental factors that increase risk of the disease (i.e. occupational hazard). There is little gender-specific data regarding other types of dystonia; however, the United Kingdom study[5] shows a slight female preponderance for generalized dystonia as well.

Ethnicity While PTD has been reported in all races, the relative distribution of PTD across racial groups is not known.[28] The methods, geographic area, ethnicity, age distribution, and case definition criteria differ considerably among the available studies. One study investigated distribution and characteristics by race and ethnicity, but obtaining prevalence and incidence data was not a primary aim.[29] In addition, the study used a preselected population and does not provide information about the distribution in an unselected population. Data from family studies indicate the prevalence of early-onset generalized dystonia is highest in Ashkenazi Jews; about 90% of these cases are due to *DYT1* mutations and an underlying founder mutation has been shown in this population.[19] Ashkenazi Jews had an earlier age at onset and greater frequency of limb onset than did non-Jewish Caucasians.[29] In the same study, African-Americans tended to have cranial and laryngeal involvement; however, only 29 cases were observed. The numbers of Hispanics and Asians in this study were too small to allow analysis. Recently, the frequency of *DYT1* mutations among primary dystonia patients in Singapore has been published, indicating such mutations are rare in this population (1%) and not significantly different than the rate reported in Western populations.[30] In a study of the Icelandic population, a haplotype of torsinA was associated with sporadic dystonia,[31] but no such correlation was evident in a group of German patients with sporadic dystonia,[32] suggesting that the former finding may be unique to the Icelandic population.

Risk factors for primary dystonia

Some of the primary dystonias are clearly familial and, for a few, a gene has been identified. However, there is

Table 2.2 Age, gender, and type of dystonia in three studies

Type of dystonia	Duffey et al, 1998[5], (record review, postal survey)			ESDE, 2000[14] (clinic study)			Dhaenens et al, 2005[23] (clinic study)		
	No. of cases	Mean age at onset	Male: female ratio	No. of cases	Mean age at onset	Male: female ratio	No. of cases	Mean age at onset	Male: female ratio
Generalized	37	16.7	1:1.3	NA	NA	NA	NA	NA	NA
Writer's cramp	19	37.9	1.4:1	79	37.9	1:0.8	9	35.8	1:1.3
Cervical	159	40.7	1:2.2	330	41.4	1:1.4	47	41.3	1:3.3
Blepharospasm	78	58.8	1:3.6	206	58.8	1:2.3	48	55.4	1:1.8

ESDE = Epidemiological Study of Dystonia in Europe.

significant phenotypic heterogeneity even within the forms with a known genetic cause. Probably, environmental factors account for at least some of this heterogeneity. The limited work to identify environmental risk factors for primary dystonia is reviewed in this section. The low penetrance and variable expressivity of *DYT1* suggest that such research is critically important to understanding the disorder. Clues to environmental causes or modifiers may be obtained from studying the function of *DYT1* or other dystonia-associated genes. Possible risk factors may also be derived from investigations of the natural history of individuals with dystonia, in an attempt to identify 'triggers' of disease. In addition, investigation of the population distribution of dystonia may provide clues to environmental determinants. These proposed risk factors must then be tested systematically in other populations, and biologic plausibility assessed in cooperation with laboratory scientists. To date, very little work has been done. However, if specific risk factors can be identified, this could improve our understanding of the pathogenesis of dystonia, and possibly provide strategies for prevention or treatment.

Antecedent illness

Because the *DYT1* gene encodes a protein in the heat-shock family, the expression of torsinA might be modulated by infection or fever.[33] Preliminary work suggests infection with fever may cause earlier onset of generalized dystonia. Comparisons of antecedent severe febrile illness and trauma in manifesting and non-manifesting *DYT1* carriers indicate that early-onset childhood illness was associated with manifesting dystonia.[33] This suggests that factors modifying metabolic pathways including torsinA may be important in DYT1 and possibly other forms of dystonia. However, more work will be needed in the laboratory and in populations.

Trauma

For more than a century, whether focal or generalized trauma can cause PTD has been controversial. Nevertheless, trauma is the most frequently proposed risk factor and is typically described as an injury to the dystonic body part, preceding dystonia onset by months or longer. Commonly reported injuries in various clinical series include 'whiplash' from a motor vehicle accident, reported in up to 20% of spasmodic torticollis patients; hand trauma, in up to 10% of those with focal hand dystonia; and ocular lesions, such as keratitis, in 10–20% of patients with blepharospasm. Sensory symptoms such as pain, discomfort, and distortion of sensory modalities have been reported as the earliest manifestations of dystonia;[34] patients with postural tremor may be more likely to develop dystonia in response to trauma.[35] The proposed pathologic mechanism for this association is injury-induced alteration of sensory input that causes central nervous system reorganization and results in a movement disorder, and data from experimental animals provide indirect support for this proposed mechanism.[36] Alternatively, torsinA expression may be modulated by trauma.[37] Since head injury has also been associated with primary dystonia, altered torsinA function might explain both focal and non-focal trauma as precipitants of dystonia. However, a recent multicenter case–control study in 177 cases with primary adult-onset cranial dystonia and 217 age- and gender-matched controls with primary hemifacial spasm did not find trauma to be associated with an increased risk of dystonia when compared with the disease control group.[38] Whether there would be a similarly negative finding if a non-affected control group were chosen must be determined by future investigations.

Occupation

Repetitive motion has been proposed as a risk factor for dystonia, but there are no epidemiologic data confirming this. Focal hand dystonias (writer's cramp, occupational dystonia) are commonly associated with tasks involving repetitive movements, such as typing or playing a musical instrument. Although musician's dystonia and other focal task-specific dystonias are generally considered sporadic conditions, study of three multiplex families suggests that an autosomally dominant genetic contribution with phenotypic variability may play a role in the development of these disorders in some cases.[39] Occupational dystonia can be devastating, often causing a career change. A study of musicians showed that anxiety disorders occurred more often in dystonic musicians and in musicians with chronic pain than in controls.[40] The authors hypothesized, however, that these psychological conditions were already present before the onset of playing-related disorders. Focal dystonia has been associated with a degradation of hand representations in the somatosensory cortex,[41] and a parallel finding of cortical reorganization has also been reported in the somatosensory areas of patients with chronic pain.[42,43] Similarly, childhood-onset DYT1 generalized dystonia frequently presents with focal signs, often manifesting only after prolonged task-specific activity (e.g. writing, running). In animal models, prolonged repetitive motions can alter central nervous system function and ultimately produce a movement disorder.[44,45] In humans, aberrant plasticity from excessive repetitive use has been thought to cause dystonia,[46,47] although a causal association of repetitive motion and dystonia has never been shown. If specific occupations, hobbies, or characteristic physical activities are shown to be associated with dystonia, avoidance of these could be important in those at risk (i.e. in non-manifesting *DYT1* carriers). Indirect support for this proposition is provided by a recent clinical study of aberrant plasticity in patients with writer's cramp.[48]

Cigarette smoking

One case–control study of adults found an inverse association of cigarette smoking with primary dystonia.[49] The magnitude of the association was similar to that observed in Parkinson's disease (PD).[50] Dystonia can occur in PD and is presumed to be mediated by the same general brain circuitry (basal ganglia and nigrostriatal pathways).[51] Alterations of central dopaminergic systems may cause both PD and dystonia,[28] and it is plausible these disorders may have common risk factors.

Thyroid disorders

Large clinical series reports indicate dystonia may be associated with autoimmune disease and thyroid disorders. Antecedent thyroid disease was observed in adults with primary torsion dystonia in Olmsted County, although only six cases were seen.[8] The high frequency of thyroid disorders among the torticollis patients in this study may only reflect the risk of thyroid disease in that community – indeed, thyroid conditions may be too prevalent in a given patient population to warrant consideration. Nevertheless, controls with peripheral sensory neuropathy had a much lower frequency of thyroid disease, and it was suggested a possible increased frequency in those with torticollis might represent an effect of an autoimmune mechanism.[8]

Hypertension

In a case–control study, primary torsion dystonia was inversely associated with hypertension in adults; however, the effect was largely due to over-representation of hypertension in a control group with hemifacial spasm.[49]

Vestibular changes

Neuro-otological tests in patients with idiopathic spasmodic torticollis often identify a breakdown of the mechanisms responsible for signaling head posture. However, there is some evidence that lesions of the VIIIth nerve may aggravate spasmodic torticollis by further disrupting processing of sensory information about head position. Thus, interventions on the vestibular system are not likely to improve the clinical condition of patients with spasmodic torticollis.[52]

EPIDEMIOLOGY OF SECONDARY DYSTONIAS

No published studies have estimated the distribution of all forms of secondary dystonia in populations. This work would be important to determine the burden of disease due to secondary dystonia, and may also provide new understandings of the pathogenesis of primary dystonia. Work has been limited for several reasons. First, describing the distribution of secondary dystonia requires a clear definition of the conditions. This is difficult to achieve given the large collection of symptoms and

Table 2.3 Age, gender, ethnicity, and other factors with neuroleptic-associated secondary dystonia syndromes

Factor	Acute dystonia	Tardive dystonia
Age	Younger	Younger
Gender	Uncertain	Men
Race		Low prevalence in Hong Kong Chinese
Antipsychotic	Higher dosage	
Birth injury		Yes
Electroconvulsive therapy		Yes
Affective disorder		Yes
Mental retardation		Yes
Temporal relationship with neuroleptic treatment	Early, first 48–72 hours	Late

dystonic syndromes that the term is used to encompass. Secondly, when dystonia is part of a more extensive syndrome, examination may be required in order to determine whether an individual is affected.

We have concentrated on:

- drug-induced dystonia due to neuroleptic exposure, acute dystonic reactions, and tardive dystonia
- dystonia associated with PD.

In each case, information is available only within the context of clinical series (Table 2.3), and is not truly population based. Although these forms of the disease are the most commonly recognized, even clinical descriptions of disease frequency are few.

Acute dystonic reactions associated with neuroleptic agents

It is difficult to clearly distinguish the incidence and prevalence of acute dystonic reactions as their duration rarely exceeds several hours, which often makes expert consultation impossible. Incidence rates vary widely from 2 to 70%[53–57] and appear to depend on the drug administered and the dose. Haloperidol therapy is generally associated with the highest incidence of acute dystonia.[56,57] Anticholinergic prophylaxis is known to reduce the likelihood of neuroleptic-induced acute dystonia[58–60] but may cause unwanted side effects and is not recommended in patients at low risk of acute dystonia.

In almost all studies, a young age of exposure appears to be an important risk factor for the development of acute dystonic reactions.[56,61,62] One small study ($n = 39$) showed a significantly higher incidence in patients <30 years old (72.2%) as compared to those >30 years old (33.3%) [$p < 0.05$].[61] In this same study, acute dystonic reactions were more frequent in men than in women,[61] although male preponderance is not consistent across all studies.[56,62] Men may be more likely to receive higher dosages of neuroleptics, and Kondo et al reported a 91.7% frequency of acute dystonic reactions in young men (11 out of 12).[61] Information about the incidence and prevalence of acute dystonic reactions among different ethnic groups is extremely scarce, with only one study including data comparing patients of different ethnic backgrounds.[62] In this study, the frequency of acute dystonic reactions was 13 out of 32 (41%) in blacks and 13 out of 41 (32%) in whites, and the difference was not statistically significant.

Tardive or persistent dystonia associated with neuroleptic agents

Tardive dystonia is a dystonic syndrome resulting from chronic neuroleptic exposure.[63] It is distinguished from acute dystonia chiefly by the duration of exposure. Tardive dystonia is differentiated from other tardive movement disorders on clinical grounds, but there is some overlap of syndromes. Although described in clinical series reports, tardive dystonia has not been studied epidemiologically. In clinical series, tardive dystonia is often a severe and disabling disorder, poorly responsive to therapy. Finding ways to prevent this iatrogenic disorder is important. Like PTD, tardive dystonia is a rare disease with considerable variation in its symptoms and presentation and requires a diagnosis by a specialist. Drawing conclusions about the relationships of age, ethnicity, or gender is difficult given the small number and highly selected ascertainment of patients studied to date.

Incidence/prevalence

There are no incidence data for tardive dystonia. The overall annual incidence for all tardive movement disorders has been reported to be 3.7–12%, and tardive dystonia would probably be a small proportion of the cases in any of these series.[64,65] Prevalence rates between 0.4 and 4% have been reported in other studies.[66–69] Table 2.4 shows prevalence data, but results should be interpreted with care, as the studies are not prospective or longitudinal, differ considerably in underlying populations, and lack information about the types and dosages of medications given.

Age and gender Several studies indicate an association between younger age and higher risk for tardive dystonia,[63,67] male preponderance,[63,69] and a younger age of onset in men,[63] but these studies did not incorporate possible confounders, so the results may be questionable. Unlike in tardive dyskinesia, neither female gender nor advanced age appears to be risk factors.[70] For example, Burke et al[63] reported an age of onset of 29.0 years old for men ($n = 26$) and 41.5 years old for women ($n = 16$), but without age at first exposure. The reported male:female ratios for tardive dystonia range from 1:1 to 1.7:1 [Chiu et al (1:1)[68]; Gimenez-Roldan et al (1.2:1)[71]; Burke et al (1.6:1)[63]; Raja (1.7:1)[69]]. Possible confounders include the age at onset of schizophrenia in men[70] and that men may develop tardive dystonia with a shorter length of exposure to neuroleptics than women.[72] The daily dosage of neuroleptics is reported to be lower in women, and the distribution of underlying psychiatric disorders may influence the likelihood of developing tardive dystonia.[69] Many of the studies cited included only referred patients; further study in unselected populations exposed to neuroleptics or in larger case–control studies are needed to confirm these observations.

Ethnicity Among the studies described above, the lowest reported prevalence of tardive dystonia was 0.4% in Chinese psychiatric inpatients.[68]

Dystonia in parkinsonism

Although dystonia in PD was first described by Charcot in 1877,[73] there is no published epidemiologic study of the incidence or prevalence of dystonic features in PD or parkinsonism; the information reviewed here has been extracted from case series and clinical descriptions. These have been derived primarily from specialty clinics. Patients in these clinics may differ from those not seeking specialty care in many ways. It would, therefore, not be appropriate to extrapolate these findings to other populations.

Dystonia in PD is most frequently described in the course of levodopa (L-dopa) treatment, although it can occur prior to the initiation of dopaminergic therapy. Dystonia is the second most common L-dopa-associated movement disorder. Dystonia associated with L-dopa treatment in PD can be maximal at the peak beneficial effect of the drug ('on') or can manifest as drug efficacy wanes (wearing 'off'). In one study, dystonic symptoms

Table 2.4 Frequency of tardive dystonia observed in selected patient surveys[a]

Study	No. of population	No. of cases	Prevalence	Comments
Yassa et al, 1986[66]	351	7	2.0%	Inpatient population, includes psychogeriatric units, meet criteria of Burke et al 1982[63]
Friedman et al, 1987[67]	331	5	1.5%	Inpatient population, complete histories not available for all patients; all were 'believed' to have had exposure to neuroleptics
Chiu et al, 1992[68]	917	4	0.4%	Inpatient population, meet criteria of Burke et al 1982[63]
Raja, 1995[69]	200	8	4.0%	Inpatient population, meet criteria of Burke et al 1982[63]

[a]Results not adjusted for differences in underlying populations.

occurred in 30% of PD patients and most often presented as early-morning foot dystonia (33 of 207 patients, 16%).[74] Biphasic 'on' dystonia was relatively rare in this study (15 of 207 patients, 7%). In another study, 46 of 56 patients also showed 'off' dystonia that tended to occur in the early morning before their first doses of L-dopa had taken effect.[75]

The frequency of dystonic symptoms in PD is linked with young age at onset. Frequency was about 50% in patients whose onset occurred before 35,[76] 40,[77] or 45[78] years of age. In our series, only 10% of patients with old-onset PD had dystonia,[79] and in another series, none of the old-onset patients had dystonia.[78] In a separate series, dystonia accompanied or preceded the onset of parkinsonism in 14% of young-onset PD patients, and early-morning dystonia occurred during treatment in 59%.[80] No information is available to judge the influences of gender or ethnicity on the development of dystonia in PD.

Risk factors for secondary dystonia

Drugs

Neuroleptic exposure causes acute and tardive dystonia.[63,81] Both 'atypical' and 'typical' neuroleptics,[81–87] as well as antiemetics blocking central dopamine receptors can cause tardive dystonia.[88] Even very short periods of exposure may cause a persistent movement disorder. Longer duration of exposure to neuroleptics does not necessarily correlate with severity of tardive dystonia.[89]

Other medications associated with tardive dystonia include some antidepressants (e.g. amoxapine,[63] amitriptyline, and doxepin[90]), and the benzamide derivative veralipride.[91]

Genetics

For some forms of secondary dystonia, the genetic background has been extensively studied and the involved genes are known (e.g. Huntington's disease and other heredodegenerative diseases). There is less information about tardive dystonia, but it has been proposed to be associated with certain *CYP2D6* genotypes that are associated with decreased drug metabolism. The results of three studies of genotyping and tardive dystonia or acute dystonic reaction were inconsistent, however, as the case numbers were small and few 'poor metabolizers' were included.[92–94] Another study in 665 schizophrenic patients analyzing dopamine (D_2) receptor subtypes did not show a significant association between any subtype and any adverse effect of neuroleptic treatment.[95] In a separate study, however, a family history of primary movement disorders was a significant predictor for development of a secondary movement disorder following neuroleptic treatment, and a positive family history of dystonia was associated with higher prevalence of acute dystonic reaction.[96] There are no data regarding family history and tardive dystonia, as family history is an exclusion in the criteria for tardive dystonia defined by Burke.[63]

Other factors

Brain injury may influence the onset of dystonia in neuroleptic-treated patients. In one study, a high frequency of lenticular or thalamic lesions was seen in patients who developed dystonia after head trauma – such associations highlight the potential importance of damage to the putaminopallidothalamic neuronal circuit in the development of dystonias.[97] Birth injury may also predispose to the development of tardive dystonia[63] and mental retardation and convulsive therapy are risk factors as well.[67]

CONCLUSIONS

Few studies have estimated the incidence of PTD and only one of these studies included all clinical subtypes – neither reported age- or gender-specific incidence. Among the studies that estimated prevalence, none has done so in age-, gender-, and race/ethnicity-specific strata, including all clinical subtypes. Despite the reduced penetrance and variable expressivity of genetic PTD, there have been few investigations of environmental risk factors, even though identifying specific risk factors is important in understanding the pathogenesis of the disease. Thus, neither the distribution nor the determinants of PTD are known. Even fewer studies have explored the epidemiology of secondary dystonia, and none has examined the combined frequency of all dystonia in a population. The overall burden of dystonia remains unknown. As has been true for many other disorders, such as cancer, observation of patterns in populations can provide important clues to potential differences in susceptibility factors – either genetic or environmental. This information may provide important clues to differential susceptibility by race or gender, leading in turn to laboratory investigations that determine underlying biologic mechanisms of these patterns. A better understanding of the incidence and prevalence of dystonia and the identification of risk factors for the disorder and its subtypes will be beneficial in healthcare planning, and may lead directly to preventive recommendations or may provide new directions for development of treatments.

ACKNOWLEDGMENTS

Michael J Fox Foundation Fellowships (Drs Chade and Kasten); NIH (NINDS) R01 NS046340 (Dr Tanner); Jennifer Wright for editorial support.

REFERENCES

1. Fahn S, Bressman SB, Marsden CD. Classification of dystonia. Adv Neurol 1998; 78: 1–10.
2. Hofman A, Mayeux R. Investigating Neurological Disease: Epidemiology for Clinical Neurology. New York: Cambridge University Press; 2001.
3. Batchelor T, Cudkowicz ME. Principles of Neuroepidemiology. Boston: Butterworth Heinemann; 2001.
4. Nelson LM, Tanner CM, Van Den Eeden SK, McGuire VM. Neuroepidemiology: From Principles to Practice. New York: Oxford University Press; 2004.
5. Duffey POF, Butler AG, Hawthorne MR, Barnes MP. The epidemiology of the primary dystonias in the north of England. In: Fahn S, Marsden CD, DeLong M, eds. Dystonia 3: Advances in Neurology, Vol. 78. Philadelphia: Lippincott-Raven Publishers; 1998: 121–5.
6. Muller J, Kiechl S, Wenning GK et al. The prevalence of primary dystonia in the general community. Neurology 2002; 59: 941–3.
7. Korczyn AD, Kahana E, Zilber N et al. Torsion dystonia in Israel. Ann Neurol 1980; 8: 387–91.
8. Nutt JG, Muenter MD, Melton LJ 3rd et al. Epidemiology of dystonia in Rochester, Minnesota. Adv Neurol 1988; 50: 361–5.
9. Erjanti HM, Martilla RJ, Rinne UK. The prevalence and incidence of cervical dystonia in south-western Finland. Mov Disord 1996; 11(Suppl 1): 215.
10. Li SC, Schoenberg BS, Wang CC et al. A prevalence survey of Parkinson's diseases and other movement disorders in the People's Republic of China. Arch Neurol 1985; 42: 655–7.
11. Nakashima K, Kusumi M, Inoue Y, Takahashi K. Prevalence of focal dystonias in the western area of Tottori prefecture in Japan. Mov Disord 1995; 10: 440–3.
12. Kandil MR, Tohamy SA, Fattah MA et al. Prevalence of chorea, dystonia, and athetosis in Assiut, Egypt: a clinical and epidemiological study. Neuroepidemiology 1994; 13: 202–10.
13. The ESDE (Epidemiological Study of Dystonia in Europe) Collaborative Group. A prevalence study of primary dystonia in eight European countries. J Neurol 2000; 247: 787–92.
14. Sex-related influences on the frequency and age of onset of primary dystonia. Neurology 1993; 53: 1871–3.
15. Castelon-Konkiewitz E, Trender-Gerhard J, Kamm C et al. Service-based study of dystonia in Munich. Neuroepidemiology 2002; 21: 202–6.
16. Butler AG, Duffy POF, Hawthorne MR, Barnes MP. An epidemiological survey of dystonia within the entire population of northeast England over the past nine years. Adv Neurol 2004; 94: 257–9.
17. Matsumoto S, Nishimura M, Shibasski H, Kaji R. Epidemiology of primary dystonias in Japan: comparison with western countries. Mov Disord 2003; 18: 1196–8.
18. Le KD, Nilsen B, Dietrichs E. Prevalence of primary focal and segmental dystonia in Oslo. Neurology 2003; 61: 1294–6.
19. Pekmezovic T, Ivanovic N, Svetel M et al. Prevalence of primary late-onset focal dystonia in the Belgrade population. Mov Disord 2003; 18: 1389–92.
20. Risch N, de Leon D, Ozelius L et al. Genetic analysis of idiopathic torsion dystonia in Ashkenazi Jews and their recent descent from a small founder population. Nat Genet 1995; 9: 152–9.
21. Defazio G, Livrea P, De Salvia R et al. Prevalence of primary blepharospasm in a community of Puglia region, Southern Italy. Neurology 2001; 56: 1579–81.
22. Zilber N, Korczyn AS, Kahana E et al. Inheritance of idiopathic torsion dystonia among Jews. J Med Gen 1984; 21: 13–20.
23. Cossu G, Mereu A, Deriu M et al. Prevalence of primary blepharospasm in Sardinia, Italy: a service-based survey. Mov Disord 2006; 21: 2005–8.
24. Dhaenens CM, Krystkowiak P, Douay X et al. Clinical and genetic evaluation in a French population presenting with primary focal dystonia. Mov Disord 2005; 20: 822–5.
25. Asgeirsson H, Jakobsson F, Hjaltason H, Jonsdottir H, Sveinbjornsdottir S. Prevalence study of primary dystonia in Iceland. Mov Disord 2006; 21: 293–8.
26. Sugawara M, Watanabe S, Toyoshima I. Prevalence of dystonia in Akita Prefecture in Northern Japan. Mov Disord 2006; 21: 1047–9.
27. Fukuda H, Kusumi M, Nakashima K. Epidemiology of primary focal dystonias in the western area of Tottori prefecture in Japan: comparison with prevalence evaluated in 1993. Mov Disord 2006; 21: 1503–6.
28. Bressman SB, de Leon D, Brin MF et al. Idiopathic dystonia among Ashkenazi Jews: evidence for autosomal dominant inheritance. Ann Neurol 1989; 26: 612–20.
29. Tanner CM. Dystonia. In: Klawans HL, Goetz CG, Tanner CM, eds. Textbook of Clinical Neuropharmacology. New York: Raven Press; 1991: 167–82.
30. Almasy L, Bressman S, de Leon D, Risch N. Ethnic variation in the clinical expression of idiopathic torsion dystonia. Mov Disord 1997; 12: 715–21.
31. Jamora RD, Tan EK, Liu CP et al. DYT1 mutations amongst adult primary dystonia patients in Singapore with review of literature comparing East and West. J Neurol Sci 2006; 247: 35–7.
32. Clarimon J, Asgeirsson H, Singleton A et al. Torsin A haplotype predisposes to idiopathic dystonia. Ann Neurol 2005; 57: 765–7.
33. Hague S, Klaffke S, Clarimon J et al. Lack of association with TorsinA haplotype in German patients with sporadic dystonia. Neurology 2006; 66: 951–2.
34. Saunders Pullman RJ. Environmental Modifiers of Genetic Dystonia: Possible Role of Infection. San Diego, CA: American Academy of Neurology; 2000.
35. Ghika J, Regli F, Growdon JH. Sensory symptoms in cranial dystonia: a potential role in the etiology? J Neurol Sci 1993; 116: 142–7.
36. Jankovic J, van der Linden C. Dystonia and tremor induced by peripheral trauma: predisposing factors. J Neurol Neurosurg Psychiatry 1988; 51: 1512–19.
37. Jankovic J. Can peripheral trauma induce dystonia and other movement disorders? Yes! Mov Disord 2001; 16: 7–12.
38. Breakefield XO, Kamm C, Hanson PI. TorsinA: movement at many levels. Neuron 2001; 31: 9–12.
39. Martino D, Defazio G, Abbruzzese G et al. Head trauma in primary cranial dystonias: a multicentre case-control study. J Neurol Neurosurg Psychiatry 2007; 78: 260–3.
40. Schmidt A, Jabusch HC, Altenmuller E et al. Dominantly transmitted focal dystonia in families of patients with musician's cramp. Neurology 2006; 67: 691–3.
41. Jabusch HC, Muller SV, Altenmuller E. Anxiety in musicians with focal dystonia and those with chronic pain. Mov Disord 2004; 19: 1169–238.
42. Elbert T, Candia V, Altenmuller E et al. Alteration of digital representations in somatosensory cortex in focal hand dystonia. Neuroreport 1998; 9: 3571–5.

43. Flor H, Braun C, Elbert T, Birbaumer N. Extensive reorganization of primary somatosensory cortex in chronic back pain patients. Neurosci Lett 1997; 224: 5–8.
44. Tinazzi M, Fisaschi A, Rosso T et al. Neuroplastic changes related to pain occur at multiple levels of the human somatosensory system: a somatosensory-evoked potentials study in patients with cervical radicular pain. J Neurosci 2000; 20: 9277–83.
45. Byl NN, Merzenich MM, Jenkins WM. A primate genesis model of focal dystonia and repetitive strain injury: I. Learning-induced dedifferentiation of the representation in the hand in the primary somatosensory cortex in adult monkeys. Neurology 1996; 47: 508–20.
46. Byl NN, Merzenich MM, Cheung S et al. A primate model for studying focal dystonia and repetitive strain injury: effects on the primary somatosensory cortex. Phys Ther 1997; 77: 269–84.
47. Byl NN. Focal hand dystonia may result from aberrant neuroplasticity. Adv Neurol 2004; 94: 19–28.
48. Zeuner KE, Shill HA, Sohn YH et al. Motor training as treatment in focal hand dystonia. Mov Disord 2005; 20: 335–41.
49. Weise D, Schramm A, Stefan K et al. The two sides of associative plasticity in writer's cramp. Brain 2006; 129: 2709–21.
50. DeFazio G, Berardelli A, Abruzzese G et al. Possible risk factors for primary adult onset dystonia: a case-control investigation by the Italian Movement Disorders Study Group. J Neurol Neurosurg Psychiatry 1998; 64: 25–32.
51. Marras C, Tanner CM. The epidemiology of Parkinson's disease. In: Watts RL, Koller WC, eds. Movement Disorders: Neurologic Principles and Practice. New York: McGraw Hill; 2002.
52. Bressman SB. Dystonia update. Clin Neuropharmacol 2000; 23: 239–51.
53. Bronstein AM, Rudge P. The vestibular system in abnormal head postures and in spasmodic torticollis. Adv Neurol 1988; 50: 493–500.
54. Ayd FJ. A survey of drug-induced extrapyramidal reactions. JAMA 1961; 175: 1054–60.
55. Keepers GA, Casey DE. Prediction of neuroleptic-induced dystonia. J Clin Psychopharmacol 1987; 7: 342–5.
56. Stern TA, Anderson WH. Benzotropine prophylaxis of dystonic reactions. Psychopharmacology (Berl) 1979; 61: 261–2.
57. Aguilar EJ, Keshavan MS, Martinez-Quiles MD et al. Predictors of acute dystonia in first-episode psychotic patients. Am J Psychiatry 1994; 151: 1819–21.
58. Donlon PT, Hopkin JT, Tupin JP et al. Haloperidol for acute schizophrenic patients. An evaluation of three oral regimens. Arch Gen Psychiatry 1980; 37: 691–5.
59. Keepers GA, Clappison VJ, Casey DE. Initial anticholinergic prophylaxis for neuroleptic-induced extrapyramidal syndromes. Arch Gen Psychiatry 1983; 40: 1113–17.
60. Sramek JJ, Simpson GM, Morrison RL, Heiser JF. Anticholinergic agents for prophylaxis for neuroleptic-induced dystonic reaction: a prospective study. J Clin Psychiatry 1986; 47: 305–9.
61. Winslow RS, Stillner V, Coons DJ, Robinson MW. Prevention of acute dystonic reactions in patients beginning high-potency neuroleptics. Am J Psychiatry 1986; 143: 706–10.
62. Kondo I, Otani K, Tokinaga N et al. Characteristics and risk factors of acute dystonia in schizophrenic patients treated with nemonapride, a selective dopamine antagonist. J Clin Psychopharmacol 1999; 19: 45–50.
63. Singh H, Levinson DF, Simpson GM et al. Acute dystonia during fixed-dose neuroleptic treatment. J Clin Psychopharmacol 1990; 10: 389–96.
64. Burke RE, Fahn S, Jankovic J et al. Tardive dystonia: late onset and persistent dystonia caused by antipsychotic drugs. Neurology (NY) 1982; 32: 1335–46.
65. Inada T, Ohnishi K, Kamisada M et al. A prospective study of tardive dyskinesia in Japan. Eur Arch Psychiatry Clin Neurosci 1991; 240: 350–4.
66. Kane JM, Woerner M, Borenstein M, Wegner J, Lieberman J. Integrating incidence and prevalence of tardive dyskinesia. Psychopharmacol Bull 1986; 22: 254–8.
67. Yassa R, Nair V, Dimitry R. Prevalence of tardive dystonia. Acta Psychiatr Scand 1986; 73: 629–33.
68. Friedman JH, Kucharski LT, Wagner RL. Tardive dystonia in a psychiatric hospital. J Neurol Neurosurg Psychiatry 1987; 50: 801–3.
69. Chiu H, Shum P, Lau J, Lam L, Lee S. Prevalence of tardive dyskinesia, tardive dystonia, and respiratory dyskinesia among Chinese psychiatric patients in Hong Kong. Am J Psychiatry 1992; 149: 1081–5.
70. Raja M. Tardive dystonia, prevalence, risk factors, and comparison with tardive dyskinesia in a population of 200 acute psychiatric inpatients. Eur Arch Psychiatry Clin Neurosci 1995; 245: 145–51.
71. Hafner HA, Riecher-Rossler A, An der Heiden W et al. Generating and testing a causal explanation of the gender difference in age at first onset of schizophrenia. Psychol Med 1993; 23: 925–40.
72. Gimenez-Roldan S, Mateo D, Bartolone P. Tardive dystonia and severe tardive dyskinesia. Acta Psychiatr Scand 1985; 71: 488–94.
73. Kiriakakis V, Bhatia KP, Quinn NP, Marsden CD. The natural history of tardive dystonia. A long-term follow-up study of 107 cases. Brain 1998; 121: 2053–66.
74. Charcot JM. Lectures on Disease of the Nervous System. London: New Sydenham Society: 1877.
75. Kidron D, Melamed E. Forms of dystonia in patients with Parkinson's disease. Neurology 1987; 37: 1009–11.
76. Poewe WH, Lees AJ, Stern GM. Dystonia in Parkinson's disease: clinical and pharmacological features. Ann Neurol 1988; 23: 73–8.
77. Gershanik OS, Leist A. Juvenile onset Parkinson's disease. In: Yahr MD, Bergmann KJ, eds. Advances in Neurology, Vol 45: Parkinson's Disease. New York: Raven Press; 1986: 213–16.
78. Gershanik OS, Nygaard TG. Parkinson's disease beginning before age 40. In: Streifler MB, Korczyn AD, Melamed E, Youdim MBH, eds. Advances in Neurology, Vol. 53: Parkinson's Disease: Anatomy, Pathology, and Therapy, New York: Raven Press; 1990: 251–8.
79. Gibb WRG, Lees AJ. A comparison of clinical and pathological features of young- and old-onset Parkinson's disease. Neurology 1988; 38: 1402–6.
80. Tanner CM, Kinori I, Goetz CG, Carvey PM, Klawans HL. Clinical course in Parkinson's disease: relationship to age at onset [Abstract]. J Neurol 1985; 232 (Suppl): 25.
81. Quinn N, Critchley P, Marsden CD. Young onset Parkinson's disease. Mov Disord 1987; 2: 73–91.
82. Yassa R, Nair V, Iskandar H. A comparison of severe tardive dystonia and severe tardive dyskinesia. Am J Psychiatry 1989; 147: 1156–63.
83. Ramos AE, Shytle RD, Silver AA, Sanberg PR. Ziprasidone-induced oculogyric crisis [Letter]. J Am Acad Child Adolesc Psychiatry 2003; 42: 1013–14.
84. Mason MN, Johnson CE, Piasecki M. Ziprasidone-induced acute dystonia. Am J Psychiatry 2005; 162: 625–6.
85. Papapetropoulos S, Wheeler S, Singer C. Tardive dystonia associated with ziprasidone. Am J Psychiatry 2005; 162: 2191.
86. Weinstein SK, Adler CM, Strakowski SM. Ziprasidone-induced acute dystonic reactions in patients with bipolar disorder. J Clin Psychiatry 2006; 67: 327–8.
87. Lohmann T, Ferbert A, Ebel H. A unique case of tardive dystonia induced by short-term therapy with perazin. Pharmacopsychiatry 1995; 28: 263–5.
88. Fdhil H, Krebs MO, Bayle F et al. Risperidone-induced tardive dystonia: a case of torticollis. Encephale 1998; 24: 581–3.
89. Factor SA, Mathews MK. Persistent extrapyramidal syndrome with dystonia and rigidity caused by combined metoclopramide and prochlorperazine therapy. South Med J 1991; 84: 626–8.
90. Adityanjee YAA, Jampala VC, Mathews T. The current status of tardive dystonia. Biol Psychiatry 1999; 45: 715–30.

91. Lee HK. Dystonic reactions to amitriptyline and doxepin [Letter]. Am J Psychiatry 1988; 145: 649.
92. Gabellini AS, Pezzoli A, de Massis P, Sacquegna T. Veralipride-induced tardive dystonia in a patient with bipolar psychosis. Ital J Neurol Sci 1992; 13: 621–3.
93. Armstrong M, Daly AK, Blennerhassett R et al. Antipsychotic drug-induced movement disorders in schizophrenics in relation to CYP2D6 genotype. Br J Psychiatry 1997; 170: 23–6.
94. Mihara K, Kondo T, Higuchi H et al. Tardive dystonia and genetic polymorphisms of cytochrome P4502D6 and dopamine D2 and D3 receptors: a preliminary finding. Am J Med Genet 2002; 114: 693–5.
95. Scordo MG, Spina E, Romeo P et al. CYP2D6 genotype and antipsychotic-induced extrapyramidal side effects in schizophrenic patients. Eur J Clin Pharmacol 2000; 56: 679–83.
96. Kaiser R, Tremblay PB, Klufmoller F et al. Relationship between adverse effects on antipsychotic treatment and dopamine D2 receptor polymorphisms in patients with schizophrenia. Mol Psychiatry 2002; 7: 695–705.
97. Lencer R, Eismann G, Kasten M et al. Family history of primary movement disorders as a predictor for neuroleptic-induced extrapyramidal symptoms. Br J Psychiatry 2004; 185: 465–71.
98. Lee MS, Rinne JO, Ceballos-Baumann A et al. Dystonia after head trauma. Neurology 1994; 44: 1374–8.

3

Overview of the genetic forms of dystonia

Thomas T Warner and Susan B Bressman

INTRODUCTION

Genetic etiologies have long been suspected for many subtypes of dystonia. Recent molecular advances have led to the identification of an increasing number of genes for primary and secondary dystonia subtypes (Table 3.1). This information has opened the way for studies aimed at characterizing basic pathogenic mechanisms, including cellular and animal models. It has also allowed for a broader analysis of phenotype and endophenotype to further characterize the spectrum of gene expression. Defining genetic etiologies has altered the way neurologists diagnose and counsel patients, including the important need to provide genetic counseling to patients and their families. Ultimately, understanding the genetic causes of dystonia, and the effects of these alterations, holds the promise of rational, targeted therapies.

There are many classification schemes to organize the causes of dystonia. Most create at least two broad categories: primary torsion dystonia (previously named idiopathic torsion dystonia) and secondary (or non-primary) dystonia (see Table 3.1 and Chapter 1). Primary torsion dystonia (PTD) is defined as a syndrome in which dystonia is the only clinical sign (except for tremor) and there is no evidence of neuronal degeneration or an acquired cause. Secondary (non-primary) dystonias include all other dystonia subtypes and can further divided into inherited, complex, and acquired etiologies.

To date 15 different (*DYT*) genetic loci have been mapped or cloned. A number of these have led to crucial advances in our understanding of molecular mechanisms underlying dystonic movements and therefore have warranted separate chapters within this book (DYT1 and non-DYT1 dystonia, dystonia-plus syndromes, paroxysmal dyskinesias). In addition, even for the common focal forms of primary torsion dystonia, such as cervical dystonia (spasmodic torticollis), blepharospasm, writer's cramp, and other limb dystonias which do not appear to have a clear genetic basis, population and family studies have found evidence for a genetic contribution to their etiology.

The dystonia genetic loci and genes are summarized in Tables 3.2–3.4. The molecular classification is somewhat complex and confusing and contains mapped loci, cloned genes including primary dystonia, dystonia-plus syndromes (dopa-responsive dystonia, myoclonus-dystonia syndrome, and rapid-onset dystonia-parkinsonism) and one heredodegenerative condition (X-linked dystonia-parkinsonism). Within this classification, two loci (*DYT2* and *DYT4*) have been assigned on the basis of clinical descriptions alone. It is clear that there are other dystonia genes yet to be discovered.

PRIMARY TORSION DYSTONIA

Early-onset autosomal dominant primary torsion dystonia (DYT1)

Early-onset PTD is 3–5 times more common in Ashkenazi Jews compared to other populations and is transmitted in an autosomal dominant fashion with reduced penetrance of 30–40% in both Ashkenazi Jews and non-Ashkenazim.[1,2] The difference in disease frequency is thought to be the result of a founder mutation in *DYT1* that was introduced into the Ashkenazi population at the time of a 'bottleneck' in the 1600s, followed by a period of tremendous population growth.[3]

The gene at locus *DYT1* was initially mapped to chromosome 9q34[4] and subsequently identified in 1997[5] and is responsible for a large proportion of early limb-onset PTD (also known as dystonia musculorum deformans or Oppenheim's disease) across many different populations.[6–8] Only one recurring mutation in *DYT1*, an in-frame GAG deletion, has been associated unequivocally with PTD. The *DYT1* gene encodes a

Table 3.1 Causes of dystonia

Primary

Autosomal dominant

Early limb (*DYT1*, other genes to be determined)
Mixed (*DYT6*, *DYT13*, other genes to be determined)
Late focal (*DYT7*, other genes to be determined)

Other genetic causes

?Autosomal recessive
Complex

Secondary

Inherited

Dystonia plus (non-degenerative):

- DRD (DYT5-GCH1, DYT14, other biopterin deficiencies, tyrosine hydroxylase deficiency)
- Myoclonus-dystonia (DYT11-ε-sarcoglycan, 18p locus)
- Rapid-onset dystonia parkinsonism (DYT12, ATP1A3)

Degenerative:

- Autosomal dominant (e.g. Huntington's disease, SCAs, especially SCA3)
- Autosomal recessive (e.g. Wilson's disease, NBIA1, GM1, GM2, parkin)
- X-linked (e.g. X-linked dystonia-parkinsonism/Lubag, DDP)
- Mitochondrial

Complex/unknown

Parkinsonism (e.g. Parkinson's disease, multisystem atrophy, progressive supranuclear palsy, corticobasal degeneration)

Acquired

For example, drug-induced, perinatal injury, head trauma, cervical trauma, peripheral trauma, infectious and post-infectious, tumor, AVM, stroke, central pontine myelinolysis, multiple sclerosis

DRD = dopa-responsive dystonia; GCH1 = GTP cyclohydrolase 1; SCA = spinocerebellar ataxia; NBIA1 = neurodegeneration with brain iron accumulation; DDP = deafness dystonia peptide; ATP1A3 = ATPase a3 subunit; GM1 and GM2 = gangliosidoses 1 and 2; AVM = arteriovenous malformation.

novel protein, torsinA, that is 332 amino acids long (~38 kD), with potential sites for glycosylation and phosphorylation, as well as an amino terminal hydrophobic leader sequence consistent with membrane translocation/targeting.[5] The GAG deletion results in the loss of one of a pair of glutamic acid residues near the carboxy terminus of the protein.

Typical DYT1 dystonia develops before the age of 28 years old, often beginning in a limb (leg >arm), often with subsequent spread to other body parts.[8] The clinical phenotype and molecular pathology of DYT1 and torsinA are described in Chapter 6.

Autosomal recessive primary torsion dystonia (DYT2)

There is limited evidence for autosomal recessive primary torsion dystonia and much of it comes from three consanguineous families of Spanish gypsies.[9] In two of the three families the phenotype resembled DYT1 dystonia and in the third family oromandibular dystonia and torticollis were the most prominent manifestations. The genetic locus is designated on the basis of the clinical description and no linkage to a chromosomal region has ever been identified. More recently, a further family of Sephardic Jewish origin has been described and purported to represent a case of DYT2 dystonia.[10] The difficulty with the description is that in the dominant form there is often reduced penetrance and it is possible that that is what these families represent.

Non-DYT1 primary torsion dystonia

There remains a large group of early-onset PTD, especially among non-Jewish populations, that is not due to the *TOR1A* GAG deletion. Two loci, *DYT6*[11] and *DYT13*,[12] have been mapped in kindreds having an average age onset in adolescence. However, neither locus has been confirmed in other families and they are suspected to account for only a minority of non-DYT1 early-onset cases. Furthermore, overall clinical features in these two families differ from DYT1 (although features in any single family member may overlap with DYT1). The family phenotypes for DYT6 and DYT13 are marked by prominent involvement of cranial and cervical muscles with variable spread; also, compared to DYT1, a greater proportion of family members have later adolescent and adult onset. To distinguish this phenotype from the typical early-onset phenotype associated with DYT1 and typical late-onset focal phenotypes, the term 'mixed' has been applied. These forms of PTD are described further in Chapter 7.

Late-onset PTD

Like early-onset PTD, late-onset PTD also appears to have autosomal dominant inheritance.[13–15] However, unlike early-onset dystonia, most studies show that penetrance is even more reduced (about 12–15% compared with 30% for early-onset dystonia); alternatively, penetrance

Table 3.2 Genetic forms of primary torsion dystonia

Type	Clinical features	Frequency	Age of onset	Inheritance and penetrance	Inheritance/ locus/gene
DYT1	Limb onset; generalized; can present as focal	50% cases; early onset in non-Jews, 90% in Ashkenazi Jews	Childhood; most present by 26 years old	Autosomal dominant with reduced penetrance (30%)	*TOR1A* gene on chromosome 9q34 Mutation: GAG deletion leading to loss of glutamate residue in protein torsinA
DYT2	Focal and generalized	Spanish gypsy families and single Iranian family	Childhood to adult	Autosomal recessive	Locus unknown
DYT4	Laryngeal and cervical, some generalize	Single Australian family	13–37 years old	Autosomal dominant	Locus unknown
DYT6	Focal or generalized; cranial, cervical, or limb	Two Mennonite Amish families	Mean age of onset 19 years old	Autosomal dominant	*DYT6* locus on chromosome 8p21-q22
DYT7	Focal dystonia; cervical and laryngeal	Single German family	28–70 years old	Autosomal dominant	*DYT7* locus on chromosome 18p
DYT13	Cranial or cervical; some generalize	Single Italian family	Childhood to adult	Autosomal dominant	*DYT13* locus on chromosome 1p36

may be higher in a subset, with the remainder sporadic. Consistent with the notion of increased penetrance in a subset of late-onset PTD, are descriptions of large families with more highly penetrant autosomal dominant disease. One such family with adult-onset torticollis was studied and resulted in the mapping of *DYT7*.[16]

Adult-onset focal primary torsion dystonia (DYT7)

This locus was originally mapped in a family from northwest Germany in which seven members were affected with late-onset torticollis, although other members had mild facial and arm involvement and spasmodic dysphonia was noted in some of the family. The gene was mapped to a 30 cM region on chromosome 18p.[16] In support of a dystonia locus on chromosome 18p is the finding that patients with the deletion of the short arm of chromosome 18 can also show dystonic symptoms.[17] Other clinically similar families have been excluded from DYT7, suggesting yet other loci for adult-onset focal PTD.[18]

The role of primary torsion dystonia genes and susceptibility loci in late-onset primary torsion dystonia

The extent to which the genes *DYT1, DYT6, DYT7*, and *DYT13* account for adult-onset, seemingly sporadic, focal dystonias is unclear. It is almost certain that there

Table 3.3 Dystonia-plus syndromes

Type	Clinical features	Age of onset	Inheritance, penetrance, and locus	Gene, protein, and mutations
DYT5: Dopa-responsive dystonia (Segawa's disease)	Dystonia, often limbs; parkinsonism; diurnal variation; dramatic response to levodopa	Usually childhood	Autosomal dominant for *DYT5* on chromosome 14q22. 1-q22.2 penetrance 30% *DYT14*: 14q13 Autosomal recessive for tyrosine hydroxylase (TH) on chromosome 11p15.5	*DYT5:* GTP-cyclohydrolase 1; biopterin synthesis – numerous point mutations *DYT14*: unknown TH: monamine synthesis
DYT11: Myoclonus-dystonia syndrome	Myoclonus of limbs and upper torso; dystonia of upper limbs and neck; alcohol responsive	Variable but usually childhood/adolescent	Autosomal dominant; incomplete penetrance, higher when inherited paternally (imprinting); *DYT11* locus 7q21-q31 *DYT15* 18p11	*DYT11*: ε-sarcoglycan; various heterozygous mutations *DYT15*: unknown
DYT12: Rapid-onset dystonia-parkinsonism	Acute or subacute onset of generalized dystonia-plus parkinsonism	Childhood to adulthood	Autosomal dominant with incomplete penetrance; locus 19q13	Na^+/K^+-ATPase α3 subunit (ATP1A3).

are other as yet unmapped genes.[19–21] The role of susceptibility loci has also been studied in cohorts of primary focal dystonia. An association has been found between a polymorphism in the dopamine D_5 receptor and patients with cervical dystonia and blepharospasm.[22,23] Although the polymorphism is not functional and therefore does not affect the receptor function, it could be linked to a nearby pathogenic mutation.

In view of the fact that the *DYT7* locus causes focal dystonia, research has looked at allelic association for several markers in the region of chromosome 18p in cases of sporadic cervical dystonia (torticollis) from northwest Germany and reported an association.[24,25] This however, was not replicated and the finding is of uncertain significance.[18,26]

More recently, an association of the single nucleotide polymorphisms within the 3-UTR of the *DYT1* gene has been found in sporadic idiopathic predominantly focal dystonia in Finland, Germany, and Austria.[27,28] However, in the Icelandic population, the rarer of the two major haplotypes was associated with dystonia risk, whereas in the German/Austrian study a strong protective effect was observed for the same haplotype.

SECONDARY DYSTONIA AND DYSTONIA-PLUS SYNDROMES (SEE TABLES 3.3 AND 3.4)

Etiological subgroups for secondary dystonias include (1) inherited causes; (2) a group of primarily parkinsonian disorders, such as Parkinson's disease, that are thought to have complex etiologies; and (3) environmental or acquired causes. In addition, most classifications also include other movement disorders that may display dystonic phenomenology such as tics and the paroxysmal dyskinesias and the pseudodystonias. The latter are not considered true dystonia but muscle contractions mimicking dystonia, such as seen in Sandifer's syndrome, orthopedic conditions, and psychogenic dystonia (see Chapter 1).

Among the inherited forms of secondary dystonia is a relatively newly defined category of dystonia-plus syndromes, consisting of three clinically defined entities:

- dopa-responsive dystonia (DRD)[29–32]
- myoclonus-dystonia (M-D)[33,34]
- rapid-onset dystonia-parkinsonism (RDP).[35–37]

Table 3.4 Other genetic forms of dystonia

Type	Clinical features	Age of onset	Inheritance, penetrance, and locus	Gene, protein, and mutations
DYT3: X-linked dystonia-parkinsonism (Lubag)	Philippino males with focal dystonia which becomes generalized; parkinsonism develops in 50%	Childhood to early adulthood	X-linked; Xq13.1; penetrance 100% by 5th decade	*TAF1* gene; encodes transcription factor, may regulate dopamine D_2 receptors
DYT8: Paroxysmal dystonic choreoathetosis (non-kinesigenic dyskinesia)	Episodic dystonia and chorea lasting hours	Childhood to early adulthood	Autosomal dominant; incomplete penetrance, 2q33-q36	*MR-1* gene; encodes myofibrillogenesis regulator 1 protein
DYT9: Paroxysmal choreoathetosis with episodic ataxia and spasticity	Chronic spastic paraplegia plus episodes of dystonia, choreoathetosis	Childhood	Autosomal dominant, 1p13.3-p21	Unknown
DYT10: Paroxysmal kinesigenic choreoathetosis	Episodes of dystonia and chorea triggered by sudden movements	Childhood	Autosomal dominant, 16p11.2-q12.1	Unknown
Deafness-dystonia syndrome; Mohr–Tranebjaerg syndrome	Dystonia, sensorineural deafness, spasticity, mental retardation, female carriers may have adult-onset focal dystonia alone	Childhood	X-linked with incomplete penetrance, Xq22	Mutations in dystonia-deafness peptide, mitochondrial protein import
Leber's hereditary optic neuropathy plus dystonia	Dystonia, optic atrophy, or both	Variable	Maternal inheritance, mitochondrial DNA	NADH dehydrogenase subunit 6, complex 1

These are further described in Chapter 12. The dystonia-plus category was distinguished from both primary dystonia and other inherited secondary dystonias because it shares some but not all features of both groups: i.e. like primary dystonia, these three syndromes do not appear to be degenerative. Although pathology is limited, evidence to date supports genetic defects that result in functional brain changes not associated with progressive neuronal death. Furthermore, unlike primary dystonia, but similar to the other degenerative secondary dystonias, the dystonia-plus group has (as characteristic clinical features) signs other than dystonia, including parkinsonism for DRD and RDP and myoclonus for M-D.

As our understanding of these syndromes is expanding, the complexity of their genetic and clinical heterogeneity is being detailed. For example, for DRD there are currently several known genetic biochemical etiologies, each with protean clinical manifestations, and for myoclonus-dystonia, there appear to be at least two genetic etiologies (see Table 3.3).[38]

PAROXYSMAL DYSTONIAS

This rare group of conditions manifests with abnormal involuntary movements that occur episodically and are of brief duration. The abnormal movements are mixed, but include dystonia, chorea, and ballism. They can be acquired or genetic in origin and the key feature is that the patient is normal between attacks. The genetic subtypes are shown in Table 3.4 and these disorders are described in more detail in Chapter 15.

CONCLUSIONS

Over the last 20 years our understanding of PTD, 'dystonia-plus', and secondary dystonia syndromes has been transformed due to the advances made in unraveling their genetic causes. The identification of genes for dystonia has already impacted dramatically both in clinical practice and research realms. It has altered the way clinicians diagnose and counsel families and their approach to therapeutics. For example, with the availability of genetic testing for DYT1, a direct diagnosis of this genetic subtype is easily made. Patients with DYT1 PTD are no longer routinely subjected to more costly and invasive investigations. In addition, because they appear to respond particularly favorably to pallidal deep brain stimulation (DBS), this form of therapy is now considered earlier in the course of disease.[39] The identification of disease genes has also opened the way for the gene-specific application of imaging, neurophysiologic, and other measures for determining phenotypic and endophenotypic expression. It has allowed for the development of disease gene-specific cellular and animal models and is revising our notions about pathogenesis. PTD due to DYT1, once considered idiopathic and due to functional brain changes, appears to be associated with anatomic brain changes, such as inclusion bodies in brainstem structures not previously considered significant in the pathogenic process. Whereas previous studies, such as therapeutics focused on dopamine transmission in PTD, it is becoming evident that motor dysfunction may also relate to other mechanisms that influence the physical foundation for corticocortical and subcorticocortical connectivity.[40] The finding of PTD genes also holds the promise of novel therapeutic strategies, such as the use of small interfering RNA to silence expression of mutant torsinA.[41]

REFERENCES

1. Bressman SB, de Leon, D, Brin MF et al. Idiopathic torsion dystonia among Ashkenazi Jews: evidence for autosomal dominant inheritance. Ann Neurol 1989; 26: 612–20.
2. Pauls DL, Korczyn AD. Complex segregation analysis of dystonia pedigrees suggests autosomal dominant inheritance. Neurology 1990; 40: 1107–10.
3. Risch N, de Leon D, Ozelius L et al. Genetic analysis of idiopathic torsion dystonia in Ashkenazi Jews and their recent descent from a small founder population. Nat Genet 1995; 9: 152–9.
4. Ozelius LJ, Kramer P, Moskowitz CB et al. Human gene for torsion dystonia located on chromosome 9q32-34. Neuron 1989; 2: 1427–34.
5. Ozelius LJ, Hewett J, Page CE et al. The early-onset torsion dystonia gene (DYT1) encodes an ATP-binding protein. Nat Genet 1997; 17: 40–8.
6. Valente EM, Warner TT, Jarman PR et al. The role of primary torsion dystonia in Europe. Brain 1998; 121: 2335–9.
7. Leube B, Kessler KR, Ferbert A et al. Phenotypic variability of the DYT1 mutation in German dystonia patients. Acta Neurol Scand 1999; 99: 248–51.
8. Bressman SB, Sabatti C, Raymond D et al. The DYT1 phenotype and guidelines for diagnostic testing. Neurology 2000; 54: 1746–52.
9. Gimenez-Roldan S, Delgado G, Marin M, Villanueva JA, Mateo D. Hereditary torsion dystonia in gypsies. Adv Neurol 1988; 50: 73–81.
10. Khan NL, Wood NW, Bhatia KP. Autosomal recessive, DYT2-like primary torsion dystonia: a new family. Neurology 2003; 61: 1801–3.
11. Almasy L, Bressman SB, Kramer PL et al. Idiopathic torsion dystonia linked to chromosome 8 in two Mennonite families. Ann Neurol 1997; 42: 670–3.
12. Valente EM, Bentivoglio AR, Cassetta E et al. DYT13, a novel primary torsion dystonia locus, maps to chromosome 1p36.13-36.32 in an Italian family with cranial-cervical or upper limb onset. Ann Neurol 2001; 49: 362–4.
13. Defazio G, Livrea P, Guanti G et al. Genetic contribution to idiopathic adult-onset blepharospasm and cranial-cervical dystonia. Eur Neurol 2003; 33: 345–50.
14. Waddy HM, Fletcher NA, Harding AE, Marsden CD. A genetic study of idiopathic focal dystonias. Ann Neurol 1991; 29: 320–4.
15. Stojanovic M, Cvetkovic D, Kostic VS. A genetic study of idiopathic focal dystonias. J Neurol 1995; 242: 508–11.
16. Leube B, Doda R, Ratzlaff T et al. Idiopathic torsion dystonia: assignment of a gene to chromosome 18p in a German family with adult onset, autosomal inheritance and purely focal distribution. Hum Mol Genet 1996; 5: 1673–7.
17. Klein C, Page CE, LeWitt P et al. Genetic analysis of three patients with an 18p syndrome and dystonia. Neurology 1999; 52: 649–51.
18. Klein C, Ozelius L, Hagenah J et al. Search for a founder mutation in idiopathic focal dystonia from Northern Germany. Am J Hum Genet 1998; 63: 1777–82.
19. Bressman SB, Warner TT, Almasy L et al. Exclusion of the DYT1 locus in familial torticollis. Ann Neurol 1996; 40: 681–4.

20. Holmgren G, Ozelius L, Forsgren L et al. Adult onset idiopathic torsion dystonia is excluded from the DYT1 region (9q34) in a Swedish family. J Neurol Neurosurg Psychiatry 1995; 59: 178–81.
21. Jarman P, delGrosso N, Valente E et al. Primary torsion dystonia: the search for genes is not over. J Neurol Neurosurg Psychiatry 1999; 67: 395–7.
22. Placzek MR, Misbahuddin A, Chaudhuri KR et al. Cervical dystonia is associated with a polymorphism in the dopamine (D5) receptor gene. J Neurol Neurosurg Psychiatry 2001; 71: 262–4.
23. Misbahuddin A, Placzec MR, Chaudhuri KR et al. A polymorphism in the dopamine receptor DRD5 is associated with blepharospasm. Neurology 2002; 58: 124–6.
24. Leube B, Hendgen T, Kessler KR et al. Evidence for DYT7 being a common cause of cervical dystonia (torticollis) in Central Europe. Am J Med Genet 1997; 74: 529–2.
25. Leube B, Hendgen T, Kessler KR et al. Sporadic focal dystonia in Northwest Germany: molecular basis on chromosome 18p. Ann Neurol 1997; 42: 111–14.
26. Leube B, Auburger G. Questionable role of adult-onset focal dystonia among sporadic dystonia patients. Ann Neurol 1998; 44: 984–5.
27. Clarimon J, Asgeirsson H, Singleton A et al. Torsin A haplotype predisposes to idiopathic dystonia. Ann Neurol 2005; 57: 765–7.
28. Kamm C, Asmus F, Mueller J et al. Strong genetic evidence for association of TOR1A-TOR1B with idiopathic dystonia. Neurology 2006; 67: 1857–9.
29. Nygaard TG, Marsden CD, Fahn S. Dopa-responsive dystonia: long-term treatment response and prognosis. Neurology 1991; 41: 174–1.
30. Segawa M, Hosaka A, Miyagawa F, Nomura Y, Imai H. Hereditary progressive dystonia with marked diurnal fluctuation. Adv Neurol 1976; 14: 215–33.
31. Furukawa Y, Land AE, Trugman JM et al. Gender-related penetrance and de novo GTP-cyclohydrolase I gene mutations in dopa-responsive dystonia. Neurology 1998; 50: 1015–20.
32. Ichinose H, Ohye T, Takahiashi E et al. Hereditary progressive dystonia with marked diurnal fluctuation caused by mutations in the GTP cyclohydrolase I gene. Nat Genet 1994; 8: 236–42.
33. Klein C, Schilling K, Saunders-Pullman RJ et al. A major locus for myoclonus-dystonia maps to chromosome 7q in eight families. Am J Hum Genet 2000; 67: 1314–19.
34. Zimprich A, Grabowski M, Asmus F et al. Mutations in the gene encoding epsilon–sarcoglycan cause myoclonus-dystonia syndrome. Nat Genet 2001; 29: 66–9.
35. Dobyns WB, Ozelius LJ, Kramer PL et al. Rapid-onset dystonia-parkinsonism. Neurology 1993; 43: 2596–602.
36. Kramer PL, Mineta M, Klein C et al. Rapid-onset dystonia-parkinsonism: linkage to chromosome 19q13. Ann Neurol 1999; 46: 176–82.
37. de Carvalho Aguiar P, Sweadner KJ, Penniston JT et al. Mutations in the Na^+/K^+-ATPase alpha3 gene ATP1A3 are associated with rapid-onset dystonia parkinsonism. Neuron 2004; 43: 169–75.
38. Grimes DA, Bulman D, George-Hyslop PS, Lang AE. Inherited myoclonus-dystonia: evidence supporting genetic heterogeneity. Mov Disord 2001; 16: 106–10.
39. Coubes P, Roubertie A, Vaysserie N, Hemm S, Echenne B. Treatment of DYT1-generalised dystonia by stimulation of internal globus pallidus. Lancet 2000; 355: 2220–1.
40. Carbon M, Kingsley PB, Su S et al. Microstructural white matter changes in carriers of the DYT1 gene mutation. Ann Neurol 2004; 56: 283–6.
41. Gonzalez-Alegre P, Bode N, Davidson BL, Paulson HL. Silencing primary dystonia: lentiviral-mediated RNA interference treatment for DYT dystonia. J Neurosci 2005; 25: 10502–9.

4

Pathophysiology of dystonia

Su Kanchana and Mark Hallett

INTRODUCTION

Dystonia is a disorder characterized by excessive movements, including sustained involuntary movements, distorted voluntary movements, and abnormal postures. Some patients may also have quick movements, called myoclonic dystonia, or tremor, but ordinarily there will have to be some sustained movements for dystonia to be recognized as such. While dystonia can be present at rest, it is brought out more by attempted voluntary movements. Dystonia movements are slow, clumsy, and characterized by overflow (excessive activity in muscles not needed for the task).

In understanding dystonia, it seems appropriate to start by examining the involuntary movements themselves. Several observations over many years have shown that dystonic movements are characterized by an abnormal pattern of electromyographic (EMG) activity with excessive co-contraction of antagonist muscles and overflow into extraneous muscles. Cohen and Hallett[1] reported detailed observations on 19 patients with focal dystonia of the hand, including writer's cramp and cramps in piano, guitar, clarinet, and organ players. Five features, identified by physiologic investigation, were indicative of impaired motor control. The first was co-contraction, which could be a brief burst or continuous. Normally, in repetitive alternating movements at a single joint, antagonist muscles alternate their firing. The dystonia patients might co-contract even with such quick movements. The second feature was prolongation of EMG bursts. EMG bursts of even a briefest movement usually last no longer than about 100 ms. Dystonia patients had bursts of 200 or 300 ms as well as very prolonged spasms. A third feature was tremor. A fourth feature was lack of selectivity in attempts to perform independent finger movements, and a fifth feature was occasional failure of willed activity to occur. All five features emphasize excessiveness of movements and lack of fine control.

The problem of excessive co-contraction could be due to deficient reciprocal inhibition. Reciprocal inhibition is represented at multiple levels in the central nervous system and can be evaluated in humans by the stimulation of the radial nerve at various times prior to producing an H-reflex with median nerve stimulation. The radial nerve afferents come from muscles that are antagonists to median nerve muscles. Via various pathways, the radial afferent traffic can inhibit motor neuron pools of median nerve muscles. Reciprocal inhibition is impaired in generalized dystonia, writer's cramp, spasmodic torticollis, and blepharospasm. Valls-Solé and Hallett[2] have evaluated the effects of radial nerve stimulation on the EMG activity of the wrist flexor muscles during a sustained contraction and showed that the first inhibitory period was reduced in patients with writer's cramp consistent with reduced reciprocal inhibition during movement. This deficit is not limited to the symptomatic body part. For example, the soleus H-reflex of the lower limb is also abnormal in patients with cervical dystonia. Additionally, the H-reflex recovery curve showed greater disinhibition in generalized dystonia compared to cervical dystonia and normal subjects during the early inhibition phase. The late facilitation phase of the recovery curve showed higher facilitation in both generalized and cervical dystonia compared with normal controls.[3]

Other spinal and brainstem reflexes have been studied, and a common result is that inhibitory processes are reduced in dystonia. Another example that has been extensively studied is the blink reflex recovery curve, evaluation of inhibition of a second blink reflex at short intervals from the first.[4] The blink reflex is generated by stimulation of the supraorbital nerve and the response measured from the orbicularis oculi muscles. Its afferent limb is mediated by the ophthalmic division of the trigeminal nerve (V_1) and the efferent limb is the facial nerve. Abnormalities of blink reflex recovery were identified for blepharospasm, generalized dystonia, spasmodic torticollis, and spasmodic dysphonia. In the last two conditions, abnormal blink reflex recovery can be seen even without clinical involvement of the eyelids. Similarly, abnormalities are seen with perioral reflexes[5] and exteroceptive silent periods, again showing a process of disinhibition common among these various types of dystonia.

A DISORDER OF SENSORY DYSFUNCTION

On first appearance, dystonia is solely a movement disorder. Its disabling characteristics of abnormal postures and movements appear entirely motor in nature. Sensation seems normal. There are clues, however, that sensory function may not be completely normal and that sensory features play an important role. In fact, it has been shown that patients with dystonia have subtle abnormalities of graphesthesia, stereognosis, and kinesthesia.

Abnormal sensory discrimination

Psychophysical studies have revealed evidence of abnormal somatosensory spatial discrimination[6,7] and temporal discrimination[8,9] in dystonia patients. Temporal discrimination is the shortest time interval for which two successive stimuli are perceived as separate. This is essential for somatosensory functions such as kinesthesia, graphesthesia, vibratory sense, and stereognosis. Temporal discrimination is impaired in patients with dystonia, and the deficit is more pronounced in focal dystonia compared with the generalized form. Fiorio et al[8] demonstrated temporal discrimination deficits not only for tactile but also for visuotactile stimuli in writer's cramp patients. The authors suggested that their finding implies dysfunction of a neural network involving the basal ganglia, which is implicated in temporal processing and integration of visuotactile stimuli. The degree of temporal discrimination impairment is positively correlated with the degree of severity of dystonia.[8,10] This discrimination deficit was identified in both the affected and unaffected hand, implying that the deficit is a result of a central process of dystonia itself, rather than a by-product of the abnormal muscle contractions.

Spatial discrimination differentiates two spatially separated stimuli and is measured as the shortest distance between the stimuli that are perceived as separate. Impaired spatial discrimination might be a clinical correlate of the abnormal finger representation in the primary somatosensory cortex (S1) seen in dystonia patients. Molloy and colleagues[7] studied spatial sensory discrimination in a wide range of focal and generalized dystonia patients. Spatial discrimination was impaired in patients with writer's cramp, as well as in the clinically normal hands of patients with spasmodic torticollis and blepharospasm, but unaffected in generalized DYT1 dystonia. The authors suggest that this latter finding implies a possibility of partially separate pathophysiologic processes in the focal and generalized subtypes of dystonia. It is also possible that the initially impaired sensorimotor integration in generalized dystonia may have been normalized by early adaptive changes or compensatory mechanisms.

Since the sensory system is an important influence on the motor system, abnormalities of the sensory system could be relevant in causing motor dysfunction. If abnormal sensory system leads to motor symptoms of dystonia, restored sensory input may at least partially reverse these motor symptoms. Indeed, when spatial acuity improved after sensory training by Braille reading, motor improvement also followed.[11] This strong influence of the sensory system to motor system functions and mechanism of dystonia is also nicely illustrated by the unique phenomenon of sensory tricks.

Sensory 'tricks'

One characteristic feature of idiopathic focal dystonia is the role of sensory feedback that manifests as the little understood phenomenon of geste antagoniste or 'tricks', which refers to various maneuvers used by patients with focal dystonia to temporarily relieve their dystonic spasms. The most commonly noted is the geste in spasmodic torticollis, where, for example, a finger placed lightly on the face will eliminate the spasm. Such tricks are seen in all forms of dystonia. Pressure on the eyelids might improve blepharospasm, a toothpick in the mouth might relieve tongue dystonia, and sensation applied to parts of the arm might improve a writer's cramp. It has been shown that the application of sensory tricks resulted in the reduction of EMG activity in the sternocleidomastoid, trapezius, and splenius capitis in patients with cervical dystonia.[12] Effects of sensory tricks on cortical activation have also been demonstrated by $H_2{}^{15}O$ positron emission tomography (PET), showing change in activation in the parietal cortex in cervical dystonia during the application of tricks.[13] Murase et al[14] suggested that in patients with writer's cramp there is a flaw in the interpretation of sensory input that occurs prior to, and perhaps during the movements, and that tricks supply this missing sensory input. The phenomenon of 'tricks' offers strong evidence that dystonia is also a sensory disorder.

A role of sensory input

On the other hand, sensory stimulation might trigger dystonia. This might be called a reverse geste.

Examples include a tart taste producing tongue dystonia or a loud noise producing spasmodic torticollis. Sensory symptoms may well precede the appearance of dystonia.[15] Common examples would be a gritty sensation in the eye preceding blepharospasm and irritation of the throat preceding spasmodic dysphonia. Photophobia is an example of distorted sensation. In some situations, patients may say that they made voluntary repetitive movements in order to relieve the sensory symptom, but the movements eventually got out of voluntary control. Abnormal sensory input might well be a trigger for dystonia. Trauma to a body part is often a precedent to dystonia of that part. A blow to the head might precede torticollis, irritations of the eye are common in blepharospasm, and a deep cut of the hand might occur just before writer's cramp develops.

There may be an important problem with processing muscle spindle input. In patients with hand cramps, vibration can induce the patient's dystonia.[16] Cutaneous input similar to that which produces the sensory trick can reverse the vibration-induced dystonia. Conversely, when muscular afferent inputs are blocked by lidocaine injections which leave the cutaneous afferents relatively unaffected, both action-induced and vibration-induced dystonia improve.

The brain response to somatosensory input is abnormal in dystonia. This can be demonstrated with PET studies[17] and evoked potential studies using electroencephalography (EEG).[14,18] In addition, studies of sensory receptive fields of thalamic neurons in humans with dystonia show expanded regions where all cells respond to the same passive movement.[19] Mapping of cortical sensory areas of the different fingers is abnormal in dystonia; this is potentially consistent with the idea that there is abnormal cortical plasticity.[20,21]

A DISORDER OF DISINHIBITION

Several studies have shown hyperexcitability of the motor cortex in dystonia. The likely explanation of the hyperexcitability is loss of inhibition. Ridding et al[22] studied intracortical inhibition with transcranial magnetic stimulation (TMS) using the 'double-pulse paradigm'. Motor evoked potentials (MEPs) are inhibited when conditioned by a subthreshold TMS stimulus given at intervals of 1–5 ms prior to the test stimulus. Inhibition was impaired in patients with focal hand dystonia in both affected and unaffected hemispheres. Decreased inhibition in writer's cramp patients can also be seen with longer interstimulus intervals (ISIs), where the most prominent decrease was identified at ISIs of 60–80 ms.[23] This deficiency was found only in the symptomatic hand and only with background contraction. This abnormality is particularly interesting since it is restricted to the symptomatic setting, as opposed to many other physiologic abnormalities in dystonia that are more generalized. Using a modified TMS double-pulse paradigm which utilized two magnetic coils and allowed for an evaluation of areas surrounding the hand motor representation and distribution of inhibition, Sommer et al[24] demonstrated deficient intracortical inhibition in the cortical hand muscle representation not only in patients with hand dystonia but also in patients with blepharospasm whose hand muscles are clinically normal. Inhibition is also found to be defective during the preparation of movement. Gilio and colleagues[25] studied motor cortex excitability before the execution of voluntary wrist extension in a mixed group of eight hand dystonia and two generalized dystonia patients. The decreased inhibition usually seen just before the EMG onset in normal subjects is absent in dystonia patients (Figures 4.1 and 4.2).

Another TMS measure that relates to intracortical inhibition is the silent period (SP), which refers to the duration of interruption of voluntary motor activity after TMS. Chen et al[23] found that the SP following an MEP was slightly shorter for the symptomatic hemisphere in patients with focal hand dystonia. Moreover, the SP is shorter during dystonic contractions than during voluntary movements with the same intensity.[26]

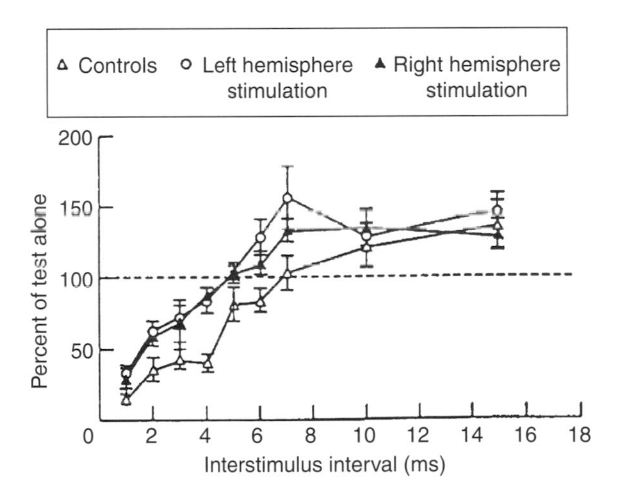

Figure 4.1 Paired-pulse TMS study of both hands of patients with hand dystonia and the dominant hand of normal controls. The percent amplitude change of the conditioned MEPs is plotted against the paired-pulse interval. Normal controls show inhibition for intervals up to 6 ms (and facilitation for intervals of 10 and 15 ms). Note the loss of inhibition in both the dystonic hand and clinically normal hand of the patients compared with normal. (Reproduced from Ridding et al,[22] with permission.)

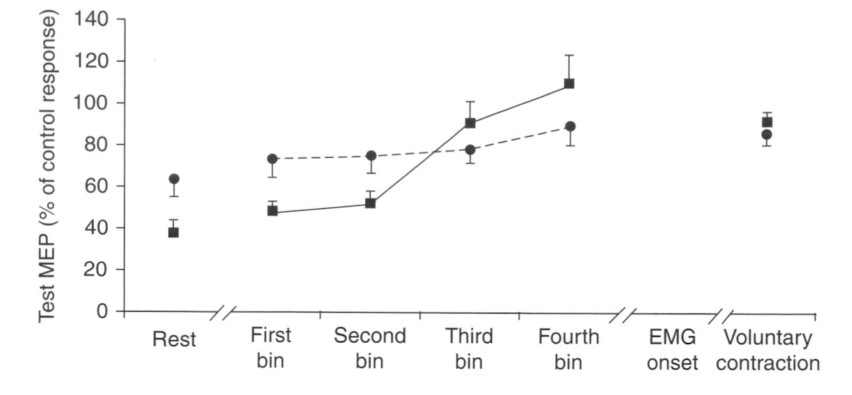

Figure 4.2 Intracortical inhibition at rest, preceding rapid wrist extension, and during contraction in healthy controls (solid line) compared with dystonia patients (dashed line). The decreased inhibition immediately prior to movement in normal subjects is absent in dystonia. The fourth bin represents 79 to 60 ms prior to movement. (Reproduced from Gilio et al,[25] with permission.)

These findings indicate a deficiency of inhibition specifically during the dystonic contraction while normal movements occur when cortical inhibition is less impaired. The implication is that the dystonic contraction is 'dystonic' because of deficient inhibition, while movements performed by the same dystonia patients when cortical inhibition was unimpaired are more normal. There is also loss of inhibition produced by cutaneous stimulation. Stimulation of the median nerve or index finger typically leads to inhibition of MEPs in hand and forearm muscles at various intervals, becoming maximal at 200 ms. This inhibition is lacking in patients with focal hand dystonia who show facilitation instead.[27] Generalized DYT1 dystonia patients have, in common with focal dystonia patients, reduced intracortical inhibition, shorter SP, and abnormal spinal reciprocal inhibition. Interestingly, carriers of the *DYT1* gene who are clinically normal were found to have abnormal intracortical inhibition and SPs, but normal reciprocal inhibition of the median H-reflex.[28] The finding of abnormal electrophysiology in non-manifesting carriers is evidence of the significant role of other modifying factors such as environmental input.

The concept of surround inhibition

Given that the central nervous system operates as a balance between excitation and inhibition, excessive movement could arise from increased excitability or reduced inhibition. Evidence has been emerging that dystonia is generated by a loss of inhibition, or, in particular, a loss of 'surround inhibition'.

Surround inhibition is a concept well accepted in sensory physiology. For example, receptive fields in the visual cortex are organized such that light in the center of the field will activate a cell, whereas light in the periphery will inhibit it. Such a pattern helps to sharpen borders and is an important step in the formation of patterns and objects. Surround inhibition is not yet well known in the motor system, but the concept is a logical one. When making a movement, the brain must activate the motor system. The brain may simply activate the specific movement, but it is more likely that when one specific movement is generated, other possible movements are suppressed simultaneously. The suppression of unwanted movements is surround inhibition. Surround inhibition should be essential for the production of precise, functional movement, just as surround inhibition in the visual system leads to more precise perceptions. If such a surround inhibition in the motor system is lacking, it is not surprising that a disorder like dystonia should emerge.

Leocani et al evaluated corticospinal excitability of both hemispheres during the auditory reaction time (RT) tasks with movement of either the right or left hand using TMS.[29] There is facilitation of MEP amplitudes on the side of movement in the 80–120 ms period before EMG onset, while the resting side showed inhibition. During the movement of the dominant hand, MEPs of contralateral hand muscles were suppressed for 60–100 ms after EMG onset, while the non-dominant hand movement failed to suppress MEPs of the dominant hand. This suppression of MEPs of the non-dominant hand by voluntary movements of a single digit in the dominant hand is not limited to the hand but also covers the proximal arm muscles that are not in any way involved in the movement, demonstrating widespread surround inhibition in normal subjects (Figure 4.3).[30] Corticospinal inhibition on the side not to be moved suggests that suppression of movement is an active process and additional proof of this comes from studies of no-go trials.[31]

A lack of surround inhibition

Liepert et al[32] used paired pulse TMS to study task-dependent modulation of cortical inhibition using muscles that act as agonist (abductor pollicis brevis, APB)-synergist (fourth dorsal interosseus muscles, 4DIO) pair in selective and non-selective tasks. Selective tasks required activation of the APB only with complete relaxation of 4DIO. In normal subjects, during selective tasks, surround inhibition could be seen as the conditioned MEP amplitudes of the agonist (APB) increased, while the conditioned MEPs of synergist were suppressed. In the non-selective task, the conditioned MEP of both muscles increased in normal and dystonia subjects. Using similar experimental design, Bütefisch et al[33] studied task-dependent modulation of inhibition in dystonia and showed that the during selective task, conditioned MEPs of both synergistic and agonist muscles increased in dystonia patients, demonstrating a disturbed surround inhibition in dystonia. Sohn and Hallett[34] were able to show an inhibition of the adductor digiti minimi (an uninvolved muscle in the 'surround') when the flexor digitorum superficialis (FDS) of the second digit is activated. This effect is less in patients with focal hand dystonia.[35]

There are also data from sensory function that are compatible with loss of inhibition. Using TMS, Tamburin et al[36] found increased intracortical inhibition 20–50 ms after cutaneous electrical stimulation to the fingers. In normal subjects, the inhibition is stronger in the finger receiving the stimulation itself, compared to an uninvolved surrounding finger. This difference in inhibition is lost in dystonia, consistent with a tendency towards fusion of finger representations as seen in earlier work. Tinazzi et al[37] studied median and ulnar nerve somatosensory evoked potentials (SEPs) in patients who had dystonia involving at least one upper limb. They compared the amplitude of spinal N13, brainstem P14, parietal N20 and P27, and frontal N30 SEPs obtained by stimulating the median and ulnar nerves simultaneously (MU), the amplitude value being obtained from the arithmetic sum of the SEPs elicited by stimulating the same nerves separately (M + U). The MU:(M + U) ratio

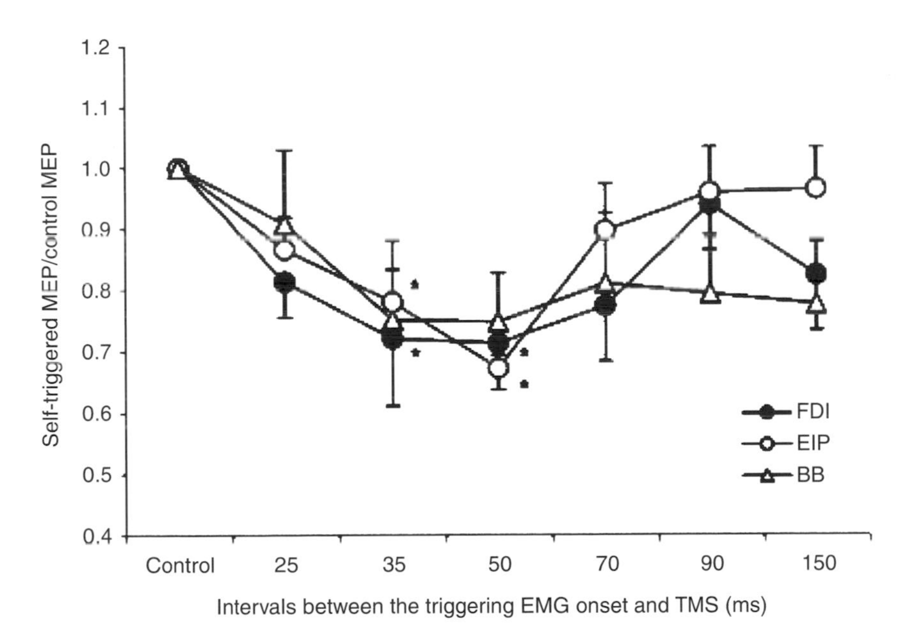

Figure 4.3 Time course changes in left sided MEPs triggered by right first dorsal interosseus (FDI) activation at stimulation intensity of 140% resting motor threshold (RMT). There is significant inhibition at intervals of 35 and 50 ms in FDI and extensor indicis proprius (EIP). There is a prominent, although not statistically significant inhibition in MEP amplitude of biceps brachii (BB) of 75% of control MEP at 35 and 50 ms, suggesting the spread of inhibition to muscles of the proximal arm not involved in the movement. (Reproduced from Sohn et al,[30] with permission.)

indicates the interaction between afferent inputs from the two peripheral nerves. No significant difference was found between SEP amplitudes and latencies for individually stimulated median and ulnar nerves in dystonic patients and normal subjects, but recordings in patients yielded a significantly higher percentage ratio for spinal N13, brainstem P14, and cortical N20, P27, and N30 components. The authors state that:

> these findings suggest that the inhibitory integration of afferent inputs, mainly proprioceptive inputs, coming from adjacent body parts is abnormal in dystonia. This inefficient integration, which is probably due to altered surrounding inhibition, could give rise to an abnormal motor output and might therefore contribute to the motor impairment present in dystonia.

A DISORDER OF CORTICAL MOTOR DYSFUNCTION

There are several abnormalities of the cortical motor system that suggest deficient function. The movement-related cortical potentials (MRCPs) begin with the Bereitschaftspotential, the slow negative shift of the EEG that start 1–2 seconds prior to self-initiated voluntary movements and is thought to reflect movement preparation. The Bereitschaftspotential consists of two components, the early part, which probably comes mainly from premotor cortex, and the later part, which adds a generator in the motor cortex. MRCPs associated with self-paced finger movement in patients with hand dystonia show a diminished late component.[38,39] A focal abnormality of the contralateral central region was confirmed with an analysis of event-related desynchronization of the EEG prior to movement, which showed a localized deficiency in desynchronization of β-frequency activity.[40] These results are consistent with reduced activation of the primary sensorimotor region. Feve et al[41] studied MRCPs in patients with symptomatic dystonia, including those with lesions in the striatum, pallidum, and thalamus. Patients with bilateral lesions showed deficient gradients for the Bereitschaftspotential. With unilateral lesions, the problem was worse for the symptomatic hand. Abnormal Bereitschaftspotential amplitude was also found preceding voluntary jaw opening in patients with oromandibular dystonia.[42] These findings confirm reduced activation of the primary sensorimotor cortex.

The contingent negative variation (CNV) is the EEG potential that appears between a warning stimulus and a go stimulus in a reaction time task. The CNV shows deficient late negativity with head turning in patients with torticollis[43] and for hand movement in patients with writer's cramp.[44] This late negativity represents motor function similar to the movement-related cortical potential. Such defective negativity in the MRCP and CNV are consistent with loss of inhibition in cortical processing.

Hyperexcitability of the motor cortex has been shown in a number of studies. Using TMS, increased excitability can be demonstrated by an abnormal increase in MEP size with increasing stimulus intensity; however, there is no change in the motor threshold, nor is there any abnormality of MEP size with increase in the level of background contraction. As mentioned earlier, abnormal intracortical inhibition in dystonia patients was seen in TMS studies using the double-pulse paradigm, as well as enlarged motor maps of dystonic muscles.

All these results fit together with the hypothesis that deficient inhibition leads to motor cortex hyperexcitability. This is a likely explanation for the excessive movement seen in patients with dystonia. Strong evidence for lack of cortical inhibition leading to a disturbance of motor function similar to dystonia was obtained by Matsumura et al in several primate studies. In the first study, local application of bicuculline, a γ-aminobutyric acid (GABA) antagonist, onto the motor cortex led to disordered movement and changed the movement pattern from reciprocal inhibition of antagonist muscles to co-contraction, the movement pattern of dystonia.[45] In the second study, the authors showed that bicuculline caused cells to lose their crisp directionality, converted unidirectional cells to bidirectional cells, and increased firing rates of most cells, including making silent cells into active ones.[46]

Origin of the abnormality in the basal ganglia

Most of the clinical evidence points to the basal ganglia as the site of pathology in dystonia. There is some evidence that the basal ganglia do affect cortical inhibition. In conditions where the basal ganglia are affected, cortical inhibition is also altered. The first line of evidence is the effect of basal ganglia disorders on the silent period following TMS. The silent period is shortened in Parkinson's disease and can be partially restored with dopaminergic treatment.[47] In Huntington's disease, the silent period is longer than normal, and this length is correlated with the degree of chorea.[48] The second line of evidence is the dopaminergic control of short-interval, intracortical inhibition. Bromocriptine given to normal subjects will increase the amount of inhibition.[49]

The third line of evidence is that thalamocortical influences on the cortex can be both excitatory and inhibitory, and, in some circumstances, the inhibitory influence is more profound. It is not unreasonable to think, therefore, that if cortical inhibition is diminished in dystonia the basal ganglia could be responsible.

The basal ganglia are anatomically organized to work in a center-surround mechanism. This idea of center-surround organization was one of the possible functions of the basal ganglia circuitry suggested by Alexander and Crutcher.[50] This was followed up by Mink, who detailed the possible anatomy.[51] The direct pathway has a focused inhibition in the globus pallidus while the subthalamic nucleus has divergent excitation. The direct pathway (with two inhibitory synapses) is a net excitatory pathway and the indirect pathway (with three inhibitory synapses) is a net inhibitory pathway (Figure 4.4). Hence the direct pathway can be the center and the indirect pathway the surround of a center-surround mechanism.

Tremblay and Filion[52] studied the reactions of single cells in the globus pallidus to stimulation in the striatum. The early inhibition was always displayed by neurons located in the center of the pallidal zone of influence of each striatal stimulation site, and was ended and often curtailed by excitation. At the periphery of the zone, excitation occurred alone or as the initial component of responses. The authors state that:

> this topological arrangement suggests that excitation is used, temporally, to control the magnitude of the central striatopallidal inhibitory signal and, spatially, to focus and contrast it onto a restricted number of pallidal neurons.

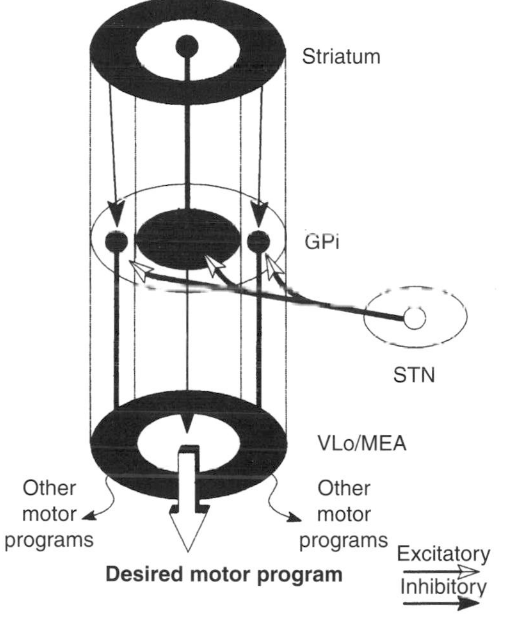

Figure 4.4 Model diagram of the basal ganglia showing possible pathways for surround inhibition. The center is the direct pathway and produces the desired movement. The periphery is the indirect pathway and functions to suppress unwanted movements. GPi is the internal division of the globus pallidus; STN is the subthalamic nucleus; VLo/MEA is the oralis portion of the ventrolateral nucleus of the thalamus and the midbrain extrapyramidal area. (Reproduced from Mink,[51] with permission.)

In interpreting these data, it is important to remember that the output of the globus pallidus is inhibitory, so that inhibition would be the 'center' signal and excitation the 'surround' signal.

The cortex also has anatomic and functional connections that allow for surround inhibition. Activation of a region gives rise to activity in short inhibitory interneurons that inhibit nearby neurons. This pattern has been well characterized in models of focal epilepsy where neurons surrounding a focus are inhibited.

GENESIS OF DYSTONIA FROM REPETITIVE ACTIVITY

Studies of focal dystonia provide a variety of lines of evidence that this form of the disorder could arise from aberrant motor learning, possibly on a substrate of an abnormal motor system produced by a genetic or other abnormality. The basic idea is that repetitive activity leads to enlargement of the regions of the brain involved with that activity. If the enlargement gets out of control, perhaps dystonia develops. Loss of inhibition might be a substrate that would permit excessive plastic changes. In an animal model, a facial palsy coupled with dopamine deficiency can produce blepharospasm.[53] The facial palsy will lead to an increased gain of eye closure, and with the appropriate background abnormality produced by the dopamine deficiency, the dystonia can develop. Facial palsy can be a precedent to blepharospasm in humans and can increase blink reflex excitability.[54] Hence, a situation similar to the animal model might exist in humans.

In another animal model, repetitive activity of the hand can induce a motor disorder akin to dystonia that is associated with enlargement of somatosensory receptive fields of neurons in primary sensory cortex.[55] As noted earlier, enlarged somatosensory fields are seen in thalamic neurons in patients with dystonia, and SEP studies are compatible with enlargement and overlap of sensory receptive fields. Thus, there can be similar pathology of sensory as well as motor function in dystonia.

PLASTICITY

The idea that repetitive activity can lead to dystonia is made more attractive by the finding that plasticity itself is abnormal. This was first found as an abnormal plasticity of the motor cortex in patients with focal hand dystonia[56] demonstrated using the technique of paired associative stimulation. In paired associative stimulation, a median nerve shock is paired with a TMS pulse to the sensorimotor cortex timed to be immediately after the arrival of the sensory volley. This intervention increases the amplitude of the MEP produced by TMS to the motor cortex. Paired associative stimulation produces motor learning similar to long-term potentiation. In patients with dystonia, paired associative stimulation produces a larger increase in the MEP than what is seen in normal subjects. These results have been confirmed.[57]

Another technique that shows increased plasticity is the pairing of high-frequency stimulation of the supraorbital nerve during the R2 of the blink reflex. This leads to an increase in the R2, and this increase is exaggerated in patients with blepharospasm.[58] There is also an abnormality in homeostatic plasticity.[59] Homeostatic plasticity is the phenomenon whereby plasticity remains within limits; this can be exceeded in dystonia.

It is probably relevant that increased plasticity may arise from decreased inhibition, so the inhibitory problem may well be more fundamental.

CONCLUSION

Evidence has accumulated showing that dystonia is a disorder of central nervous system inhibition that affects sensory as well as motor function. A model of dystonia as a disease with abnormal 'surround inhibition' may explain the generation of uncontrolled excessive movements. Dystonia could result from dysfunction of the basal ganglia which fails to focus movement. Focal hand dystonia appears to be caused by repetitive use of the dystonic body parts, and this suggests an important role for plasticity. Clearly, dystonia also has some hereditary component. There appears to be a requirement for a combination of a background central nervous system abnormality, perhaps genetically based, and a genetic modifier, such as an environmental influence.

ACKNOWLEDGMENT

This chapter is extensively modified, revised, and updated from:

Hallett M. Dystonia: abnormal movements result from loss of inhibition. In: Fahn S, Hallett M, DeLong M, eds. Dystonia 4. Advances in Neurology, Volume 94. Philadelphia: Lippincott, Williams and Wilkins; 2003: 1–9.

REFERENCES

1. Cohen LG, Hallett M. Hand cramps: clinical features and electromyographic patterns in a focal dystonia. Neurology 1988; 38: 1005–12.
2. Valls-Solé J, Hallett M. Modulation of electromyographic activity of wrist flexor and extensor muscles in patients with writer's cramp. Mov Disord 1995; 10: 741–8.
3. Sabbahi M, Etnyre B, Al-Jawayed I, Jankovic J. Soleus H-reflex measures in patients with focal and generalized dystonia. Clin Neurophysiol 2003; 114(2): 288–94.
4. Berardelli A, Rothwell JC, Day BL, Marsden CD. Pathophysiology of blepharospasm and oromandibular dystonia. Brain 1985; 108: 593–608.
5. Topka H, Hallett M. Perioral reflexes in orofacial dyskinesia and spasmodic dysphonia. Muscle Nerve 1992; 15: 1016–22.
6. Bara-Jimenez W, Shelton P, Hallett M. Spatial discrimination is abnormal in focal hand dystonia. Neurology 2000; 55(12): 1869–73.
7. Molloy FM, Carr TD, Zeuner KE, Dambrosia JM, Hallett M. Abnormalities of spatial discrimination in focal and generalized dystonia. Brain 2003; 126(Pt 10): 2175–82.
8. Fiorio M, Tinazzi M, Bertolasi L, Aglioti SM. Temporal processing of visuotactile and tactile stimuli in writer's cramp. Ann Neurol 2003; 53(5): 630–5.
9. Tinazzi M, Fiorio M, Bertolasi L, Aglioti SM. Timing of tactile and visuo-tactile events is impaired in patients with cervical dystonia. J Neurol 2004; 251(1): 85–90.
10. Bara-Jimenez W, Shelton P, Sanger TD, Hallett M. Sensory discrimination capabilities in patients with focal hand dystonia. Ann Neurol 2000; 47(3): 377–80.
11. Zeuner KE, Bara-Jimenez W, Noguchi PS et al. Sensory training for patients with focal hand dystonia. Ann Neurol 2002; 51(5): 593–8.
12. Muller J, Wissel J, Masuhr F et al. Clinical characteristics of the geste antagoniste in cervical dystonia. J Neurol 2001; 248(6): 478–82.
13. Naumann M, Magyar-Lehmann S, Reiners K, Erbguth F, Leenders KL. Sensory tricks in cervical dystonia: perceptual dysbalance of parietal cortex modulates frontal motor programming. Ann Neurol 2000; 47(3): 322–8.
14. Murase N, Kaji R, Shimazu H et al. Abnormal premovement gating of somatosensory input in writer's cramp. Brain 2000; 123(Pt 9): 1813–29.
15. Ghika J, Regli F, Growdon JH. Sensory symptoms in cranial dystonia: a potential role in the etiology? J Neurol Sci 1993; 116: 142–7.
16. Kaji R, Rothwell JC, Katayama M et al. Tonic vibration reflex and muscle afferent block in writer's cramp: implications for a new therapeutic approach. Ann Neurol 1995; 38: 155–62.
17. Tempel LW, Perlmutter JS. Abnormal cortical responses in patients with writer's cramp. Neurology 1993; 43: 2252–7.
18. Reilly JA, Hallett M, Cohen LG, Tarkka IM, Dang N. The N30 component of somatosensory evoked potentials in patients with dystonia. Electroencephalogr Clin Neurophysiol 1992; 84: 243–7.
19. Lenz FA, Byl NN. Reorganization in the cutaneous core of the human thalamic principal somatic sensory nucleus (Ventral caudal) in patients with dystonia. J Neurophysiol 1999; 82(6): 3204–12.
20. Bara-Jimenez W, Catalan MJ, Hallett M, Gerloff C. Abnormal somatosensory homunculus in dystonia of the hand. Ann Neurol 1998; 44: 828–31.
21. Butterworth S, Francis S, Kelly E et al. Abnormal cortical sensory activation in dystonia: an fMRI study. Mov Disord 2003; 18(6): 673–82.
22. Ridding MC, Sheean G, Rothwell JC, Inzelberg R, Kujirai T. Changes in the balance between motor cortical excitation and

inhibition in focal, task specific dystonia. J Neurol Neurosurg Psychiatry 1995; 59: 493–8.
23. Chen R, Wassermann E, Caños M, Hallett M. Impaired inhibition in writer's cramp during voluntary muscle activation. Neurology 1997; 49: 1054–9.
24. Sommer M, Ruge D, Tergau F et al. Intracortical excitability in the hand motor representation in hand dystonia and blepharospasm. Mov Disord 2002; 17(5): 1017–25.
25. Gilio F, Curra A, Inghilleri M et al. Abnormalities of motor cortex excitability preceding movement in patients with dystonia. Brain 2003; 126(Pt 8): 1745–54.
26. Filipovic SR, Ljubisavljevic M, Svetel M et al. Impairment of cortical inhibition in writer's cramp as revealed by changes in electromyographic silent period after transcranial magnetic stimulation. Neurosci Lett 1997; 222(3): 167–70.
27. Abbruzzese G, Marchese R, Buccolieri A, Gasparetto B, Trompetto C. Abnormalities of sensorimotor integration in focal dystonia: a transcranial magnetic stimulation study. Brain 2001; 124(Pt 3): 537–45.
28. Edwards MJ, Huang YZ, Wood NW, Rothwell JC, Bhatia KP. Different patterns of electrophysiological deficits in manifesting and non-manifesting carriers of the DYT1 gene mutation. Brain 2003; 126(Pt 9): 2074–80.
29. Leocani L, Cohen LG, Wassermann EM, Ikoma K, Hallett M. Human corticospinal excitability evaluated with transcranial magnetic stimulation during different reaction time paradigms. Brain 2000; 123(Pt 6): 1161–73.
30. Sohn YH, Jung HY, Kaelin-Lang A, Hallett M. Excitability of the ipsilateral motor cortex during phasic voluntary hand movement. Exp Brain Res 2003; 148(2): 176–85.
31. Sohn YH, Wiltz K, Hallett M. Effect of volitional inhibition on cortical inhibitory mechanisms. J Neurophysiol 2002; 88(1): 333–8.
32. Liepert J, Classen J, Cohen LG, Hallett M. Task-dependent changes of intracortical inhibition. Exp Brain Res 1998; 118(3): 421–6.
33. Bütefisch CM, Boroojerdi B, Chen R, Battaglia F, Hallett M. Task-dependent intracortical inhibition is impaired in focal hand dystonia. Mov Disord 2005; 20(5): 545–51.
34. Sohn YH, Hallett M. Surround inhibition in human motor system. Exp Brain Res 2004; 158(4): 397–404.
35. Sohn YH, Hallett M. Disturbed surround inhibition in focal hand dystonia. Ann Neurol 2004; 56(4): 595–9.
36. Tamburin S, Manganotti P, Marzi CA, Fiaschi A, Zanette G. Abnormal somatotopic arrangement of sensorimotor interactions in dystonic patients. Brain 2002; 125(Pt 12): 2719–30.
37. Tinazzi M, Priori A, Bertolasi L et al. Abnormal central integration of a dual somatosensory input in dystonia. Evidence for sensory overflow. Brain 2000; 123(Pt 1): 42–50.
38. Deuschl G, Toro C, Matsumoto J, Hallett M. The movement related cortical potential is abnormal is patients with writer's cramp. Mov Disord 1992; 7(Suppl 1): 127.
39. van der Kamp W, Rothwell JC, Thompson PD, Day BL, Marsden CD. The movement related cortical potential is abnormal in patients with idiopathic torsion dystonia. Mov Disord 1995; 5: 630–3.
40. Toro C, Deuschl G, Hallett M. Movement-related EEG desynchronization in patients with hand cramps: evidence for cortical involvement in focal dystonia. Neurology 1993; 43(Suppl 2): A379.
41. Feve A, Bathien N, Rondot P. Abnormal movement related potentials in patients with lesions of basal ganglia and anterior thalamus. J Neurol Neurosurg Psychiatry 1994; 57: 100–4.
42. Yoshida K, Kaji R, Kohara N et al. Movement-related cortical potentials before jaw excursions in oromandibular dystonia. Mov Disord 2003; 18(1): 94–100.
43. Kaji R, Ikeda A, Ikeda T et al. Physiological study of cervical dystonia. Task-specific abnormality in contingent negative variation. Brain 1995; 118: 511–22.
44. Ikeda A, Shibasaki H, Kaji R et al. Abnormal sensorimotor integration in writer's cramp: study of contingent negative variation. Mov Disord 1996; 11: 638–90.
45. Matsumura M, Sawaguchi T, Oishi T, Ueki K, Kubota K. Behavioral deficits induced by local injection of bicuculline and muscimol into the primate motor and premotor cortex. J Neurophysiol 1991; 65: 1542–53.
46. Matsumura M, Sawaguchi T, Kubota K. GABAergic inhibition of neuronal activity in the primate motor and premotor cortex during voluntary movement. J Neurophysiol 1992; 68: 692–702.
47. Priori A, Berardelli A, Inghilleri M, Accornero N, Manfredi M. Motor cortical inhibition and the dopaminergic system. Pharmacological changes in the silent period after transcranial brain stimulation in normal subjects, patients with Parkinson's disease and drug-induced parkinsonism. Brain 1994; 117: 317–23.
48. Roick H, Giesen HJ, Lange HW, Benecke R. Postexcitatory inhibition in Huntington's disease. Mov Disord 1992; 7: 27.
49. Ziemann U, Tergau F, Bruns D, Baudewig J, Paulus W. Changes in human motor cortex excitability induced by dopaminergic and anti-dopaminergic drugs. Electroencephalogr Clin Neurophysiol 1997; 105(6): 430–7.
50. Alexander GE, Crutcher MD. Functional architecture of basal ganglia circuits: neural substrates of parallel processing. Trends Neurosci 1990; 13: 266–71.
51. Mink JW. The basal ganglia: focused selection and inhibition of competing motor programs. Prog Neurobiol 1996; 50: 381–425.
52. Tremblay L, Filion M. Responses of pallidal neurons to striatal stimulation in intact waking monkeys. Brain Res 1989; 498(1): 1–16.
53. Schicatano EJ, Basso MA, Evinger C. Animal model explains the origins of the cranial dystonia benign essential blepharospasm. J Neurophysiol 1997; 77(5): 2842–6.
54. Syed NA, Delgado A, Sandbrink F et al. Blink reflex recovery in facial weakness: an electrophysiologic study of adaptive changes. Neurology 1999; 52(4): 834–8.
55. Byl N, Merzenich MM, Jenkins WM. A primate genesis model of focal dystonia and repetitive strain injury: I. Learning-induced dedifferentiation of the representation of the hand in the primary somatosensory cortex in adult monkeys. Neurology 1996; 47: 508–20.
56. Quartarone A, Bagnato S, Rizzo V et al. Abnormal associative plasticity of the human motor cortex in writer's cramp. Brain 2003; 126(Pt 12): 2586–96.
57. Weise D, Schramm A, Stefan K et al. The two sides of associative plasticity in writer's cramp. Brain 2006; 129(Pt 10): 2709–21.
58. Quartarone A, Sant'Angelo A, Battaglia F et al. Enhanced long-term potentiation-like plasticity of the trigeminal blink reflex circuit in blepharospasm. J Neurosci 2006; 26(2): 716–21.
59. Quartarone A, Rizzo V, Bagnato S et al. Homeostatic-like plasticity of the primary motor hand area is impaired in focal hand dystonia. Brain 2005; 128(Pt 8): 1943–50.

5

Functional imaging in primary dystonia

Maren Carbon-Correll, Kotaro Asanuma and David Eidelberg

INTRODUCTION

Primary torsion dystonia (PTD) has been generally conceptualized as a functional disorder of the basal ganglia and its output. Electrophysiologic studies have revealed abnormal input from the thalamus to the premotor cortex (PMC) attributable to alterations in the activity of pallidal projections to the ventral tier and intralaminar thalamic nuclei,[1] as well as to overexcitability of PMC regions.[2,3] By contrast, postmortem studies have failed to reveal substantial structural or neurochemical changes in the brains of PTD patients.[4–6] In this context, functional imaging can provide a unique in-vivo tool to expand the current understanding of the pathophysiology of PTD and related disorders.

In this chapter we review imaging studies on resting state metabolism in PTD as well as in dopamine-responsive dystonia (DRD). We further discuss the impact of these changes on regional activation responses during motor, sensory, and cognitive tasks. Additionally, we present data on dopamine metabolism and discuss the potential relevance of these findings to the pathophysiology of the dystonias.

PRIMARY TORSION DYSTONIA

Abnormal resting state metabolism

Despite the promising nature of in-vivo functional imaging, investigations of resting regional metabolism in dystonia have yielded conflicting results, particularly in the highly relevant corpus striatum and globus pallidus. Positron emission tomography (PET) with [^{18}F]-fluorodeoxyglucose (FDG) in the resting state is an indicator of local synaptic activity in the brain tissue.[7,8] This versatile imaging method does not require a simultaneous behavioral challenge, and has the advantages of high-signal, technical simplicity, and increasingly widespread availability. While some studies using radiolabeled FDG have reported increased striatal glucose utilization in PTD,[9–11] other studies have demonstrated decreased striatal metabolism.[12,13] Because the heterogeneity of dystonia cohorts could potentially confound imaging results, we have focused our studies on genotypically and phenotypically homogeneous groups. Using a novel regional network analytical approach in PTD patients,[9,14] we identified a reproducible pattern of abnormal regional glucose utilization in two independent cohorts of clinically non-manifesting *DYT1* carriers.[15,16] We found that these subjects express a specific metabolic topography characterized by increases in the posterior putamen/globus pallidus, cerebellum, and supplementary motor area (SMA).[16] In an ancillary study, we demonstrated that this abnormal torsion dystonia-related pattern (TDRP) was also present in clinically affected patients, persisting even following the suppression of involuntary dystonic movements by sleep induction.[15,17] Moreover, abnormal TDRP expression proved not to be specific for the *DYT1* genotype: it was also detected in a cohort of manifesting and non-manifesting carriers of the *DYT6* dystonia mutation (North American Mennonites), but not in DRD patients.[16] In summary, these findings suggest that TDRP expression is a feature of certain primary dystonia genotypes and is not only linked to the presence of clinical manifestations.

Despite the presence of a distinct metabolic network as a shared trait feature in manifesting and non-manifesting *DYT1* and *DYT6* mutation carriers, functional activity within TDRP nodes may differ across genotypes (*DYT1* and *DYT6*) and phenotypes (manifesting and non-manifesting). Manifesting carriers of both genotypes exhibited hypermetabolism in the

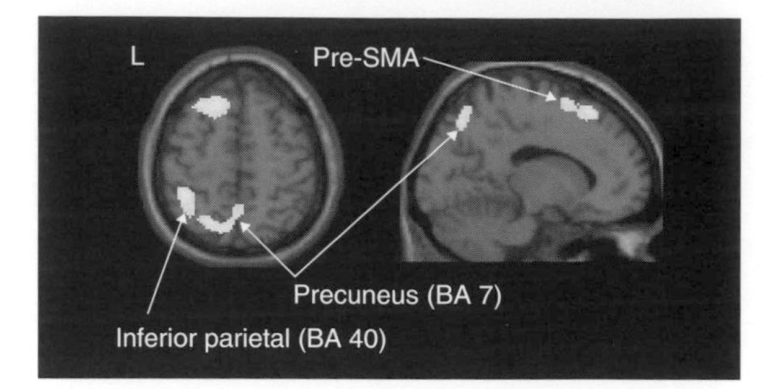

Figure 5.1 Statistical parametric map (SPM) comparing resting state FDG PET scans in manifesting and non-manifesting gene carriers. Significant metabolic differences were detected in the Pre-SMA and posterior parietal areas (arrows). In these regions, metabolism was increased in affected *DYT1* and *DYT6* gene carriers compared with their non-manifesting counterparts. (Differences in voxel intensity were thresholded at $T = 3.3$, $p < 0.001$; SPM 99.)

pre-supplementary motor area (Pre-SMA, BA 6) and parietal association cortices (BA 40/7) compared to their non-manifesting counterparts. These regional changes were also present when compared to age-matched gene-negative controls (Figure 5.1;[18]). The Pre-SMA is thought to be in a key function in higher-order motor planning, while the superior parietal cortices function as visuomotor integrators. Therefore, these observations support the notion of dystonia as a syndrome of abnormal movement preparation caused by defective sensorimotor integration.[19] In addition, regardless of clinical penetrance, genotype-specific metabolic increases in *DYT1* carriers were present in the putamen and cerebellar hemispheres bilaterally. By contrast, *DYT6* carriers have relative hypometabolism of the putamen, associated with hypermetabolism in the middle temporal gyrus (BA 21;[18]). Thus, the neocortical changes in Pre-SMA and parietal cortex may be a constant feature of the phenomenology of dystonia; the subcortical metabolic changes may relate to the underlying pathologic mechanisms associated with different PTD muations. The genotype-specific differences in local metabolic activity suggest that primary dystonia may be mediated by a variety of biologic mechanisms depending on the nature of the underlying mutation.

Abnormal motor activation patterns

The presence of an abnormal resting metabolic topography may affect the functional activity of key nodes of the motor cortico-striato-pallido-thalamo-cortical (CSPTC) loops and related cerebellar pathways.[14,20,21] Activation studies are usually performed with ^{15}O-water ($H_2{}^{15}O$) and PET to describe changes in regional cerebral blood flow (rCBF). Alternatively, functional magnetic resonance imaging (fMRI) measures the blood oxygenation level dependent (BOLD) response. The meaning of this signal is not yet clearly understood, but it is believed to reflect changes in local hemodynamics.[22] Overall, activation studies in dystonia have demonstrated differences in brain activation responses mainly in the prefrontal cortex and the sensorimotor cortex (SMC). However, these results have largely differed regarding the amount and the direction of these differences. In idiopathic generalized dystonia, simple motor execution was related to relative activation increases in the prefrontal cortex, PMC,[23–25] and putamen[23,24] concomitant with relatively decreased activation of the SMC.[23,24] Studies into writers' cramp have been more conflicting. Some studies showed SMC overactivation during symptom-provoking writing tasks[26–28] or during simple motor execution.[29] Yet others demonstrated relatively decreased activity in the SMC during writing[23] or during sustained contraction[30,31] as well as during relaxation.[31] Additionally, increased activity was found in PMC[26,27,32] and the cerebellum[26,27,32] as well as in the thalamus[26,27] and parietal association cortices.[32] Contrasting with the results in writers' cramp as one form of task-induced hand dystonia, musicians' dystonia studied in fMRI[33] was characterized by the reverse pattern, i.e. an overactivity of the primary motor cortex concomitant to an underactivation of PMC. Importantly, recent studies have demonstrated somatotopic disorganization of motor activiation in writers' cramp with impaired segregation of cortical[34] and putamenal[35] activation. Similarly, Blood and colleagues[29] recently reported putamenal dysfunction in focal hand dystonia. They found abnormally persistent activation of the putamen during rest periods after tapping and suggested that these elevations reflected impaired inhibitory control within the basal ganglia.

Similar to the results in focal hand dystonia, studies into orofacial dystonia have yielded heterogeneous results. Blepharospasm was related to dysfunction of the putamen during eyelid spasm periods.[36] Symptom-provoking vocal tasks demonstrated marked activation deficits of the SMC[37] and PMC[37,38] in orofacial dystonia. In addition, relatively increased activation of the SMA and somatosensory cortex was found independent of the affected body part during whistling.[37]

Activation studies in affected dystonia subjects may be confounded by the epiphenomena of abnormal movement, such as smaller ranges of motion, or by harder button presses. In our studies, we therefore chose to use kinematically controlled tasks[39] and to focus our investigations on non-manifesting *DYT* gene carriers. We used a simple motor task that required subjects to reach for radially arrayed targets in a predictable order with their right hand. Compared to controls, *DYT1* carriers had increased activation in the right SMA, the left lateral PMC, and inferior parietal cortex (BA 40).[40] By contrast, a relative reduction in motor activation was present in *DYT1* carriers in the left posterior medial cerebellum, possibly reflecting the functional consequences of increased deposition of torsin A in this region.[41,42] Notably, these abnormalities in regional activation were present in carriers, despite normal movement trajectories.[40]

As the basal ganglia have been shown to mediate specific aspects of motor learning, especially the process of combining individual movements into sequences,[43] we selected motor sequence learning as a behavioral paradigm to study brain-performance relationships in *DYT1* carriers.[44] Interestingly, non-manifesting *DYT1* gene carriers, despite being otherwise highly functional, exhibited a striking deficit in motor sequence learning performance: the mean learning index across cycles[39,45] was only 17.5 in *DYT1* gene carriers as compared to 42 in controls ($p < 0.008$). As mentioned above, movements to predictable targets were unimpaired in the *DYT1* carriers as well as movements to random, unpredictable targets. In ancillary studies, we found that the deficit in sequence learning was not specific for motor functioning, but was also evident in a purely observational sequence learning paradigm.

To assess brain activation responses during task performance, we scanned seven *DYT1* gene carriers and seven age-matched controls with $H_2{}^{15}O$ and PET while they performed two kinematically controlled sequence-learning tasks. Similar to the simple motor execution task, which served as the control, subjects had to reach for eight radially arrayed targets. However, in the motor sequence learning task (MSEQ), the eight targets appeared in an unknown, but repeating order over the 90s trial block. Additionally, in a trial-and-error guided sequence learning task (TE-SEQ), subjects had to detect the sequence order by reaching for the targets (video clips of all tasks are available at http://feinsteinneuroscience.org).[46,47]

Activation patterns during MSEQ and TE-SEQ showed significant group differences. During MSEQ, non-manifesting *DYT1* carriers displayed significantly greater activation than controls in the right pre-SMA and posterior parietal cortex, the right anterior cerebellum, and the left prefrontal cortex.[40] Nonetheless, this overactivation did not result in normal learning performance. For the analyses of TE-SEQ we used a parametric design[48] and compared the two groups at

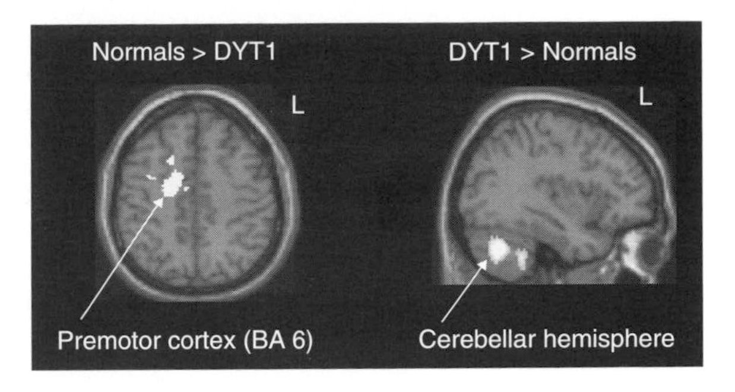

Figure 5.2 Comparison of *DYT1* carriers and control subjects performing a trial-and-error motor sequence learning task (TE-SEQ); see text. This analysis was performed using a parametric design[48] to compare the two groups at equiperformance. *DYT1* carriers achieved an accuracy of 58.3% correct hit rate, with a group mean of 5.7 targets. Accordingly, we matched this group to healthy age-matched volunteers who performed this task at the same level of accuracy. To achieve control performance levels, the *DYT1* carriers utilized more activation (right) in the cerebellar hemispheres, with comparatively less activation (left) in the premotor region (p <0.001, uncorrected).

equiperformance. *DYT1* carriers achieved an accuracy of 58.3% correct hit rate, with a group mean of 5.7 targets, and were accordingly matched to a group of healthy age-matched volunteers who performed TE-SEQ at the same level of accuracy. To achieve control performance levels, the *DYT1* carriers utilized more activation in the cerebellar hemispheres with comparatively less activation in the prefrontal cortices (Figure 5.2). These findings indicate that sequence processing is impaired in clinically non-manifesting *DYT1* carriers. However, further studies are needed to characterize the effects of resting state metabolic changes on sequence processing in *DYT6* to determine whether the sequence-learning deficit is a general feature of idiopathic dystonia.

In order to expand these observations, we used network analysis to study the relationship between learning performance and patterns of brain activation in *DYT1* gene carriers. In previous $H_2{}^{15}O$ studies of sequence learning,[49] we identified a specific regional covariance pattern involving caudate, prefrontal, and posterior parietal activation that was highly correlated with the learning achieved during imaging in both healthy volunteers and in patients with Parkinson's disease. While reproducible in three independent populations,[45] this learning network failed to predict performance in the *DYT1* carrier group. To detect an alternative network that mediates sequence learning in mutation carriers, we performed an exploratory analysis restricted only to gene-positive subjects.[50] Indeed, a significant network with novel topography was identified in the $H_2{}^{15}O$ PET data of these subjects scanned during motor sequence learning. This learning-related pattern was associated with activation in regions not generally employed by control subjects performing the same task. In particular, significant contributions to the network ($p < 0.01$) were detected in the cerebellar cortex and dentate nucleus, as well as in the ventral prefrontal cortex. Interestingly, the caudate nucleus and the premotor regions contributed significantly to the learning network in normals,[45,49] but not in *DYT1* carriers.

The presence of a different learning network in non-manifesting gene carriers raises the possibility of functional reorganization of frontostriatal pathways in these subjects, perhaps on a genetic and/or developmental basis. Indeed, using diffusion tensor MRI, we have recently detected impaired integrity of the subgyral white matter of the SMC in *DYT1* gene carriers.[51] Abnormal anatomic connectivity of the SMC may contribute to the vulnerability of *DYT1* gene carriers for the development of torsion dystonia. Additionally, metabolic changes in the basal ganglia may lead to the shift from striatal to cerebellar processing as a feature of the *DYT1* carrier state. Notably, while activation changes during the simple execution task can be effective in compensating for resting metabolic pathology in non-manifesting carriers, such changes appear to be inadequate to achieve a normal degree of sequence learning performance. The presence of dystonic manifestations in select gene carriers may reflect an upper bound ('ceiling effect') for compensatory brain activation that is exceeded in a subset of individuals at risk.

Abnormal sensory activation patterns

Impaired sensory integration has also been discussed as a pathologic mechanism in dystonia.[19,52] Experimental animal data[53] have suggested that focal dystonias can result from dysfunctional remodeling of sensory cortical areas after peripheral distress. However, even in the absence of precipitating peripheral strain, abnormalities in sensorimotor integration have been illustrated by electrophysiologic means.[54–57] To date, a line of neuroimaging research provides substantial evidence for impaired sensorimotor information processing in focal dystonias. Subjects with focal hand dystonia showed decreased responses to vibration in the hand region of the primary sensorimotor area and SMA of the affected or unaffected hand.[58] Similarly, they also showed altered processing of simultaneous sensory stimuli.[59] Expanding on these observations, impaired sensorimotor[60] and somatosensory[61] activation during sensory stimulation was also seen in subsequent cohorts. Feiwell and colleagues[60] proposed a region-specific processing deficit in blepharospasm subjects, as the activation differences were most pronounced when the stimulus was localized to the face, while responses to vibrotactile stimulation of the hands only showed subthreshold differences. Taking advantage from the high resolution in MRI[61] and stable source localization in magnetoencephalography,[34,62] researchers were able to demonstrate differences in the cortical separation of digit representation in focal hand dystonia. Cortical representations of digits were clearly separated in controls but showed substantial overlap[61] or reduced distances[34,62] in affecteds. Whereas this line of research has established impaired somatosensory cortical processing, only one recent study (interestingly) identified altered basal ganglia activation in the context of sensory discrimination.[63]

It has long been recognized that the so-called geste antagoniste, consisting of a sensory stimulation of the affected body part or an adjacent area, can effectively alleviate dystonic symptoms. Naumann et al[64] demonstrated decreases in the ipsilateral SMA and sensorimotor cortex activation along with increases in the parietal cortex with the geste antagoniste. Although activation changes were not compared to controls in this study, the reported changes probably reflect a normalization of activation, as increased SMA metabolism is a characteristic of dystonic symptomatology in other rCBF studies.[23,24,37,40]

Treatment effects on brain activation

To date, imaging studies have not played a major role in measuring treatment effects. Although botulinum toxin is the most effective therapy for focal dystonias, Ceballos-Baumann and colleagues[32,37] demonstrated that the alleviating effect is symptomatic but does not reverse the cortical dysfunction associated with dystonia. Utilizing $H_2{}^{15}O$ PET, they showed that brain activation responses increased during writing after botulinum toxin treatment in the parietal cortex and, importantly, in the SMA. Because these areas exhibit overactivation in writers' cramp without treatment, it is conceivable that botulinum toxin treatment leads to compensatory brain activation rather than supporting adaptive changes by normalizing rCBF. Nonetheless, activation in the primary sensory cortex was facilitated by treatment, whereas it was inhibited relative to controls without therapy.

Deep brain stimulation (DBS) of the internal globus pallidus (GPi) has recently been found to be safe and effective in the treatment of PTD patients with medically intractable symptoms, especially *DYT1* carriers.[65] The mechanism by which this intervention alleviates dystonia is not known, although a reduction in the noise of pallidal output pathways with restoration of a more tonic pattern has been suggested.[1] In a single case report,[66] GPi DBS in dystonia was associated with comparatively reduced brain activation during joystick movements in the lateral and medial premotor cortices, SMC, anterior cingulate, and prefrontal cortices. By contrast, no motor activation increases with GPi DBS were found in a more recent study.[25] In this study on six patients with primary generalized dystonia, unilateral GPi DBS induced relative decreases in motor activation in the prefrontal and temporal cortex as well as in the putamen and thalamus. Notably, the prefrontal cortex was the only region where abnormally increased motor activation at baseline was reversed by the treatment intervention. Thus, to date, imaging studies on the treatment effects in dystonia have failed to support the idea of a treatment-induced normalization of activation patterns.

Dopamine metabolism

PET also provides valuable measures on neurochemical changes in vivo. Early studies on the presynaptic dopaminergic function in PTD using [^{18}F]-dopa PET found only slight uptake reductions in the putamen.[67] Playford et al concluded that these mild reductions were unlikely to represent the major mechanism of pathology, although uptake in the three most severely affected subjects was outside the 2 SD ranges of normal controls.[67] By contrast, Perlmutter et al,[68] using [^{18}F]-spiperone, showed a significantly decreased D_2 receptor availability. We studied nine non-manifesting *DYT1* gene carriers using [^{11}C]-raclopride and PET to measure D_2 receptor binding, and found a 14% reduction in both the putamen and caudate ($p < 0.01$).[69] The magnitude of this estimated striatal reduction was less pronounced than the 29% reduction reported previously in focal dystonia.[68] These data suggest that a threshold of D_2 receptor availability may exist for the development of dystonic manifestations to appear. In other words, a subthreshold reduction of D_2 receptor availability as seen in our cohort of non-manifesting *DYT1* gene carriers may represent a genetically mediated 'at risk' state, while a more pronounced reduction may be needed for the development of actual clinical manifestations. However, to date, a marked reduction of dopamine content in the rostral putamen and caudate (54% and 50% of age-matched control values) has been reported in only one DYT1 autopsy case.[70] An increase in dopamine turnover with trends toward D_1 and D_2 neuroreceptor binding loss was subsequently reported,[71] without reduction in dopamine content. The role of dopaminergic transmission in DYT1 dystonia remains unclear. Indeed, the reported decrements in [^{11}C]-raclopride binding in DYT1 dystonia may represent an effect of increased dopamine turnover alone, or in the company of D_2 neuroreceptor loss.

DOPAMINE-RESPONSIVE DYSTONIA

Dopamine-responsive dystonia is an autosomal dominant inherited dystonia caused by mutation in the gene of the GTP cyclohydrolase 1 (*GCH1*).[75] This mutation induces a dopaminergic deficit in the absence of histopathologic changes.[76–78] A partial deficiency of tetrahydrobiopterin (BH_4) affects the function of tyrosine hydroxylase, the rate-limiting enzyme of dopamine synthesis. DRD is characterized by childhood onset and marked diurnal fluctuation.[76] Although sharing the symptoms of dystonic impairment with primary torsion dystonia, DRD is distinguished from other early-onset dystonias by its profound and sustained response to low-dose L-dopa.

Dopamine metabolism

Although the rate of dopamine synthesis is impaired, presynaptic nigrostriatal dopamine function assessed by PET imaging appears to be only mildly impaired in DRD. Snow et al[79] used [^{18}F]-fluoro-L-dopa (F-DOPA) PET measures and reported normal striatal tracer uptake in DRD patients. By contrast, Sawle and colleagues[80] found a mild but significant striatal F-DOPA uptake reduction. These finding suggest that L-dopa uptake, decarboxylation, and storage mechanisms are generally intact in DRD, as opposed to juvenile Parkinson's disease (JPD). Other studies have demonstrated that dopamine transporter (DAT) density measured with [^{123}I]-β-CIT SPECT,[81] as well as with [^{123}I]-2β-carbomethoxy-3β-(4-iodophenyl)-*N*-(3-fluoropropyl)- nortropane (FP-CIT),[82] was normal in DRD. Particular emphasis should be paid to the differentiation of JPD and clinical atypical DRD. Normal striatal DAT binding in a young parkinsonian patient points to a non-degenerative cause of parkinsonism and differentiates DRD from JPD. Similarly, postsynaptic dopaminergic function also appears to be minimally altered in DRD. Putamen and caudate D_2 receptor binding was found to be mildly increased in [^{11}C]-raclopride PET studies.[83,84] The mild elevation of tracer uptake could possibly be due to compensatory up-regulation of dopamine D_2 receptor density. Alternatively, the increased D_2 binding could also reflect low synaptic dopamine concentration, which in turn leads to diminished binding competition with [^{11}C]-raclopride at postsynaptic receptor sites. Kishore and colleagues found elevated striatal D_2 receptor binding in six DRD patients as well as in five asymptomatic gene carriers, all over 30 years old.[84] Additionally, these authors argued against treatment-induced D_2 receptor changes, and demonstrated elevated D_2 binding in one drug-naïve symptomatic subject at baseline and after 7 months of treatment. In conclusion, the increased striatal D_2 receptor binding in DRD possibly reflects a homeostatic response to the dopamine-deficient state.

In summary, these imaging studies have indicated that, despite the partial down-regulation of dopamine synthesis in DRD, the downstream functions of dopamine metabolism are generally preserved.

Glucose metabolism in DRD

To examine the possibility that dopaminergic dysfunction in DRD is reflected by downstream changes in regional glucose utilization, we used FDG PET to assess metabolic network activity: specifically, we explored the possibility that the clinical distinction from other early-onset dystonias is linked to a parallel difference in resting glucose metabolism. Prospectively calculated network expression of the TDRP (see above) in a cohort of DRD subjects confirmed that the latter group does not express the abnormal increases seen in PTD mutation carriers.[16] Similarly, the DRD group did not express the previously described metabolic network associated with Parkinson's disease.[21,85] Network analysis of DRD patients and controls did, however, reveal a distinct disease-related pattern accurately discriminating the two groups ($p < 0.005$).[86] This DRD-related pattern was characterized by bilateral metabolic increases in the supplemental motor areas and cerebellar hemispheres, associated with bilateral decrements in primary motor cortex and PMC, as well as ventral prefrontal cortex (BA 10/11). In a final analytical step, we found that *DYT1* carriers, even if affected, did not express this pattern, confirming both a unique clinical and metabolic phenotype.

In summary, functional imaging in dystonia can broaden our understanding of the pathologic mechanisms underlying clinically different subgroups within the dystonia spectrum. The identification of abnormal brain metabolism in dystonia has several practical implications. The presence of genotype-specific metabolic changes can possibly support linkage studies. Additionally, disease-related networks can prove useful for assessing mechanisms of therapeutic interventions, as has been demonstrated in Parkinson's disease.[87,88] A combined network-performance approach may be especially relevant in characterizing the effects of treatment on higher-order motor functioning.[21,45]

ACKNOWLEDGMENTS

This work was supported by the National Institutes of Health (NIH RO1 NS 37564) and the Dystonia Medical Research Foundation. Dr Eidelberg was supported by NIH K24 NS 02101. In particular, the authors wish to thank Mr Nathaniel Brown and Mrs Toni Flanagan for valuable editorial assistance.

REFERENCES

1. Vitek JL. Pathophysiology of dystonia: a neuronal model. Mov Disord 2002; 17(Suppl 3): S49–62.
2. Hanajima R, Ugawa Y, Terao Y et al. Cortico-cortical inhibition of the motor cortical area projecting to sternocleidomastoid muscle in normals and patients with spasmodic torticollis or essential tremor. Electroencephalogr Clin Neurophysiol 1998; 109: 391–6.
3. Siebner HR, Auer C, Conrad B. Abnormal increase in the corticomotor output to the affected hand during repetitive transcranial magnetic stimulation of the primary motor cortex in patients with writer's cramp. Neurosci Lett 1999; 262: 133–6.
4. Zeman W. Pathology of the torsion dystonias (dystonia musculorum deformans). Neurology 1970; 20: 79–88.
5. Zweig RM, Hedreen JC, Jankel WR et al. Pathology in brainstem regions of individuals with primary dystonia. Neurology 1988; 38: 702–6.
6. Walker R, Brin M, Sandu D et al. TorsinA immunoreactivity in brains of patients with DYT1 and non-DYT1 dystonia. Neurology 2002; 58: 120–4.
7. Jueptner M, Weiller C. Review: does measurement of regional cerebral blood flow reflect synaptic activity? Implications for PET and fMRI. Neuroimage 1995; 2: 148–56.
8. Eidelberg D, Moeller JR, Kazumata K et al. Metabolic correlates of pallidal neuronal activity in Parkinson's disease. Brain 1997; 120: 1315–24.
9. Eidelberg D, Moeller JR, Ishikawa T et al. The metabolic topography of idiopathic torsion dystonia. Brain 1995; 118: 1473–84.
10. Galardi G, Perani D, Grassi F et al. Basal ganglia and thalamocortical hypermetabolism in patients with spasmodic torticollis. Acta Neurol Scand 1996; 94: 172–6.
11. Magyar-Lehmann S, Antonini A, Roelcke U et al. Cerebral glucose metabolism in patients with spasmodic torticollis. Mov Disord 1997; 12: 704–8.
12. Karbe H, Holthoff VA, Rudolf J et al. Positron emission tomography demonstrates frontal cortex and basal ganglia hypometabolism in dystonia. Neurology 1992; 42: 1540–4.
13. John B, Klemm E, Haverkamp F. Evidence for altered basal ganglia and cortical functions in transient idiopathic dystonia. J Child Neurol 2000; 15: 820–2.
14. Eidelberg D. Brain networks and clinical penetrance: lessons from hyperkinetic movement disorders. Curr Opin Neurol 2003; 16: 471–4.
15. Eidelberg D, Moeller JR, Antonini A et al. Functional brain networks in DYT1 dystonia. Ann Neurol 1998; 44: 303–12.

16. Trošt M, Carbon M, Edwards C et al. Primary dystonia: is abnormal functional brain architecture linked to genotype? Ann Neurol 2002; 52: 853–6.
17. Hutchinson M, Nakamura T, Moeller JR et al. The metabolic topography of essential blepharospasm: a focal dystonia with general implications. Neurology 2000; 55: 673–7.
18. Carbon M, Su S, Dhawan V et al. Regional metabolism in primary torsion dystonia: effects of penetrance and genotype. Neurology 2004; 62: 1384–90.
19. Hallett M. Disorder of movement preparation in dystonia. Brain 2000; 123: 1765–6.
20. Wichmann T, DeLong MR. Functional and pathophysiological models of the basal ganglia. Curr Opin Neurobiol 1996; 6: 751–8.
21. Carbon M, Eidelberg D. Modulation of regional brain function by deep brain stimulation: studies with positron emission tomography. Curr Opin Neurol 2002; 15: 451–5.
22. Heeger DJ, Ress D. What does fMRI tell us about neuronal activity? Nat Rev Neurosci 2002; 3: 142–51.
23. Ceballos-Baumann AO, Passingham RE, Warner T et al. Overactive prefrontal and underactive motor cortical areas in idiopathic dystonia. Ann Neurol 1995; 37: 363–72.
24. Playford ED, Passingham RE, Marsden CD, Brooks DJ. Increased activation of frontal areas during arm movement in idiopathic torsion dystonia. Mov Disord 1998; 13: 309–18.
25. Detante O, Vercueil L, Thobois S et al. Globus pallidus internus stimulation in primary generalized dystonia: a $H_2{}^{15}O$ PET study. Brain 2004; 127: 1899–908.
26. Preibisch C, Berg D, Hofmann E et al. Cerebral activation patterns in patients with writer's cramp: a functional magnetic resonance imaging study. J Neurol 2001; 248: 10–17.
27. Odergren T, Stone-Elander S, Ingvar M. Cerebral and cerebellar activation in correlation to the action-induced dystonia in writer's cramp. Mov Disord 1998; 13: 497–508.
28. Lerner A, Shill H, Hanakawa T et al. Regional cerebral blood flow correlates of the severity of writer's cramp symptoms. Neuroimage 2004; 21: 904–13.
29. Blood AJ, Flaherty AW, Choi JK et al. Basal ganglia activity remains elevated after movement in focal hand dystonia. Ann Neurol 2004; 55: 744–8.
30. Ibanez V, Sadato N, Karp B, Deiber MP, Hallett M. Deficient activation of the motor cortical network in patients with writer's cramp. Neurology 1999; 53: 96–105.
31. Oga T, Honda M, Toma K et al. Abnormal cortical mechanisms of voluntary muscle relaxation in patients with writer's cramp: an fMRI study. Brain 2002; 125: 895–903.
32. Ceballos-Baumann AO, Sheean G, Passingham RE et al. Botulinum toxin does not reverse the cortical dysfunction associated with writer's cramp. A PET study. Brain 1997; 120: 571–82.
33. Pujol J, Roset-Llobet J, Rosines-Cubells D et al. Brain cortical activation during guitar-induced hand dystonia studied by functional MRI. Neuroimage 2000; 12: 257–67.
34. Braun C, Schweizer R, Heinz U et al. Task-specific plasticity of somatosensory cortex in patients with writer's cramp. Neuroimage 2003; 20: 1329–38.
35. Delmaire C, Krainik A, Tezenas du Montcel S et al. Disorganized somatotopy in the putamen of patients with focal hand dystonia. Neurology 2005; 64: 1391–6.
36. Schmidt KE, Linden DE, Goebel R et al. Striatal activation during blepharospasm revealed by fMRI. Neurology 2003; 60: 1738–43.
37. Dresel C, Haslinger B, Castrop F, Wohlschlaeger AM, Ceballos-Baumann AO. Silent event-related fMRI reveals deficient motor and enhanced somatosensory activation in orofacial dystonia. Brain 2006; 129: 36–46.
38. Haslinger B, Erhard P, Dresel C et al. "Silent event-related" fMRI reveals reduced sensorimotor activation in laryngeal dystonia. Neurology 2005; 65: 1562–9.
39. Ghilardi MF, Eidelberg D, Silvestri G, Ghez C. The differential effect of PD and normal aging on early explicit sequence learning. Neurology 2003; 60: 1313–19.
40. Ghilardi MF, Carbon M, Silvestri G et al. Impaired sequence learning in carriers of the DYT1 dystonia mutation. Ann Neurol 2003; 54: 102–9.
41. Augood SJ, Martin DM, Ozelius LJ et al. Distribution of the mRNAs encoding torsinA and torsinB in the normal adult human brain. Ann Neurol 1999; 46: 761–9.
42. Konokova M, Huynh DP, Yong W, Pulst SM. Cellular distribution of torsin A and torsin B in normal human brain. Arch Neurol 2001; 58: 921–7.
43. Soliveri P, Brown RG, Jahanshahi M et al. Learning manual pursuit tracking skills in patients with Parkinson's disease. Brain 1997; 120: 1325–37.
44. Ghilardi MF, Ghez C, Eidelberg D. Visuospatial learning may be impaired in non-manifesting carriers of the DYT1 mutation. Neurology 1999; 52: A516.
45. Carbon M, Ghilardi MF, Feigin A et al. Learning networks in health and Parkinson's disease: reproducibility and treatment effects. Hum Brain Mapp 2003; 19: 197–211.
46. Krakauer JW, Ghilardi MF, Ghez C. Independent learning of internal models for kinematic and dynamic control of reaching. Nat Neurosci 1999; 2: 1026–31.
47. Ghilardi MF, Ghez C, Dhawan V et al. Patterns of regional brain activation associated with different forms of motor learning. Brain Res 2000; 871: 127–45.
48. Mentis MJ, Dhawan V, Nakamura T et al. Enhancement of brain activation during trial-and-error sequence learning in early PD. Neurology 2003; 60: 612–19.
49. Nakamura T, Ghilardi MF, Mentis M et al. Functional networks in motor sequence learning: abnormal topographies in Parkinson's disease. Hum Brain Mapp 2001; 12: 42–60.
50. Carbon M, Ghilardi MF, Dhawan V et al. Abnormal brain networks in primary torsion dystonia. Adv Neurol 2004; 94: 155–61.
51. Carbon M, Kingsley PB, Su S et al. Microstructural white matter changes in carriers of the DYT1 gene mutation. Ann Neurol 2004; 56: 283–6.
52. Hallett M. Is dystonia a sensory disorder? Ann Neurol 1995; 38: 139–40.
53. Byl NN, Merzenich MM, Cheung S et al. A primate model for studying focal dystonia and repetitive strain injury: effects on the primary somatosensory cortex. Phys Ther 1997; 77: 269–84.
54. Reilly JA, Hallett M, Cohen LG et al. The N30 component of somatosensory evoked potentials in patients with dystonia. Electroencephalogr Clin Neurophysiol 1992; 84: 243–7.
55. Toro C, Deuschl G, Hallett M. Movement-related electroencephalographic desynchronization in patients with hand cramps: evidence for motor cortical involvement in focal dystonia. Ann Neurol 2000; 47: 456–61.
56. Abbruzzese G, Marchese R, Buccolieri A et al. Abnormalities of sensorimotor integration in focal dystonia: a transcranial magnetic stimulation study. Brain 2001; 124: 537–45.
57. Tamburin S, Manganotti P, Marzi CA et al. Abnormal somatotopic arrangement of sensorimotor interactions in dystonic patients. Brain 2002; 125: 2719–30.
58. Tempel LW, Perlmutter JS. Abnormal cortical responses in patients with writer's cramp. Neurology 1993; 43: 2252–7.
59. Sanger TD, Pascual-Leone A, Tarsy D, Schlaug G. Nonlinear sensory cortex response to simultaneous tactile stimuli in writer's cramp. Mov Disord 2002; 17: 105–11.

60. Feiwell RJ, Black KJ, McGee-Minnich LA et al. Diminished regional cerebral blood flow response to vibration in patients with blepharospasm. Neurology 1999; 52: 291–7.
61. Butterworth S, Francis S, Kelly E et al. Abnormal cortical sensory activation in dystonia: an fMRI study. Mov Disord 2003; 18: 673–82.
62. Elbert T, Candia V, Altenmuller E et al. Alteration of digital representations in somatosensory cortex in focal hand dystonia. Neuroreport 1998; 9: 3571–5.
63. Peller M, Zeuner KE, Munchau A et al. The basal ganglia are hyperactive during the discrimination of tactile stimuli in writer's cramp. Brain 2006; 129: 2697–708.
64. Naumann M, Magyar-Lehmann S, Reiners K et al. Sensory tricks in cervical dystonia: perceptual dysbalance of parietal cortex modulates frontal motor programming. Ann Neurol 2000; 47: 322–8.
65. Vercueil L, Pollak P, Fraix V et al. Deep brain stimulation in the treatment of severe dystonia. J Neurol 2001; 248: 695–700.
66. Kumar R, Dagher A, Hutchison WD et al. Globus pallidus deep brain stimulation for generalized dystonia: clinical and PET investigation. Neurology 1999; 53: 871–4.
67. Playford ED, Fletcher NA, Sawle GV et al. Striatal [^{18}F]dopa uptake in familial idiopathic dystonia. Brain 1993; 116: 1191–9.
68. Perlmutter JS, Stambuk MK, Markham J et al. Decreased [^{18}F]spiperone binding in putamen in idiopathic focal dystonia. J Neurosci 1997; 17: 843–50.
69. Asanuma K, Ma Y, Okulski J et al. Decreased striatal D_2 receptor binding in non-manifesting carriers of the DYT1 mutation. Neurology 2005; 64: 347–9.
70. Furukawa Y, Hornykiewicz O, Fahn S et al. Striatal dopamine in early-onset primary torsion dystonia with the DYT1 mutation. Neurology 2000; 54: 1193–5.
71. Augood SJ, Hollingsworth Z, Albers DS et al. Dopamine transmission in DYT1 dystonia: a biochemical and autoradiographical study. Neurology 2002; 59: 445–8.
72. Saint-Cyr JA. Frontal-striatal circuit functions: context, sequence, and consequence. J Int Neurophyschol Soc 2003; 9: 103–27.
73. Carbon M, Ma Y, Barnes A et al. Caudate nucleus: influence of dopaminergic input on sequence learning and brain activation in Parkinsonism. Neuroimage 2004; 21: 1497–507.
74. Carbon M, Feigin A, Ghilardi MF et al. Longitudinal changes in the relationship between striatal D_2 receptor binding and brain activation in preclinical Huntington's disease. Neurology 2003; 60S1: A247–8.
75. Ichinose H, Ohye T, Takahashi E et al. Hereditary progressive dystonia with marked diurnal fluctuation caused by mutations in the GTP cyclohydrolase I gene. Nat Genet 1994; 8: 236–42.
76. Segawa M, Hosaka A, Miyagawa F et al. Hereditary progressive dystonia with marked diurnal fluctuation. Adv Neurol 1976; 14: 215–33.
77. Rajput AH, Gibb WR, Zhong XH et al. Dopa-responsive dystonia: pathological and biochemical observations in a case. Ann Neurol 1994; 35: 396–402.
78. Furukawa Y, Kish SJ. Dopa-responsive dystonia: recent advances and remaining issues to be addressed. Mov Disord 1999; 14: 709–15.
79. Snow BJ, Nygaard TG, Takahashi H, Calne DB. Positron emission tomographic studies of dopa-responsive dystonia and early-onset idiopathic parkinsonism. Ann Neurol 1993; 34: 733–8.
80. Sawle GV, Leenders KL, Brooks DJ et al. Dopa-responsive dystonia: [^{18}F]dopa positron emission tomography. Ann Neurol 1991; 30: 24–30.
81. Jeon BS, Jeong JM, Park SS et al. Dopamine transporter density measured by [^{123}I]beta-CIT single-photon emission computed tomography is normal in dopa-responsive dystonia. Ann Neurol 1998; 43: 792–800.
82. O'Sullivan JD, Costa DC, Gacinovic S et al. SPECT imaging of the dopamine transporter in juvenile-onset dystonia. Neurology 2001; 56: 266–7.
83. Kunig G, Leenders KL, Antonini A et al. D_2 receptor binding in dopa-responsive dystonia. Ann Neurol 1998; 44: 758–62.
84. Kishore A, Nygaard TG, de la Fuente-Fernandez R et al. Striatal D_2 receptors in symptomatic and asymptomatic carriers of dopa-responsive dystonia measured with [^{11}C]-raclopride and positron-emission tomography. Neurology 1998; 50: 1028–32.
85. Moeller JR, Nakamura T, Mentis MJ et al. Reproducibility of regional metabolic covariance patterns: comparison of four populations. J Nucl Med 1999; 40: 1264–9.
86. Asanuma K, Ma Y, Huang C et al. The metabolic pathology of dopa-respomsive dystonia. Ann Neurol 2005; 57: 596–600.
87. Fukuda M, Mentis MJ, Ma Y et al. Networks mediating the clinical effects of pallidal brain stimulation for Parkinson's disease: a PET study of resting-state glucose metabolism. Brain 2001; 124: 1601–9.
88. Feigin A, Ghilardi MF, Fukuda M et al. Effects of levodopa infusion on motor activation responses in Parkinson's disease. Neurology 2002; 59: 220–6.

6

DYT1 dystonia

Laurie J Ozelius and Susan B Bressman

INTRODUCTION

In 1908, Schwalbe described an Eastern European family of Ashkenazi Jewish descent in which three siblings were affected with childhood-onset dystonia.[1] The term dystonia was not yet coined and Schwalbe called them chronic cramps; he also described the movements as hysterical. Three years later, Oppenheim reported the same disorder,[2] invented the term dystonia, argued for an organic basis, and named the condition dystonia musculorum deformans. Because of his contribution characterizing this form of dystonia, DYT1 dystonia has also been named 'Oppenheim's dystonia'. But Oppenheim didn't recognize that the disorder was inherited; that was considered in yet another report.[3] Thus, within its very first descriptions, lay important clues to the etiology of DYT1 dystonia. But for over half a century progress was stymied. In part this was due to nosologic confusion and the lumping of what we now categorize as primary and secondary dystonias. Racist political doctrine also contributed. In 1944 Herz resurrected primary dystonia as a distinct condition,[4] but he chose to ignore its predilection to affect Jews. He wrote:

> I have not elaborated on the possible prevalence of dystonia in any one group . . . recent experiences with *Rassebiologie* have been so depressing and grotesque that they do not encourage speculations.

The changing political and scientific environments over the last 30 years have, thankfully, led to a flourishing in our knowledge. Astute clinical observation and disease classification, led by David Marsden[5,6] and Stanley Fahn,[7] along with the application of genetic epidemiologic tools and molecular advances, have been critical to progress in our understanding of both primary dystonia and secondary dystonias. This chapter provides an overview of dystonia caused by mutations in the *DYT1* gene, describing clinical and genetic aspects as well as current knowledge of the encoded protein, torsinA.

EARLY-ONSET PRIMARY DYSTONIA AND IDENTIFYING DYT1

As alluded to above, early-onset primary dystonia was first described by Schwalbe and Oppenheim and its familial nature was noted. Over 50 years later, in a hallmark paper, Zeman and Dyken[8] analyzed pedigrees of 253 primary dystonia cases and concluded that the disorder was inherited as an autosomal trait with reduced penetrance; they also estimated a fivefold increased gene frequency in Ashkenazi Jews compared to non-Jews. Subsequent systematic family studies confirmed autosomal dominant transmission with reduced penetrance of 30–40% in Ashkenazi Jews and non-Ashkenazim[9–11] and confirmed a higher prevalence in Jews.[12,13]

Because of the reduced penetrance, large multiplex families with this phenotype are uncommon. Using one such large North American non-Jewish family with 13 affected members, a gene for early-onset primary dystonia (*DYT1*) was mapped to chromosome 9q32-34 in 1989.[14] Clinically similar Ashkenazi and non-Jewish families were subsequently also found to be linked to the same 9q region.[15,16] A common haplotype spanning about 2 cM indicative of linkage disequilibrium was then identified among Ashkenazi Jews.[13,17,18] The finding of linkage disequilibrium supported the idea posited earlier by Risch et al[10] that a single mutational event is responsible for most early-onset primary dystonia in the Ashkenazi population. Using haplotype data across this 2 cM interval, Risch and colleagues calculated that the mutation was introduced into the Ashkenazi population about 350 years ago and probably originated in Lithuania or Byelorussia.[13] They also argued that the current high prevalence of the disease in Ashkenazim (estimated to be about 1:3000–1:9000, with a gene frequency of about 1:2000–1:6000) is due to the tremendous growth of that population in the 18th century from a small reproducing founder population.[13] A founder mutation and genetic drift (changes in gene frequency due to chance events such as migrations, population expansions), rather than a heterozygote advantage (i.e. non-penetrant *DYT1* carriers have some advantage that leads to carriers being more prevalent), is probably responsible for the high frequency of DYT1 dystonia in Ashkenazim.

Examining the haplotypes for the markers in linkage disequilibrium, evolutionary recombination events were identified among Ashkenazi families that defined the candidate gene to a 150 kb region containing four genes.[19] An in-frame deletion of three base pairs (GAG) was identified in the coding sequence of one of these genes, *DYT1*; it was present in affected members from both Ashkenazi and non-Jewish primary dystonia families, but not controls.[20] Subsequently, this same mutation was found in families of diverse ethnic backgrounds.[21–25] Haplotype analysis indicated that deletions in the non-Ashkenazi population originated from multiple independent mutation events, including de-novo mutations.[26] In contrast, among the great majority of Ashkenazi Jews, the GAG deletion derives from the same founder mutation. The reason for the GAG deletion's singular disease-causing status is not known but it is hypothesized that genetic instability due to an imperfect tandem 24 bp repeat in the region of the deletion leads to an increased frequency of the mutation.[26]

Despite extensive screening[27–29] the GAG deletion is the only definitive *DYT1* disease-producing mutation identified to date. Three other variations in *DYT1* have been found that change the amino acid sequence, but none have been unequivocally associated with disease. First, an 18 bp deletion causes loss of residues 323–328[28] and was identified in a family that included affected individuals with both dystonia and myoclonus. This family was later found to have a mutation in the ε-sarcoglycan gene,[30] thus casting doubt on whether the 18 bp deletion contributes to disease. A second deletion of 4 bp was identified which causes a frameshift and truncation starting at residue 312; however, this was found in a single control blood donor who was not examined neurologically.[31] Finally, a polymorphism in the coding sequence for residue 216 encodes aspartic acid in 88% and histidine in 12% of alleles in control populations[20] and its disease-modifying effects are discussed below.

GENE AND PROTEIN PROPERTIES

The *DYT1* (also known as *TOR1A*) cDNA is 998 bp long and encodes two ubiquitously expressed messages on Northern blot analysis of 1.8 kb and 2.2 kb.[20] These two messages are a consequence of two poly-A addition sites in the 3′ untranslated region of the gene. Sequence analysis of the human genome reveals three other genes that are highly homologous to *DYT1*: *TOR1B*, *TOR2A*, and *TOR3A*. *TOR1B* is 70% identical to *DYT1* at both the DNA and protein level. The two genes each have five exons with their splice sites conserved. They are located in a tail-to-tail orientation adjacent to each other on chromosome 9q34 and presumably arose from a tandem duplication of an evolutionary precursor gene.[27] *TOR2A* and *TOR3A*, share about 50% homology with *DYT1* at the amino acid level (References 27 and 32, unpublished results). *TOR2A* also has a similar structure, with five exons encoding a 321 amino acid protein. It is located about 10 cM centromeric to *DYT1* and *TOR1B* on chromosome 9q34. *TOR3A* is also known as *ADIR1* (ATP-dependent interferon responsive gene), as it was independently cloned by virtue of transcriptional regulation in response to α-interferon.[32] It is located on chromosome 1q24 and has alternative splicing of a sixth exon, resulting in two protein products of 397 amino acids or 336 amino acids (*ADIR2*).[32] All three *DYT1* homologs, *TOR1B*, *TOR2A*, and *TOR3A*, are ubiquitously expressed by Northern blot analysis.[20,32] Comparative sequence analyses have revealed torsin-like genes, in mouse, rat, nematode, fruit fly, pig, cow, zebrafish, chicken, hamster, and *Xenopus*.[27]

The *DYT1* gene encodes a 332 amino acid (37 kDa) protein called torsinA. The protein has a signal sequence and membrane-spanning region in the *N*-terminus as well as a glycosylation site and putative phosphorylation sites.[20] The 3 bp GAG deletion in the *DYT1* gene results in the loss of one of a pair of glutamic acid residues in the C-terminal region of the protein.[20] Analysis of torsinA protein sequence reveals that it is a novel member of a superfamily of ATPases associated with a variety of cellular activities (AAA^+).[20,33,34] These proteins typically possess Mg^{++}-dependent ATPase activity, form six-membered homomeric ring structures, and share a secondary structure.[34] This superfamily of chaperone proteins mediates conformational changes in target proteins and performs a variety of functions, including degradation of denatured proteins, membrane trafficking, vesicle fusion and organelle movement, cytoskeletal dynamics, and correct folding of nascent proteins.[35,36] Studies carried out both in vivo and in vitro and documented below suggest several of these are plausible functions for torsinA.

TorsinA is widely expressed in most cells in the body. In normal adult brain, torsinA is widely distributed with intense expression in substantia nigra dopamine neurons, cerebellar Purkinje cells, thalamus, globus pallidus, hippocampal formation, and cerebral cortex.[37–41]

Both the mRNA and protein are localized to neurons and not to glia, and protein studies also showed torsinA in neuronal processes. Labeling is predominantly present in cytoplasm with some perinuclear staining.[40,41] A similar widespread pattern of expression is seen in mouse[42] and rat[40,43] brains. Ultrastructural studies in human adult and macaque striatum demonstrate torsinA immunostaining of small vesicles in the presynaptic terminals, consistent with a role in modulating striatal signaling.[39]

Because clinical expression of DYT1 dystonia is generally limited to a 'window' of susceptibility, with onset in most patients between 4 and 21 years old, the developmental expression of torsinA has particular import. In humans, torsinA immunoreactivity is first seen 4–8 weeks postnatal in the four regions tested – cerebellum, substantia nigra, hippocampus, and basal ganglia.[44] In both mice and rats, torsinA is most highly expressed during prenatal and early postnatal development.[45,46] Significant regional differences are noted, with the highest level of expression in the cerebral cortex from embryonic day 15 (E15) to E17, in the striatum from E17 to P7, in the thalamus from P0 to P7, and in the cerebellum from P7 to P14.[45,46]

Finally, two studies have found co-localization of torsinA and α-synuclein immunoreactivity in Lewy bodies, implicating torsinA in dopamine transmission.[47,48]

NEUROPATHOLOGY

Early studies on brains from patients with primary dystonia reported no consistent neuropathologic changes.[49,50] With the identification of the *DYT1* gene, researchers are now able to screen brains for the 3 bp deletion and identify those with the *DYT1* GAG deletion. In a study of a single *DYT 1*-positive (i.e. with the *DYT1* GAG deletion) brain, nigral cellularity was normal as were striatal dopamine and homovanillic acid levels, except in the rostral portions of the putamen and caudate nucleus, where they were slightly decreased compared with controls.[51] Although this suggests that the *DYT1* GAG deletion mutation is not associated with significant damage to the nigrostriatal dopaminergic system, an increase in the ratio of dopamine metabolites to dopamine compared to controls was reported in a second study of four *DYT1* brains, consistent with increased dopamine turnover.[52] At the protein level, several studies have not found torsinA immunostaining pattern differences between *DYT1*-positive, *DYT1*-negative, and control brains.[53,54] However, comparing *DYT1*-positive and *DYT1*-negative brains to controls, larger and more closely spaced nigral dopaminergic neurons were identified in *DYT1*-positive dystonia brains as compared to controls. However, no evidence was found for neuronal loss, suggesting a functional rather than degenerative etiology.[54] A further study examining four *DYT1*-positive brains found ubiquitin-positive perinuclear inclusions in the midbrain reticular formation and the periaqueductal gray but not in the substantia nigra, striatum, hippocampus, or select regions of the cerebral cortex.[55] Although this finding has not been replicated in human brains, similar inclusions have been reported in several DYT1 mouse models.[56,57]

CELLULAR AND ANIMAL MODELS OF DISEASE

In vitro

Cellular studies indicate that the majority of torsinA is in the lumen of the endoplasmic reticulum (ER), consistent with its deduced signal sequence and the observed high mannose content.[58,59] Several studies suggest torsinA is associated with the ER membrane through its hydrophobic *N*-terminal region.[58-61] However, according to a recent report, torsinA appears to be associated peripherally with the ER membrane, possibly through an interaction with an integral membrane protein.[62] In cellular models with GAG-deleted torsinA there is a striking redistribution of torsinA from the ER to the nuclear envelope (NE). This also occurs with the introduction of an E171Q mutation in the ATP-binding domain, which does not allow ATP hydrolysis. This enrichment is presumably due to prolonged interaction of torsinA with substrate(s) at the NE.[63,64] Possible substrates include LAP1, an NE localized protein that interacts to a greater extent with GAG-deleted torsinA rather than wild-type protein, and a novel lumenal ER membrane protein that is related to LAP1, named LULL1.[65] Mutant torsinA expression is associated with abnormal morphology and apparent thickening of the NE, including altered connections between the inner and outer membranes, as well as generation of whorled membrane inclusions, which appear to 'spin off' the ER/NE.[63,64,66,67] In addition, further relating torsinA to dopamine, VMAT2, a protein important for bioactive monoamines in neurons, is associated with the membrane inclusions.[68]

TorsinA extends to the ends of processes and is also found associated with vesicles and neurite varicosities.[58,69] This is supported by work in human and non-human primate brain where torsin has been localized in neuronal processes and at synaptic endings in association with vesicles.[39] TorsinA has also been shown to interact with the kinesin light chain 1 (KLC1)[70] as well as vimentin (VIM)[71] and to regulate the cellular trafficking of the dopamine transporter and other polytopic membrane-bound proteins,[72] all of which are consistent with a role for torsinA in intracellular trafficking and an association with the cytoskeleton.

The role of torsinA in cellular stress has been examined by several different groups. Overexpression of wild-type but not mutant torsinA suppresses α-synuclein aggregation in cells.[73] In PC12 cells, levels of endogenous torsinA increase and the protein redistributes in response to oxidative stress.[74] Furthermore, overexpression of torsinA in both COS-1 and PC12 cells protects against cell death when cells are exposed to a variety of toxic insults.[75,76] Taken together with the in-vivo experiments described below[77,78] these studies point to a chaperone function for torsinA.

Non-mammalian models

In addition to the mammalian torsin family members, there are several torsin orthologs, including a single torsin-like gene in *Drosophila* and zebrafish and three torsin-related genes in nematodes.[27] One of the nematode genes, *OOC-5*, is critical for rotation of the nuclear–centrosome complex during embryogenesis and, when defective, leads to misorientation of the mitotic spindle and disruption of asymmetric cell division and cell fate determination.[79] Taken together with the information that torsinA interacts with KLC1[70] and VIM,[71] this provides additional evidence that torsinA interacts with the cytoskeleton and has a role in membrane movement. The OOC-5 protein is also found in the ER, suggesting that some essential ER-related function has been conserved throughout evolution in the torsin proteins.

Studies involving a second *Caenorhabditis elegans* torsin-like gene, *TOR-2*, show that wild-type torsin but not mutant torsin, has the ability to suppress polyglutamine-induced protein aggregation[77] as well as protect dopaminergic neurons from cellular stress after treatment with the neurotoxin 6-hydroxydopamine (6- OHDA).[78] Similarly, treatment with another dopaminergic toxin, MPTP, resulted in a significant increase in torsinA expression in the brains of mice several hours post treatment.[80] These results are reminiscent of cell culture studies described above[73,75,76] and provide evidence that torsinA has a role in protein folding and degradation.

Two *Drosophila* models of torsin have been described. In the first, overexpression of mutant human torsinA but not wild-type protein elicited locomotor defects in the flies.[81] In neurons they identified enlarged synaptic boutons of irregular shape with reduced vesicle content; they also found dense torsinA-immunoreactive bodies associated with synaptic densities and nuclear envelope changes consistent with the increased perinuclear staining seen in cultured cells overexpressing this protein (see above).[63,64] Both the locomotor and cellular defects could be suppressed with overexpression of human or fly Smad2, a downstream effector of the transforming growth factor-β (TGF-β) signaling pathway, suggesting that TGF-β signaling might be involved in early-onset dystonia.[81] The second *Drosophila* model used overexpression and RNA interference (RNAi) to analyze the function of torp4a, the endogenous fly torsin. Using the eye as a model, overexpression protected the retina from age-related neural degeneration, while down-regulation of torp4a caused degeneration of the retina.[82] Consistent with both cellular and mouse studies, torp4a was largely expressed in the ER but also found at the NE. A genetic screen to identify enhancers of torp4a demonstrated an association with components of the AP-3 adaptor complex, a protein related to myosin II function, and the superoxide dismutase 1 (*SOD1*) gene.[82]

Mouse

A number of genetic models are available for DYT1 dystonia in mice, including both engineered lines where the endogenous mouse locus (*Tor1a*) has been modified, as well as overexpressing transgenic models, where the human gene has been randomly inserted into the mouse genome (for review see Reference 83).

In one transgenic model, human mutant torsinA is overexpressed using the neuron-specific enolase (NSE) promoter; in this model about 40% of the mice show hyperactivity, circling, and abnormal movement.[56] These mice also demonstrate abnormal levels of dopamine metabolites as well as aggregates in the brainstem similar to those reported in *DYT1* human brains.[56] A second transgenic model expressing human mutant torsinA under the control of the CMV promoter does not show an overt movement disorder; these animals do, however, exhibit impaired motor sequence learning on the rotorod[84] reminiscent of the motor learning difficulties reported in human *DYT1* non-manifesting mutation carriers discussed below.[85] Recordings of the activity of striatal cholinergic interneurons in slice preparations from these animals in the presence of quinpirole, demonstrate an increase in firing rate that was mediated by a greater inhibition of N-type calcium currents.[86] An imbalance between striatal dopaminergic and cholinergic signaling in DYT1 dystonia is suggested by this study.

Three different types of engineered mice have been published to date. Knock-in (KI) mice bearing the 3 bp deletion in the heterozygous state, analogous to the human DYT1 dystonia, manifest hyperactivity in the open field, difficulty in beam walking, and possess abnormal levels of dopamine metabolites, but no overt dystonic posturing.[57] These mice also have brainstem neuronal aggregates consistent with human pathologic data.[55] In contrast, mice that are either homozygous KI or knock-out (KO) for the deletion die at birth with apparently normal morphology, but with postmigratory neurons showing abnormalities of the nuclear membranes.[87] The fact that both the homozygous KO and KI animals display the same lethal phenotype suggests that DYT1 dystonia results from a loss of function of the torsinA protein. The knock-down (KD) mouse model in which a reduced level of torsinA protein is expressed, displays a phenotype very similar to the heterozygous KI mice, showing both deficits in motor control as well as dopamine metabolite levels.[88] This mouse also supports a loss of function model because no deleted torsinA is necessary to produce the phenotype; this loss of function could be due to a dominant negative effect whereby the mutant protein interferes with the wild-type protein.

Although the exact function of torsinA remains elusive, the evidence presented above suggests a role in protein folding and degradation[72–78] and/or membrane movement within cells.[70,71,79] It seems clear from both the cellular and animal models that DYT1 dystonia results from a loss of function.[72,87,88] Although DYT1 dystonia is inherited as a dominant trait, this loss of function may occur through a dominant negative mechanism as a result of the fact that AAA+ proteins usually form oligomeric complexes. The carboxy terminus of AAA+ proteins is important for both the binding of interacting proteins[89,90] and for oligomerization.[91] If mutant torsinA interacts with wild-type torsinA, forming inactive multimers,[92] then suboptimal levels of functional torsinA might result. Alternatively, mutant torsinA could block binding to interacting partners or bind to and sequester partner proteins – either way, interfering with their functions. RNAi has been used in cell culture systems overexpressing the mutant torsin protein to block aggregate formation and restore normal distribution of wild-type torsinA.[93,94] These results support the dominant negative model for torsinA function and suggest RNAi could be used therapeutically.

DYT1 ROLE IN FOCAL DYSTONIA

Recent studies implicate involvement of other variations in the *DYT1/TORB* genomic region in late-onset, mainly focal dystonias. In dystonia patients from Iceland, a significant association was observed with a haplotype spanning the *DYT1* gene.[95] Two studies from Germany failed to replicate this association.[96,97] However, a study involving Italian and North American cohorts revealed an association in the Italian group with the same risk allele as was seen in Iceland but no association in the American group.[98] Finally, a group of Austrian and German patients with predominantly focal dystonia showed a strong association with two single nucleotide polymorphisms (SNPs) in the 3′ untranslated region of the gene (Figure 6.1C). However, rather than being a risk haplotype, as shown in the previous populations, the SNPs showed a strong protective effect.[99] Whether these opposing results reflect population difference or, instead, indicate that the tested SNPs are in strong linkage disequilibrium with a real causal variant(s), is unknown. Nevertheless, the combined results support a role for genetic variability in the *DYT1* genomic region as a contributing factor in the risk of developing late-onset, focal dystonia.

OTHER DYT1 VARIANTS AND THEIR ROLE IN DISEASE

As discussed above, when mutant torsinA is overexpressed in cells, it forms membrane inclusions that are thought to derive from the ER/NE.[63,64,66,67] The only identified non-synonymous coding variant in the *DYT1* gene is located in exon 4 and replaces an aspartic acid (D) at position 216 with a histidine (H) in about 12% of normal alleles.[20] It has recently been shown that when the H allele is overexpressed in cells, similar membrane inclusions result.[100] However, when the H allele is co-overexpressed with a construct carrying the GAG-deleted torsinA, fewer inclusions are formed (Figure 6.1). This suggests that the two alleles jointly have a canceling effect.[100] This finding raises the possibility that this variant may play a role in the reduced penetrance associated with DYT1 dystonia or in causing other forms of dystonia. Regarding the latter, there have been two studies examining the role of the D216H SNP in focal dystonia, and in both no associations were identified.[96,99]

Regarding the role of the D216H allele in modifying penetrance of DYT1, a recent study assessed 119 GAG deletion carriers with signs of dystonia ('manifesting'), 113 considered to be 'non-manifesting' carriers and 197 controls.[101] There was a significantly increased frequency of the 216H allele in non-manifesting deletion carriers and a decreased frequency in manifesting carriers compared to the controls. Analysis of haplotypes demonstrated a highly protective effect of the H allele in *trans* with the GAG deletion; there was also suggestive evidence that the D216 allele in *cis* is required for disease to be penetrant. Although these results support this variant as a potent intragenic modifier, it has a relatively small role in explaining reduced penetrance because the H allele is not common (at most, occurring in 20% of the population).

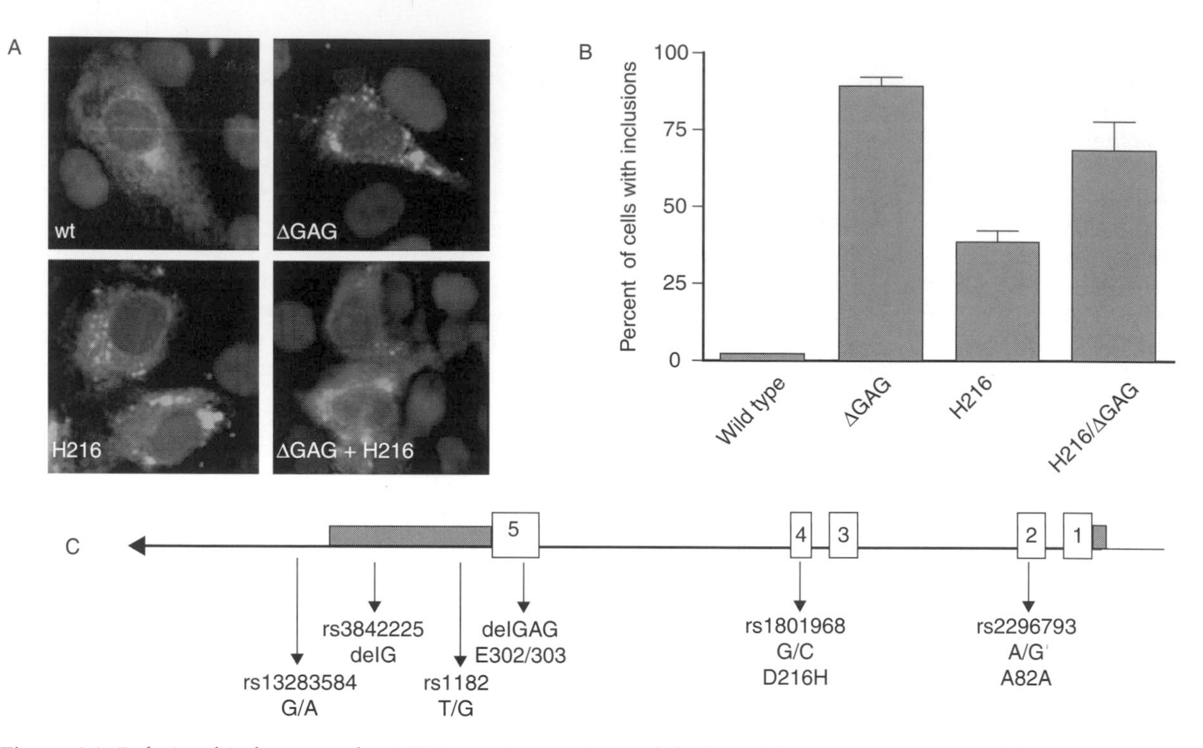

Figure 6.1 Relationship between the *DYT1* GAG mutation and the D216H polymorphism. (A) U2OS cells transiently transfected with plasmids, encoding torsinA-His_6myc containing the indicated mutation(s). Green shows torsinA and blue shows DAPI. (B) Quantitation of proportion of transfected U2OS cells with torsinA-positive inclusions. (Reproduced from Kock et al[100] with permission.) (C) A schematic (not drawn to scale) of the exon:intron structure of *DYT1* showing the position of the GAG deletion in exon 5, the D216H single nucleotide polymorphism (SNP), and several SNPs used in association and functional studies described in the text. (Modified from Risch et al,[101] with permission.)

DYT1 PHENOTYPE AND ENDOPHENOTYPE

With the identification of the *DYT1* gene, it has become possible to return to the clinical domain to determine the phenotypic spectrum and role of *DYT1* in the dystonia population. Clinical expression is extraordinarily broad, even within families; 70% of gene carriers have no definite signs of dystonia and among the remaining 30% dystonia ranges from focal to severe generalized.[102,103] There are, however, common DYT1 clinical characteristics that have been described across ethnic groups.[22,104–108] The vast majority of people with dystonia due to the *DYT1* mutation have a 'window' of early onset (starting after age 3 years and before 26 years), with dystonia first affecting an arm or leg. About 65% progress over 5–10 years to a generalized or multifocal distribution, the rest having segmental (10%) or only focal (25%) involvement. When viewed in terms of body regions ultimately involved, one or more limbs are almost always affected (over 95% have an affected arm) and the dystonia can be jerky or tremulous, mimicking myoclonus-dystonia. The trunk and neck may also be affected (about 25–35%) and they may be the regions producing the greatest disability.[109] The cranial muscles are less likely to be involved (<15–20%), and in one study of early-onset primary dystonia cranial involvement was the best clinical predictor of non-*DYT1* status.[110] Rarely, affected family members have been identified with late-onset (up to 64 years) dystonia.[103] These individuals are generally identified in the course of family studies and often do not seek medical attention. Also, although the arm is the body region most commonly affected in those with focal disease, the neck or cranial muscles have been reported as isolated affected sites;[29,104,111] however this is quite rare. Indeed, one study of patients with early-onset cervical dystonia failed to find any patients with the *DYT1* GAG deletion[112] and DYT1 very rarely causes adult focal dystonia, which constitutes the great majority of primary dystonia.[113]

The *DYT1* GAG deletion is more important in the Ashkenazi population, because of the founder effect, where it accounts for about 80% of early-onset (<26 years) cases;[18,104] this compares with 16–53% in early-onset non-Jewish populations (Figure 6.2).[22–24,104,114,115] The frequency of DYT1 dystonia among Ashkenazi Jews was estimated in one study,[13] using the founder haplotype. The mutation frequency was 1/6000–1/2000 (giving a carrier frequency of 1/3000–1/1000), which translates into a disease frequency of 1/3000–1/9000 (based on a penetrance of 30%). A recent study from south-eastern France, using direct genotyping of 12 000 newborn dried blood samples, identified one disease allele.[116] This carrier incidence of 1 in 12 000 is consistent with the approximately fivefold increased frequency of early-onset dystonia in Ashkenazim compared to non-Jews advanced in older studies, prior to gene identification.[8] These studies also imply that a significant proportion of early-onset cases, especially among non-Ashkenazim, are not due to *DYT1*, and other causes, including autosomal dominant and recessive genes, have been implicated.[105,117]

Another avenue opened by *DYT1* identification is a further exploration of its range of expression, and also an exploration of DYT1 endophenotypes that use imaging, electrophysiologic, and other techniques to measure subclinical traits. Non-manifesting family members (i.e. those without overt dystonia), a group constituting 70% of mutation carriers, can be studied; they can be compared to their non-carrier family members as well as those manifesting dystonia. Psychiatric expression of *DYT1* was investigated using this strategy. *Both* manifesting and non-manifesting gene carriers had the same increased risk for early-onset recurrent major depression when compared to their non-carrier-related family members;[118] differences in OCD (obsessive-compulsive disorder) frequency, a psychiatric feature associated with other movement disorders such as tics and myoclonus-dystonia, were not observed.[119] Other subtle clinical abnormalities noted in non-manifesting carriers are deficiencies in sequence learning[85] and probable dystonia. The latter, although increased in carriers compared to non-carriers, is not 100% specific, raising concerns about using family members with only probable dystonia in genetic linkage studies.[120]

DYT1 endophenotypes have been investigated using various imaging and neurophysiologic approaches. Eidelberg and colleagues demonstrated a characteristic pattern of glucose utilization with [^{18}F]-fluorodeoxyglucose (FDG) positron emission tomography (PET) and network analysis. There are covarying metabolic increases in the basal ganglia, cerebellum, and supplementary motor area (SMA) in both 'manifesting' and 'non-manifesting' gene carriers.[121,122] Other imaging studies of *DYT1* gene carriers, including

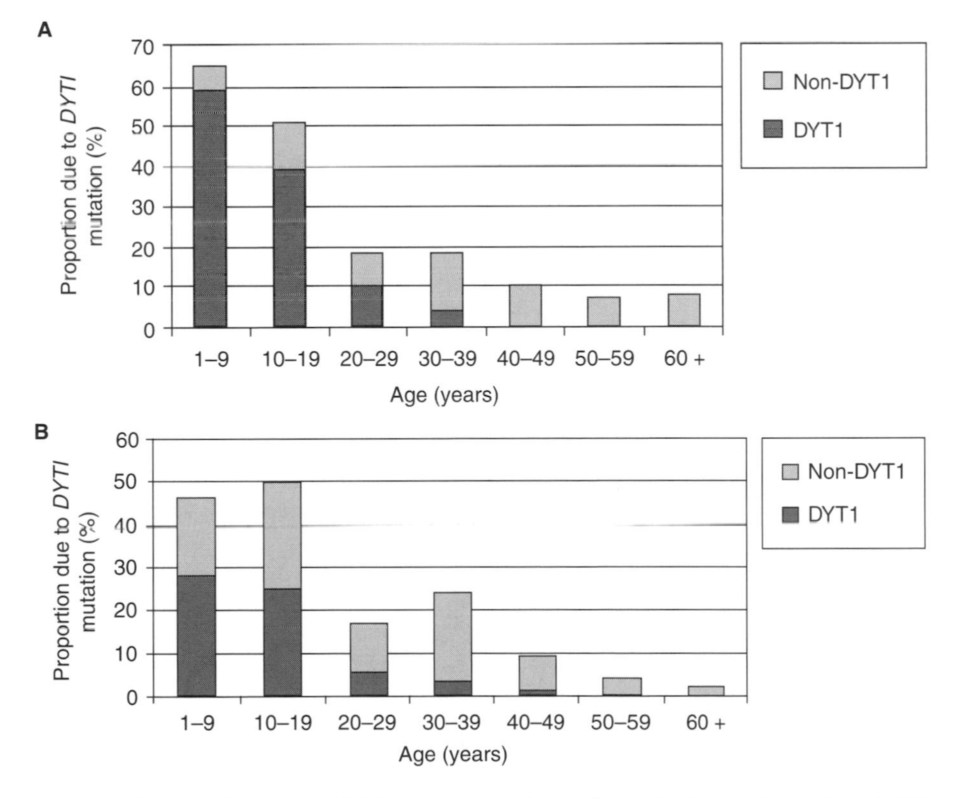

Figure 6.2 Proportion of dystonia due to *DYT1* mutation in the Ashkenazim (A) and non-Jewish (B) population.

non-manifesting carriers, have found decreased striatal D_2 receptor binding,[123] and microstructural changes involving the subgyral white matter of the sensorimotor cortex.[122] Electrophysiologic analyses have also identified genotype-associated abnormalities – namely, reduced intracortical inhibition and a shortened cortical silent period[124] – as well as higher tactile and visuotactile temporal discrimination thresholds and temporal order judgments.[125] These studies strongly support the presence of wider clinical gene expression, abnormal brain processing, and associated structural brain changes in gene carriers regardless of overt motor signs of dystonia, expanding the notion of penetrance and phenotype.

GENETIC COUNSELING AND TESTING

As described above, many studies have assessed the frequency of the *DYT1* GAG deletion in different clinical and ethnic populations. All studies confirm a very low rate of positive cases in adult-onset and focal primary dystonia populations and those suspected of having a secondary etiology. Two studies have formulated testing guidelines to help clinicians decide whom to screen. One study assessed 180 Ashkenazi and non-Jewish individuals with primary dystonia ascertained for diagnosis and treatment.[104] Features of dystonia in *DYT1* GAG deletion carriers and non-carriers were compared to determine a classification scheme that optimized prediction of carriers. The optimal algorithm for classification was disease onset before age 24 years in a limb. Although application of this classification scheme provided good separation among Ashkenazim (sensitivity, 96%; specificity, 88%), as well as in the group overall, it was less specific in discriminating non-Jewish mutation carriers from non-carriers (sensitivity, 94%; specificity, 69%). Using age 26 years as the cut-off, any site at onset gave a sensitivity of 100%, although specificity decreased to 54%. Based on these findings, diagnostic *DYT1* testing in conjunction with genetic counseling was recommended for primary dystonia patients (regardless of family history) with onset before age 26 years (Table 6.1). However, using this cut-off could miss the rare mutation carrier with later onset. Thus, a caveat was added advising that older-onset patients, especially those with writer's cramp and an early-onset blood relative, should be considered for screening. In another summary report,[126] *DYT1* testing in conjunction with genetic counseling was recommended for patients with primary dystonia with onset before age 30 years and in those with an affected relative with early onset. In both recommendations genetic counseling is an integral component. Counseling provides a format to explain the implications of both a positive and negative test. For instance, if a test is negative, a genetic etiology is not necessarily excluded and this needs to be explained. If the test is positive, a diagnosis is secured but this diagnosis impacts on other at-risk family members. These members, even if asymptomatic, may wish carrier testing, and genetic counseling for all asymptomatic family members is imperative before testing is performed. The psychological and social implications of autosomal dominant disorders with markedly reduced penetrance and very variable expression are complicated and require considerable time for patient and family education and counseling.

To obtain up-to-date information regarding genetic testing sites, a highly recommended on-line resource is www.geneclinics.org.

Table 6.1 ***DYT1*** **testing guidelines based on screening 180 medically diagnosed cases, including 89** ***DYT1*** **gene carriers**[a]

	AJ (n = 126)	NJ (n = 54)	All (n = 180)
Age onset < 26 years	Sensitivity = 100% Specificity = 63% PPV = 80%	Sensitivity = 100% Specificity = 43% PPV = 38%	Sensitivity = 100% Specificity = 54% PPV = 64%
Onset in a limb and age onset <24 years	Sensitivity = 96% Specificity = 88%	Sensitivity = 94% Specificity = 69%	Sensitivity = 95% Specificity = 80%
Two or more limbs	Sensitivity = 95% Specificity = 98%	Sensitivity = 93% Specificity = 53%	Sensitivity = 95% Specificity = 79%

[a]AJ = Ashkenazi Jews; NJ = non-Jewish; PPV = positive predictive value. Modified from Bressman et al,[104] with permission.

SUMMARY AND FUTURE DIRECTIONS

There has been a veritable explosion in our understanding of the genetic underpinnings of that form of primary dystonia, termed dystonia musculorum deformans, first described by Oppenheim almost 100 years ago. This condition results from a single and recurring GAG deletion in the *DYT1* gene which codes for a neuronal protein, torsinA, that appears to have many functions. Our understanding of normal and mutated torsinA is widening and no doubt will continue to progress along current paths, as cellular and animal models are further explored. Especially important will be investigations that not only focus on the striatum but also assess anatomic and functional changes elsewhere in the brain. Various lines of study suggest that the brainstem and cerebellum[55,127] need closer scrutiny. Also, there are only a handful of human DYT1 neuropathologic studies, and confirmation and elaboration of the crucial findings of McNaught et al[55] are needed. Other lines of investigation that hold great promise include additional search for DYT1 modifiers, genetic and environmental. Only 30% of GAG deletion carriers ever manifest dystonia, and clinical expression ranges from severe generalized dystonia to barely discernible action dystonias. The recent finding that a *trans* variation within *DYT1* itself is highly protective against clinical expression is an important step in illuminating factors involved in disease expression. Understanding the naturally occurring modulators of disease expression will shed light on the mechanism of torsinA pathogenesis and the steps that take human motor control across a threshold into clinical dysfunction.

Finally, new avenues of research that hold the promise for targeted treatments of *DYT1* dystonia are just being initiated. These derive from several different approaches, including the search for DYT1 modifiers, better understanding of the neurophysiologic correlates of DYT1, and cellular and animal models that not only shed light on disease mechanism but also allow for drug or other interventional screening. One such novel approach uses RNAi in cell culture systems overexpressing the mutant torsin protein to block aggregate formation and restore normal distribution of wild-type torsinA.[93,94] These results support the dominant negative model for torsinA function but also suggest RNAi could be used therapeutically.

REFERENCES

1. Schwalbe W. Eine eigentumliche tonische Krampform mit hysteriscehn Symptomen. Medicin and chirurgie. Berlin: Universitats-Buchdrukerei von Gustav Schade; 1908.
2. Oppenheim H. Uber eine eigenartige Krampfkrankheit des kindlichen und jugendlichen. Alters (dysbasia lordotica progressiva, dystonia musculorum deformans). Neurol Centralbr 1911; 75: 323–45.
3. Flateau E, Sterlinge W. Progressiver Torsionspasms bie Kindern. Z Gesamte Neurol Psychiatr 1911; 7: 586–612.
4. Herz E. Dystonia, Part 2 (clinical classification). Arch Neurol Psychiat 1944; 51: 319–55.
5. Marsden CD, Harrison MJ. Idiopathic torsion dystonia (dystonia musculorum deformans). A review of forty-two patients. Brain 1974; 97(4): 793–810.
6. Marsden CD, Harrison MJG, Bundey S. Natural history of idiopathic torsion dystonia. Adv Neurol 1976; 14: 177–87.
7. Fahn S. Concept and classification of dystonia. Adv Neurol 1988; 50: 1–8.
8. Zeman W, Dyken P. Dystonia musculorum deformans. Clinical, genetic and pathoanatomical studies. Psychiatr Neurol Neurochir 1967; 70(2): 77–121.
9. Bressman SB, de Leon D, Brin MF et al. Idiopathic torsion dystonia among Ashkenazi Jews: evidence for autosomal dominant inheritance. Ann Neurol 1989; 26: 612–20.
10. Risch NJ, Bressman SB, deLeon D et al. Segregation analysis of idiopathic torsion dystonia in Ashkenazi Jews suggests autosomal dominant inheritance. Am J Hum Genet 1990; 46(3): 533–8.
11. Pauls DL, Korczyn AD. Complex segregation analysis of dystonia pedigrees suggests autosomal dominant inheritance. Neurology 1990; 40(7): 1107–10.
12. Zilber N, Korczyn AD, Kahana E, Fried K, Alter M. Inheritance of idiopathic torsion dystonia among Jews. J Med Genet 1984; 21(1): 13–20.
13. Risch N, de Leon D, Ozelius L et al. Genetic analysis of idiopathic torsion dystonia in Ashkenazi Jews and their recent descent from a small founder population. Nat Genet 1995; 9: 152–9.
14. Ozelius LO, Kramer PL, Moskowitz CB et al. Human gene for torsion dystonia located on chromosome 9q32-q34. Neuron 1989; 2: 1427–34.
15. Kramer PL, deLeon D, Ozelius LO et al. Dystonia gene in Ashkenazi Jewish population located on chromosome 9q32-34. Ann Neurol 1990; 27: 114–20.
16. Kramer PL, Heiman G, Gasser T et al. The DYT1 gene on 9q34 is responsible for most cases of early-onset idiopathic torsion dystonia in non-Jews. Am J Hum Genet 1994; 55: 468–75.
17. Ozelius LJ, Kramer PL, de Leon D et al. Strong allelic association between the torsion dystonia gene (DYT1) and loci on chromosome 9q34 in Ashkenazi Jews. Am J Hum Genet 1992; 50(3): 619–28.
18. Bressman SB, de Leon D, Kramer PL et al. Dystonia in Ashkenazi Jews: clinical characterization of a founder mutation. Ann Neurol 1994; 36(5): 771–7.
19. Ozelius LJ, Hewett J, Kramer P et al. Fine localization of the torsion dystonia gene (DYT1) on human chromosome 9q34: YAC map and linkage disequilibrium. Genome Res 1997; 7(5): 483–94.
20. Ozelius LJ, Hewett J, Page C et al. The early-onset torsion dystonia gene (*DYT1*) encodes an ATP-binding protein. Nat Genet 1997; 17: 40–8.
21. Ikeuchi T, Shimohata T, Nakano R et al. A case of primary torsion dystonia in Japan with the 3-bp (GAG) deletion in the DYT1 gene with a unique clinical presentation. Neurogenetics 1999; 2(3): 189–90.
22. Valente EM, Warner TT, Jarman PR et al. The role of primary torsion dystonia in Europe. Brain 1998; 121: 2335–9.
23. Slominsky PA, Markova ED, Shadrina MI et al. A common 3-bp deletion in the DYT1 gene in Russian families with early-onset torsion dystonia. Hum Mutat 1999; 14(3): 269.

24. Lebre AS, Durr A, Jedynak P et al. DYT1 mutation in French families with idiopathic torsion dystonia. Brain 1999; 122(Pt 1): 41–5.
25. Major T, Svetel M, Romac S, Kostic VS. DYT1 mutation in primary torsion dystonia in a Serbian population. J Neurol 2001; 248(11): 940–3.
26. Klein C, Pramstaller PP, Castellan CC et al. Clinical and genetic evaluation of a family with a mixed dystonia phenotype from South Tyrol. Ann Neurol 1998; 44(3): 394–8.
27. Ozelius LJ, Page CE, Klein C et al. The TOR1A (DYT1) gene family and its role in early onset torsion dystonia. Genomics 1999; 62: 377–84.
28. Leung JC, Klein C, Friedman J et al. Novel mutation in the TOR1A (DYT1) gene in atypical early onset dystonia and polymorphisms in dystonia and early onset parkinsonism. Neurogenetics 2001; 3(3): 133–43.
29. Tuffery-Giraud S, Cavalier L, Roubertie A et al. No evidence of allelic heterogeneity in DYT1 gene of European patients with early onset torsion dystonia. J Med Genet 2001; 38: e35.
30. Klein C, Hedrich K, Kabakci K et al. Exon deletions in the GCHI gene in two of four Turkish families with dopa-responsive dystonia. Neurology 2002; 59(11): 1783–6.
31. Kabakci K, Hedrich K, Leung JC et al. Mutations in DYT1: extension of the phenotypic and mutational spectrum. Neurology 2004; 62(3): 395–400.
32. Dron M, Meritet JF, Dandoy-Dron F et al. Molecular cloning of ADIR, a novel interferon responsive gene encoding a protein related to the torsins. Genomics 2002; 79: 315–25.
33. Lupas A, Flanagan JM, Tamura T, Baumeister W. Self-compartmentalization proteases. Trends Biochem Sci 1997; 22: 399–404.
34. Neuwald AF, Aravind L, Spouge JL, Koonin EV. AAA+: a class of chaperone-like ATPases associated with the assembly, operation, and disassembly of protein complexes. Genome Res 1999; 9: 27–43.
35. Vale RD. AAA proteins: Lords of the ring. J Cell Biol 2000; 150: F13–F19.
36. Hanson PI, Whiteheart SW. AAA+ proteins: have engine, will work. Nat Rev Mol Cell Biol 2005; 6: 519–29.
37. Augood SJ, Penney JB, Friberg I et al. Expression of the early-onset torsion dystonia gene (DYT1) in human brain. Ann Neurol 1998; 43: 669–73.
38. Augood SJ, Martin DM, Ozelius LJ et al. Distribution of the mRNAs encoding torsinA and torsinB in the adult human brain. Ann Neurol 1999; 46: 761–9.
39. Augood SJ, Keller-McGandy CE, Siriani A et al. Distribution and ultrastructural localization of torsinA immunoreactivity in the human brain. Brain Res 2003; 986: 12–21.
40. Shashidharan P, Kramer C, Walker R, Olanor CW, Brin MF. Immunohistochemical localization and distribution of torsinA in normal human and rat brain. Brain Res 2000; 853: 197–206.
41. Konakova M, Huynh DP, Yong W, Pulst SM. Cellular distribution of torsin A and torsin B in normal human brain. Arch Neurol 2001; 58: 921–7.
42. Konakova M, Pulst SM. Immunocytochemical characterization of torsin proteins in mouse brain. Brain Res 2001; 922: 1–8.
43. Walker RH, Brin MF, Sandu D et al. Distribution and immunohistochemical characterization of torsinA immunoreactivity in rat brain. Brain Res 2001; 900: 348–54.
44. Siegert S, Bahn E, Kramer M et al. TorsinA expression is detectable in human infants as old as four weeks old. Brain Res Dev Brain Res 2005; 157: 19–26.
45. Vasudevan A, Breakefield XO, Bhide PG. Developmental patterns of torsinA and torsinB expression. Brain Res 2006; 1073–4: 139–45.
46. Xiao J, Gong S, Zhao Y, LeDoux MS. Developmental expression of rat torsinA transcript and protein. Brain Res Dev Brain Res 2004; 152: 47–60.
47. Shashidharan P, Good PF, Hsu A et al. TorsinA accumulation in Lewy bodies in sporadic Parkinson's disease. Brain Res 2000; 877: 379–381.
48. Sharma N, Hewett J, Ozelius LJ et al. A close association of torsinA and alpha-synuclein in Lewy bodies: a fluorescence resonance energy transfer study. Am J Pathol 2001; 159: 339–44.
49. Zeman W. Pathology of the torsion dystonias (dystonia musculorum deformans). Neurology 1970; 20(No. 11 Part 2): 79–88.
50. Hedreen JC, Zweig RM, DeLong MR, Whitehouse PJ, Price DL. Primary dystonias: a review of the pathology and suggestions for new directions of study. Adv Neurol 1988; 50: 123–32.
51. Furukawa Y, Hornykiewicz O, Fahn S, Kish SJ. Striatal dopamine in early-onset primary torsion dystonia with the DYT1 mutation. Neurology 2000; 54: 1193–5.
52. Augood SJ, Hollingsworth Z, Albers D et al. Dopamine transmission in DYT1 dystonia: a biochemical and autoradiographical study. Neurology 2002; 59: 445–8.
53. Walker RH, Brin MF, Sandu D, Good PF, Shashidharan P. TorsinA immunoreactivity in brains of patients with DYT1 and non-DYT1 dystonia. Neurology 2002; 58: 120–4.
54. Rostasy K, Augood SJ, Hewett JW et al. TorsinA protein and neuropathology in early onset generalized dystonia with GAG deletion. Neurobiol Dis 2003; 12: 11–24.
55. McNaught KS, Kapustin A, Jackson T et al. Brainstem pathology in DYT1 primary torsion dystonia. Ann Neurol 2004; 56: 540–7.
56. Shashidharan P, Sandu D, Potla U et al. Transgenic mouse model of early-onset DYT1 dystonia. Hum Mol Genet 2005; 14: 125–33.
57. Dang MT, Yokoi F, McNaught KS et al. Generation and characterization of Dyt1 DeltaGAG knock-in mouse as a model for early-onset dystonia. Exp Neurol 2005; 196: 452–63.
58. Hewett J, Gonzalez-Agosti C, Slater D et al. Mutant torsinA, responsible for early onset torsion dystonia, forms membrane inclusions in cultured neural cells. Hum Mol Genet 2000; 22: 1403–13.
59. Kustedjo K, Bracey MH, Cravatt BF. Torsin A and its torsion dystonia-associated mutant forms are lumenal glycoproteins that exhibit distinct subcellular localizations. J Biol Chem 2000; 275: 27933–9.
60. Kustedjo K, Deechongkit S, Kelly JW, Cravatt BF. Recombinant expression, purification, and comparative characterization of torsinA and its torsin dystonia-associated variant Delta E-torsinA. Biochemistry 2003; 42: 15333–41.
61. Liu Z, Zolkiewska A, Zolkiewska M. Characterization of human torsinA and its dystonia-associated mutant form. Biochem J 2003; 374: 117–22.
62. Callan AC, Bunning S, Jones OT, High S, Swanton E. Biosynthesis of the dystonia-associated AAA+ ATPase torsinA at the endoplasmic reticulum. Biochem J 2007; 401: 607–12.
63. Naismith TV, Heuser JE, Breakefield XO, Hanson PI. TorsinA in the nuclear envelope. Proc Natl Acad Sci USA 2004; 101: 7612–17.
64. Goodchild RE, Dauer WT. Mislocalization of the nuclear envelope: an effect of the dystonia-causing torsinA mutation. Proc Natl Acad Sci USA 2004; 1001: 847–52.
65. Goodchild RE, Dauer WT. The AAA+ protein torsinA interacts with a conserved domain present in LAP1 and a novel ER protein. Cell Biol 2005; 168: 855–62.
66. Bragg DC, Kaufman CA, Kock N, Breakefield XO. Inhibition of N-linked glycosylation prevents inclusion formation by the dystonia-related mutant form of torsinA. Mol Cell Neurosci 2004; 27: 417–26.

67. Gonzalez-Alegre P, Paulson HL. Aberrant cellular behavior of mutant torsinA implicates nuclear envelope dysfunction in DYT1 dystonia. J Neurosci 2004; 24: 2593–601.
68. Misbahuddin A, Placzek MR, Taanman JW et al. Mutant torsinA, which causes early-onset primary torsion dystonia, is redistributed to membranous structures enriched in vesicular monoamine transporter in cultured human SH-SY5Y cells. Mov Disord 2005; 20: 432–40.
69. Ferrari-Toninelli G, Paccioretti S, Francisconi S, Uberti D, Memo M. TorsinA negatively controls neurite outgrowth of SH-SY5Y human neuronal cell line. Brain Res 2004; 1012(1–2): 75–81.
70. Kamm C, Boston H, Hewett J et al. The early onset dystonia protein torsinA interacts with kinesin light chain 1. J Biol Chem 2004; 279: 19882–92.
71. Hewett JW, Zeng J, Niland BP, Bragg DC, Breakefield XO. Dystonia-causing mutant torsinA inhibits cell adhesion and neurite extension through interference with cytoskeletal dynamics. Neurobiol Dis 2006; 22: 98–111.
72. Torres GE, Sweeney AL, Beaulieu JM, Shashidharan P, Caron MG. Effect of torsinA on membrane proteins reveals a loss of function and a dominant negative phenotype of the dystonia-associated DeltaE-torsinA mutant. Proc Natl Acad Sci USA 2004; 101: 15650–5.
73. McLean PJ, Kawamata H, Shariff S et al. TorsinA and heat shock proteins act as molecular chaperones: suppression of alpha-synuclein aggregation. J Neurochem 2002; 83: 846–54.
74. Hewett J, Ziefer P, Bergeron D et al. TorsinA in PC12 cells: localization in the endoplasmic reticulum and response to stress. J Neurosci Res 2003; 72: 158–68.
75. Kuner R, Teismann P, Trutzel A et al. TorsinA protects against oxidative stress in COS-1 and PC12 cells. Neurosci Lett 2003; 350: 153–6.
76. Shashidharan P, Paris N, Sandu D et al. Overexpression of torsinA in PC12 cells protects against toxicity. J Neurochem 2004; 88: 1019–25.
77. Caldwell GA, Cao S, Sexton EG et al. Suppression of polyglutamine-induced protein aggregation in Caenorhabditis elegans by torsin proteins. Hum Mol Genet 2003: 12: 307–19.
78. Cao S, Gelwix CC, Caldwell KA, Caldwell GA. Torsin-mediated protection from cellular stress in the dopaminergic neurons of *Caenorhabditis elegans*. J Neurosci 2005; 25: 3801–12.
79. Basham SE, Rose LS. The Caenorhabditis elegans polarity gene ooc-5 encodes a Torsin-related protein of the AAA ATPase superfamily. Development 2001; 128: 4645–56.
80. Kuner R, Teismann P, Trutzel A et al. TorsinA, the gene linked to early-onset dystonia, is upregulated by the dopaminergic toxin MPTP in mice. Neurosci Lett 2004; 355: 126–30.
81. Koh YH, Rehfeld K, Ganetzky B. A Drosophila model of early onset torsion dystonia suggests impairment in TGF-beta signaling. Hum Mol Genet 2004; 13: 2019–30.
82. Muraro NI, Moffat KG. Down-regulation of torp4a, encoding the Drosophila homologue of torsinA, results in increased neuronal degeneration. J Neurobiol 2006; 66: 1338–53.
83. Jinnah HA, Hess EJ, Ledoux MS et al. Rodent models for dystonia research: characteristics, evaluation, and utility. Mov Disord 2005; 20: 283–92.
84. Sharma N, Baxter MG, Petravicz J et al. Impaired motor learning in mice expressing torsinA with the DYT1 dystonia mutation. J Neurosci 2005; 25: 5351–5.
85. Ghilardi MR, Carbon M, Silvestri G et al. Impaired sequence learning in carriers of the DYT1 dystonia mutation. Ann Neurol 2003: 54: 102–19.
86. Pisani A, Martella G, Tscherter A et al. Altered responses to dopaminergic D2 receptor activation and N-type calcium currents in striatal cholinergic interneurons in a mouse model of DYT1 dystonia. Neurobiol Dis 2006; 24: 318–25.
87. Goodchild RE, Kim CE, Dauer WT. Loss of the dystonia-associated protein torsinA selectively disrupts the neuronal nuclear envelope. Neuron 2005; 48: 923–32.
88. Dang MT, Yokoi F, Pence MA, Li Y. Motor deficits and hyperactivity in Dyt1 knockdown mice. Neurosci Res 2006; 56: 470–4.
89. Missiakas D, Schwager F, Betton J-M, Georgopoulos C, Raina J. Identification and characterization of HS1V HS1U (ClpQ ClpY) proteins involved in overall proteolysis of misfolded proteins in Eschericia coli. EMBO J 1996; 15: 6899–909.
90. Akiyama Y, Shirai Y, Ito K. Involvement of FtsH in protein assembly into and through the membrane. J Biol Chem 1994; 269: 5225–9.
91. Whiteheart SW, Rossnagel K, Buhrow SA et al. N–ethylmaleimide-sensitive fusion protein: a trimeric ATPase whose hydrolysis of ATP is required for membrane fusion. J Cell Biol 1994; 125: 945–54.
92. Breakefield XO, Kamm C, Hanson PI. TorsinA: movement at many levels. Neuron 2001; 31: 9–12.
93. Gonzalez-Alegre P, Bode N, Davidson BL, Paulson HL. Silencing primary dystonia: lentiviral-mediated RNA interference therapy for DYT1 dystonia. J Neurosci 2005; 25: 10502–9.
94. Kock N, Allchorne AJ, Sena-Esteves M, Woolf CJ, Breakefield XO. RNAi blocks DYT1 mutant torsinA inclusions in neurons. Neurosci Lett 2006; 395: 201–5.
95. Clarimon J, Asgeirsson H, Singleton A et al. TorsinA haplotype predisposes to idiopathic dystonia. Ann Neurol 2005; 57: 765–7.
96. Sibbing D, Asmus F, Konig IR et al. Candidate gene studies in focal dystonia. Neurology 2003; 61: 1097–101.
97. Hague S, Klaffke S, Clarimon J et al. Lack of association with TorsinA haplotype in German patients with sporadic dystonia. Neurology 2006; 66: 951–2.
98. Clarimon J, Brancati F, Peckham E et al. Assessing the role of DRD5 and DYT1 in two different case-control series with primary blepharospasm. Mov Disord 2007; 22: 162–6.
99. Kamm C, Asmus F, Mueller J et al. Strong genetic evidence for association of TOR1A/TOR1B with idiopathic dystonia. Neurology 2006; 67: 1857–9.
100. Kock N, Naismith TV, Boston HE et al. Effects of genetic variations in the dystonia protein torsinA: identification of polymorphism at residue 216 as protein modifier. Hum Mol Genet 2006; 15: 1355–64.
101. Risch NJ, Bressman SB, Senthil G, Ozelius LJ. Intragenic cis and trans modification of genetic susceptibility in DYT1 torsion dystonia. Am J Hum Genet 2007; 80: 1188–93.
102. Gasser T, Windgassen K, Bereznai B, Kabus C, Ludolph AC. Phenotypic expression of the DYT1 mutation: a family with writer's cramp of juvenile onset. Ann Neurol 1998; 44(1): 126–8.
103. Opal P, Tintner R, Jankovic J et al. Intrafamilial phenotypic variability of the DYT1 dystonia: from asymptomatic TOR1A gene carrier status to dystonic storm. Mov Disord 2002; 17(2): 339–45.
104. Bressman SB, Sabatti C, Raymond D et al. The DYT1 phenotype and guidelines for diagnostic testing. Neurology 2000; 54: 1746–52.
105. Gambarin M, Valente EM, Liberini P et al. Atypical phenotypes and clinical variability in a large Italian family with DYT1-primary torsion dystonia. Mov Disord 2006; 21(10): 1782–4.
106. Im JH, Ahn TB, Kim KB, Ko SB, Jeon BS. DYT1 mutation in Korean primary dystonia patients. Parkinsonism Relat Disord 2004; 10(7): 421–3.
107. Lin YW, Chang HC, Chou YH et al. DYT1 mutation in a cohort of Taiwanese primary dystonias. Parkinsonism Relat Disord 2006; 12(1): 15–19.

108. Yeung WL, Lam CW, Cheng WT et al. Early-onset primary torsional dystonia in a 4-generation Chinese family with a mutation in the DYT1 gene. Chin Med J (Engl) 2005; 118(10): 873–6.
109. Chinnery PF, Reading PJ, McCarthy EL, Curtis A, Burn DJ. Late-onset axial jerky dystonia due to the DYT1 deletion. Mov Disord 2002; 17(1): 196–8.
110. Fasano A, Bentivoglio AR, Ialongo T, Soleti F, Evoli A. Non-DYT1 early-onset primary torsion dystonia: comparison with DYT1 phenotype and review of the literature. Mov Disord 2006; 21(9): 1411–18.
111. Leube B, Kessler KR, Ferbert A et al. Phenotypic variability of the DYT1 mutation in German dystonia patients. Acta Neurol Scand 1999; 99: 248–51.
112. Koukouni V, Martino D, Arabia G, Quinn NP, Bhatia KP. The entity of young onset primary cervical dystonia. Mov Disord 2007; 22: 843–7.
113. Jamora RD, Tan EK, Liu CP et al. DYT1 mutations amongst adult primary dystonia patients in Singapore with review of literature comparing East and West. J Neurol Sci 2006; 247(1): 35–7.
114. Brassat D, Camuzat A, Vidailhet M et al. Frequency of the DYT1 mutation in primary torsion dystonia without family history. Arch Neurol 2000; 57(3): 333–5.
115. Zorzi G, Garavaglia B, Invernizzi F et al. Frequency of DYT1 mutation in early onset primary dystonia in Italian patients. Mov Disord 2002; 17(2): 407–8.
116. Frederic M, Lucarz E, Monino C et al. First determination of the incidence of the unique TOR1A gene mutation, c.907delGAG, in a Mediterranean population. Mov Disord 2007; 22: 884–6.
117. Moretti P, Hedera P, Wald J, Fink J. Autosomal recessive primary generalized dystonia in two siblings from a consanguineous family. Mov Disord 2005; 20(2): 245–7.
118. Heiman GA, Ottman R, Saunders-Pullman RJ et al. Increased risk for recurrent major depression in DYT1 dystonia mutation carriers. Neurology 2004; 63(4): 631–7
119. Heiman GA, Ottman R, Saunders-Pullman RJ et al. Obsessive-compulsive disorder is not a clinical manifestation of the DYT1 dystonia gene. Am J Med Genet B Neuropsychiatr Genet 2007; 144: 361–4.
120. Bressman SB, Raymond D, Wendt K et al. Diagnostic criteria for dystonia in DYT1 families. Neurology 2002; 59: 1780–82.
121. Eidelberg D, Moeller JR, Antonini A et al. Functional brain networks in DYT1 dystonia. Ann Neurol 1998; 44: 303–12.
122. Carbon M, Kingsley PB, Su S et al. Microstructural white matter changes in carriers of the DYT1 gene mutation. Ann Neurol 2004; 56(2): 283–6.
123. Asanuma K, Ma Y, Huang C et al. Decreased striatal D_2 receptor binding in non-manifesting carriers of the DYT1 dystonia mutation. Neurology 2005; 64: 347–9.
124. Edwards MJ, Huang YZ, Wood NW, Rothwell JC, Bhatia KP. Different patterns of electrophysiological deficits in manifesting and non-manifesting carriers of the DYT1 gene mutation. Brain 2003; 126: 2074–80.
125. Fiorio M, Gambarin M, Valente EM et al. Defective temporal processing of sensory stimuli in DYT1 mutation carriers: a new endophenotype of dystonia? Brain 2007; 130(Pt 1): 134–42.
126. Albanese A, Barnes MP, Bharia KP et al. A systematic review on the diagnosis and treatment of primary (idiopathic) dystonia and dystonia plus syndromes: report of an EFNS/MDS-ES Task Force. Eur J Neurol 2006; 13(5): 433–44.
127. Jinnah HA, Hess EJ. A new twist on the anatomy of dystonia: the basal ganglia and the cerebellum? Neurology 2006; 67(10): 1740–1.

7

Other primary generalized dystonias

Antonio E Elia, Anna Rita Bentivoglio, Enza Maria Valente, and Alberto Albanese

INTRODUCTION

Dystonia is the only clinical sign of primary torsion dystonias (PTDs) and there is no identifiable exogenous cause or other inherited or degenerative disease.[1] The best-known PTD is DYT1 dystonia,[2] but PTDs encompass several other genetically determined forms, none of which has been characterized. DYT1 dystonia was first identified among Ashkenazi Jews[3,4] and was then recognized as a possible cause of early-onset generalized PTD in populations of any ethnic origin.[5–7] Clinical observations have reported that DYT1 dystonia can have heterogeneous phenotypic expressions,[8–10] making it difficult to differentiate DYT1 and non-DYT1 patients on clinical grounds.[11]

This chapter revises the evidence collected during the last decade, in order to report the phenotype of non-DYT1 generalized PTD families either linked or unlinked to known loci, and to characterize the clinical features of non-DYT1 early-onset dystonia in sporadic and familial PTD patients.

EPIDEMIOLOGY

The available evidence suggests that non-DYT1 PTDs are by far more prevalent in the general population than DYT1 cases. In a large series of Italian PTD patients, it has been observed that DYT1 cases accounted for 41% of the patients with generalized dystonia and for only 5.4% of all PTD cases.[12] A large Italian study on early-onset (<21 years) PTD showed that non-DYT1 cases account for 75% of all early-onset cases.[11] This finding is consistent with previous data showing that DYT1 cases account for only 7.9% of total PTDs in Serbia,[13] for 15% in Denmark,[14] and for 16% in Italy.[15]

There are no published data on the prevalence of generalized (or early-onset) non-DYT1 dystonia in the general population, because most epidemiologic studies were service-based rather than community-based and were performed before DYT1 testing became available.[16,17] Early-onset cases account for about 15% of all PTDs, the majority of which are represented by non-DYT1 late-onset (focal or segmental) cases.[18]

CLINICAL FEATURES

Familial dystonias have been listed with progressive numbering preceded by the DYT code (meaning 'dystonia'; Table 3.2). This list was originally supposed to include only primary dystonias, but currently encompasses several heterogeneous conditions, such as unmapped PTD familial loci (e.g. *DYT2* and *DYT4*), heredodegenerative dystonias (e.g. *DYT3*), dystonia-plus syndromes (*DYT5* and *DYT11*, *DYT12*, *DYT14*), and paroxysmal dyskinesias or choreoathetosis (*DYT8*, *DYT9*, *DYT10*). Therefore, of the 15 *DYT* loci, only six refer to PTDs, namely those marked as *DYT1*, *DYT2*, *DYT4*, *DYT6*, *DYT7*, and *DYT13*. With the exception of *DYT2*, all PTDs are inherited as a dominant trait with reduced penetrance.

Monogenic primary torsion dystonias

Four PTD genotypes have been identified, three of which present with generalized phenotypes.

DYT1 phenotype

A common cause of generalized PTD is the GAG deletion in the *DYT1* gene encoding the protein torsinA.[4] The disease was originally described among Ashkenazi Jews with a relatively homogeneous phenotype characterized by early limb-onset generalized dystonia.[3,19]

It was later reported that, particularly in Caucasian patients,[5] the DYT1 phenotype is broader than originally thought. The 'classical' DYT1 phenotype is characterized by early onset in a limb, generalization without spread to the craniocervical region.[5] In a series of patients with early-onset PTD it has been confirmed that dystonia never starts in the craniocervical region in *DYT1* carriers, but it has been shown that craniocervical sites can be involved in later stages.[11] It is remarkable that DYT1 patients who develop severe generalized involvement may carry out their daily activities with significant adaptation in many cases. Extreme cases have also been observed, ranging from asymptomatic status to craniocervical involvement or even to status dystonicus.[9,20–22]

Atypical DYT1 phenotypes can be grouped in five main types.[23]

1. Generalized dystonia with cranial–cervical involvement, more frequent in Europe than in North America, with a record prevalence of 80% in DYT1 patients of a French series.[7]
2. The generalized myoclonus-dystonia phenotype which is more severe than that observed in DYT11 myoclonus-dystonia.[10]
3. Focal dystonia with slow progression; in these cases spread may occasionally occur several years after onset.[24,25]
4. Late-onset DYT1.[9]
5. Non-limb (cervical, laryngeal, or trunk) onset[6,26] dystonia DYT1 dystonia.

Regardless of onset, positron emission tomography (PET) studies have shown that DYT1 dystonia is associated with abnormal movement preparation due to defective sensorimotor integration. These features are genotype-specific, as putaminal metabolism is increased in DYT1 patients, but decreased, for example, in DYT6 patients.[27] Since clinical criteria can hardly distinguish DYT1 from non-DYT1 patients, the identification of endophenotypes associated with *DYT1* carriers (either affected or non-affected) provides a new potential diagnostic tool. Striatal D_2 receptor binding is reduced in manifesting as well as in non-manifesting *DYT1* carriers.[28] Another possible endophenotype of *DYT1* carriers is the finding of higher tactile and visuotactile temporal discrimination thresholds or temporal order judgments.[29]

DYT6 phenotype

The *DYT6* locus has been mapped in two Mennonite families, where dystonia was inherited as an autosomal dominant trait with an estimated penetrance of 30%.[30] The locus was mapped to 8p21-q22 and a founder effect was supported by the observation that haplotypes across the candidate region were identical in the affected members of the two families, suggesting a common underlying mutation. A total of 15 definitely affected individuals were identified among 220 family members.

The DYT6 phenotype has been described as 'mixed type', characterized by early or adult onset and prevalent segmental (craniocervical) distribution, with presentation at onset equally involving limb, cervical, and cranial muscles. Four patients presented generalized dystonia, and some had a classical DYT1 phenotype. DYT6 patients with generalized phenotype had (on average) an older age at disease onset than DYT1 patients (18.9 ± 11.9 years; range: 5–38 years); in addition, they commonly had craniocervical involvement either at onset or later during disease progression. Many DYT6 patients were remarkably disabled in their living activities by this craniocervical involvement. It has been shown that manifesting *DYT6* gene carriers have bilateral hypermetabolism in the supplementary motor area and the temporoparietal cortex, and bilateral hypometabolism in the putamen.[27]

DYT7 phenotype

The *DYT7* locus mapping to the short arm of chromosome 18 was identified in a large German family with autosomal dominant focal dystonia.[31] The mean age of disease onset was 40 years and no patient had generalized dystonia.

DYT13 phenotype

The *DYT13* locus was mapped in a family with prominent upper body involvement (craniocervical and upper limb), the majority of whom had onset in infancy or adolescence.[32,33] Disease progression was evaluated for 6 years in this family.[34] There were 11 definitely affected individuals, two of whom had generalized dystonia with early onset in the upper limb or in the cervical region. The peculiar features of the DYT13 phenotype are prominent cervical or upper limb involvement; disability is mild, even in generalized cases.

The first patient with generalized PTD was a woman who presented postural tremor of the upper limbs at age 5. The tremor rapidly spread to involve the whole body and did not aggravate. Upon observation in her sixties, the patient had generalized dystonia with prominent action tremor affecting the larynx, limbs, and trunk. Despite this widespread involvement, her disability was mild. Being a housekeeper, she could run her daily duties without help. The second patient with generalized dystonia was a man, who had cervical onset at age 20. This did not progress for the following 30 years. In his fifties, dystonia spread to the right hand, then to both upper limbs, and to the head. He was last examined at age 56, when he had a generalized dystonia involving the neck and all the limbs. Similar to the other patient, his disability was mild: he could still work on a farm and was engaged in full-time labor.

PTD pedigrees

Two familial PTD phenotypes with occasional generalization have been coded. In addition, several other pedigrees, many of which with generalization, have also been described.

DYT2 phenotype

This is a recessive dystonia locus originally described in three consanguineous pedigrees of Spanish Gypsies. The disease was named 'autosomal recessive dystonia in Gypsies' and listed as DYT2.[35,36] In two of the families, the phenotype was similar to that of DYT1 dystonia, consisting of early limb onset and progression to generalization; in the third family, dystonia presented with prominent oromandibular and cervical dystonia.[36]

A Sephardic Jewish Iranian family with a similar phenotype and autosomal recessive inheritance has been described more recently.[37] Three siblings in this family had PTD with limb onset in childhood, and slow progression to generalized dystonia with predominant craniocervical involvement. Two patients first developed in-turning of the foot with gait abnormalities, and all had cervical involvement, facial grimacing, blepharospasm, and involvement of the upper and lower limbs. Two patients also had dystonic dysphagia. It was hypothesized that this Sephardic family originating from Spain could be related to the DYT2 Gypsy family, but this possibility appears unlikely, also because most Iranian Jews do not originate from Spain or Portugal.[38]

A third family with childhood-onset, generalized dystonia, and autosomal recessive inheritance was also classified as DYT2.[39]

Overall, the DYT2 phenotype is consistent in the three families described and is characterized by early onset, generalization, and autosomal recessive transmission. DYT2 dystonia should be considered in every family with such features, particularly if there is prominent craniocervical involvement. Unfortunately, DYT2 dystonia has not been mapped to a genetic locus yet.

DYT4 phenotype

A large Australian pedigree had 20 members affected by dystonia in at least five consecutive generations and autosomal dominant inheritance.[40] This PTD pedigree was classified as DYT4. Penetrance was complete in all the examined obligate gene carriers; age at onset varied from 13 to 37 years. Many of the patients presented with 'whispering dysphonia', others had cervical dystonia; most eventually developed generalized dystonia. Wilson's disease coexisted in the same pedigree, but was excluded as a cause of dystonia in the affected individuals.[41] The DYT4 phenotype has not been observed in other families or individual cases.

Non-coded pedigrees

In some PTD families not carrying the *DYT1* mutation, the phenotype has been described in the affected individuals. Linkage studies have not been performed in these small pedigrees, which have remained unclassified.

A non-Jewish American family presented with adult-onset *DYT1*-negative PTD.[42] The disease started in the neck in six cases and in a leg in one. All patients developed cervical dystonia, and language impairment (dysarthria or dysphonia) occurred in five patients. Four patients developed generalization of symptoms. In another Swedish family, transmission was autosomal dominant with variable phenotype.[43] There was involvement of the face and larynx, and generalization occurred in three of the 10 patients. A family from South Tyrol had six affected individuals, four of whom developed generalization approximately 5 years after onset.[44] Limbs were involved at onset in all but one patient, who started with cervical dystonia. Upper body involvement was observed in three of the four generalized cases. An Italian family had six affected individuals, one of whom had severe segmental dystonia.[45] The prevalent phenotype was with adult-onset craniocervical dystonia with occasional axial involvement but no generalization.

Table 7.1 provides a synopsis of unclassified PTD pedigrees with a generalized phenotype.

Non-DYT1 early-onset PTD cases

The observation that early-onset dystonia cases progress to severe forms has been reported since the first descriptions of dystonia.[46,47] In their seminal description of the natural history of PTD, Marsden et al[48] identified age at onset as one of the most important features in determining outcome. A consensus meeting later identified three age groups for PTD onset: childhood (0–12 years), adolescent (13–20 years), and adult (>20 years).[49] Based on this consensus, cases with early onset (encompassing onset in childhood or in adolescence) were distinguished from those with adult onset by the threshold age of 21 years. Later retrospective series have confirmed that patients with early onset are more likely to have

Table 7.1 Clinical features of unclassified PTD pedigrees with generalized dystonia; cases without generalization are not listed

No. of patients	Mean age at onset (years, range)	Site of onset: number	Progression: number	Cranial involvement: number	Additional features	Reference
7	28.4 (7–50)	Neck: 6 Leg: 1	Generalized: 4 Segmental: 3	Yes: 7	Tongue involvement in 4 patients. Family with AD inheritance	42
7	27.3 (17–50)	Face: 4 Arm: 2 Unknown: 1	Generalized: 3 Multifocal: 3 Focal: 1	Yes: 4	Prominent cranial involvement. Family with AD inheritance	43
6	23.3 (4–50)	Cervical: 1 Arm: 3 Leg: 2	Generalized: 4 Segmental: 2	Yes: 2	Prominent cervical involvement. Family with AD inheritance	44
16 probands	The proband with generalized dystonia was early onset	NA	Generalized: 1 Segmental: 7 Focal: 8	NA	At least one early-onset patient in each family	13
25 patients	7.7 (1.5–15)	Cranial: 1 Neck: 1 Arm: 12 Trunk: 2 Leg: 9	Generalized: 22 Segmental: 3	Yes: 16	Series of both sporadic and familial patients	15
1	2	Leg: 1	Generalized: 1	No	Myoclonus dystonia-like phenotype with familial occurrence. AD inheritance	54
7 probands	13.9 (1–17)	Cervical: 3 Arm: 2 Leg: 2	Generalized: 3 Multifocal: 1 Segmental: 2 Focal: 1	Yes: 2	The proband of DYT13 family is included	11

AD = autosomal dominant; NA = not available.

a generalized form than those with older age at onset and that there is a bimodal curve representing the frequency distribution of age at disease onset, with a nadir separating two clusters of patients.[50,51]

Later series described the frequency distribution of ages at onset and attempted to identify the predictive value of early vs adult age at disease onset for the probability of developing a generalized form of dystonia.[3,51] In a North American series (characterized by a predominance of Ashkenazi Jewish patients), a threshold age at disease onset of more than 26 years indicated a low probability of being carrier of a *DYT1* mutation,[26] but this was not confirmed in other series based on different populations.[52] Thus, while all retrospective series confirm a bimodal distribution of age at onset for PTD, with a higher likelihood of generalization for the early age group, the measured predictive value of the age thresholds vary based on the populations considered.

In a large Italian series, encompassing a majority of non-DYT1 patients, the frequency distribution of the ages at onset was a bimodal curve with modes at 9 and 57 years and a nadir at 21 years.[12] The sensitivity and specificity of age at onset to predict generalization were calculated for all patients with a follow-up observation of at least 5 years. Receiver operating characteristic (ROC) curves were plotted and the best trade-off threshold predicting generalization was found at 32 years, yielding sensitivity and specificity of 83% (Figure 7.1). The negative predictive value was 99%, indicating a negligible probability that patients with age at onset higher than 32 years would progress to generalization.

The phenotype of non-DYT1 early-onset PTD cases is not completely characterized, but several series remarked differences from the DYT1 phenotype that may be unapparent in individual cases. In a French study of 100 patients with sporadic PTD,[7] 10 were affected by generalized dystonia, and five of them carried the *DYT1* mutation. The phenotype of generalized dystonia in non-carriers was not described in detail, but it was reported that age at onset was higher in non-carriers. In a series of 30 Italian patients with early-onset sporadic PTD, 25 were not *DYT1* carriers: 22 of them had generalized dystonia, and 16 presented oromandibular or laryngeal involvement.[15]

A series of 57 consecutive genetically characterized patients with early-onset PTD was recently reported.[11] The majority of these patients (43 (75%), 27 men, 16 women; ratio, 1.7: 1) did not carry the *DYT1* mutation. Twenty-nine non-DYT1 patients eventually developed generalized dystonia, with notable oromandibular involvement in 17 and laryngeal involvement in four. The remaining 14 non-DYT1 patients developed segmental (eight), multifocal (one), or focal (five) forms. Non-DYT1 patients with generalized dystonia had earlier onset than those without generalization.

The same series showed that sporadic non DYT1 patients had cranial involvement and earlier generalization more often than DYT1 patients. By contrast, familial non-DYT1 cases had older age at onset and older age at generalization, more frequent cervical involvement, and less common limb onset. Progression was more rapid in sporadic non-DYT1 patients than in familial non-DYT1 patients, suggesting that the latter may belong to a different phenotype (Figure 7.2). In keeping with this, familial non-DYT1 cases of this Italian series had a relatively homogeneous phenotype, similar to the so-called 'mixed phenotype',[30,34] with cervical involvement, frequent non-limb onset, relatively benign disease

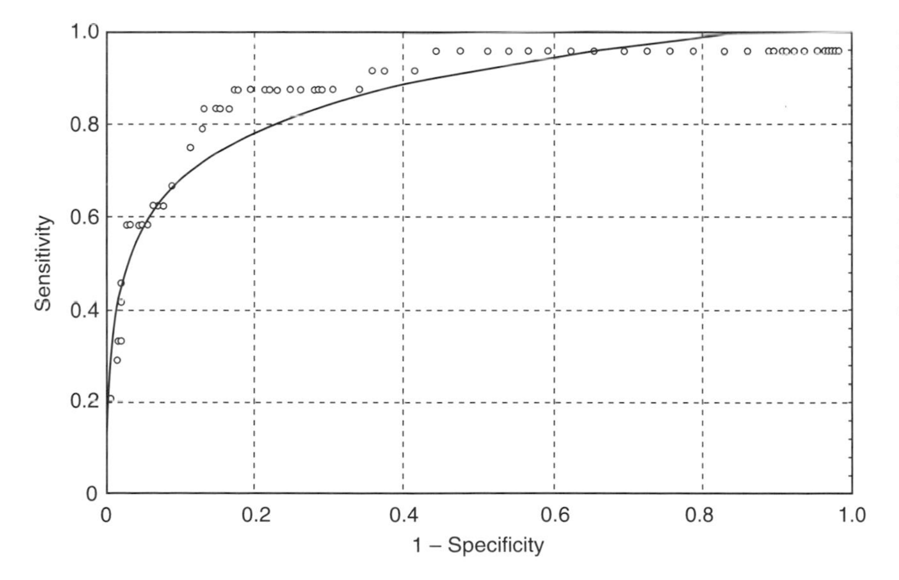

Figure 7.1 ROC curve plotting sensitivity and specificity for the prediction of dystonia generalization in 443 patients followed up for more than 5 years.[12] Age at disease onset of 32 years predicts generalization with sensitivity and specificity of 83%.

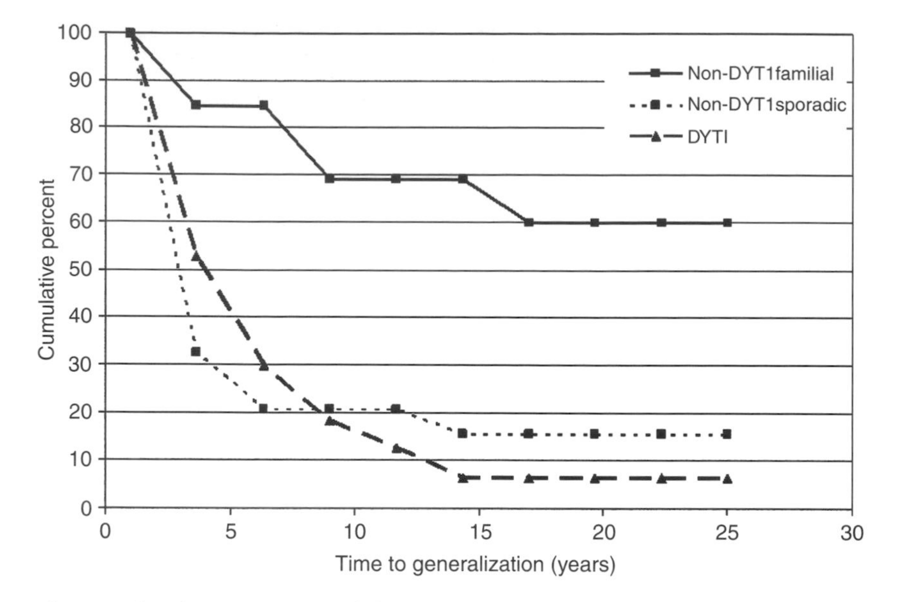

Figure 7.2 Survival curves for the progression of dystonia measured by the time to generalization. DYT1 patients are compared to familial and sporadic non-DYT1 cases. It is shown that familial non-DYT1 cases have less severe progression than DYT1 or sporadic non-DYT1 patients. (Reproduced from Fasano et al,[11] with permission.)

course, and uncommon generalization. This finding suggests that these non-DYT1 Italian families may share a common genetic defect.

CONCLUSIONS AND OUTLOOK

Generalized dystonias represent a heterogeneous group encompassing sporadic and familial cases with overlapping clinical features. A certain number of still unmapped genes are certainly responsible for these cases. Since large families suitable for linkage analysis are rare, it is useful to classify patients into homogeneous phenotypic groups and to look for endophenotypic markers before planning new linkage studies. The available data on familial PTD cases suggest that the traditional classification of 'predominantly generalized' and 'predominantly focal' forms[53] may be reductive. Indeed, regardless of the predominant familial phenotype, generalized and focal PTDs often coexist in the same pedigree, making clinical heterogeneity a cardinal feature of inherited dystonias.

REFERENCES

1. Albanese A, Barnes MP, Bhatia KP et al. A systematic review on the diagnosis and treatment of primary (idiopathic) dystonia and dystonia plus syndromes: report of an EFNS/MDS-ES Task Force. Eur J Neurol 2006; 13: 433–44.
2. Bressman S, Ozelius L. Oppenheim's generalised dystonias (DYT1 dystonia). In: Warner TT, Bressman S, eds. Dystonia: Clinical Diagnosis and Management. London: Martin Dunitz; 2007.
3. Bressman SB, de Leon D, Kramer PL et al. Dystonia in Ashkenazi Jews: clinical characterization of a founder mutation. Ann Neurol 1994; 36: 771–7.
4. Ozelius LJ, Hewett JW, Page CE et al. The early-onset torsion dystonia gene (DYT1) encodes an ATP-binding protein. Nat Genet 1997; 17: 40–8.
5. Valente EM, Warner TT, Jarman PR et al. The role of DYT1 in primary torsion dystonia in Europe. Brain 1998; 121: 2335–9.
6. Ikeuchi T, Shimohata T, Nakano R et al. A case of primary torsion dystonia in Japan with the 3-bp (GAG) deletion in the DYT1 gene with a unique clinical presentation. Neurogenetics 1999; 2: 189–90.
7. Brassat D, Camuzat A, Vidailhet M et al. Frequency of the DYT1 mutation in primary torsion dystonia without family history. Arch Neurol 2000; 57: 333–5.
8. Jarman PR, Del Grosso N, Valente EM et al. Primary torsion dystonia: the search for genes is not over. J Neurol Neurosurg Psychiatry 1999; 67: 395–7.
9. Opal P, Tintner R, Jankovic J et al. Intrafamilial phenotypic variability of the DYT1 dystonia: from asymptomatic TOR1A gene carrier status to dystonic storm. Mov Disord 2002; 17: 339–45.
10. Gatto EM, Pardal MM, Micheli FE. Unusual phenotypic expression of the DYT1 mutation. Parkinsonism Relat Disord 2003; 9: 277–9.
11. Fasano A, Nardocci N, Elia AE et al. Non-DYT1 early-onset primary torsion dystonia: comparison with DYT1 phenotype and review of the literature. Mov Disord 2006; 21: 1411–18.
12. Elia AE, Filippini G, Bentivoglio AR et al. Onset and progression of primary torsion dystonia in sporadic and familial cases. Eur J Neurol 2006; 13: 1083–8.
13. Major T, Svetel M, Romac S, Kostic VS. DYT1 mutation in primary torsion dystonia in a Serbian population. J Neurol 2001; 248: 940–3.

14. Hjermind LE, Werdelin LM, Sorensen SA. Inherited and de novo mutations in sporadic cases of DYT1-dystonia. Eur J Hum Genet 2002; 10: 213–16.
15. Zorzi G, Garavaglia B, Invernizzi F et al. Frequency of DYT1 mutation in early onset primary dystonia in Italian patients. Mov Disord 2002; 17: 407–8.
16. Nutt JG, Muenter MD, Aronson A, Kurland LT, Melton LJ 3rd. Epidemiology of focal and generalized dystonia in Rochester, Minnesota. Mov Disord 1988; 3: 188–94.
17. The Epidemiological Study of Dystonia in Europe (ESDE) Collaborative Group. A prevalence study of primary dystonia in eight European countries. J Neurol 2000; 247: 787–92.
18. Defazio G, Abbruzzese G, Livrea P, Berardelli A. Epidemiology of primary dystonia. Lancet Neurol 2004; 3: 673–8.
19. Bressman SB, de Leon D, Brin MF et al. Idiopathic dystonia among Ashkenazi Jews: evidence for autosomal dominant inheritance. Ann Neurol 1989; 26: 612–20.
20. Bentivoglio AR, Loi M, Valente EM et al. Phenotypic variability of DYT1-PTD: does the clinical spectrum include psychogenic dystonia? Mov Disord 2002; 17: 1058–63.
21. Gambarin M, Valente EM, Liberini P et al. Atypical phenotypes and clinical variability in a large Italian family with DYT1-primary torsion dystonia. Mov Disord 2006; 21: 1782–4.
22. Kostic VS, Svetel M, Kabakci K et al. Intrafamilial phenotypic and genetic heterogeneity of dystonia. J Neurol Sci 2006; 250: 92–6.
23. Fasano A, Elia A, Albanese A. Early onset primary torsion dystonia. In: Fernández-Alvarez E, Arzimanoglou A, Tolosa E, eds. Paediatric Movement Disorders. Esher: John Libbey; 2005: 31–55.
24. Chinnery PF, Reading PJ, McCarthy EL, Curtis A, Burn DJ. Late-onset axial jerky dystonia due to the DYT1 deletion. Mov Disord 2002; 17: 196–8.
25. Edwards M, Wood N, Bhatia K. Unusual phenotypes in DYT1 dystonia: a report of five cases and a review of the literature. Mov Disord 2003; 18: 706–11.
26. Bressman SB, Sabatti C, Raymond D et al. The DYT1 phenotype and guidelines for diagnostic testing. Neurology 2000; 54: 1746–52.
27. Carbon M, Su S, Dhawan V et al. Regional metabolism in primary torsion dystonia: effects of penetrance and genotype. Neurology 2004; 62: 1384–90.
28. Asanuma K, Ma Y, Okulski J et al. Decreased striatal D_2 receptor binding in non-manifesting carriers of the DYT1 dystonia mutation. Neurology 2005; 64: 347–9.
29. Fiorio M, Gambarin M, Valente EM et al. Defective temporal processing of sensory stimuli in DYT1 mutation carriers: a new endophenotype of dystonia? Brain 2007; 130: 134–42.
30. Almasy L, Bressman SB, Raymond D et al. Idiopathic torsion dystonia linked to chromosome 8 in two Mennonite families. Ann Neurol 1997; 42: 670–3.
31. Leube B, Rudnicki D, Ratzlaff T et al. Idiopathic torsion dystonia: assignment of a gene to chromosome 18p in a German family with adult onset, autosomal dominant inheritance and purely focal distribution. Hum Mol Genet 1996; 5: 1673–7.
32. Bentivoglio AR, Del Grosso N, Albanese A et al. Non-DYT1 dystonia in a large Italian family. J Neurol Neurosurg Psychiatry 1997; 62: 357–60.
33. Valente EM, Bentivoglio AR, Cassetta E et al. DYT13, a novel primary torsion dystonia locus, maps to chromosome 1p36.13–36.32 in an Italian family with cranial-cervical or upper limb onset. Ann Neurol 2001; 49: 362–6.
34. Bentivoglio AR, Ialongo T, Contarino MF, Valente EM, Albanese A. Phenotypic characterization of DYT13 primary torsion dystonia. Mov Disord 2004; 19: 200–6.
35. Gimenez-Roldan S, Delgado G, Marin M, Villanueva JA, Mateo D. Hereditary torsion dystonia in gypsies. Adv Neurol 1988; 50: 73–81.
36. Gimenez-Roldan S, Lopez-Fraile IP, Esteban A. Dystonia in Spain: study of a Gypsy family and general survey. Adv Neurol 1976; 14: 125–36.
37. Khan NL, Wood NW, Bhatia KP. Autosomal recessive, DYT2-like primary torsion dystonia: a new family. Neurology 2003; 61: 1801–3.
38. Zlotogora J. Autosomal recessive, DYT2-like primary torsion dystonia: a new family. Neurology 2004; 63: 1340.
39. Moretti P, Hedera P, Wald J, Fink J. Autosomal recessive primary generalized dystonia in two siblings from a consanguineous family. Mov Disord 2005; 20: 245–7.
40. Parker N. Hereditary whispering dysphonia. J Neurol Neurosurg Psychiatry 1985; 48: 218–24.
41. Ahmad F, Davis MB, Waddy HM et al. Evidence for locus heterogeneity in autosomal dominant torsion dystonia. Genomics 1993; 15: 9–12.
42. Bressman SB, Heiman GA, Nygaard TG et al. A study of idiopathic torsion dystonia in a non Jewish family: evidence for genetic heterogeneity. Neurology 1994; 44: 283–7.
43. Holmgren G, Ozelius L, Forsgren L et al. Adult onset idiopathic torsion dystonia is excluded from the DYT 1 region (9q34) in a Swedish family. J Neurol Neurosurg Psychiatry 1995; 59: 178–81.
44. Klein C, Pramstaller PP, Castellan CC et al. Clinical and genetic evaluation of a family with a mixed dystonia phenotype from South Tyrol. Ann Neurol 1998; 44: 394–8.
45. Albanese A, Bentivoglio AR, Del Grosso N et al. Phenotype variability of dystonia in monozygotic twins. J Neurol 2000; 247: 148–50.
46. Herz E. Dystonia. I. Historical review: analysis of dystonic symptoms and physiologic mechanisms involved. Arch Neurol Psychiat (Chicago) 1944; 51: 305–18.
47. Cooper IS. Involuntary movement disorders. New York: Evanston; 1969.
48. Marsden CD, Harrison MJ, Bundey S. Natural history of idiopathic torsion dystonia. Adv Neurol 1976; 14: 177–87.
49. Fahn S, Marsden CD, Calne DB. Classification and investigation of dystonia. In: Marsden CD, Fahn S, eds. Movement Disorders 2. London: Butterworths; 1987: 332–58.
50. Fahn S. Generalized dystonia: concept and treatment. Clin Neuropharmacol 1986; 9(Suppl 2): S37-S48.
51. Bressman SB, de Leon D, Brin MF et al. Inheritance of idiopathic torsion dystonia among Ashkenazi Jews. Adv Neurol 1988; 50: 45–56.
52. Klein C, Friedman J, Bressman S et al. Genetic testing for early-onset torsion dystonia (DYT1): introduction of a simple screening method, experiences from testing of a large patient cohort, and ethical aspects. Genet Test 1999; 3: 323–8.
53. Nemeth AH. The genetics of primary dystonias and related disorders. Brain 2002; 125: 695–721.
54. Kock N, Kasten M, Schule B et al. Clinical and genetic features of myoclonus-dystonia in 3 cases: a video presentation. Mov Disord 2004; 19: 231–4.

8

Cervical dystonia

Cynthia L Comella

DEFINITION AND CLINICAL FEATURES

Cervical dystonia (CD) is a focal dystonia of the cervical muscles that causes abnormal postures of the head, neck, and shoulders[1] (Table 8.1). In the past, CD was considered a psychiatric disorder, and terms such as 'torticollis mentalis' were used to describe the condition.[2] The reasons for this misconception arise from its unusual movements, worsening with certain actions or postures, enhancement by stress, improvement by touches or 'tricks' and the lack of anatomic, physiologic, and biochemical abnormalities.[3] Patients were referred to psychiatrists, some receiving inpatient psychiatric treatment, counseling, and electroconvulsive therapy for 'hysteria'.[4] Subsequently, the neurologic basis of CD was recognized, it was redefined as a subtype of focal dystonia and is now referred to as cervical dystonia.[3,5]

CD is marked by deviation of the head around horizontal (torticollis), coronal (retrocollis, anterocollis), and vertical axis (laterocollis), often associated with reduced range of motion in the direction contralateral to the movement.[6] CD has been categorized into three types associated with dystonic muscle activation: tonic, phasic, and tremulous.[7] Horizontal rotation is the most common abnormal movement, present in approximately 80% of patients. Electromyography in superficial neck muscles showed that this posture typically arises from activity of the sternocleidomastoid muscle contralateral to the turn and splenius capitis muscle ipsilateral to the direction of turn. Deeper muscles, including the longissimus capitis, splenius cervices, longus capitis, and obliquus capitis, can also be involved. Laterocollis is seen in 10–20% of patients, and is associated with electromyographic activity in ipsilateral splenius, sternocleidomastoid, and levator scapulae muscles. Retrocollis and anterocollis are less frequent, and involve bilateral posterior and anterior muscles, respectively. In most patients, these movements are not present in pure form, with combinations of torticollis and laterocollis. Shoulder involvement is present in approximately half of the patients.

Approximately 70–75% of patients have pain associated with CD. Pain occurs mostly with more severe head turn and spasm, and contributes to a greater degree of disability.[8] CD-related pain could be due to involuntary muscle contractions or to secondary phenomenan such as cervical arthritis or nerve root compression with radicular symptoms.[9] Premature arthritic changes have been observed in approximately 24% in small series and primarily affect the cervical spine ipsilateral to the direction of turn or tilt.[10]

One of the distinctive features of CD is the presence of a trick (geste antagoniste) that effectively alleviates symptoms. Although sometimes consisting of a forceful counterpressure that offsets the abnormal head posture,[11] often the trick is related solely to sensory input that effectively reduces abnormal dystonic muscle activity.[12] Common sensory tricks are touching the back of the head, cheek, or temple. Other tricks, such as chewing a toothpick, wrapping the head, or pulling the ear, can

Table 8.1 Common clinical features of cervical dystonia

- Movement of head, neck, and shoulders:
  - Horizontal (torticollis)
  - Sagittal
  - Coronal (retrocollis, anterocollis)
  - Lateral (laterocollis)
  - Shoulder elevation, anterior deviation
- Neck pain, stiffness
- Reduced range of motion
- Overlying spasms
- Sensory tricks (geste antagoniste)

also be present. Most patients will have more than one effective trick.[13] The effect of the sensory trick may be in the movement of the arm or in the touch itself.[14] In some CD patients, the mental imagery of a sensory trick may be as effective as the physical performance.[15] The presence of a trick is more common in younger-onset CD patients and in most the effect of a trick is maintained throughout the course of disease.[16]

The symptoms of focal CD usually begin in adulthood in the fifth decade.[8] The initial symptoms of CD are diverse, with neck pain and head posturing being the most frequent.[17] In some patients, there may be overlying muscle spasms causing quick, repetitive jerking movements that may resemble essential tremor, but can be differentiated by the directional preponderance of the movements.[18] Head tremor in the horizontal axis ('no-no' tremor) may be an initial manifestation of CD.[19]

Although variable, CD symptoms tend to worsen for the first 5 years and then stabilize.[20] Focal dystonia may spread from the neck to contiguous body areas including the face and arm, but seldom generalizes.[21,22] Spontaneous remission of symptoms can occur in up to 20% of CD patients, typically within 1–3 years of symptom onset.[20,21] The remissions may last up to 20 years, but almost all patients relapse.[23] The long-term complications of CD include cervical spine degeneration, spondylosis, disk herniation, vertebral subluxations and fractures, radiculopathies, and myelopathies. These complications are more frequent in generalized dystonia and cerebral palsy than focal dystonia and may affect from 20 to 40% of patients.[24]

Although not life threatening, CD can be disabling, affecting employability and negatively affecting quality of life.[25] In addition to the physical manifestations, CD patients have a variety of associated psychosocial issues, including a greater frequency of depression and an increased inability to maintain full-time employment.[26,27] These issues are improved if CD symptoms are alleviated by effective treatment.[28]

CD is the most common focal dystonia,[29] with a crude incidence of 10.9 per million person-years, and a crude prevalence rate of 88.6 per million persons in Rochester, Minnesota and an incidence of 1.2 per 100 000 person-years.[30] A cross-sectional study of dystonia conducted by the Epidemiologic Study of Dystonia in Europe found that CD constituted almost half of the cases of focal dystonia identified.[31] CD is more common in women, with a ratio of women to men of 1.4–1.6 to 1.[8,31]

Factors that predispose to the development of CD have not been identified. Scoliosis, defined as a lateral curvature of the spine exceeding 10° on radiography, is common in CD, affecting up to 39%.[9] The increased frequency of scoliosis in CD has been suggested to be a manifestation of more widespread dystonic involvement of paraspinal muscles,[32] extending from the neck into the back. Alternatively, it may be that spinal curvature arises secondary to the abnormal postures of the head and neck.[9] A recent case–control study suggests that childhood scoliosis may increase the risk of developing CD in adulthood.[33]

Although trauma has been hypothesized to be a risk factor for the development of CD, the role of trauma in the pathogenesis of CD has been controversial. In one study, CD patients with symptoms occurring within 4 weeks of a traumatic event had an increased frequency of laterocollis, pain, and depression,[34] and a minimal response to treatment with botulinum toxin.[35] In contrast, another report of CD occurring within 1 year of neck trauma showed no distinctive clinical features.[36] It has been suggested that CD related to acute trauma may arise secondary to peripheral muscle spasms and not to central mechanisms that underlie true dystonia.[35] A third study demonstrated that patients with post-traumatic CD had an increase in psychological factors and associated non-neurologic features such as give-away weakness and distractibility.[37] In all studies, post-traumatic CD patients were more likely to be involved in litigation or compensation issues.The association of trauma to dystonia remains an unsettled issue.

CD is a dynamic disorder that varies in severity depending on posture, activity, sensory input, presence of compensatory head postures, and the presence of dystonic spasms or tremor.[38] These qualities make CD problematic to evaluate utilizing rating scales. The Tsui rating scale is a six-item scale that assesses amplitude and duration of involuntary neck movements, shoulder elevation, and head tremor. This scale was utilized in early studies of botulinum toxin and had excellent inter-rater reliability, but was limited by discrepancies between rating scores and patient assessments of severity.[39,40] The Cervical Dystonia Severity Scale (CDSS) uses a protractor and wall chart to rate the severity of the head's deviation from neutral in each of three planes of motion (rotation, laterocollis, anterocollis/retrocollis).[41] Although the CDSS has excellent inter-rater agreement, validity has not been assessed and the need to perform the measures in a fixed, seated position may not reflect the dynamic qualities of CD. The Toronto Western Spasmodic Torticollis Rating Scale (TWSTRS) consists of three subscales to assess motor severity, pain, and disability of CD. The motor subscale of the TWSTRS has good to excellent inter-rater reliability, and a published teaching tape.[42,43] It has been utilized extensively in recent clinical trials of CD. The pain and disability subscales of the TWSTRS have not been adequately assessed for psychometric properties. Recently, a disease-specific quality of life rating scale for blepharospasm and cervical dystonia has been published.

Consisting of 24 items, the CDQ-24 was found to be a reliable and valid instrument that was sensitive to change following treatment.[44] The CDQ-24 may be useful in future studies of CD. A description and comparison of these, and other rating scales, is described in Chapter 23.

In addition to clinical rating scales, numerous electrophysiologic techniques have been developed to quantify the positional aspects of CD utilizing three-dimensional motion detection and computer analysis.[45,46] Although these may provide a more precise measurement of postural deviations, use in a clinical setting is currently limited due to the additional equipment and training needed for implementation.[47,48]

The pathophysiology of CD is not known. CD patients have abnormal orienting and postural responses to vibratory input and spatial perturbations that may increase with advancing disease.[49] Abnormalities of spatial orientation,[50,51] shifting of the perception of 'straight ahead' from the head to the trunk,[52] and abnormal sway deviation[53] have been described. Vestibular abnormalities have also been reported, although whether these are primary to the disorder or secondary to the chronic abnormal posture of the head have not been determined.

CD often occurs as a sporadic dystonia, without a major genetic contribution. However, twin pairs and families with non-progressive CD have been described.[54] The familial occurrence of CD is probably underestimated. This may be due, in part, to inaccuracies in identifying affected relatives on the part of the probands,[55] or failure to diagnose dystonia on the part of clinicians.[56] A recent study found that 19% of probands with craniocervical dystonia had a family member with definite dystonia, and as many as 33% had definite or probable dystonia,[57] suggesting that the genetic contribution in adult-onset CD may in fact be larger than anticipated from prior studies. Some investigators have suggested an autosomal dominant mode of inheritance with reduced penetrance.[58] Others have found evidence for genetic anticipation in CD.[59] The *DYT1* gene has largely been excluded in sporadic CD.[60] The *DYT7* locus linked to chromosome 18 has been reported to be associated with familial CD, and may be a common etiology in families in central Europe.[61–63] This locus has been excluded as a cause of adult-onset focal dystonia in other families.[64,65] As with other forms of dystonia, CD is likely to be a heterogeneous disorder.

Although in most adult patients, CD is a primary disorder without a defined etiology, secondary or symptomatic CD can occur and should be suspected, particularly if CD begins in infancy, or childhood, or is associated other physical findings (Table 8.2). Symptomatic CD is distinguished from primary CD by the presence of additional neurologic, orthopedic, or medical disorders or a history of drug exposure or trauma prior to onset.

Table 8.2 Clues that cervical dystonia is secondary

Sudden onset of dystonia
Severe pain
Rapid progression of symptoms
Fixed postures
Onset in an infant or child
Additional neurologic abnormalities

The differential diagnosis of secondary CD is extensive (Table 8.3). CD rarely occurs as a primary dystonia in children. Congenital muscular torticollis[66] is the most frequent underlying etiology in infants and is the sequela of an intrauterine or perinatal compartment syndrome.[67] Congenital torticollis, also called sternomastoid pseudotumor, typically presents with a shortened, tightened sternocleidomastoid muscle, an ipsilateral head tilt, and reduced range of motion. It is most frequently associated with a breech birth, hip dysplasia, and craniofacial asymmetry. If diagnosed and treated at an early age, congenital muscular torticollis has an excellent prognosis with manual stretching therapy or partial sectioning of the sternocleidomastoid muscle.[68–70]

Benign paroxysmal torticollis in infancy is a self-limiting condition that appears in early infancy before the age of 1 year and disappears spontaneously before the age of 5 years. The infant demonstrates recurrent episodes of sudden, stereotypic torticollis, that usually alternates from side to side and lasts from hours to days.[71] The infant may also show pallor, vomiting, and ataxia during the episodes. Recently, two patients in a family with familial hemiplegic migraine linked to *CACNA1A* mutation were described with this syndrome, suggesting an association with the calcium channelopathies.[72]

Atlantoaxial subluxation occurs with excessive ligamentous laxity found in some children, and has also been observed in Marfan's syndrome. Presenting symptoms include pain, abnormal posturing of the head ('cock-robin' position), and diminished range of motion of the neck. The onset is spontaneous and usually occurs following minor trauma.[73] Another cause of atlantoaxial subluxation in children is Grisel's syndrome, consisting of atlantoaxial subluxation associated with an inflammatory or infectious process, such as pharyngitis, mastoiditis, or a retropharyngeal abscess. These children may present with neck pain, fever, sore throat, a neck mass, and respiratory distress or stridor.[74] Acute torticollis in children can also result from an inflammatory process that irritates the cervical muscles, nerves, or vertebrae, causing spasm of cervical muscles, in particular

Table 8.3 Causes of cervical dystonia associated with age of onset

Infants and children	Cerebral palsy
	Congenital muscular torticollis
	Focal spasm
	Trauma
	Benign paroxysmal torticollis in infancy
	Oculogyric crisis
	Atantoaxial subluxation
	Grisel's syndrome
	Ocular disorders:
	Oculomotor palsies
	Brachial plexus palsies
	Anoxia
	Central nervous system lesions
	Intervertebral disc calcification
	Chiari type 1 malformations
	Chordoma of the clivus
	Sandifer's syndrome
Adults	Primary dystonia
	Drug-induced dystonic reactions:
	Acute
	Tardive
	Associated with other neurologic disorders:
	Parkinsonism
	Dystonia
	Huntington's disease
	Trauma

the sternocleidomastoid muscle, in the absence of a subluxation.[75]

A survey study of 288 pediatric patients with torticollis showed that 18% had a non-muscular etiology for their torticollis. Of these, Klippel–Feil anomalies and neurologic disorders were frequent. These neurologic conditions included ocular disorders in 23%, brachial plexus palsies in 17%, and lesions involving the central nervous system in 11% of the children.[76]

The diagnostic evaluation of an infant or child with torticollis includes cervical radiographs, cervical tomography, dynamic computed tomography, and magnetic resonance imaging.[77] If a subluxation is present, treatment approaches vary. In early cases (within 3 months of onset), analgesics, cervical traction, and immobilization are often effective.[78] In chronic or severe cases, spinal fusion may be required.[79] In cases secondary to infection or inflammation, treatment of the subluxation is combined with appropriate treatment of the inflammatory process.[80]

Other disorders that can cause abnormal head postures in children that are mistaken for CD include intervertebral disc calcification[81] and Chiari type 1 malformations.[82] Abnormal head posturing can also arise from superior oblique muscle palsy,[83] chordoma of the clivus,[84] and Sandifer's syndrome with gastric reflux into the esophagus.[85]

Both children and adults may develop CD following treatment with dopamine receptor antagonist drugs, usually psychotropic or antiemetic medications. Dystonia may occur as an acute reaction or after months to years of chronic treatment. Acute dystonic symptoms may present as oculogyric crisis, which includes symptoms of retrocollis associated with ocular deviation (oculogyric reaction). CD can also be the only manifestation of an acute drug reaction. Acute dystonic reactions can develop following the first dose of drug after increasing the dose and respond well to anticholinergic administration or discontinuation of the offending drug.

Tardive CD occurs following chronic treatment (defined as 3 months) with dopamine receptor antagonists, and may be differentiated from primary dystonia by the presence of extracervical involvement, retrocollis, spasmodic head movements, and the absence of an effective sensory trick or family history.[86] Although tardive dystonia typically begins as a focal dystonia, involving the craniocervical area in over 80% of cases, in most patients it progresses over months to years into generalized dystonia. The phenomenology of tardive dystonia may be indistinguishable from that of primary dystonia, although retrocollis and anterocollis are more common in tardive dystonia. Tardive CD is a persistent disorder, with less than 20% having a remission. Discontinuation of dopamine receptor antagonists increases the chance of remission but in many patients, tardive CD is irreversible and may not respond well to treatment.[87]

In adults, secondary CD may arise as a part of a more extensive neurologic disorder. CD has been described in association with multiple system atrophy (MSA), Parkinson's disease, and progressive supranuclear palsy.[88] Structural lesions usually localized to the brainstem and cerebellum can be associated with cervical dystonia. Lesions of the cervical spinal cord and basal ganglia have also been reported. Typically, other neurologic abnormalities are also present in patients with CD secondary to a degenerative neurologic disease or to a structural lesion.[89]

The extent of the diagnostic evaluation for CD depends on its presentation. In infants and children, the work-up can be extensive, as indicated above. In adults, if CD is typical and not associated with other abnormalities, no additional laboratory assessments are required. If CD is atypical at presentation, further evaluation for structural or metabolic abnormalities is indicated.

TREATMENT OF CERVICAL DYSTONIA

The treatment of CD has undergone important change in the past two decades. Oral pharmacologic agents used to date have not been adequately assessed and are of limited use for most patients with CD. A variety of agents have been tried, including drugs affecting cholinergic, dopaminergic, serotonergic, and γ-aminobutyric acid systems.[90] Anticholinergic drugs, while useful for treatment of generalized dystonia, provide symptom relief for a limited number of patients with focal dystonia.[91] A retrospective analysis of 71 CD patients reported 39% with a good response to anticholinergic agents, with women improving more than men.[92] Peripheral side effects, such as dry mouth, blurred vision, and urinary retention, are frequent, but may be reversed using a peripheral cholinesterase inhibitor (glycopyrrolate). The central side effects of sedation and memory loss are dose limiting.

Other drugs that can be of benefit in some CD patients include carbidopa/levodopa, clonazepam, and baclofen. Although dopamine receptor antagonists can improve symptoms of CD, the potential adverse effects, including tardive dystonia, limit the usefulness of this class of drugs. Although also reported to be sometimes helpful, dopamine receptor blocking agents are discouraged. Tetrabenazine, a monoamine-depleting and a dopamine-receptor-blocking drug,[93] is useful, but as many as 30% of patients will experience sedation, parkinsonism, depression, anxiety, or akathisia with treatment. Tetrabenazine is currently not generally available in the USA. Oral mexiletine was assessed in one open-label study of nine CD patients, and showed improvement in motor symptoms, with electrophysiologic dampening of dystonic activity in the sternocleidomastoid muscle. This effect persisted for the 6 months of the study, but these results have not been confirmed in a controlled study.[94]

Botulinum toxin injections have largely supplanted other treatment modalities for CD. Botulinum toxin type A is effective for the treatment of CD as has been demonstrated in both double-blind and open-label studies.[95] Approximately 60–85% of patients improve, with reduced head movement and pain, and increased range of motion and quality of life. The adverse effects from botulinum toxin are frequent, affecting up to 30%. The most common adverse effects include dysphagia and neck weakness, which are related to the local effects of the toxin,[96] and are usually mild and transient. A small percent of patients receiving repeated injections develop resistance to the effect of botulinum toxin type A. The development of new types of botulinum toxin provides an alternative for CD patients with resistance to type A. Controlled clinical trials using botulinum toxin type B show significant improvement in CD patients with and without resistance to type A.[97–99]

Phenol is a neurolytic agent that has been used in a limited number of CD patients. Although initial results are promising,[100,101] this agent requires specific training in its application and can cause serious adverse effects if used inappropriately.

Surgical treatments for CD are reserved for patients with disabling symptoms that fail to benefit from drug treatments and botulinum toxin. Chronic spinal cord stimulation, although initially promising in an open-label study,[102] was not found to be an effective treatment for dystonia in a small, double-blind study.[103] Rhizotomy and myectomy have, likewise, not been successful. Selective peripheral denervation, with specific lesion of the branch of the spinal accessory nerve to the sternocleidomastoid muscle and a selective ramisectomy of the branches serving the posterior neck muscles, is promising, but is often an extensive surgery with a prolonged recovery time requiring intensive rehabilitation.[104] The success rate in carefully selected patients operated on by experienced surgeons is over 80% and the complication rate is low. The surgical technique has recently been modified to reduce the occurrence of postoperative numbness in the C2 distribution and lessen the frequency of postoperative occipital neuralgia.[105]

Deep brain stimulation (DBS) is successful for the treatment of primary generalized dystonia.[106] Preliminary results in a small number of CD patients show that pallidal DBS can be very effective.[107] However, larger controlled clinical trials are needed.

REFERENCES

1. Fahn S, Bressman SB, Marsden CD. Classification of dystonia. Adv Neurol 1998; 78: 1–10.
2. Podivinsky F. Torticollis. In: Vinken RA, Bruyn GW, eds. Handbook of Clinical Neurology. Amsterdam: North Holland Publishing; 1968: 567–603.
3. Marsden CD. The problem of adult-onset idiopathic torsion dystonia and other isolated dyskinesias in adult life (including blepharospasm, oromandibular dystonia, dystonic writer's cramp, and torticollis, or axial dystonia). Adv Neurol 1976; 14: 259–76.
4. Matthews WB, Beasley P, Parry-Jones W, Garland G. Spasmodic torticollis: a combined clinical study. J Neurol Neurosurg Psychiatry 1978; 41: 485–92.

5. Marsden CD. Dystonia: the spectrum of the disease. Res Publ Assoc Res Nerv Ment Dis 1976; 55: 351–67.
6. Caputi F, Nashold BS Jr, Spaziante R. Analysis of static and kinetic abnormalities typical of torticollis, and postoperative changes. Stereotact Funct Neurosurg 1995; 64: 16–31.
7. Deuschl G, Heinen F, Kleedorfer B et al. Clinical and polymyographic investigation of spasmodic torticollis. J Neurol 1992; 239: 9–15.
8. Chan J, Brin MF, Fahn S. Idiopathic cervical dystonia: clinical characteristics. Mov Disord 1991; 6: 119–26.
9. Jankovic J, Leder S, Warner D, Schwartz K. Cervical dystonia: clinical findings and associated movement disorders. Neurology 1991; 41: 1088–91.
10. Chawda SJ, Munchau A, Johnson D et al. Pattern of premature degenerative changes of the cervical spine in patients with spasmodic torticollis and the impact on the outcome of selective peripheral denervation. J Neurol Neurosurg Psychiatry 2000; 68: 465–71.
11. Stejskal L. Counterpressure in torticollis. J Neurol Sci 1980; 48: 9–19.
12. Buchman AS, Comella CL, Leurgans S et al. The effect of changes in head posture on the patterns of muscle activity in cervical dystonia (CD). Mov Disord 1998; 13: 490–6.
13. Muller J, Wissel J, Masuhr F et al. Clinical characteristics of the geste antagoniste in cervical dystonia. J Neurol 2001; 248: 478–82.
14. Wissel J, Muller J, Ebersbach G, Poewe W. Trick maneuvers in cervical dystonia: investigation of movement- and touch-related changes in polymyographic activity. Mov Disord 1999; 14: 994–9.
15. Greene PE, Bressman S. Exteroceptive and interoceptive stimuli in dystonia. Mov Disord 1998; 13: 549–51.
16. Filipovic SR, Jahanshahi M, Viswanathan R et al. Clinical features of the geste antagoniste in cervical dystonia. Adv Neurol 2004; 94: 191–201.
17. Van Zandijcke M. Cervical dystonia (spasmodic torticollis). Some aspects of the natural history. Acta Neurol Belg 1995; 95: 210–15.
18. Bressman SB. Dystonia update. Clin Neuropharmacol 2000; 23: 239–51.
19. Rivest J, Marsden CD. Trunk and head tremor as isolated manifestations of dystonia. Mov Disord 1990; 5: 60–5.
20. Lowenstein DH, Aminoff MJ. The clinical course of spasmodic torticollis. Neurology 1988; 38: 530–2.
21. Jahanshahi M, Marion MH, Marsden CD. Natural history of adult-onset idiopathic torticollis. Arch Neurol 1990; 47: 548–52.
22. Greene P, Kang UJ, Fahn S. Spread of symptoms in idiopathic torsion dystonia. Mov Disord 1995; 10: 143–52.
23. Friedman A, Fahn S. Spontaneous remissions in spasmodic torticollis. Neurology 1986; 36: 398–400.
24. Konrad C, Vollmer-Haase J, Anneken K, Knecht S. Orthopedic and neurological complications of cervical dystonia – review of the literature. Acta Neurol Scand 2004; 109: 369–73.
25. Ben-Shlomo Y, Camfield L, Warner T. What are the determinants of quality of life in people with cervical dystonia? J Neurol Neurosurg Psychiatry 2002; 72: 608–14.
26. Jahanshahi M, Marsden CD. Personality in torticollis: a controlled study. Psychol Med 1988; 18: 375–87.
27. Jahanshahi M. Psychosocial factors and depression in torticollis. J Psychosom Res 1991; 35: 493–507.
28. Jahanshahi M, Marsden CD. Psychological functioning before and after treatment of torticollis with botulinum toxin. J Neurol Neurosurg Psychiatry 1992; 55: 229–31.
29. Nutt JG, Muenter MD, Aronson A et al. Epidemiology of focal and generalized dystonia in Rochester, Minnesota. Mov Disord 1988; 3: 188–94.
30. Claypool DW, Duane DD, Ilstrup DM, Melton LJ 3rd. Epidemiology and outcome of cervical dystonia (spasmodic torticollis) in Rochester, Minnesota. Mov Disord 1995; 10: 608–14.
31. Sex-related influences on the frequency and age of onset of primary dystonia. Epidemiologic Study of Dystonia in Europe (ESDE) Collaborative Group. Neurology 1999; 53: 1871–3.
32. O'Riordan S, Lynch T, Hutchinson M. Familial adolescent-onset scoliosis and later segmental dystonia in an Irish family. J Neurol 2004; 251: 845–8.
33. Defazio G, Abbruzzese G, Girlanda P et al. Primary cervical dystonia and scoliosis: a multicenter case-control study. Neurology 2003; 60: 1012–15.
34. O'Riordan S, Hutchinson M. Cervical dystonia following peripheral trauma – a case-control study. J Neurol 2004; 251: 150–5.
35. Tarsy D. Comparison of acute- and delayed-onset posttraumatic cervical dystonia. Mov Disord 1998; 13: 481–5.
36. Samii A, Pal PK, Schulzer M et al. Post-traumatic cervical dystonia: a distinct entity? Can J Neurol Sci 2000; 27: 55–9.
37. Sa DS, Mailis-Gagnon A, Nicholson K, Lang AE. Posttraumatic painful torticollis. Mov Disord 2003; 18: 1482–91.
38. Fahn S. Assessment of the primary dystonias. In: Munsat T, ed. Quantification of Neurologic Deficit. London: Butterworths; 1989: 241–70.
39. Tsui JK, Eisen A, Stoessl AJ et al. Double-blind study of botulinum toxin in spasmodic torticollis. Lancet 1986; 2: 245–7.
40. Tarsy D. Comparison of clinical rating scales in treatment of cervical dystonia with botulinum toxin. Mov Disord 1997; 12: 100–2.
41. O'Brien C, Brashear A, Cullis P et al. Cervical dystonia severity scale reliability study. Mov Disord 2001; 16: 1086–90.
42. Consky E, Lang, AE. Clinical assessments of patients with cervical dystonia. In: Jankovic J, Hallett M, ed. Therapy with Botulinum Toxin. New York: Marcel Dekker; 1994: 211–37.
43. Comella CL, Stebbins GT, Goetz CG et al. Teaching tape for the motor section of the Toronto Western Spasmodic Torticollis Scale. Mov Disord 1997; 12: 570–5.
44. Muller J, Wissel J, Kemmler G et al. Craniocervical dystonia questionnaire (CDQ-24): development and validation of a disease-specific quality of life instrument. J Neurol Neurosurg Psychiatry 2004; 75: 749–53.
45. Albani G, Bulgheroni MV, Mancini F et al. The position of the head in space: a kinematic analysis in patients with cervical dystonia treated with botulinum toxin. Funct Neurol 2001; 16: 135–41.
46. Galardi G, Micera S, Carpaneto J et al. Automated assessment of cervical dystonia. Mov Disord 2003; 18: 1358–67.
47. Dykstra D, Ellingham C, Belfie A et al. Quantitative measurement of cervical range of motion in patients with torticollis treated with botulinum A toxin. Mov Disord 1993; 8: 38–42.
48. Carpaneto J, Micera S, Galardi G et al. A protocol for the assessment of 3D movements of the head in persons with cervical dystonia. Clin Biomech (Bristol, Avon) 2004; 19: 659–63.
49. Bove M, Brichetto G, Abbruzzese G, Marchese R, Schieppati M. Neck proprioception and spatial orientation in cervical dystonia. Brain 2004; 127(Pt 12): 2764–78.
50. Muller SV, Glaser P, Troger M et al. Disturbed egocentric space representation in cervical dystonia. Mov Disord 2005; 20(1): 58–63.
51. Anastasopoulos D, Bhatia K, Bisdorff A et al. Perception of spatial orientation in spasmodic torticollis. Part I: The postural vertical. Mov Disord 1997; 12: 561–9.
52. Anastasopoulos D, Nasios G, Psilas K et al. What is straight ahead to a patient with torticollis? Brain 1998; 121(Pt 1): 91–101.

53. Lekhel H, Popov K, Anastasopoulos D et al. Postural responses to vibration of neck muscles in patients with idiopathic torticollis. Brain 1997; 120(Pt 4): 583–91.
54. Uitti RJ, Maraganore DM. Adult onset familial cervical dystonia: report of a family including monozygotic twins. Mov Disord 1993; 8: 489–94.
55. Martino D, Aniello MS, Masi G et al. Validity of family history data on primary adult-onset dystonia. Arch Neurol 2004; 61: 1569–73.
56. Logroscino G, Livrea P, Anaclerio D et al. Agreement among neurologists on the clinical diagnosis of dystonia at different body sites. J Neurol Neurosurg Psychiatry 2003; 74: 348–50.
57. Defazio G, Abbruzzese G, Girlanda P et al. Does sex influence age at onset in cranial-cervical and upper limb dystonia? J Neurol Neurosurg Psychiatry 2003; 74: 265–7.
58. Waddy HM, Fletcher NA, Harding AE, Marsden CD. A genetic study of idiopathic focal dystonias. Ann Neurol 1991; 29: 320–4.
59. Cheng JT, Liu A, Wasmuth J et al. Clinical evidence of genetic anticipation in adult-onset idiopathic dystonia. Neurology 1996; 47: 215–19.
60. Sessa M, Galardi G, Agazzi E, Casari G. Sporadic idiopathic cervical dystonia: exclusion of the DYT1 deletion. J Neurol 2001; 248: 812–13.
61. Leube B, Rudnicki D, Ratzlaff T et al. Idiopathic torsion dystonia: assignment of a gene to chromosome 18p in a German family with adult onset, autosomal dominant inheritance and purely focal distribution. Hum Mol Genet 1996; 5: 1673–7.
62. Leube B, Hendgen T, Kessler KR et al. Evidence for DYT7 being a common cause of cervical dystonia (torticollis) in Central Europe. Am J Med Genet 1997; 74: 529–32.
63. Jarman PR, del Grosso N, Valente EM et al. Primary torsion dystonia: the search for genes is not over. J Neurol Neurosurg Psychiatry 1999; 67: 395–7.
64. Brancati F, Defazio G, Caputo V et al. Novel Italian family supports clinical and genetic heterogeneity of primary adult-onset torsion dystonia. Mov Disord 2002; 17: 392–7.
65. Munchau A, Valente EM, Davis MB et al. A Yorkshire family with adult-onset cranio-cervical primary torsion dystonia. Mov Disord 2000; 15: 954–9.
66. Morrison DL, MacEwen GD. Congenital muscular torticollis: observations regarding clinical findings, associated conditions, and results of treatment. J Pediatr Orthop 1982; 2: 500–5.
67. Davids JR, Wenger DR, Mubarak SJ. Congenital muscular torticollis: sequela of intrauterine or perinatal compartment syndrome. J Pediatr Orthop 1993; 13: 141–7.
68. Cheng JC, Tang SP, Chen TM. Sternocleidomastoid pseudotumor and congenital muscular torticollis in infants: a prospective study of 510 cases. J Pediatr 1999; 134: 712–16.
69. Akazawa H, Nakatsuka Y, Miyake Y, Takahashi Y. Congenital muscular torticollis: long-term follow-up of thirty-eight partial resections of the sternocleidomastoid muscle. Arch Orthop Trauma Surg 1993; 112: 205–9.
70. Yu SW, Wang NH, Chin LS, Lo WH. Surgical correction of muscular torticollis in older children. Zhonghua Yi Xue Za Zhi (Taipei) 1995; 55: 168–71.
71. Kimura S, Nezu A. Electromyographic study in an infant with benign paroxysmal torticollis. Pediatr Neurol 1998; 19: 236–8.
72. Giffin NJ, Benton S, Goadsby PJ. Benign paroxysmal torticollis of infancy: four new cases and linkage to CACNA1A mutation. Dev Med Child Neurol 2002; 44: 490–3.
73. Muniz AE, Belfer RA. Atlantoaxial rotary subluxation in children. Pediatr Emerg Care 1999; 15: 25–9.
74. Craig FW, Schunk JE. Retropharyngeal abscess in children: clinical presentation, utility of imaging, and current management. Pediatrics 2003; 111: 1394–8.
75. Bredenkamp JK, Maceri DR. Inflammatory torticollis in children. Arch Otolaryngol Head Neck Surg 1990; 116: 310–13.
76. Ballock RT, Song KM. The prevalence of nonmuscular causes of torticollis in children. J Pediatr Orthop 1996; 16: 500–4.
77. Maheshwaran S, Sgouros S, Jeyapalan K et al. Imaging of childhood torticollis due to atlanto-axial rotatory fixation. Childs Nerv Syst 1995; 11: 667–71.
78. Subach BR, McLaughlin MR, Albright AL, Pollack IF. Current management of pediatric atlantoaxial rotatory subluxation. Spine 1998; 23: 2174–9.
79. Lee SC, Lui TN, Lee ST. Atlantoaxial rotatory subluxation in skeletally immature patients. Br J Neurosurg 2002; 16: 154–7.
80. Mathern GW, Batzdorf U. Grisel's syndrome. Cervical spine clinical, pathologic, and neurologic manifestations. Clin Orthop Relat Res 1989; 224: 131–46.
81. Hahn YS, McLone DG, Uden D. Cervical intervertebral disc calcification in children. Childs Nerv Syst 1987; 3: 274–7.
82. Dure LS, Percy AK, Cheek WR, Laurent JP. Chiari type I malformation in children. J Pediatr 1989; 115: 573–6.
83. Nemet P, Godel V, Baruch E, Lazar M. Pitfall of acquired ocular torticollis. J Pediatr Ophthalmol Strabismus 1980; 17: 310–11.
84. Nolte K. Malignant intracranial chordoma and sarcoma of the clivus in infancy. Pediatr Radiol 1979; 8: 1–6.
85. Werlin SL, D'Souza BJ, Hogan WJ et al. Sandifer syndrome: an unappreciated clinical entity. Dev Med Child Neurol 1980; 22: 374–8.
86. Molho ES, Feustel PJ, Factor SA. Clinical comparison of tardive and idiopathic cervical dystonia. Mov Disord 1998; 13: 486–9.
87. Kiriakakis V, Bhatia KP, Quinn NP, Marsden CD. The natural history of tardive dystonia. A long-term follow-up study of 107 cases. Brain 1998; 121(Pt 11): 2053–66.
88. Rivest J, Quinn N, Marsden CD. Dystonia in Parkinson's disease, multiple system atrophy, and progressive supranuclear palsy. Neurology 1990; 40: 1571–8.
89. LeDoux MS, Brady KA. Secondary cervical dystonia associated with structural lesions of the central nervous system. Mov Disord 2003; 18: 60–9.
90. Lal S. Pathophysiology and pharmacotherapy of spasmodic torticollis: a review. Can J Neurol Sci 1979; 6: 427–35.
91. Lang AE, Sheehy MP, Marsden CD. Anticholinergics in adult-onset focal dystonia. Can J Neurol Sci 1982; 9: 313–19.
92. Greene P, Shale H, Fahn S. Analysis of open-label trials in torsion dystonia using high dosages of anticholinergics and other drugs. Mov Disord 1988; 3: 46–60.
93. Jankovic J, Beach J. Long-term effects of tetrabenazine in hyperkinetic movement disorders. Neurology 1997; 48: 358–62.
94. Ohara S, Hayashi R, Momoi H et al. Mexiletine in the treatment of spasmodic torticollis. Mov Disord 1998; 13: 934–40.
95. Jankovic J. Treatment of cervical dystonia with botulinum toxin. Mov Disord 2004; 19 (Suppl 8): S109–15.
96. Comella CL, Tanner CM, DeFoor-Hill L, Smith C. Dysphagia after botulinum toxin injections for spasmodic torticollis: clinical and radiologic findings. Neurology 1992; 42: 1307–10.
97. Lew MF. Duration of effectiveness of botulinum toxin type B in the treatment of cervical dystonia. Adv Neurol 2004; 94: 211–15.
98. Brashear A, Lew MF, Dykstra DD et al. Safety and efficacy of NeuroBloc (botulinum toxin type B) in type A-responsive cervical dystonia. Neurology 1999; 53: 1439–46.
99. Brin MF, Lew MF, Adler CH et al. Safety and efficacy of NeuroBloc (botulinum toxin type B) in type A-resistant cervical dystonia. Neurology 1999; 53: 1431–8.
100. Takeuchi N, Chuma T, Mano Y. Phenol block for cervical dystonia: effects and side effects. Arch Phys Med Rehabil 2004; 85: 1117–20.
101. Massey JM. Treatment of spasmodic torticollis with intramuscular phenol injection. J Neurol Neurosurg Psychiatry 1995; 58: 258–9.

102. Waltz JM, Scozzari CA, Hunt DP. Spinal cord stimulation in the treatment of spasmodic torticollis. Appl Neurophysiol 1985; 48: 324–38.
103. Goetz CG, Penn RD, Tanner CM. Efficacy of cervical cord stimulation in dystonia. Adv Neurol 1988; 50: 645–9.
104. Bertrand CM. Selective peripheral denervation for spasmodic torticollis: surgical technique, results, and observations in 260 cases. Surg Neurol 1993; 40: 96–103.
105. Taira T, Kobayashi T, Takahashi K, Hori T. A new denervation procedure for idiopathic cervical dystonia. J Neurosurg Spine 2002; 97: 201–6.
106. Krauss JK, Yianni J, Loher TJ, Aziz TZ. Deep brain stimulation for dystonia. J Clin Neurophysiol 2004; 21: 18–30.
107. Eltahawy HA, Saint-Cyr J, Poon YY et al. Pallidal deep brain stimulation in cervical dystonia: clinical outcome in four cases. Can J Neurol Sci 2004; 31: 328–32.

9

Cranial dystonia

Dirk Dressler and Fereshte Adib Saberi

INTRODUCTION

Cranial muscles form a highly complex network that provides an amazing multitude of different functions, including some of the most sophisticated functions that muscles can perform. This complexity is reflected by the overproportional size of their motor cortical representation, as suggested by Penfield and Rasmussen's homunculus.[1] Cranial muscles are involved in psychomotor communication, in speech articulation, in exploration, intake, processing, transport and swallowing of food and liquids, in affective exploration, in eye movements, in vision control, in eye protection and in hearing.

With the exception of vision control and hearing, all of their functions can be impaired by dystonia. However, dystonia is just one of many disorders affecting cranial muscles, including other disorders of the basal ganglia, disorders of the limbic system, the frontal lobe, the pyramidal tract, the peripheral nervous system, and the cranial muscles themselves.

Cranial dystonia can be part of a complex movement disorder where dystonia occurs together with other abnormal movements, as in Huntington's disease (see Chapter 2). Sometimes cranial dystonia can be the presenting feature of those complex movement disorders, as in neurodegeneration with brain accumulation of iron (NBAI) or in neuroacanthocytosis. Cranial dystonia can also be part of a widespread dystonic syndrome, as in Oppenheim's dystonia. Sometimes, cranial dystonia is the predominant manifestation of those dystonic syndromes, as in tardive dystonia. Cranial dystonia can also occur in isolation, as in blepharospasm. There is reason to believe that the different context in which cranial dystonia occurs reflects different pathophysiologic and etiologic entities.

ANATOMY

As shown in Table 9.1, the cranial muscles comprise at least 58 paired muscles and 1 unpaired muscle and connect the skull and its associated structures, such as the mandible, the os hyoideum, the cranial and nuchal skin, the tongue, the pharynx, the eyes, and the ears. Muscles originating on those associated structures and inserting elsewhere are not considered cranial muscles.

Mimic muscles are cranial muscles originating from the skull and the jaw and inserting into the facial or nuchal skin or into aponeuroses. They form a highly complex functional network. Originating from the second visceral arch, they are all innervated by the facial nerve. Inserting into the skin, all mimic muscles lack a fascia, thus making them prone to transdermal infections. Figure 9.1 shows the mimic muscles. Mimic muscles model the skin and moving structures imbedded into the skin, such as the eyebrows, the mouth, and the eyelids. Activation of mimic muscles is performed with enormous precision and velocity. Mimic muscles are one of the main psychomotor output channels. Estimated by the amount of information transmitted, psychomotor communication is probably the most important output channel available to humans. Other mimic muscle functions include eye protection, exploratory lip movements, and food and liquid intake. Because of the functional complexity of the mimic muscle network, therapeutic interventions, such as botulinum toxin therapy or surgery, are complicated and often impair the fragile balance of agonistic and antagonistic muscle activity.

The orbicularis oculi muscle consists of the palpebral part covering the eyelids, the orbital part surrounding the palpebral part and connecting it to the surrounding mimic muscles, and the lacrimal part controlling

Table 9.1 Cranial muscles

Mimic muscles	
Epicranium	M. occipitofrontalis
	M. temoroparietalis (not to be mistaken for M. temporalis)
Ear	M. auricularis anterior
	M. auricularis superior
	M. auricularis posterior
Eye lid	M. orbicularis oculi
	M. corrugator supercilii
	M. levator palpebrae
Nasal	M. procerus (non-paired)
	M. nasalis
	M. levator labii superioris alaeque
Neck	Platysma
Mouth	M. orbicularis oris
	M. buccinator
	M. zygomaticus major
	M. zygomaticus minor
	M. risorius
	M. levator labii superioris
	M. levator anguli oris
	M. depressor labii inferioris
	M. depressor anguli oris
	M. mentalis
Jaw muscles	M. masseter
	M. temporalis
	M. pterygoideus lateralis
	M. pterygoid medialis
Floor of the mouth	M. mylohyoideus
	M. geniohyoideus
	M. stylohoideus
	M. digastricus
Pharynx	M. tensor veli palatini
	M. levator veli palatini
	M. palatoglossus
	M. palatopharyngeus
	M. uvulae
	M. constrictor pharyngis superior
	M. constrictor pharyngis medius
	M. constrictor pharyngis inferior
	M. stylopharyngeus
	M. palatopharyngeus
Tongue	
internal	M. longitudinalis superior
	M. longitudinalis inferior
	M. transversus linguae
	M. verticalis linguae
external	M. genioglossus
	M. hyoglossus
	M. styloglossus
	M. palatoglossus
Eye	
external	M. rectus superior
	M. rectus inferior
	M. rectus lateralis
	M. rectus medialis
	M. obliqus superior
	M. obliqus inferior
internal	M. sphincter pupillae
	M. dilatator pupillae
	M. cilaris
Tympanon	M. tensor tympani
	M. stapedius

Cranial muscles connect the skull, the jaw, the os hyoideum, the cranial skin, the eyes, the tympanon, the tongue, and the pharynx. Muscles originating in those elements and inserting elsewhere are not considered cranial muscles.

tear drainage. The fiber architecture of the orbicularis oculi muscle is shown in Figure 9.2. Figure 9.3 shows its complex movement sequence, producing eyelid closure, initiating tear drainage, and achieving foreign body removal. The orbicularis oris muscle is densely interconnected with the overlaying skin. Because of its fiber architecture it is able to produce complex modeling of the lips. It is held in place entirely by its surrounding muscles. The depressor anguli oris muscle depresses the corner of the mouth and stabilizes the lower lip. The mentalis muscle forms the chin dimples. It also stabilizes the lower lip, however, to a lesser degree than the depressor anguli oris muscle. The risorius muscle abducts the corner of the mouth. The muscles above the dividing line between the lower lip and the upper lip – i.e. the levator anguli oris, levator labii superioris, zygomaticus major, zygomaticus minor, and levator labii superioris alaeque nasi muscles – fixate the orbicularis oris muscle

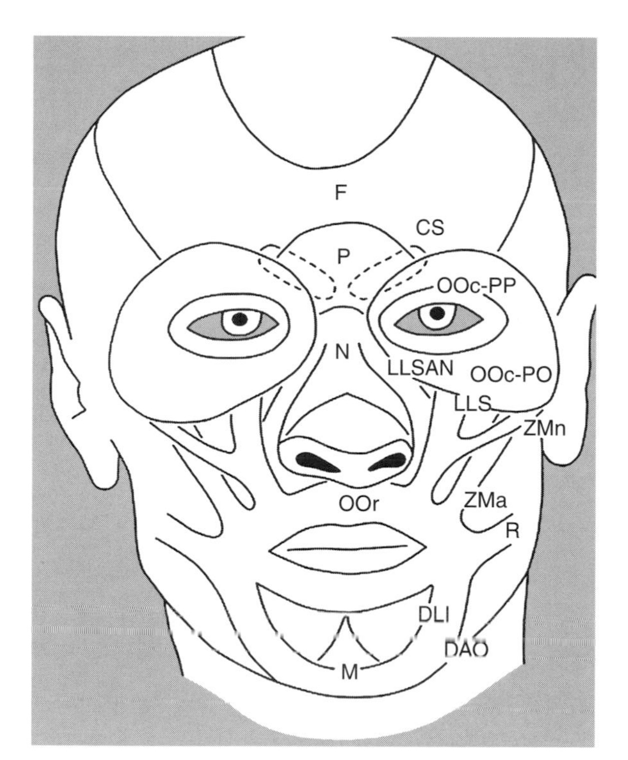

Key

CS	corrugator supercilii
DAO	depressor anguli oris
F	frontalis
LLS	levator labii superioris
LLSAN	levator labii superioris alaeque nasi
N	nasalis
OOc-PO	orbicularis oculi, orbital part
OOc-PP	orbicularis oculi, palpebral part
OOr	orbicularis oris
P	procerus
R	risorius
Zma	zygomaticus major
Zmn	zygomaticus minor

Figure 9.1 Mimic muscles. (Reproduced from Dressler,[2] with permission.)

against gravity. Therapeutic interventions in these muscles frequently induce a drop of the corner of the mouth.

Jaw muscles connect the jaw with the skull. They originate from the first visceral arch and are innervated by the trigeminal nerve. They provide jaw closure, jaw protrusion, jaw retraction, and lateral jaw movements and, together with the muscles of the floor of the mouth and the infrahyal muscles, are involved in jaw opening. The jaw muscles stabilize the mandibular joint, which is otherwise a joint with an extreme degree of freedom. The masseter and the pterygoideus medialis muscles close the jaw, the pterygoideus lateralis muscle, the muscles of the floor of the mouth, and the infrahyal muscles open the jaw, the pterygoideus lateralis muscle supported by superficial fibers of the masseter and the medial pterygoideus muscles protrude the jaw, unilateral activation of the lateral pterygoideus muscle moves the jaw to one side, and the temporalis muscle retracts the jaw.

Tongue muscles form the shape of the tongue and move it around. The shape of the tongue is modeled by the internal tongue muscles. The tongue is shortened by the longitudinal tongue muscles, it is flattened by the vertical tongue muscles, and narrowed and rounded by the transversal tongue muscles. The external tongue muscles move the tongue. The styloglossus and the hyoglossus muscles retract the tongue and the genioglossus muscle moves the tongue forward.

Muscles of the floor of the mouth close the intermandibular space and are involved in jaw opening.

Pharynx muscles form the introitus to the esophagus and to the trachea, and are involved in food and liquid transport.

DEFINITIONS

Cranial dystonias are dystonias that affect the cranial muscles. Blepharospasm or periocular dystonia describes dystonia in the orbicularis oculi and – facultatively – its adjacent muscles, including the corrugator supercilii, procerus, nasalis, and levator labii superioris alaeque nasi muscles. When blepharospasm occurs in isolation, it is called essential blepharospasm or – slightly misleadingly – benign essential blepharospasm. Perioral dystonia refers to dystonia of the orbicularis oris and its adjacent muscles, orofacial dystonia to dystonia in the orbicularis oris and in other mimic muscles. Oromandibular dystonia describes dystonia in the orbicularis oris and its adjacent mimic muscles, in the jaw muscles, and in the floor of the mouth. Frequently, dystonia in the tongue and in the pharyngeal muscles is associated.

Orobuccolingual dystonia is dystonia in the orbicularis oris, its adjacent mimic muscles, and in the tongue. Meige syndrome, named after the French neurologist Henry Meige (1866–1940), describes the combination of facial and oromandibular dystonia.[4] The term Brueghel's syndrome was suggested by C David Marsdens[5] for the combination of blepharospasm and oromandibular dystonia. It was named after the

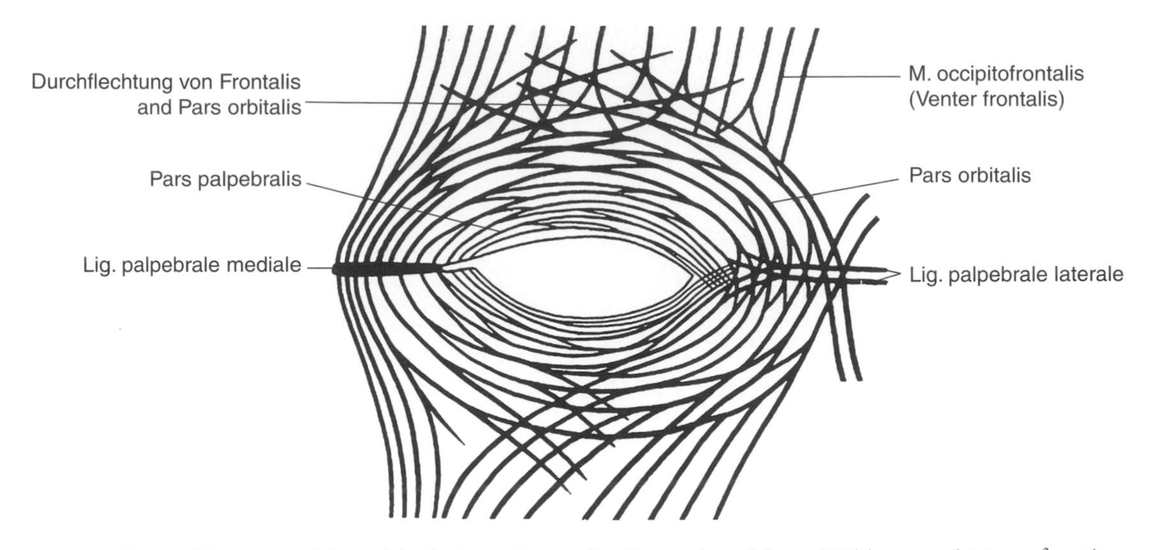

Figure 9.2 Fiber architecture of the orbicularis oculi muscle. (Reproduced from Waldeyer and Mayet,[3] with permission.)

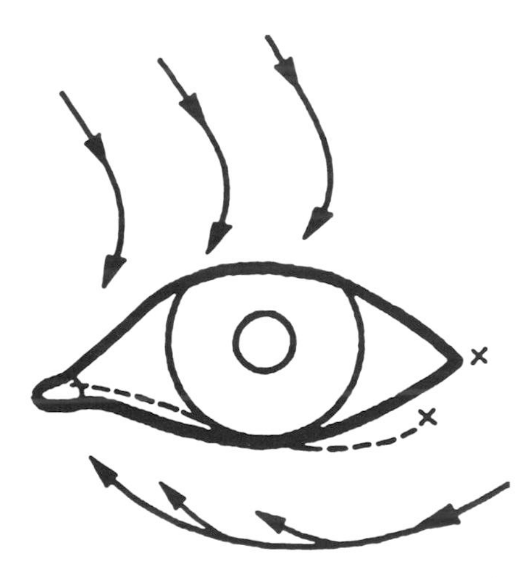

Figure 9.3 Movement sequence producing eyelid closure. (Reproduced from Waldeyer and Mayet,[3] with permission.)

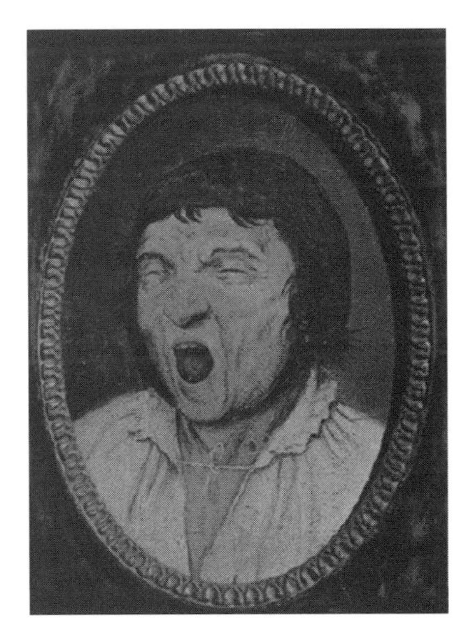

Figure 9.4 'De Gaper' ('The Yawner') (1558) by Pieter Brueghel the Elder (1525–1569).

painting 'De Gaper' ('The Yawner') by Pieter Brueghel the Elder (1525–1569) (Figure 9.4), but was never widely accepted. We suggest describing cranial dystonia according to its localization as periocular (blepharospasm), perioral, facial (periocular and perioral), oromandibular and faciomandibular (Meige syndrome, Brueghel's syndrome).

Sometimes the term dyskinesia is used to describe a mixture of choriform and dystonic cranial muscle hyperactivities usually as the result of chronic neuroleptic medication.

DIFFERENTIAL DIAGNOSES

Clinical conditions resembling cranial dystonia are numerous. In hemifacial spasm, involuntary muscle activity is virtually always unilateral, although bilateral cases have been reported.[6–8] Hemifacial spasm produces a typical electromyographic pattern with brief high-frequency discharges occurring simultaneously in several mimic muscles. In advanced cases, perioral facial weakness becomes frequent. Reinnervation synkinesias can occur after facial nerve lesions when aberrant nerve sprouting produces mismatched innervation of mimic muscles. Reinnervation synkinesias do not occur at rest. Usually, eyelid closure occurs when perioral activation is intended and vice versa. Tics consist of complex muscle activation patterns. Eye blinking is a common manifestation.[9] Almost all idiopathic tics manifest before age 11 years.[10] Frequently, vocal tics and obsessive-compulsive behavior are associated. Myasthenia gravis used to be a frequent misdiagnosis of blepharospasm before the concept of cranial dystonia received more widespread attention. Now, ocular myasthenia gravis, with all its diagnostic pitfalls, has to be considered in patients with lack of orbicularis oculi muscle hyperactivity and more pronounced diurnal fluctuations.[11] Facial weakness in Lambert–Eaton myasthenic syndrome can be reminiscent of blepharospasm.[12] Its diagnostic hallmarks include the typical increment of electromyographic responses to serial stimulation and antibodies against presynaptic calcium channels. Depression can produce a facial expression vaguely resembling blepharospasm. Again, no muscle hyperactivity in the orbicularis oculi muscle is detected by electromyography. Psychogenic dystonia has always to be considered. Typically, it has an abrupt onset, varies in localization and severity, and frequently consists of movement sequences rather than dystonic movement fragments. Stereotypies are repetitive movements in patients with psychosis or obsessive-compulsive behavior. They can consist of grimacing and eye blinking. Levodopa-induced dyskinesias usually produce choreiform rather than dystonic facial movements. Benign hereditary chorea is a childhood-onset disorder predominantly affecting axial and limb muscles.[13,14] Hemimasticatory spasms are a rare disorder presenting with frequent paroxysmal unilateral jaw muscle hyperactivity, leading to painful forced jaw closures. It is believed to be caused by demyelinating lesions of the peripheral trigeminal motor fibers producing ephaptic neural activities similar to those seen in hemifacial spasm.[15–17] Hemifacial atrophy is frequently associated and possibly causes the trigeminal nerve lesion.[17–19] Senile perioral dyskinesias or benign senile chorea, perioral choreiform movements, more often affect women than men. With a prevalence of 1.5% in individuals aged 67–87 years old,[20] they are rarer than generally believed. They may include minor tardive syndromes, unusual cases of Huntington's disease,[21] or may be associated with Alzheimer's disease.[22] In non-dystonic blepharospasm, increased blinking and/or closure of the eyelids is caused by local eye irritation, as in conjunctival or corneal infection, foreign body entrapment, senile entropion, or use of personal defense sprays.[23]

In some patients, eyelid opening is impaired not by hyperactivity of the orbicularis oculi muscle closing the eyelid but by the patient's inability to activate the levator palpebrae muscle. This condition is called apraxia of eyelid opening or levator inhibition. It typically occurs in progressive supranuclear palsy,[24] but also in idiopathic Parkinson's disease.[25] Electromyography demonstrates lack of orbicularis oculi muscle hyperactivity, delayed activation of the levator palpebrae muscle, and an impaired coordination between both muscles. It can occur in combination with blepharospasm.

Rare differential diagnoses of cranial dystonias include facial myokymia with clinically and electromyographically typical undulatory muscle activity due to demyelinating brainstem lesions or potassium channel abnormalities, Isaacs' syndrome with its typical continuous muscle fiber activity, Schwartz–Jampel syndrome[26] with continuous muscle fiber activity, and additional dysmorphic features.

ETIOLOGY

Cranial dystonias can occur isolated or as part of segmental, axial, or generalized dystonia. When they occur as part of a more widespread dystonia, they can be caused by the full spectrum of etiologies so far identified as producing dystonia; these are discussed in Chapter 1. Apart from a primary or idiopathic etiology with all its genetic options, cranial dystonias can be part of a dystonia-plus syndrome, i.e. dystonia with parkinsonism or dystonia with myoclonus, a secondary or symptomatic dystonia, and a dystonia in heredodegenerative or other degenerative disorders. When cranial dystonia is the prominent feature in a widespread dystonia, NBAI, neuroacanthocytosis, and tardive dystonia have to be considered.

ESSENTIAL BLEPHAROSPASM

Prevalence

Blepharospasm is the most common form of cranial dystonia. After cervical dystonia, it is the second most common form of focal dystonia. Its exact prevalence is not known. Service-based surveys indicate a prevalence of 3.1 in 100 000.[27] Other data suggest a prevalence of 13.3 in 100 000.[28] The sex ratio ranges from 1.8 females to 1 male[29] to 2.5 females to 1 male.[30]

Clinical features

Essential blepharospasm starts in adult life, most commonly in the sixth or seventh decade. Its onset is insidious. Usually both eyes are affected equally, although unilateral onset has been described. Its first symptoms are often soreness of the eyes or the eyelids or dryness or excessive watering of the eyes. Later, excessive blinking occurs, especially on exposure to bright light or drafts, or when reading small texts, watching television, or when embarrassment, emotional tension, or fatigue occurs. Figure 9.5 gives an example of a patient with severe blepharospasm with additional perioral involvement. Frequently, patients wear dark glasses to protect their eyes from bright light and from drafts. Some patients avoid outdoor activities for these reasons. At this point, vision is impaired by losing text lines or focus during the blinking. Despite the relative mild vision impairment, patients are often severely disturbed, because of the constant additional effort to counteract blepharospasm. Socially, patients become stigmatized since the psychomotor communication with their environment becomes impaired and the increased blinking frequency is often misinterpreted as emotional instability or as a sign of substance abuse. Although increased blinking initially occurs only during certain periods, those periods later become prolonged and occur more frequently. The intensity of the blinking increases, so that eventually the eyelid closure is forced, and so prolonged that the patient is rendered functionally blind for long periods of the day. At this point, tension-type headache frequently occurs. During sleep, the condition disappears and in the morning the patient often feels relieved for the first few hours. Involvement of extraocular eye muscles does not occur. Some patients use tricks to open the eyes, such as forced jaw opening, yawning, neck extension, pressure with one finger against the temple bone, and preferentially using downward gaze. It is important to distinguish between primary dystonic muscle hyperactivity and secondary tricks to overcome it. Many patients experience corneal and conjunctival irritation due to impaired tear drainage. After prolonged courses, dehiscences of the eyelids can occur. In the upper eyelid, connective tissue may bulge over the pupil and may further impair vision. In the lower eyelid, entropion can develop with additional irritation of the cornea. One study suggested that Obsessive-compulsive symptoms are an associated feature of blepharospasm.[31]

Course

Essential blepharospasm usually begins insidiously. It slowly progresses to reach a plateau after some years. Once the condition has been stable for several years, further progress is rare. Spontaneous remissions are reported to occur in 10% of the patients within the first 5 years.[32] According to our experience, this rate is lower. When essential blepharospasm progresses, it can expand into adjacent body areas, i.e. into other cranial muscles and into the neck muscles. Figure 9.6 shows a patient with Meige syndrome. Generalization is exceedingly rare.

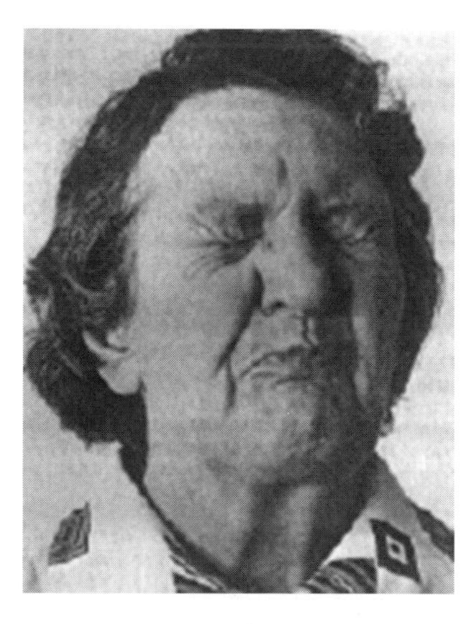

Figure 9.5 Blepharospasm with additional perioral involvement. (Reproduced from Marsden,[5] with permission.)

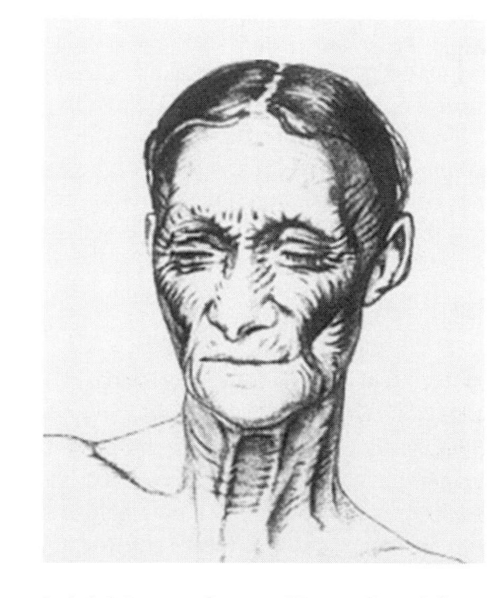

Figure 9.6 Meige syndrome. (Reproduced from Curshmann and Kramer,[33] with permission.)

Apraxia of eyelid opening

In some patients with essential blepharospasm, additional apraxia of eyelid opening can be detected by simultaneous electromyography of the orbicularis oculi and the levator palpebrae.[8,25,34–36] Pure essential blepharospasm and pure apraxia of eyelid opening may be extremes of a spectrum, with some patients presenting with a mixture of both elements.

Etiology

Essential blepharospasm is considered a focal dystonia since the pivotal studies of C David Marsden.[5] Its etiology is probably multifactorial, consisting of a genetic predisposition and additional factors. Occurrence of focal dystonia amongst first-degree relatives of patients with essential blepharospasm is reported to be about 6%.[37] Special forms of inheritance have also been reported.[38] Additional etiologic factors include basal ganglia or rostral brainstem lesions[30,39,40] preceding eyelid or ocular surface irritation, including dry eye problems,[41] and functional brainstem abnormalities.[42]

Treatment

Treatment of cranial dystonia consists of botulinum toxin therapy, drugs, surgery, and additional measures. Sometimes it may be necessary to combine different therapeutic regimens.

Drugs

Drug treatment of essential blepharospasm is usually frustrating. As shown in Table 9.2, there are a large number of drugs with occasional positive effects reported in the literature. All drugs suggested to treat other focal or generalized dystonias can be used for essential blepharospasm as well. Chances of improvement after drug treatment, however, are poor. Times to gradually build up the dose of each of the potentially antidystonic drugs are long. Frequently, severe adverse reactions occur, including dryness of mouth, drowsiness, concentration difficulties, agitation, and accommodation difficulties. The best therapeutic effects are seen with trihexyphenidyl, probably followed by baclofen, clonazepam, and tetrabenazine.

Table 9.2 Drugs used to treat dystonia

Anticholinergics	Trihexyphenidyl
	Biperiden
D_2 receptor blocking agents	Sulpiride
Dopamine depletors	Tetrabenazine
Benzodiazepines	Clonazepam
GABA agonists	Baclofen
Anticonvulsants	Carbamazepine
	Phenytoin
Others	Tizanidine

GABA = γ-aminobutyric acid.

Surgery

Traditional treatment of blepharospasm is the eyelid protractor myectomy procedure, including excision of the orbicularis oculi, the corrugator supercilii, and the procerus muscles.[43] Reported results indicate subjective improvement with long-term benefit in most of the patients treated. Consecutive tissue defects can be compensated by muscle grafts.[44] Additional application of botulinum toxin is possible. More recently, selective peripheral denervation procedures, so-called facial nerve avulsions, have been suggested.[45,46] The main problem with this operation is to control the degree of denervation in the target muscles, partly because the facial nerve branches form a complex nerve plexus.[47] Insufficient denervation produces suboptimal therapeutic effects and excessive denervation adverse effects, including ectropion and facial asymmetries. Reoperations to adjust the therapeutic effect, therefore, become frequently necessary.[48] Reinnervation and facial pain are other frequent side effects. For the frontalis suspension operation,[49,50] the upper eyelid is connected with subcutaneous strings to the frontalis muscle to facilitate eyelid opening. This operation is successful in apraxia of eyelid opening. In patients with apraxia of eyelid opening and blepharospasm, it should be combined with botulinum toxin therapy. In pure blepharospasm, it is not successful, since the eyelid closing forces may damage the string fixation. Pallidal stimulation has recently been tried for blepharospasm and Meige syndrome.[51]

Botulinum toxin

Botulinum toxin is by far the most successful treatment of cranial dystonias. When injected into muscle tissue, i.e. the target muscle, botulinum toxin produces a well-controllable paresis by blocking the neuromuscular junction. Apart from some minor spread into muscles adjacent to the target muscle it does not participate in general metabolism and thus does not produce adverse effects otherwise frequently seen with antidystonic drugs.

The botulinum toxin effect usually starts after 3–5 days and lasts for up to 4 months. The therapeutic effect of botulinum toxin is caused by relaxation of the dystonic muscle, thus reducing functional impairment and pain. Early application of botulinum toxin can avoid secondary complications of dystonia. Additional effects of botulinum toxin on muscle spindles and on the central nervous system have been described; a contribution to the therapeutic effect, however, remains unclear. Direct analgesic effects of botulinum toxin have been hypothesized, but their relevance in clinical practice is unclear. In order to achieve optimal therapeutic effects, dystonic muscles need to be identified and their dystonic involvement needs to be established so that they can be injected with adequate doses and unaffected muscles can be spared. Botulinum toxin drugs include Botox (Allergen Inc., Irvine, CA, USA), Dysport (Ipsen Ltd, Slough, Berks, UK), NeuroBloc/Myobloc (Solstice, Malvern, PA, USA), and Xeomin (Merz Pharmaceuticals, Frankfurt, Germany). Whereas Botox and Xeomin doses can be converted on a 1:1 basis, the conversion ratio between Botox and Dysport has been a matter of debate. Currently a 1:2 to 1:3 conversion rate seems to be most appropriate. The conversion ratio between Botox and NeuroBloc/Myobloc seems to be in the order of 1:40.

Possible target muscles and botulinum toxin doses for the treatment of blepharospasm are shown in Table 9.3. The primary target muscle is the orbicularis oculi, which is usually injected in three or four sites between its orbital and its tarsal part. Sparing of the muscle part covering the levator palpebrae muscle helps to avoid ptosis. Botulinum toxin injections into the pretarsal parts of the orbicularis oculi can be used to intensify the therapeutic effect. They seem to be particularly helpful in patients with components of apraxia of eyelid opening.[52,53] Mimic muscles adjacent to the orbicularis oculi, such as the procerus, the corrugator supercilii and the nasalis muscles, may also be used as target muscles. Injection of the frontalis muscle should be avoided because of its function as an auxiliary eyelid opening muscle. Botulinum toxin therapy of blepharospasm has a high success rate. Primary therapy failure is extremely rare and can be due to the presence of apraxia of eyelid opening and non-dystonic blepharospasm, excessive lid edema, eyelid dehiscences, doubled eyelids (shuang yan pi or dan yan pi) in Chinese patients,[54] and to concomitant entropion. In some patients, blepharospasm is associated with intense sensory irritations that may persist despite botulinum toxin-induced reduction of dystonic muscle hyperactivity. Secondary therapy failure can be due to the formation of neutralizing antibodies against botulinum neurotoxin. It is, however, exceedingly rare.[2] Side effects include hematoma, diplopia, ptosis, and ectropion. With the exception of hematoma, other side effects are rare and may be influenced by the botulinum toxin preparation used.[55]

Additional measures

Dark glasses may reduce the facilitating effects of bright light and drafts. Wire springs attached to spectacle frames have been suggested to push up the upper eyelids. When blepharospasm is severe, this approach is not effective; in minor cases or when eyelid dehiscences are present, it may have some effect. The use of adhesive tapes may be temporarily effective in mild cases, but frequently causes skin lacerations. Sensory tricks, such as touching skin of the temporal bone, may be partially effective. When blepharospasm has existed for a prolonged period of time, sometimes eyelid dehiscences can occur. When botulinum toxin injections are applied, they may be mobilized and may impair vision. Eyelid lifting operations can correct them. They are not effective to treat the muscle hyperactivity of blepharospasm. Application of artificial tears may compensate impaired lacrimal drainage.

Table 9.3 Possible target muscles and dose ranges for botulinum toxin therapy of blepharospasm

Muscle	Function	Botulinum toxin dose (100 MU Botox in 2.5 ml NaCl/H_2O) [MU Botox]
Orbicularis oculi	Eyelid closing	18–36
Procerus	Formation of transversal nasal root fold	6–12
Corrugator supercilii	Eyebrow adduction	6–12
Nasalis	Formation of nasal dorsum fold	4–8

Modified from Dressler.[2]

OROMANDIBULAR DYSTONIA

Prevalence

Oromandibular dystonia is substantially less common than cervical dystonia and may have similar prevalence to blepharospasm.[56] Valid data on the epidemiology, however, are lacking. There is a female preponderance of about 2:1.[6]

Clinical features

Oromandibular dystonia presents as a jaw opening type, jaw closing type, and as a mixed type. Most of the patients suffer from the jaw closing type.[6] Figure 9.7 shows a patient with oromandibular dystonia of the mixed type. Figure 9.8 shows two patients with oromandibular dystonia of the jaw opening type. Usually, oromandibular dystonia presents bilaterally, but side predominances may occur. Unilateral manifestations are very rare, but have been reported.[57] Associated features can include tongue protrusion, tongue twisting, and involvement of facial, neck, and pharyngeal muscles. Frequently, dysarthria and relative hypersalivation develops. Dysphagia and dyspnea are less frequent. In advanced cases, the condition is extremely stigmatizing and patients try to hide the jaw opening, tongue protrusion, and hypersalivation with their hands or with

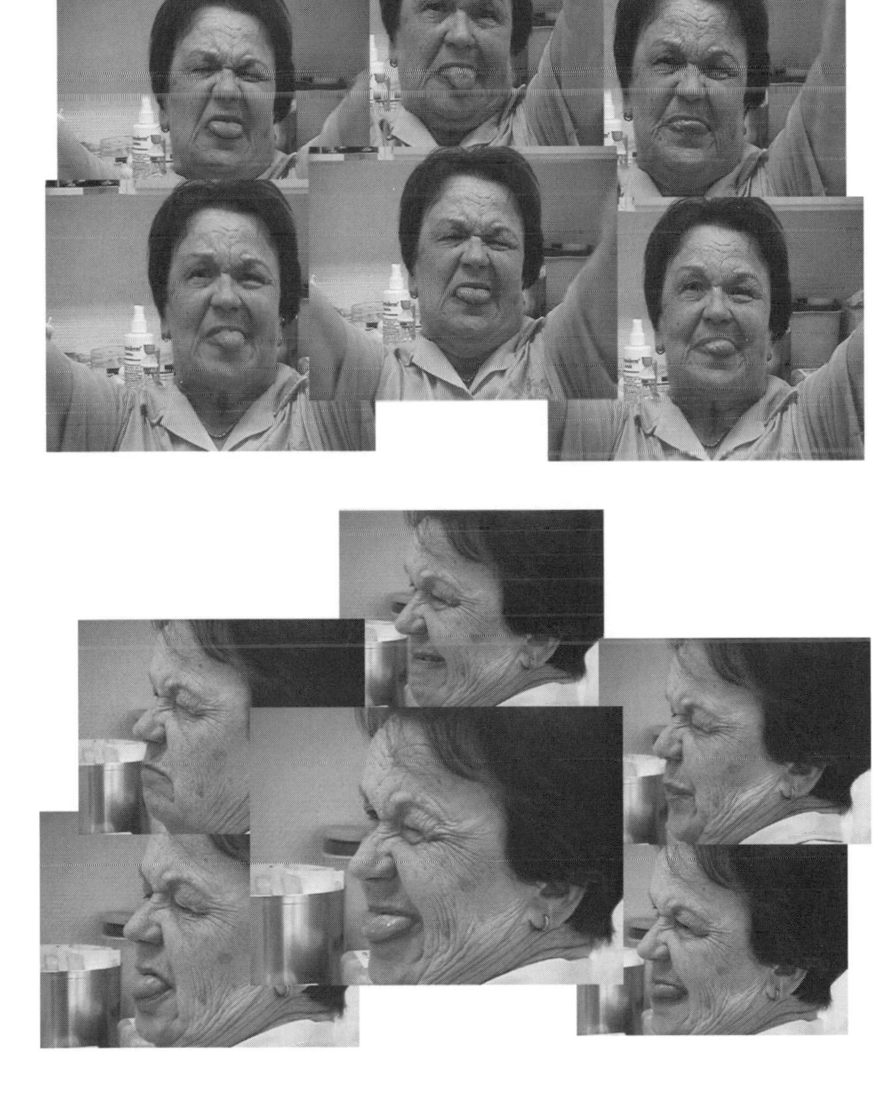

Figure 9.7
Orofaciomandibular dystonia with oromandibular dystonia of the mixed type and blepharospasm.

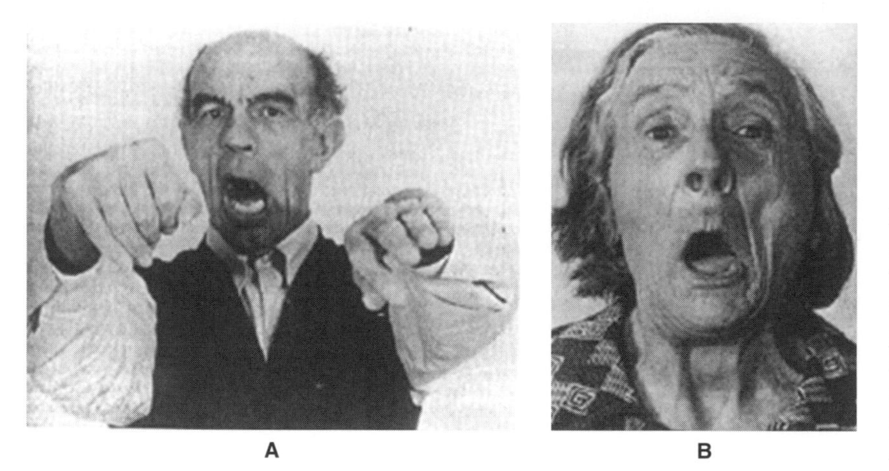

Figure 9.8 Oromandibular dystonia of the jaw opening type. (A) The cranial dystonia is probably facilitated by physical activity, such as holding the arms outstretched or by repetitively forming a fist. (Reproduced from Marsden,[5] with permission.)

towels. After a prolonged duration, temporomandibular joint impairment and muscular pain frequently occur. Jaw and tongue movements may loosen natural and artificial teeth.

Primary oromandibular dystonia

As with other primary focal dystonias, the onset of oromandibular dystonia is insidious. It usually reaches a plateau after several years. Further exacerbations are then rare. Oromandibular dystonia can spread into adjacent body parts. Generalization, however, is exceedingly rare.

Tardive oromandibular dystonia

Tardive oromandibular dystonia seems to have a more acute onset than idiopathic oromandibular dystonia. In one study it developed around six years after onset of D_2 blocking agent administration.[58] In some patients this latency may be as short as 4 days or as long as 23 years.[58] In 87% of patients with tardive muscle hyperactivity disorders, the first and predominant manifestation is in craniocervical muscles.[58] Oromandibular involvement often presents with typical complex licking and smacking movements. Additionally, cervical involvement with a high rate of antecollis and retrocollis[58] can be observed. Seven percent of patients present with respiratory problems,[59] including shortness of breath, irregular breathing patterns, and involuntary grunting and gasping noises.[60] Associated features include tremor, parkinsonian syndromes, akathisia, and limb stereotypies.[6] Numerous medicolegal problems are associated with tardive oromandibular dystonia, including obtaining informed consent in psychotic patients and properly balancing risks and benefits of D_2 receptor blocking agent therapy. Use of D_2 receptor blocking agents for treatment of minor depression, anxiety, or psychosomatic disorders may constitute medical malpractice.

Etiology

Oromandibular dystonia can occur as part of a more severe dystonia phenotype. When it is the predominant manifestation, a tardive etiology has to be considered. Pathophysiology of tardive oromandibular dystonia is still not fully understood. Evidence for a causal role of D_2 receptor blocking agents is compelling.[58] A number of lines of evidence suggest a key role for dopamine receptor hypersensitivity in the pathogenesis.[61] However, the effects of D_2 receptor blocking agents on other transmitter systems may also play a role in the pathophysiology of tardive dystonia. In some patients, oromandibular-facial trauma, including dental procedures, may precipitate the onset of oromandibular dystonia.[62,63]

Treatment

The decision to initiate treatment of oromandibular dystonia depends on the severity of the symptomatology. Especially in tardive oromandibular dystonia, some patients only have minor perioral muscle hyperactivities not requiring treatment.

Drugs

Drug treatment for primary oromandibular dystonia is similar to that for periocular or other dystonias. In tardive oromandibular dystonia, discontinuation of the causative agent provides a chance for spontaneous

Table 9.4 Possible target muscles and dose ranges for botulinum toxin therapy of oromandibular dystonia

Muscle	Function	Botulinum toxin dose (100 MU Botox in 2.5 ml $NaCl/H_2O$) [MU Botox]
Masseter	Jaw closing	40–60
Temporalis	Jaw closing	40–80
Pterygoidei	Jaw protrusion	20–60
	Jaw closing	
	Jaw lateralization	
	Jaw opening	
Mylohyoideus	Jaw opening	20–40
Mentalis	Formation of chin dimple	6–12
Depressor anguli oris	Depression of the corner of the mouth	4–8
Risorius	Abduction of the corner of the mouth	4–8
Platysma		16–32
Infrahyal muscles	Jaw opening	40–60

Modified from Dressler,[2] with permission.

remission. Debate is still open as to the percentage of patients improving. Whereas some authors report improvement in about half of their patients,[64–66] others have seen improvement in only 14% of patients.[58] On average, improvement occurs after 2.6 years, with some patients improving after 1 month, and others up to 9 years later.[58] When discontinuation is contraindicated because of the psychiatric diagnosis, atypical neuroleptics should be used. Benzodiazepines, such as clonazepam, may be helpful in minor cases for reduction of dystonia and of associated anxiety. Tetrabenazine is also effective and does not bear the risk of further aggravating the dystonic symptomatology. However, it has a significant risk of causing parkinsonism. As a last resort, D_2 blocking agents may be used successfully supporting the D_2 hypersensitivity hypothesis. However, they are said to reinforce the underlying pathophysiologic process and the dystonic symptomatology.

Botulinum toxin

Botulinum toxin therapy of oromandibular dystonia focuses on the jaw muscles. In the jaw closing type, botulinum toxin injections can be performed in the masseter bilaterally (Table 9.4). Rarely, additional botulinum toxin injections of the temporalis muscles are necessary. If there is remaining pain and jaw protrusion, botulinum toxin injections of the pterygoid muscles can also be performed. The therapeutic outcome of botulinum toxin therapy of jaw closing oromandibular dystonia is excellent. Apart from chewing fatigue, which can occur on prolonged chewing, adverse effects are rare. The jaw opening type is considerably more difficult to treat, since jaw opening is performed by numerous muscles in the front of the neck also involved in swallowing. The primary target muscles for jaw opening dystonia are the pterygoid muscles bilaterally.

Whereas the medial pterygoid is a jaw closing muscle, the lateral pterygoid is involved in all jaw movements, including jaw opening. For jaw opening dystonia, the lateral pterygoid should therefore be the primary target muscle. However, separation of both pterygoids would require electromyography and would, thus, complicate the elegant transcutaneous approach through the incisura mandibulae. Since isolated involvement of the lateral pterygoid has not been demonstrated anyway, transcutaneous injection of both pterygoids seems to be a practical approach. Often pain reduction and reduction of the jaw opening force is achieved. Additional injection of the mylohyoid muscles bilaterally and the infrahyoid muscles bilaterally can be tried. Swallowing difficulties, however, may be triggered. Botulinum toxin injections of the platysma can improve the cosmetic appearance, but have minor functional relevance. Botulinum toxin injections of perioral muscles are difficult because of a high risk of functional and cosmetically disturbing facial weakness. For this reason, botulinum toxin injections above the line between the upper and the lower lips should be avoided. Below this line, the depressor anguli oris muscle can be targeted.

Occasionally, instability of the lower lip may result. Botulinum toxin injections of the mentalis muscle have minor functional relevance, but improve cosmetic appearance considerably. Rarely, they produce side effects. Genioglossal muscle injections may reduce tongue protrusion. Botulinum toxin injections into the parotid gland bilaterally are effective to reduce drooling and to alleviate stigmatization of the patient.

Additional measures

Splints have been used for many years to treat jaw closing oromandibular dystonia by diverting the jaw closing force to a larger area, and thus protecting the teeth. They may also reduce the generation of dystonic muscle hyperactivity by changing the jaw position and the jaw mechanics. In severe cases, application of a percutaneous endoscopic gastrostomy may become necessary.

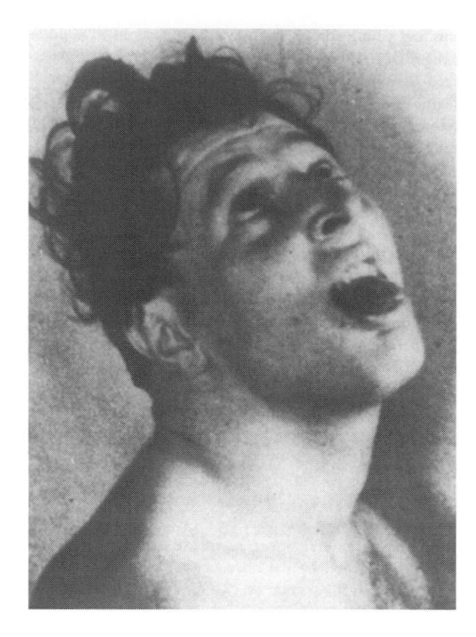

Figure 9.9 Acute dystonic reaction to application of dopamine D_2 blocking agents with oculogyric crisis, retrocollis, right torticollis, jaw opening, and tongue protrusion. (Reproduced from Delay and Deniker,[76] with permission.)

OTHER CRANIAL DYSTONIAS

Bruxism

Bruxism is used to describe forceful jaw closures producing grinding or clenching of the teeth. Bruxism can be part of a more widespread oromandibular dystonia. It can also be an isolated occurrence. Isolated bruxism usually presents at night, justifying the term sleep bruxism. It is produced by a relatively typical electromyographic pattern.[67] The prevalence of bruxism may be as high as 8% of the general population.[68] In children and young adults, its prevalence may be considerably higher.[69] Sex differences seem not to exist.[67] The etiology of bruxism is not clear. Dopaminergic mechanisms may be involved, as suggested by the frequent association between isolated bruxism and periodic movements in sleep.[70] Bruxism may also present exaggerated physiologic jaw movements.[68] Facilitation of bruxism by emotional stress has been debated controversely. It becomes a pathologic condition in a minority of individuals affected, when tooth problems, jaw muscle pain, temporomandibular joint impairment, and non-restorative sleep occurs. Spouses may also be disturbed in their night sleep. Alcohol, amphetamine, cocaine, and tricyclic antidepressants can exacerbate isolated bruxism.[71,72] Oral splinting has been used for decades and seems to help.[73] It protects the teeth and may reduce bruxism's intensity and frequency. Botulinum toxin therapy may also be tried in more severe cases.

Acute dystonic reactions

Acute dystonic reactions are tonic muscles hyperactivities induced by application of D_2 receptor blocking agents. They most often affect the external eye muscles, producing the clinical picture of oculogyric crisis with gaze deviation upward or sideward first described as sequalae of encephalitis lethargica.[74] They also affect mimic muscles and jaw, tongue, and pharyngeal muscles, typically producing forced mouth opening and tongue protrusion. Extracranial manifestations include the neck and trunk muscles and less frequently the limb muscles, producing head tilt backward or sideways and trunk arching.[75] Figure 9.9 shows a patient with an acute dystonic reaction with oculogyric crisis, retrocollis, right torticollis, jaw opening, and tongue protrusion. Often, muscle hyperactivities seen in acute dystonic reactions are so forceful that acute pain occurs. Pharyngeal involvement may trigger anxiety. Acute dystonic reactions mostly occur in males and in young patients.[77] Previous acute dystonic reactions are an additional predictor for additional acute dystonic reactions.[78] Half of the patients develop their acute dystonic reactions within 2 days and 90% within 5 days after initiation of D_2 receptor blocking agent treatment.[79,80] The frequency of acute dystonic reactions varies according to the type of D_2 receptor blocking agent used. Highly potent D_2 blocking agents such as haloperidol and fluphenazine may produce acute dystonic reactions in more than 50% of patients treated,[81] whereas low-potency D_2 blocking agents like thioridazine and chlorpromazine bear a lower risk.[78,82] Acute dystonic reactions can also be triggered by risperidone,[83,84] clozapine,[85] tetrabenazine,[86] and serotonergics,[87,88] probably by side effects or indirect effects on D_2 receptors.

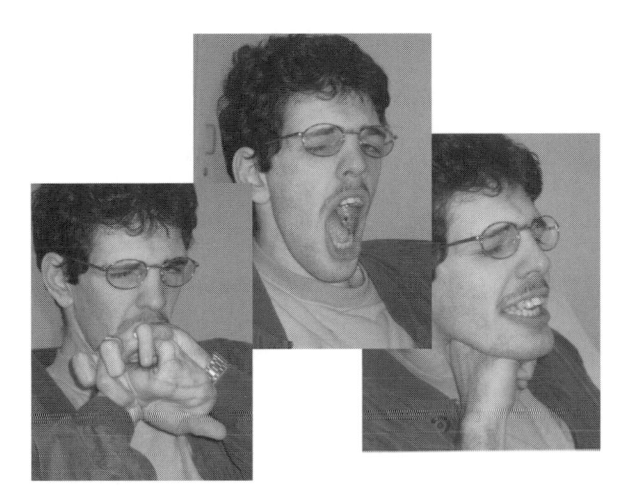

Figure 9.10 Neurodegeneration with brain accumulation of iron. The patient presents with severe oromandibular dystonia of the jaw opening type with temporomandibular joint subluxation. External pressure is used to keep the mouth shut. Additional features include blepharospasm and voluntary hyperextension of the finger joints. Later, the patient developed severe bilateral extensor type leg dystonia.

D_2 blocking agents are also used in antiemetics, such as metoclopramide and prochlorperazine, both of which can cause acute dystonic reactions.[89] Applied to children, metoclopramide can trigger acute dystonic reactions in up to one-third of the patients.[90] The pathophysiology of acute dystonic reactions is complex and not fully understood. A dysbalance between dopaminergic and cholinergic functions seems to be involved. Postacute D_2 receptor sensitivity changes may also play a role. Application of anticholinergics, such as biperiden or benztropine, or of antihistamines, such as diphenhydramine, almost invariably produces relief within 15–30 minutes.[91] Occasionally, repeated application may become necessary. Without therapy, acute dystonic reactions resolve within 12–48 hours. Acute dystonic reactions should be prevented by using D_2 receptor blocking agents in the lowest effective doses only. Contrary to antiquated belief, extrapyramidal side effects are not necessary to produce antipsychotic effects. Therefore, handwriting tests to monitor parkinsonism for optimal dose adjustment of neuroleptics are obsolete. In at-risk populations, prophylactic application of anticholinergics is justified.

Neurodegeneration with brain accumulation of iron (Hallervorden–Spatz syndrome)

NBAI is an autosomal recessive disorder characterized by dystonia, parkinsonism, and iron accumulation in the brain. Typically, it presents with predominant oromandibular dystonia.[92] Figure 9.10 shows a patient with NBAI with severe oromandibular dystonia of the

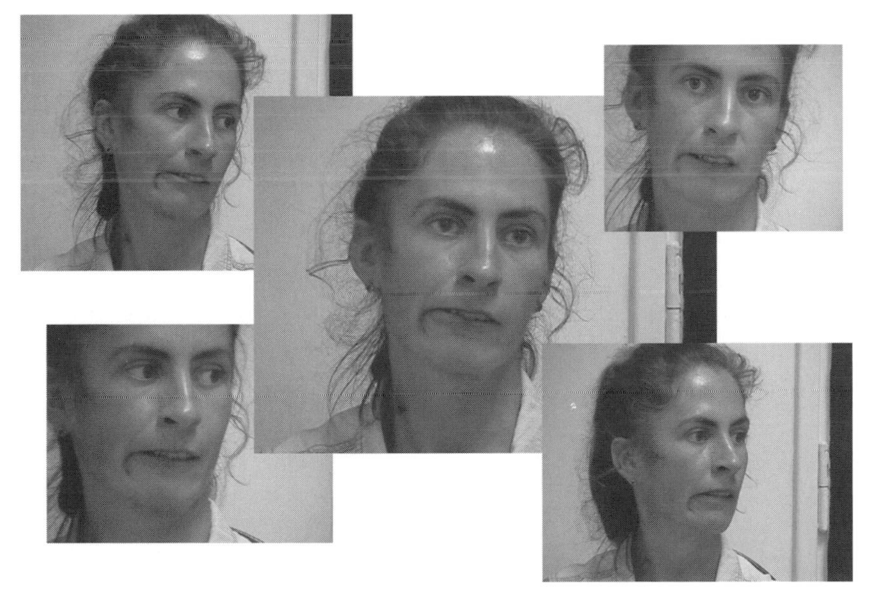

Figure 9.11 Wilson's disease. The patient presents with oromandibular dystonia of the jaw closing type with typical abduction of the corners of the mouth (risus sardonicus).

jaw opening type. Classically, the syndrome starts in childhood and deteriorates rapidly. Atypical cases have a later onset and a slower progression.[93] T2-weighted magnetic resonance imaging reveals a specific pattern of hyperintensity within the hypointense medial globus pallidus, the eye-of-the-tiger sign.[94] A defect in the pantothenate kinase gene (*PANK2*) can be detected in a large number of patients. Botulinum toxin therapy applied to jaw muscles is helpful.[95] In advanced cases, botulinum toxin injections into the neck, axial, and limb muscles may be applied.

Neuroacanthocytosis

Neuroacanthocytosis consists of a group of three inherited disorders presenting with abnormal erythrocyte configuration and different neurologic symptoms. In chorea-acanthocytosis, an autosomal recessive condition, oromandibular dystonia with typical lip and tongue biting is the predominant clinical feature.[96,97]

Risus sardonicus in Wilson's disease

The risus sardonicus of Wilson's disease, a jaw closing oromandibular dystonia with typical abduction of the corners of the mouth, is usually preceded by gait ataxia, dysarthria, and limb tremor, which can be of the highly typical wing-flapping type. Figure 9.11 shows a patient with Wilson's disease and risus sardonicus. Frequently, hepatic manifestations are present. Chelating compounds are highly effective when used early in the disease. Botulinum toxin injections can also be tried for remaining symptomatologies.

Auctioneer's jaw

Auctioneer's jaw is an extremely rare task-specific dystonic muscle hyperactivity in the jaw muscles, exclusively and predictably triggered by the typical auctioneer's selling 'patter'.[98] Botulinum toxin injections are helpful.

Trismus

Trismus, forced and painful jaw closure, is one of the predominant manifestations of tetanus.[99] Symptomatic treatment can include botulinum toxin therapy.[100]

Familial nocturnal faciomandibular myoclonus

Familial nocturnal faciomandibular myoclonus is an extremely rare condition characterized by nocturnal tongue biting with bleeding. Muscle activities originate in the masseters and spread to the orbicularis oris and orbicularis oculi muscles. They only occur at sleep and seem to be familial.[101] The term myoclonus may be misleading.

REFERENCES

1. Penfield W, Rasmussen T. The Cerebral Cortex of Man. New York: Macmillan; 1950.
2. Dressler D. Botulinum Toxin Therapy. Stuttgart: Thieme; 2000.
3. Waldeyer A, Mayet A. Anatomie des Menschen. 16. Auflage. Berlin: Walter de Gruyter; 1993.
4. Meige H. Les convulsions de la face, une forme clinique de convulsion faciale, bilatérale et médiane. Rev Neurologique (Paris) 1910; 20: 437–43.
5. Marsden CD. Blepharospasm-oromandibular dystonia syndrome (Brueghel's syndrome). A variant of adult-onset torsion dystonia? J Neurol Neurosurg Psychiatry 1976; 39: 1204–9.
6. Tan EK, Jankovic J. Botulinum toxin A in patients with oromandibular dystonia: long-term follow-up. Neurology 1999; 53: 2102–7.
7. Machado FC, Fregni F, Campos CR, Limongi JC. [Bilateral hemifacial spasm: case report]. Arq Neuropsiquiatr 2003; 61: 115–18. [in Portuguese].
8. Boghen DR. Disorders of facial motor function. Curr Opin Ophthalmol 1996; 7: 48–52.
9. Tatlipinar S, Iener EC, Ilhan B, Semerci B. Ophthalmic manifestations of Gilles de la Tourette syndrome. Eur J Ophthalmol 2001; 11: 223–6.
10. Robertson MM. The Gilles de la Tourette syndrome: the current status. Br J Psychiatry 1989; 154: 147–9.
11. Roberts ME, Steiger MJ, Hart IK. Presentation of myasthenia gravis mimicking blepharospasm. Neurology 2002; 58: 150–1.
12. Kanzato N, Motomura M, Suehara M, Arimura K. Lambert–Eaton myasthenic syndrome with ophthalmoparesis and pseudoblepharospasm. Muscle Nerve 1999; 22: 1727–30.
13. Schrag A, Quinn NP, Bhatia KP, Marsden CD. Benign hereditary chorea – entity or syndrome? Mov Disord 2000; 15: 280–8.
14. Breedveld GJ, Percy AK, MacDonald ME et al. Clinical and genetic heterogeneity in benign hereditary chorea. Neurology 2002; 59: 579–84.
15. Thompson PD, Carroll WM. Hemimasticatory and hemifacial spasm: a common pathophysiology? Clin Exp Neurol 1983; 19: 110–19.
16. Esteban A, Traba A, Prieto J, Grandas F. Long term follow up of a hemimasticatory spasm. Acta Neurol Scand 2002; 105: 67–72.
17. Cruccu G, Inghilleri M, Berardelli A et al. Pathophysiology of hemimasticatory spasm. J Neurol Neurosurg Psychiatry 1994; 57: 43–50.
18. Ebersbach G, Kabus C, Schelosky L, Terstegge L, Poewe W. Hemimasticatory spasm in hemifacial atrophy: diagnostic and therapeutic aspects in two patients. Mov Disord 1995; 10: 504–7.
19. Kim HJ, Jeon BS, Lee KW. Hemimasticatory spasm associated with localized scleroderma and facial hemiatrophy. Arch Neurol 2000; 57: 576–80.
20. D'Alessandro R, Benassi G, Cristina E, Gallassi R, Manzaroli D. The prevalence of lingual-facial-buccal dyskinesias in the elderly. Neurology 1986; 36: 1350–1.
21. Warren JD, Firgaira F, Thompson EM et al. The causes of sporadic and 'senile' chorea. Aust N Z J Med 1998; 28: 429–31.

22. Delwaide PJ, Hurlet A. Bromocriptine and buccolinguofacial dyskinesias in patients with senile dementia. A quantitative study. Arch Neurol 1980; 37: 441–3.
23. Lee RJ, Yolton RL, Yolton DP, Schnider C, Janin ML. Personal defense sprays: effects and management of exposure. J Am Optom Assoc 1996; 67: 548–60.
24. Macia F, Ballan G, Yekhlef F et al. [Progressive supranuclear palsy: a clinical, natural history and disability study]. Rev Neurol (Paris) 2003; 159: 31–42. [in French]
25. Lamberti P, De Mari M, Zenzola A, Aniello MS, Defazio G. Frequency of apraxia of eyelid opening in the general population and in patients with extrapyramidal disorders. Neurol Sci 2002; 23(Suppl 2): S81–2.
26. Topaloglu H, Serdaroglu A, Okan M, Gucuyener K, Topcu M. Improvement of myotonia with carbamazepine in three cases with the Schwartz–Jampel syndrome. Neuropediatrics 1993; 24: 232–4.
27. Castelon Konkiewitz E, Trender-Gerhard I, Kamm C et al. Service-based survey of dystonia in Munich. Neuroepidemiology 2002; 21(4): 202–6.
28. Defazio G, Livrea P, De Salvia R et al. Prevalence of primary blepharospasm in a community of Puglia region, Southern Italy. Neurology 2001; 56: 1579–81.
29. Grandas F, Elston J, Quinn N, Marsden CD. Blepharospasm: a review of 264 patients. J Neurol Neurosurg Psychiatry 1988; 51: 767–72.
30. Defazio G, Lamberti P, Lepore V, Livrea P, Ferrari E. Facial dystonia: clinical features, prognosis and pharmacology in 31 patients. Ital J Neurol Sci 1989; 10: 553–60.
31. Broocks A, Thiel A, Angerstein D, Dressler D. Higher prevalence of obsessive-compulsive symptoms in patients with blepharospasm than in patients with hemifacial spasm. Am J Psychiatry 1998; 155: 555–7.
32. Castelbuono A, Miller NR. Spontaneous remission in patients with essential blepharospasm and Meige syndrome. Am J Ophthalmol 1998; 126: 432–5.
33. Curshmann H, Kramer F. Lehrbuch der Nervenkrankheiten. 2. Auflage. Berlin: Springer; 1925.
34. Krack P, Marion MH. "Apraxia of lid opening," a focal eyelid dystonia: clinical study of 32 patients. Mov Disord 1994; 9: 610–15.
35. Aramideh M, Ongerboer de Visser BW, Devriese PP, Bour LJ, Speelman JD. Electromyographic features of levator palpebrae superioris and orbicularis oculi muscles in blepharospasm. Brain 1994; 117: 27–38.
36. Tozlovanu V, Forget R, Iancu A, Boghen D. Prolonged orbicularis oculi activity: a major factor in apraxia of lid opening. Neurology 2001; 57: 1013–18.
37. Elston JS. Botulinum toxin for blepharospasm. In: Jankovic J, Hallett M, eds. Therapy with Botulinum Toxin. New York: Marcel Dekker; 1994: 191–7.
38. Defazio G, Brancati F, Valente EM et al. Familial blepharospasm is inherited as an autosomal dominant trait and relates to a novel unassigned gene. Mov Disord 2003; 18: 207–12.
39. Jankovic J. Blepharospasm with basal ganglia lesions. Arch Neurol 1986; 43: 866–8.
40. Gibb WR, Lees AJ, Marsden CD. Pathological report of four patients presenting with cranial dystonias. Mov Disord 1988; 3: 211–21.
41. Elston JS, Marsden CD, Grandas F, Quinn NP. The significance of ophthalmological symptoms in idiopathic blepharospasm. Eye 1988; 2: 435–9.
42. Hasan SA, Baker RS, Sun WS et al. The role of blink adaptation in the pathophysiology of benign essential blepharospasm. Arch Ophthalmol 1997; 115: 631–6.
43. Chapman KL, Bartley GB, Waller RR, Hodge DO. Follow-up of patients with essential blepharospasm who underwent eyelid protractor myectomy at the Mayo Clinic from 1980 through 1995. Ophthal Plast Reconstr Surg 1999; 15: 106–10.
44. Yen MT, Anderson RL, Small RG. Orbicularis oculi muscle graft augmentation after protractor myectomy in blepharospasm. Ophthal Plast Reconstr Surg 2003; 19: 287–96.
45. Bates AK, Halliday BL, Bailey CS, Collin JR, Bird AC. Surgical management of essential blepharospasm. Br J Ophthalmol 1991; 75: 487–90.
46. Fante RG, Frueh BR. Differential section of the seventh nerve as a tertiary procedure for the treatment of benign essential blepharospasm. Ophthal Plast Reconstr Surg 2001; 17: 276–80.
47. Nemoto Y, Sekino Y. Anatomical reasons for problems after neurectomy for blepharospasm: a study in cadavers. Scand J Plast Reconstr Surg Hand Surg 2000; 34: 21–5.
48. McCord CD Jr, Coles WH, Shore JW, Spector R, Putnam JR. Treatment of essential blepharospasm. I. Comparison of facial nerve avulsion and eyebrow-eyelid muscle stripping procedure. Arch Ophthalmol 1984; 102: 266–8.
49. Roggenkamper P, Nussgens Z. Frontalis suspension in the treatment of essential blepharospasm unresponsive to botulinum-toxin therapy: long-term results. Graefes Arch Clin Exp Ophthalmol 1997; 235: 486–9.
50. De Groot V, De Wilde F, Smet L, Tassignon MJ. Frontalis suspension combined with blepharoplasty as an effective treatment for blepharospasm associated with apraxia of eyelid opening. Ophthal Plast Reconstr Surg 2000; 16: 34–8.
51. Capelle HH, Weigel R, Krauss JK. Bilateral pallidal stimulation for blepharospasm-oromandibular dystonia (Meige syndrome). Neurology 2003; 60: 2017–18.
52. Boghen D, Tozlovanu V, Iancu A, Forget R. Botulinum toxin therapy for apraxia of lid opening. Ann NY Acad Sci 2002; 956: 482–3.
53. Forget R, Tozlovanu V, Iancu A, Boghen D. Botulinum toxin improves lid opening delays in blepharospasm-associated apraxia of lid opening. Neurology 2002; 58: 1843–6.
54. Dressler D. Complete secondary botulinum toxin therapy failure in blepharospasm. J Neurol 2000; 247: 809–10.
55. Dressler D. Dysport produces intrinsically more swallowing problems than Botox: unexpected results from a conversion factor study in cervical dystonia. J Neurol Neurosurg Psychiatry 2002; 73: 604.
56. Nutt JG, Muenter MD, Melton LJ 3rd, Aronson A, Kurland LT. Epidemiology of dystonia in Rochester, Minnesota. Adv Neurol 1988; 50: 361–5.
57. Thompson PD, Obeso JA, Delgado G, Gallego J, Marsden CD. Focal dystonia of the jaw and the differential diagnosis of unilateral jaw and masticatory spasm. J Neurol Neurosurg Psychiatry 1986; 49: 651–6.
58. Kiriakakis V, Bhatia KP, Quinn NP, Marsden CD. The natural history of tardive dystonia. A long-term follow-up study of 107 cases. Brain 1998; 121: 2053–66.
59. Yassa R, Lal S. Respiratory irregularity and tardive dyskinesia. A prevalence study. Acta Psychiatr Scand 1986; 73: 506–10.
60. Weiner WJ, Goetz CG, Nausieda PA, Klawans HL. Respiratory dyskinesias: extrapyramidal dysfunction and dyspnea. Ann Intern Med 1978; 88: 327–31.
61. Kane JM. Tardive dyskinesia. In: Joseph AB, Young RR, eds. Movement Disorders in Neurology and Neuropsychiatry. Malden, MA: Blackwell Science; 1999: 31–5.
62. Sankhla C, Lai EC, Jankovic J. Peripherally induced oromandibular dystonia. J Neurol Neurosurg Psychiatry 1998; 65: 722–8.
63. Schrag A, Bhatia KP, Quinn NP, Marsden CD. Atypical and typical cranial dystonia following dental procedures. Mov Disord 1999; 14: 492–6.

64. Gimenez-Roldan S, Mateo D, Bartolome P. Tardive dystonia and severe tardive dyskinesia. A comparison of risk factors and prognosis. Acta Psychiatr Scand 1998; 71: 488–94.
65. Itoh H, Yagi G. Reversibility of tardive dyskinesia. Folia Psychiatr Neurol Jpn 1979; 33: 43–54.
66. Mauriello JA Jr, Carbonaro P, Dhillon S, Leone T, Franklin M. Drug-associated facial dyskinesias – a study of 238 patients. J Neuroophthalmol 1998; 18: 153–7.
67. Hartmann E. Alcohol and bruxism. N Engl J Med 1979; 301: 333–4.
68. Lavigne GJ, Kato T, Kolta A, Sessle BJ. Neurobiological mechanisms involved in sleep bruxism. Crit Rev Oral Biol Med 2003; 14: 30–46.
69. Wigdorowicz-Makowerowa N, Grodzki C, Panek H et al. Epidemiologic studies on prevalence and etiology of functional disturbances of the masticatory system. J Prosthet Dent 1979; 41: 76–82.
70. Montplaisir J, Godbout R, Boghen D et al. Familial restless legs with periodic movements in sleep: electrophysiologic, biochemical, and pharmacologic study. Neurology 1985; 35: 130–4.
71. Hartmann E, Mehta N, Forgione A. Bruxism: effects of alcohol. Sleep Res 1987; 16: 185–388.
72. Ehrenberg BL. Sleep bruxism. In: Joseph AB, Young RR, eds. Movement Disorders in Neurology and Neuropsychiatry, 2nd edn. Malden, MA: Blackwell Science; 1999: 594–6.
73. Sheikholeslam A, Holmgren K, Riise C. Therapeutic effects of the plane occlusal splint on signs and symptoms of craniomandibular disorders in patients with nocturnal bruxism. J Oral Rehabil 1993; 20: 473–82.
74. Von Economo C. Encephalitis Lethargica: Its Sequelae and Treatment. London: Oxford University Press; 1931.
75. Rupniak NM, Jenner P, Marsden CD. Acute dystonia induced by neuroleptic drugs. Psychopharmacology (Berl) 1986; 88: 403–19.
76. Delay J, Deniker P. Drug-induced extrapyramidal syndromes. In: Vincken PJ, Bruyn GW, eds. Handbook of Clinical Neurology, Vol. 6. Diseases of the Basal Ganglia. Amsterdam: North Holland Publishing, 1968: 248–66.
77. Aguilar EJ, Keshavan MS, Martinez-Quiles MD et al. Predictors of acute dystonia in first-episode psychotic patients. Am J Psychiatry 1994; 151: 1819–21.
78. Keepers GA, Casey DE. Prediction of neuroleptic-induced dystonia. J Clin Psychopharmacol 1987; 7: 342–5.
79. Ayd FJ. A survey of drug-induced extrapyramidal reactions. JAMA 1961; 75: 1054–60.
80. Garver DL, Davis DM, Dekirmenjian H et al. Dystonic reactions following neuroleptics: time course and proposed mechanisms. Psychopharmacologia 1976; 47: 199–201.
81. Boyer WF, Bakalar NH, Lake CR. Anticholinergic prophylaxis of acute haloperidol-induced acute dystonic reactions. J Clin Psychopharmacol 1987; 7: 164–6.
82. Keepers GA, Clappison VJ, Casey DE. Initial anticholinergic prophylaxis for neuroleptic-induced extrapyramidal syndromes. Arch Gen Psychiatry 1983; 40: 1113–17.
83. Brody AL. Acute dystonia induced by rapid increase in risperidone dosage. J Clin Psychopharmacol 1996; 16: 461–2.
84. Simpson GM, Lindenmayer JP. Extrapyramidal symptoms in patients treated with risperidone. J Clin Psychopharmacol 1997; 17: 194–201.
85. Kastrup O, Gastpar M, Schwarz M. Acute dystonia due to clozapine. J Neurol Neurosurg Psychiatry 1994; 57: 119.
86. Burke RE, Reches A, Traub MM et al. Tetrabenazine induces acute dystonic reactions. Ann Neurol 1985; 17: 200–2.
87. Olivera AO. Sertraline and akathisia: spontaneous resolution. Biol Psychiatry 1997; 41: 241–2.
88. Madhusoodanan S, Brenner R. Reversible choreiform dyskinesia and extrapyramidal symptoms associated with sertraline therapy. J Clin Psychopharmacol 1997; 17: 138–9.
89. Bateman DN, Darling WM, Boys R, Rawlins MD. Extrapyramidal reactions to metoclopramide and prochlorperazine. Q J Med 1989; 71: 307–11.
90. Kris MG, Tyson LB, Gralla RJ et al. Extrapyramidal reactions with high-dose metoclopramide. N Engl J Med 1983; 309: 433–4.
91. Keepers GA, Casey DE. Clinical management of acute neuroleptic-induced extrapyramidal syndromes. Curr Psychiatr Ther 1986; 23: 139–57.
92. Angelini L, Nardocci N, Rumi V et al. Hallervorden–Spatz disease: clinical and MRI study of 11 cases diagnosed in life. J Neurol 1992; 239: 417–25.
93. Hayflick SJ, Westaway SK, Levinson B et al. Genetic, clinical, and radiographic delineation of Hallervorden–Spatz syndrome. N Engl J Med 2003; 348: 33–40.
94. Guillerman RP. The eye-of-the-tiger sign. Radiology 2000; 217: 895–6.
95. Dressler D, Wittstock M, Benecke R. Botulinum toxin for treatment of jaw opening dystonia in Hallervorden–Spatz syndrome. Eur Neurol 2001; 45(4): 287–8.
96. Estes JW, Morley TJ, Levine IM, Emerson CP. A new hereditary acanthocytosis syndrome. Am J Med 1967; 42: 868–81.
97. Rampoldi L, Danek A, Monaco AP. Clinical features and molecular bases of neuroacanthocytosis. J Mol Med 2002; 80: 475–91.
98. Scolding NJ, Smith SM, Sturman S, Brookes GB, Lees AJ. Auctioneer's jaw: a case of occupational oromandibular hemidystonia. Mov Disord 1995; 10: 508–9.
99. Lau LG, Kong KO, Chew PH. A ten-year retrospective study of tetanus at a general hospital in Malaysia. Singapore Med J 2001; 42: 346–50.
100. Andrade LA, Brucki SM. Botulinum toxin A for trismus in cephalic tetanus. Arq Neuropsiquiatr 1994; 52: 410–13.
101. Vetrugno R, Provini F, Plazzi G et al. Familial nocturnal faciomandibular myoclonus mimicking sleep bruxism. Neurology 2002; 58: 644–7.

10

Writer's cramp, limb dystonia, and other task-specific dystonias

Jörg Müller and Werner Poewe

INTRODUCTION

The dystonias have been classified by a variety of criteria, including age at onset, anatomic distribution, etiology, and, most recently, genetics. One of the most striking and puzzling features of certain types of dystonia has been the selective involvement of certain motor programs where dystonic muscle contractions are restricted to specific tasks or motor acts while the same muscles can be activated normally with most or all other activities. Writer's cramp is the most common and prominent example of the task-specific dystonias, but selective hand dystonia can also affect a variety of other manual skills such as typing, sorting, and painting; playing string or keyboard instruments; or engaging in sports like tennis, golf, or snooker. The common theme to all task-specific dystonias is that they selectively affect highly overlearned and automated types of movement and that treatment often fails to restore the premorbid level of function for the tasks involved. This chapter reviews the clinical features, pathophysiology, prognosis, and treatment of the task-specific dystonias as well as other limb-selective dystonias.

WRITER'S CRAMP

Writer's cramp is the most common type of task-specific dystonia. The reported frequency among the focal dystonias ranges from 5% to 19% in different epidemiologic studies[1–5] and a European medical record-based study found a prevalence of 1.4 per 100 000.[2] Recent epidemiologic studies suggest that the prevalence of primary focal dystonia, including writer's cramp, in the general population may be much higher than assumed from hospital-based series.[6,7]

Clinical features

Writer's cramp, typically, is a disorder of mid-adulthood affecting patients between the third and fifth decade, with a mean age at onset in the mid thirties or mid forties.[8–10] There is no specific precipitant in most cases, but occasional patients may report a history of trauma or strain to the affected limb,[8,9] and, in historical series of patients with writer's cramp, office clerks engaged in professional handwriting were over-represented.[11,12] Initial symptoms may be feelings of tension in the fingers or forearms that interfere with the fluency of writing; a minority may also experience pain.[8] The pen is held abnormally forcefully due to dystonic contraction of the hand and/or forearm muscles, causing different patterns of deviation from the normal or premorbid pen grip and hand posture (Figures 10.1 and 10.2). A common pattern involves excessive flexion of the thumb and index finger, with pronation of the hand and ulnar deviation of the wrist.[10] Other patients may have abnormal activation of wrist flexors, with supination of the hand and flexion of the wrist. Individual patients may experience involuntary lifting off of the index or thumb from the pen or isolated extension of other fingers as well. When dystonic cramps affect up to three fingers only, Cohen and Hallett have suggested the term of 'localized' (vs non-localized) writer's cramp.[9] The forearm muscles most often involved in writer's cramp are the flexor carpi ulnaris and radialis, flexor digitorum superficialis, flexor pollicis longus, and extensor digitorum communis muscles.[13–16]

Up to 50% of patients with writer's cramp may also show upper limb tremor.[8] Like the dystonic movements themselves, tremor in writer's cramp can be task specific,[17] whereas in other instances it may resemble typical essential tremor.[18] Several reports have emphasized the occurrence of task-specific tremor without

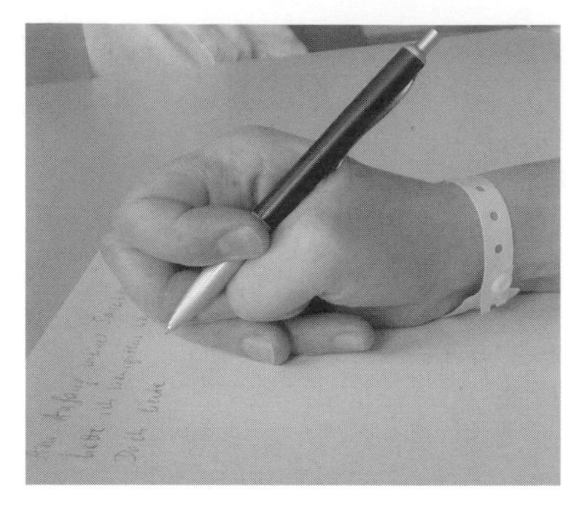

Figure 10.1 Patient with localized writer's cramp affecting the first three fingers of the right hand.

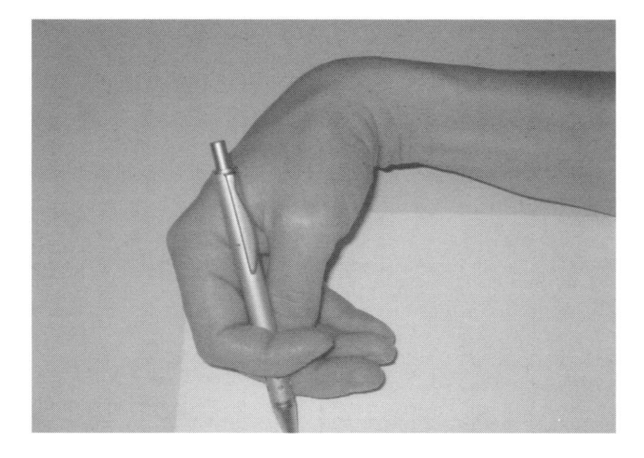

Figure 10.2 Patient with simple writer's cramp showing involuntary flexion of the wrist and dystonic posturing of the thumb and index finger during writing.

associated dystonic features when writing and termed this condition primary writing tremor. Although possibly related to writer's cramp, writing tremor is currently classified among tremor disorders rather than dystonias.[17]

Although sensations of strain and aching in dystonic forearm muscles are common in writer's cramp, pain – unlike in cervical dystonia – is rarely a prominent feature, presumably due to the task-specific and intermittent nature of the disorder where the build-up of pain would normally stop individuals from performing the task.

Course and prognosis

About a third of patients initially note intermittent problems and at the beginning of their illness may be able to write short stretches of text normally before dystonic cramping starts to interfere with their script. Such patients generally note progressive shortening of the time during which they can write without onset of dystonic finger or hand movements. A majority of patients with writer's cramp, however, complain of difficulties with holding a pen and impaired script as soon as they start writing already at disease onset.[8–10]

A minority of individuals with writer's cramp also have dystonia when engaging their affected hand in other manual tasks, such as opening the lid of a jar or manipulating a variety of objects (shaving, brushing teeth, handling a knife and fork). Sheehy and Marsden[8] have suggested the term 'dystonic writer's cramp' to differentiate such patients from the majority where dystonia is selective for the act of writing ('simple writer's cramp'). These authors found that a proportion (8 of 21 in their series) of patients may progress from simple to dystonic writer's cramp within months or years.[8]

Whereas progression of writer's cramp to involve other manual tasks is not uncommon, spontaneous remissions are rare and have only exceptionally been described.[18] Many patients with writer's cramp develop strategies by which they try to overcome their writing problems. These include changes in the way they hold their pen, often supported by adaptations to the shape and size of the pen to support changes in finger and hand positions to the pen.

Some 50% of patients who are no longer able to write intelligibly attempt to learn to write with the contralateral unaffected hand and a proportion of these will develop similar difficulties in this hand over periods as short as a few months to many years. About 5% of patients who have relearned to write with their non-dominant hand will display dystonic mirror movements of their initially affected hand when writing.[19]

Investigations

Writer's cramp is a straightforward clinical diagnosis in cases with typical onset and presentation. Neurophysiologic studies reveal a number of abnormalities but are not strictly necessary in clinical routine. While routine electromyography (EMG) and nerve conduction studies of forearm muscles and nerves are usually normal, polymyographic recordings during writing show deficient reciprocal inhibition with co-contraction of antagonistic muscles, prolonged EMG bursts with or without tremor, and pathologic build up of co-contracting muscle activity ('crescendo-phenomenon', Figure 10.3).[9,20]

Investigations of reciprocal inhibition of H-reflexes in forearm flexor muscles in patients with writer's cramp and other task-specific dystonias show a normal disynaptic phase but a reduction in the amount of

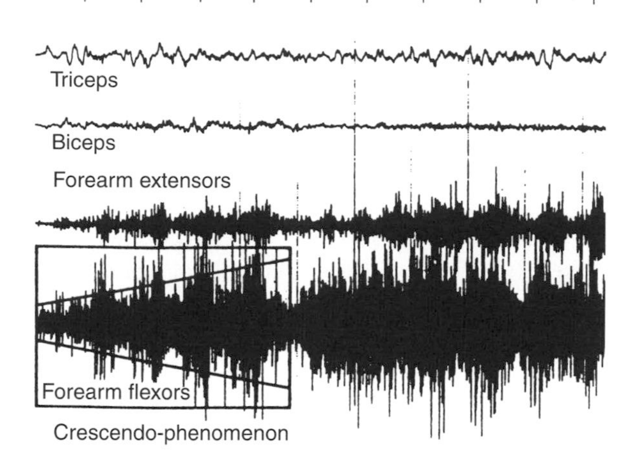

Figure 10.3 Surface EMG recordings from elbow and forearm muscles during a standardized writing task in a patient with writer's cramp. Surface EMG recordings show increased tonic activation with disturbed reciprocal inhibition and co-contraction of forearm flexor and extensor muscles in a patient with simple writer's cramp. Crescendo phenomenon during build-up of tonic contraction is a characteristic sign of dystonic activity in writer's cramp.

presynaptic inhibition.[21] Cutaneous silent periods and cortical inhibitory mechanisms are abnormal, as shown by several findings, including decreased silent periods following transcranial magnetic stimulation (TMS) in writer's cramp and other task-specific dystonias.[22,23] Siebner et al have shown reduced corticocortical inhibition in the primary motor cortex regions by using a repetitive TMS technique in patients with writer's cramp,[24] and TMS mapping procedures revealed displacement and distortion of cortical hand muscle representation in the primary motor cortex of patients with writer's cramp.[25] Routine imaging studies using computed tomography (CT) or magnetic resonance imaging (MRI) are typically normal, but may serve to exclude rare symptomatic forms of writer's cramp in patients with contralateral basal ganglia pathology and in cases with atypical presentation or associated non-dystonic features like rigidity, akinesia, myoclonus, apraxia, or sensory loss (Table 10.1).

Functional imaging studies in patients with writer's cramp using [^{18}F]fluorodeoxyglucose positron emission tomography (FDG-PET) or functional magnetic resonance imaging (fMRI) have revealed conflicting results. Earlier data in patients with writer's cramp consistently showed an overactivity of the prefrontal motor planning areas and underactivation of the primary sensorimotor cortex during passive vibrotactile stimulation of the hand,[26] while writing a stereotyped word[27] and during sustained contraction of the affected hand.[28] In addition, Ceballos-Baumann et al reported a similar activation pattern during freely selected joystick movements in patients with focal and generalized dystonia.[29] However, two more recent functional neuroimaging studies showed contradictory findings, with underactivity of prefrontal motor areas and overactivity of the primary sensorimotor cortex in patients with writer's and musician's cramp during full expression of their task-specific dystonia.[30,31] Pujol et al suggested that these conflicting findings might result from different test conditions.[31] Therefore, reduced activation of the primary sensorimotor cortex might result from a strategy used to circumvent dystonia, in which overactivity of premotor areas represents the attempt of the patient to suppress the unwanted dystonic movements.[32]

Writer's cramp can be a rare manifestation of DYT1 dystonia. The *DYT1* GAG deletion was found to be responsible for juvenile onset writer's cramp in a German family with five affected patients without further spread of symptoms.[33] Additionally, in early-onset, DYT1 positive segmental and generalized cases, symptoms frequently start in an upper limb and *DYT1* GAG deletion carriers with isolated writer's cramp have been described in different families. However, the *DYT1* GAG deletion was not found in a larger series of middle European patients with sporadic and familial writer's cramp.[34] In addition, Gasser et al did not find the *DYT1* mutation in a series of Ashkenazi Jewish patients with isolated musician's and writer's cramp.[35] These results indicate that task-specific limb dystonia is only in rare cases a phenotypic manifestation of the *DYT1* mutation, and testing for *DYT1* mutations is only recommended for patients with onset before age 26 years or in older patients having an affected relative with early-onset primary dystonia.[36]

Occasional reports have described writer's cramp as a presenting symptom in untreated Parkinson's disease[37,38] and this may be less rare in parkin disease. When there is reasonable suspicion, dopamine transporter single-photon emission computed tomography (DAT-SPECT) imaging may aid in the differential diagnosis vs primary dystonia.

Treatment

Behavioral therapies

On the basis of the hypothesis that abnormal sensory processing could cause a motor disorder, Zeuner et al have studied the efficacy of learning to read Braille as a method of sensory training for patients with focal hand dystonia.[39] After 8 weeks of daily practice, focal dystonia

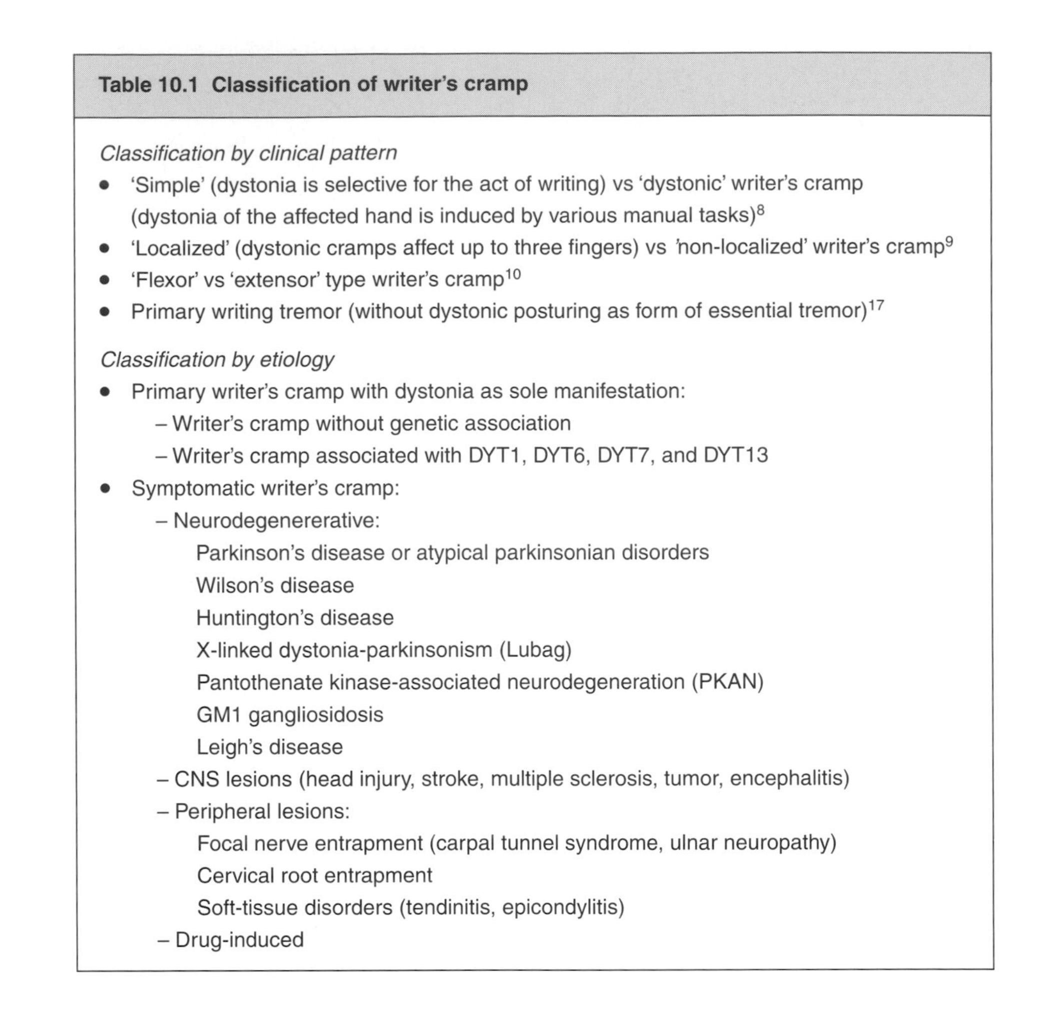

Table 10.1 Classification of writer's cramp

Classification by clinical pattern

- 'Simple' (dystonia is selective for the act of writing) vs 'dystonic' writer's cramp (dystonia of the affected hand is induced by various manual tasks)[8]
- 'Localized' (dystonic cramps affect up to three fingers) vs 'non-localized' writer's cramp[9]
- 'Flexor' vs 'extensor' type writer's cramp[10]
- Primary writing tremor (without dystonic posturing as form of essential tremor)[17]

Classification by etiology

- Primary writer's cramp with dystonia as sole manifestation:
  - Writer's cramp without genetic association
  - Writer's cramp associated with DYT1, DYT6, DYT7, and DYT13
- Symptomatic writer's cramp:
  - Neurodegenererative:
    - Parkinson's disease or atypical parkinsonian disorders
    - Wilson's disease
    - Huntington's disease
    - X-linked dystonia-parkinsonism (Lubag)
    - Pantothenate kinase-associated neurodegeneration (PKAN)
    - GM1 gangliosidosis
    - Leigh's disease
  - CNS lesions (head injury, stroke, multiple sclerosis, tumor, encephalitis)
  - Peripheral lesions:
    - Focal nerve entrapment (carpal tunnel syndrome, ulnar neuropathy)
    - Cervical root entrapment
    - Soft-tissue disorders (tendinitis, epicondylitis)
  - Drug-induced

improved in 50% of patients and spatial acuity also improved significantly in patients and controls.[39] In addition, Byl and McKenzie have combined sensory discriminative training with traditional fitness exercises to improve sensory processing and motor control of the hand affected by dystonia and reported gains in motor control, sensory discrimination, and physical performance.[40]

In conclusion, behavioral treatments to restore normal fine motor activities may be effective in some patients with writer's cramp. However, the most effective form and necessary duration of these therapies as well as their long-term stability remain to be established.

Systemic drug treatment

Systemic drug treatment, including anticholinergics, benzodiazepines, baclofen, or atypical neuroleptics, may provide some benefit in patients with writer's cramp but their usefulness is limited by low response rates and disproportionate side effects.[41] Localized injections with botulinum toxin are generally far more effective.

Botulinum toxin treatment

Botulinum toxin (BTX) treatment is considered the treatment of choice for most patients with focal dystonia, including writer's cramp. Double-blind and open trials have shown the efficacy of local BTX injections for writer's cramp. However, the complex functional anatomy of finger and forearm muscles and their sensitivity to even very low doses of BTX indicate that task-specific dystonias should perhaps be treated only by neurologists with special experience in this field.

BTX has proven efficacy in improving function (Figure 10.4), relieving dystonic muscle overactivity, abnormal postures, and associated pain in patients with writer's cramp and other task-specific dystonias[10,13,14–16,42–49] as well as in secondary limb dystonia in atypical parkinsonian disorders.[50]

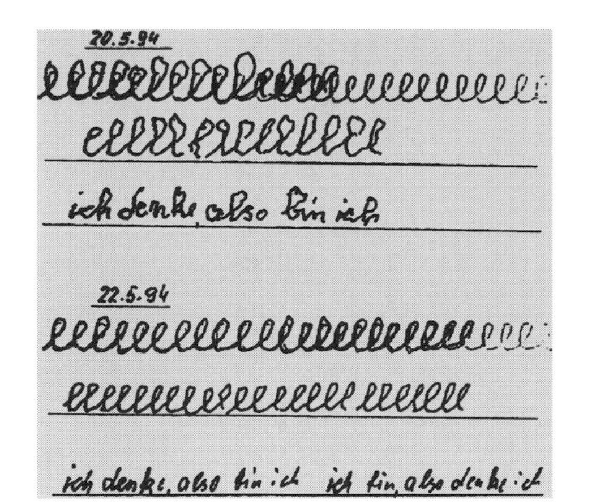

Figure 10.4 Writing in a patient with writer's cramp before and after local botulinum toxin therapy.

Except for pregnancy and lactation, there are no absolute contraindications to using BTX; relative contraindications include significant peripheral nerve or muscle disease, particularly disorders of the neuromuscular junction.

Botulinum toxin trials In open and double-blind studies, BTX injections have been shown to be effective in 50–85% of patients with writer's and musician's cramp[10,13,14–16,42–49] (Table 10.2).

In many studies, muscle selection for BTX injections is based on clinical examinations. However, surface, wire, or needle EMG is also used for muscle selection (see Table 10.2). The majority of studies have utilized global response ratings and assessments of script quality to evaluate treatment results. Some trials have included response measures such as blinded video ratings of writing performance[10,45,49] or measurements of either pen control[15] or writing speed.[10]

Muscle selection and injection technique Selection of muscles for BTX injection requires examination of the act of writing or playing an instrument. During a standard writing or drawing task, dystonic postures of the fingers and wrist may be identified. Additional palpation of the muscles during activation of the dystonic posture may be helpful to detect overactive and painful muscles.

Common patterns in writer's cramp include flexion of the wrist, often accompanied by ulnar deviation, involuntary flexion of one or more fingers, or of the thumb. Corresponding extensor patterns are also common.[51] However, it is important to distinguish involuntary muscle activity from compensatory activity that patients have developed to prevent dystonic posturing. Patients may begin to perform these tasks using an altered writing technique: e.g. hyperflexion of the thumb and index finger in extensor writer's cramp. Proximal abnormal postures may also occur, such as shoulder abduction. This may be attributed to a spread of dystonia to proximal limb muscles or represent a compensatory activity to counteract the dystonic posture.[51]

Based on clinical observation, the muscles considered overactive are injected with low initial doses to avoid excessive weakness. BTX doses may be increased gradually, with subsequent injection sessions, until optimal subjective benefit is obtained. BTX dose recommendations for selected upper limb muscles are given in Table 10.3.

The number of muscles and the anatomic complexity of the forearm require EMG guidance or electrical stimulation for accurate BTX injection into most distal upper limb muscles (see Table 10.3). The injection is given with a Teflon-coated hollow needle. EMG guidance may be limited by the inability of some patients with task-specific dystonia to voluntary contract one muscle or finger without co-activation of adjacent structures. In these cases, electrical stimulation may be used for accurate placement of BTX into the target muscle (Figure 10.5).

Outcome measures Outcome measures for clinical use may include handwriting examples (see Figure 10.4), a clinical measure of dystonic posturing and muscle strength (Medical Research Council 0–5 scale), as well as the patient's overall confidence with BTX therapy. For objective evaluation, the writer's cramp rating scale (WCRS) was developed to assess the degree of dystonic writing movement, posture, and impaired writing speed.[10] The WCRS consists of two subscales: part A describes the writing movement and posture, while part B assesses writing speed. Part A allows the writing position of the elbow, wrist, and fingers I, II, and III each to be described separately, and includes an evaluation of the latency of dystonia onset and the degree of tremor present during writing.[10] More comprehensive measures include EMG of stereotyped writing (Figure 10.6), computational analysis of handwriting,[52] or spiral drawing[53] on a digitizing tablet using specialized computer software.

Surgery

Single reports in patients with writer's cramp suggest that stereotactic nucleus ventrooralis thalamotomy may improve focal hand dystonia.[54] Recently, a small series of eight patients with medically intractable writer's cramp were reported to show immediate postoperative disappearance of dystonic symptoms which

Table 10.2 Studies of botulinum toxin in the treatment of writer's cramp and other task-specific dystonias

Author	Diagnosis (*n*)	Muscle selection	Assessment
Brin (1987)[42]	Limb dystonia (3)	Clinical + EMG	Global rating scale
Cohen (1989)[13]	Writer's cramp (14) + others (5)	Clinical + EMG	Global rating scale
Jankovic (1990)[43]	Writer's cramp + others (28)	Clinical	Global rating scale
Rivest (1991)[14]	Writer's cramp (12)	Clinical	Global rating scale, pain rating
Poungvarin (1991)[44]	Writer's cramp (21)	Clinical	Global rating scale, pain rating
Yoshimura (1992)[45]	Writer's cramp (9) + others (8)	Clinical + EMG	Subjective response, video rating
Tsui (1993)[15]	Writer's cramp (20)	Clinical + EMG	Pen control, writing speed
Karp (1994)[16]	Writer's cramp (32) + others (21)	Clinical + EMG	Global rating scale
Cole (1995)[46]	Writer's cramp (6) + others (4)	Clinical	Global rating scale, video rating, subjective response
Pullman (1996)[47]	Focal dystonia (91)	Clinical + EMG	Level of disability, pain rating, subjective response
Wissel (1996)[10]	Writer's cramp (31)	Clinical + EMG	Writer's cramp rating scale, writing speed, video rating
Turjanski (1996)[98]	Writer's cramp (44) + musician's cramp	Clinical	Global rating scale, pain rating
Ross (1997)[48]	Writer's cramp (29) + musician's cramp (11)	Clinical	Global rating scale
Chen (1999)[49]	Writer's cramp (9)	Clinical	Video rating, WCRS

EMG = electromyography; WCRS = writer's cramp rating scale.

persisted in all except one patient during the follow-up period of 3–29 months.[55] So far, there are no reports of deep brain stimulation (DBS) of the globus pallidus internus specifically in patients with writer's cramp. However, the first sham-stimulation-controlled DBS study indicates that pallidal DBS may have differential effects on writer's cramp in patients with generalized dystonia.[56]

OTHER TASK-SPECIFIC DYSTONIAS

Although writer's cramp is the most common form of focal task-specific dystonia, similar abnormalities with involuntary muscle contractions and loss of movement speed or fluency can also develop in the context of other highly learned motor skills. Such occupational cramps most commonly occur in professional musicians, craftsmen, or sportsmen whose work or hobby activity involves frequent, repetitive movements of particular muscle groups.

Clinical features

Task-specific dystonia may develop in about 0.5–1% of professional musicians[57,58] and focal dystonia occurs more frequently in male musicians. The symptoms displayed depend mainly upon the type of instrument

Table 10.3 Botulinum toxin dose recommendations for selected upper limb muscles in dystonia

Muscle	BOTOX (BTX-A), units	Dysport (BTX-A), units	EMG – control or stimulation recommended
Biceps brachii	50–80	150–300	–
Triceps brachii	50–80	150–300	–
Pronator teres	15–30	40–80	×
Flexor carpi radialis	15–30	40–80	×
Flexor carpi ulnaris	15–30	40–80	–
Extensor carpi radialis	7.5–20	20–60	×
Extensor carpi ulnaris	7.5–20	20–60	×
Flexor digitorum superficialis	10–30	30–80	×
Flexor digitorum profundus	10–30	30–80	×
Extensor digitorum communis	7.5–20	20–60	×
Flexor pollicis longus	7.5–15	20–40	×
Flexor pollicis brevis	5–10	15–30	×
Extensor pollicis longus	7.5–15	20–40	×
Abductor pollicis longus	5–10	15–30	×
Adductor pollicis	5–10	15–30	×

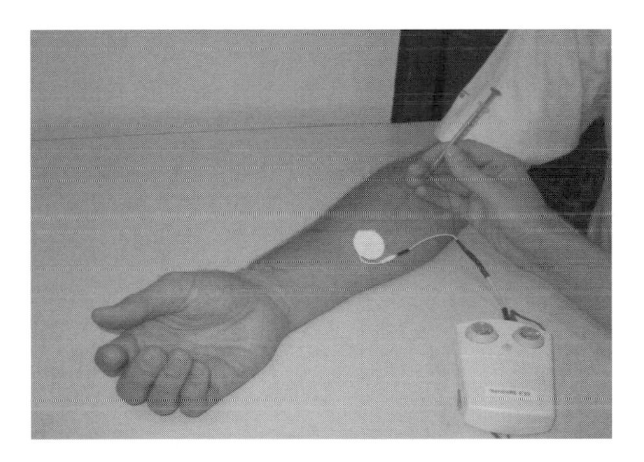

Figure 10.5 Botulinum toxin (BTX) injection given with a Teflon-coated hollow needle using electrical stimulation for accurate placement of BTX into the target muscle.

rather than hand dominance.[58,59] Dystonia occurs more frequently in pianists and guitarists, particularly in the fourth and fifth fingers of the right hand in pianists, and in the third finger of the right hand of guitarists.[59,60] For flutists, involuntary movements more often occur in the left hand, whereas for clarinettists and violinists, either hand is likely to be affected.[57–59]

In wind instrument players, the hand supporting the instrument and doing the fingering at the same time is the most affected. Rarely, wind instrument players also develop orofacial dystonia with involuntary movements of the lower face like lip pursing or jaw opening.

Tremor accompanies task-specific dystonia in about 30–40% of the patients[8,10] and hand dystonia can also affect a variety of other manual skills such as typing, sorting, and painting; playing string or keyboard instruments; or engaging in sports like tennis, golf, or snooker.[61,62]

Course and prognosis

In task-specific dystonia, the symptoms typically do not generalize. Only in rare cases, task-specific limb dystonia is a phenotypic manifestation of the *DYT1* mutation.[63,64]

Some patients report remissions after prolonged pauses in their professional or hobby musical activities, but these are rare and almost never sustained. The typical fate of musicians with task-specific dystonia is having to give up their performing career and to resort to other types of musical activities such as conducting or teaching.[19]

Symptomatic treatment with botulinum toxin is less effective in musicians than in patients with writer's cramp, which may be because of the musician's

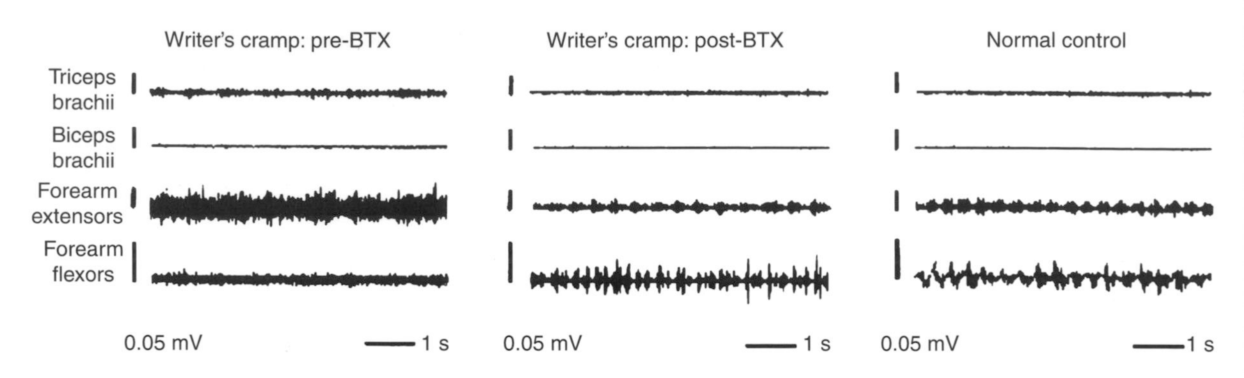

Figure 10.6 Surface EMG pattern of stereotyped poly-L-writing in a patient with writer's cramp before (left) and after local botulinum toxin (BTX) therapy (middle) and in a healthy control (right).

high demand for perfect performance so that anything less than a complete response is considered unsatisfactory.[65]

Investigations

In patients with task-specific dystonia, inflammation, damage, or strain of peripheral tissue such as tendinitis and tenosynovitis as potential sensory triggers should be excluded. Likewise, nerve conduction studies and ultrasound of the nerves and surrounding tissue may be applied to exclude peripheral nerve lesions. A possible relationship between ulnar neuropathy and focal dystonia was assumed by Ross and coworkers, who found EMG burst pattern abnormalities similar to those observed in focal dystonia in the majority of musicians with ulnar neuropathy.[66] In addition, the same group reported ulnar neuropathy in 40% of their cases with musician's cramp,[67] while another more recently published study by Lederman did not find an association between focal nerve entrapment and dystonia in a large group of instrumental musicians with neuromuscular and musculoskeletal problems.[68] Investigations of reciprocal inhibition in patients with different types of task-specific dystonia show a normal disynaptic phase but a reduction in the amount of presynaptic inhibition.[21] Cutaneous silent periods and cortical inhibitory mechanisms are also abnormal in different types of task-specific dystonia.[22,23] Magnetic source imaging in patients with musician's cramp shows alterations of digital representations in the somatosensory cortex,[69] and magnetoencephalographic (MEG) studies have shown a fusion with shorter distance between the representations of the digits of the affected hand in the primary somatosensory cortex of patients with musician's cramp[69] and focal hand dystonia.[70] In addition, Byl and coworkers were able to demonstrate anatomic and function degradation in the hand representation area of a flutist with focal hand dystonia[71] and a study by Meunier et al showed a bilateral disorganization of somatic hand representation in patients with unilateral task-specific dystonia using MEG.[72]

Routine neuroimaging studies in patients with task-specific dystonia are usually normal and cerebral MRI is only necessary in cases with additional neurologic symptoms to exclude a suspected structural brain pathology. Functional neuroimaging studies in task-specific dystonia have been mainly focused on writer's cramp. However, Pujol and coworkers have studied cortical activation during guitar-induced hand dystonia by fMRI and found underactivity of prefrontal motor areas and overactivity of the primary sensorimotor cortex during full expression of the task-specific dystonia.[31]

Treatment

Behavioral therapies

Different types of behavioral treatment, with the goal of sensory motor retuning, have been applied to patients with task-specific dystonia. Priori et al have reported that simple limb immobilization of the forearm and hand with a plastic splint for 4–5 weeks may improve musician's cramp for at least 6 months.[73] Candia et al have shown the efficacy of constraint-induced movement therapy in patients with musician's cramp. These authors have used splints to immobilize digits other than the fingers affected by dystonia while the dystonic finger performed systematic training with the respective musical instrument.[74,75] All patients showed improvement in clinical rating scales and computer-based measurements of fine finger movements.[74,75] The clinical improvement was accompanied by functional reorganization of the somatosensory cortex as measured by whole-head magnetoencephalography.[76,77]

Botulinum toxin treatment

Botulinum toxin is considered the treatment of choice for most patients with task-specific dystonia. BTX has proven efficacy in improving function, relieving muscle overactivity, abnormal postures, and associated pain in patients with different types of task-specific dystonia.[13,16,42–49] (For further details, see Chapter 18 and Tables 10.2 and 10.3.)

However, BTX treatment is consistently less efficacious in patients with musician's cramp than with writer's cramp. The most likely explanation is that professional musicians require optimum fine motor control without any muscle weakness, which is hardly achievable with BTX treatment. The best results are obtained in patients with isolated task-induced flexion of single fingers. Treatment of complex postures or tremor with the need to inject several muscles is usually associated with a mild degree of muscle weakness, which interferes with high levels of musical performance. Finger extensor muscles are particularly sensitive to BTX and even the smallest amount of BTX required for control of dystonic movements may be associated with some degree of muscle weakness.

LIMB DYSTONIA

The reported relative frequency of focal limb dystonia (excluding writer's cramp) is between 2.1% and 3.5% of all focal dystonias.[2,3] In addition, limb-onset dystonia with non-task-specific dystonia is common in several of the childhood- or juvenile-onset primary dystonias, whereas limb-onset dystonia in adults should raise a suspicion of secondary causes (see Table 10.1).

Clinical features

Limb dystonia in primary hereditary dystonia

In 94% of DYT1 patients, dystonia primarily affects a limb (arm and leg equally), and over 70% of carriers progress to a generalized or multifocal distribution.[36] Initially, upper limb dystonia may present as distal focal task-specific dystonia, with subsequent progression to a more sustained and fixed dystonic posture. Foot dystonia in DYT1 frequently starts insidiously as clumsiness in one leg while walking or running. With disease progression, limb dystonia with flexion and inversion of the affected foot and crural involvement develops.

Adult-onset idiopathic torsion dystonia of mixed type (dystonia 6; gene locus *DYT6*) may show a phenotype indistinguishable from DYT1 with limb-onset dystonia. However, the site of onset was cranial or cervical in about half of the reported patients.[78] Autosomal dominant adult-onset focal dystonia (dystonia 7; gene locus *DYT7*) has been linked to chromosome 18p in a large German family with a mean disease onset at age 43 years.[79] One of the family members had writer's cramp and several were affected by wrist tremor in addition to other types of focal dystonia. Valente and coworkers recently reported a large Italian family with predominant craniocervical or upper limb onset (dystonia 13; gene locus *DYT13*).[80] About 25% of affected individuals had upper limb-onset dystonia, which either remained focal or showed occasional generalization.[80]

Limb dystonia is also a key feature of dopa-responsive dystonia (DRD). Onset of dystonia in DRD occurs during childhood and nearly always involves the legs, progressing to other body parts in the majority of patients, with some features of parkinsonism such as bradykinesia and postural instability later in the course of the disease. Foot dystonia in DRD is characterized by equinovarus deformity and toe flexion plus extension of the great toe. Symptoms worsen significantly during the course of the day and improve after sleep.[81]

Limb dystonia in paroxysmal dyskinesias

Paroxysmal dyskinesias are characterized by involuntary, intermittent limb movements consisting of dystonia alone or a combination of hyperkinetic movement disorders. Four categories of paroxysmal dyskinesias have been classified:

1. Paroxysmal kinesigenic dyskinesia (PKD), induced by sudden movement.
2. Paroxysmal non-kinesigenic dyskinesia (PNKD), occurring spontaneously.
3. Paroxysmal exertion-induced dyskinesia (PED), induced after prolonged exercise.
4. Paroxysmal hypnogenic dyskinesia (PHD).[82]

PED consists mainly of attacks of dystonia, sometimes combined with chorea or athetosis. Attacks of PED are triggered by prolonged exertion and involve the lower limbs; the distribution is often bilateral, but can also be unilateral. The frequency of attacks in PED ranges from 1–2/day to 1–5/month, a single attack usually lasting 5–30 minutes.[82]

Limb dystonia in neurodegenerative disorders

Limb dystonia may occur as a presenting feature of untreated Parkinson's disease (PD) and as a late complication of levodopa treatment.[83] Writer's cramp and exercise-induced painful foot dystonia may be a rare presentation of PD that may precede the onset of parkinsonism by years.[37,84] Dystonia as a presenting symptom has been found in 25% of patients with onset before age 45 years but was markedly more common (42%) in those early-onset PD patients carrying a *parkin* mutation.[85] Dystonia in levodopa-treated PD develops during sustained levodopa treatment and can be classified as off-period, biphasic, or peak-dose dystonia. Off-period dystonia in PD primarily affects the feet and is characterized by equinovarus deformity and toe flexion plus extension of the great toe with calf stiffening and pain and occurs typically as early morning dystonia.[37] Biphasic dystonia is characterized by dystonic symptoms both during the onset and end-of-dose phases of an individual dose. Biphasic dystonia is predominantly unilateral with involvement of the foot in an identical manner to that seen in off-period dystonia and frequent involvement of the ipsilateral arm and leg.[37] Peak-dose involuntary movements may include both cranial dystonia and limb chorea.[37]

Unilateral upper limb dystonia is common in the early course of corticobasal degeneration (CBD) and is observed in about 70% of patients in the late course of the disease.[86] Non-task-specific upper limb dystonia in CBD is frequently accompanied by bradykinesia, rigidity, and alien limb syndrome, which may allow a clinical differentiation from other disorders associated with limb dystonia. Limb dystonia is also present in up to 30% of patients with progressive supranuclear palsy with hemidystonia as the most frequent distribution.[87]

Limb dystonia associated with neurodegenerative disorders may also be observed in Wilson's and Huntington's disease as well as in multiple system atrophy and panthotenate kinase-associated neurodegeneration.[88,89]

Symptomatic limb dystonia

Secondary dystonia due to contralateral structural basal ganglia pathology may rarely present as focal task-specific dystonia. This type of symptomatic dystonia typically occurs as non-task-specific dystonia and is frequently associated with additional neurologic symptoms. About 75% of patients with hemidystonia show contralateral basal ganglia lesions on CT or MRI. Infarction or hemorrhage involving the basal ganglia, particularly the putamen, is the most frequent cause of hemidystonia.[90] Dystonia induced by drugs or toxins may also involve the limbs: acute dystonic reactions caused by neuroleptics, calcium channel blockers, tetrabenazine, or methamphetamine typically involve the craniocervical region but may also involve the trunk and limbs. Tardive dystonia induced by drugs interfering with dopaminergic transmission most commonly affects the craniocervical region; the upper and lower limbs are only rarely involved.[91] Manganese intoxication may induce a characteristic type of foot dystonia with 'cock gait'.[92]

Psychogenic dystonia

Whereas lower limb onset is common in childhood dystonias and particularly in DYT1-positive patients, it is uncommon in primary adult-onset dystonia. In adult patients with isolated leg dystonia in whom secondary causes have been excluded, psychogenic dystonia may be considered.

Less than 5% of patients with dystonia are considered to have psychogenic dystonia.[93] In a sample of 21 patients with psychogenic dystonia, 90% were women and 67% had limb onset.[94] Clues to the diagnosis of psychogenic dystonia include abrupt onset, early fixed postures, foot/leg involvement in adults, paroxysmal symptoms, and complete remissions. By contrast, adult patients with organic dystonia usually report gradual onset, fixed postures develop late, foot or leg involvement as well as paroxysmal symptoms are rare, and complete remissions are uncommon. The clinical investigation of patients with psychogenic dystonia may show false weakness, false sensory symptoms, inconsistent movements, decreasing movements with distraction, increasing movements with attention, or responsiveness to placebo.

Course and prognosis

Dystonia in the childhood- or juvenile-onset primary dystonias tends to progress to a generalized or multifocal distribution in the majority of patients, whereas limb dystonia in adults usually remains focal or segmental.[36] The course and prognosis of limb dystonia in dystonia-plus syndromes and heredodegenerative diseases is variable. Dopa-responsive dystonia shows an excellent and sustained response to levodopa therapy and off-period dystonia in Parkinson's disease may be effectively treated with levodopa or dopamine agonists. Limb dystonia in neurodegenerative disorders is frequently associated with other disabling neurologic symptoms and prognosis depends largely on the course of the underlying disorder.

Investigations

In all cases with a possible secondary cause of dystonia, a thorough clinical examination together with neuroradiologic biochemical, or genetic testing should be performed depending on the suspected etiology.

Genetic testing for *DYT1* mutations is recommended for patients with onset before age 26 years or in older patients having an affected relative with early-onset primary dystonia.[36] Genetic testing is also indicated in suspected DRD and Huntington's disease. Diagnostic testing for Wilson's disease includes serum ceruloplasmin, 24-hour urinary copper excretion, slit-lamp examination, and perhaps liver biopsy as the most sensitive test. DAT-SPECT is indicated when Parkinson's disease is suspected. Routine imaging studies using CT or MRI may serve to exclude symptomatic forms of limb dystonia due to contralateral basal ganglia pathology or CBD, where MRI may demonstrate asymmetric pericentral cortical atrophy.

Treatment

A specific pharmacotherapy directed at the underlying biochemical defect exists only for a limited number of symptomatic limb dystonias.[95] Wilson's disease is effectively treated with drugs that deplete copper or interfere with copper absorption such as penicillamine or trientene. Patients with dopa responsive dystonia show an excellent and sustained response to low-dose levodopa therapy.[81] In patients with Parkinson's disease, dopaminergic treatment should be optimized to handle off-period dystonia and prevent levodopa-induced dyskinesia.

In primary torsion dystonia, chronic bilateral globus pallidus internus stimulation seems to be the most effective treatment for limb dystonia.[56,96,97] Patients with PKD may respond to treatment with anticonvulsants, those with PNKD to acetazolamide.[82]

For the remaining patients with focal limb dystonia, symptomatic treatment with botulinum toxin is the therapy of choice (see Chapter 18). Additional pharmacologic therapies, including anticholinergics, benzodiazepines, baclofen, or atypical neuroleptics, may also be tried similar to other types of dystonia.

REFERENCES

1. Nutt JG, Muenter MD, Aronson A, Kurland LT, Melton LJ. Epidemiology of focal and generalized dystonia in Rochester, Minnesota. Mov Disord 1988; 3: 188–94.
2. Epidemiological Study of Dystonia in Europe (ESDE) Collaborative Group. A prevalence study of primary dystonia in eight European countries. J Neurol 2000; 247: 787–92.
3. Duffey PO, Butler AG, Hawthorne MR, Barnes MP. The epidemiology of the primary dystonias in the North of England. Adv Neurol 1998; 78: 121–5.
4. Nakashima K, Kusumi M, Inoue Y, Takahashi K. Prevalence of focal dystonias in the western area of Tottori prefecture in Japan. Mov Disord 1995; 10(4): 440–3.
5. Soland VL, Bhatia KP, Marsden CD. Sex prevalence of focal dystonias. J Neurol Neurosurg Psychiatry 1996; 60: 204–5.
6. Mueller J, Kiechl S, Wenning GK et al. The prevalence of primary dystonia in the general community. Neurology 2002; 59: 941–3.
7. Defazio G, Livrea P, De Salvia R et al. Prevalence of primary blepharospasm in a community of Puglia region, Southern Italy. Neurology 2001; 56: 1579–81.
8. Sheehy MP, Marsden CD. Writer's cramp – a focal dystonia. Brain 1982; 105: 461–80.
9. Cohen LG, Hallett M. Hand cramps: clinical features and electromyographic patterns in a focal dystonia. Neurology 1988; 38: 1005–12.
10. Wissel J, Kabus C, Wenzel R et al. Botulinum toxin in writer's cramp: objective response evaluation in 31 patients. J Neurol Neurosurg Psychiatry 1996; 61: 172–5.
11. Solly S. Scrivener's palsy, or the paralysis of writers. Lancet 1864; 2: 709–11.
12. Poore GV. An analysis of 75 cases of writer's cramp and impaired writing power. Trans Roy Med Chir Soc 1878; 61: 111–45.
13. Cohen LG, Hallett M, Geller BD, Hochberg F. Treatment of focal dystonias of the hand with botulinum toxin injections. J Neurol Neurosurg Psychiatry 1989; 52: 355–63.
14. Rivest J, Lees AJ, Marsden CD. Writer's cramp: treatment with botulinum toxin injections. Mov Disord 1991; 6: 55–9.
15. Tsui JKC, Bhatt M, Calne S, Calne DB. Botulinum toxin in the treatment of writer's cramp: a double blind study. Neurology 1993; 43: 183–5.
16. Karp BI, Cole RA, Cohen LG et al. Long-term botulinum toxin treatment of focal hand dystonia. Neurology 1994; 44: 70–6.
17. Deuschl G, Bain P, Brin M. Consensus statement of the Movement Disorder Society on Tremor. Ad Hoc Scientific Committee. Mov Disord 1998; 13(Suppl 3): 2–23.
18. Marsden CD, Sheehy MP. Writer's cramp. Trends Neurosci 1990; 13(4): 148–53.
19. Sheehy MP, Rothwell JC, Marsden CD. Writer's cramp. Adv Neurol 1988; 50: 457–72.
20. Marsden CD, Rothwell JC. The physiology of idiopathic dystonia. Can J Neurol Sci 1987; 14: 521–7.
21. Nakashima K, Rothwell JC, Day BL et al. Reciprocal inhibition between forearm muscles in patients with writer's cramp and other occupational cramps, symptomatic hemidystonia and hemiparesis due to stroke. Brain 1989; 112: 681–97.
22. Pullman SL, Ford B, Elibol B et al. Cutaneous electromyographic silent period findings in brachial dystonia. Neurology 1996; 46: 503–8.
23. Filipovic SR, Ljubisavljevic M, Svetel M et al. Impairment of cortical inhibition in writer's cramp as revealed by changes in electromyographic silent period after transcranial magnetic stimulation. Neurosci Lett 1997; 222: 167–70.
24. Siebner HR, Tormos JM, Ceballos-Baumann AO et al. Low-frequency repetitive transcranial magnetic stimulation of the motor cortex in writer's cramp. Neurology 1999; 52: 529–37.
25. Byrnes ML, Thickbroom GW, Wilson SA et al. The corticomotor representation of upper limb muscles in writer's cramp and changes following botulinum toxin injection. Brain 1998; 121: 977–88.
26. Tempel LW, Perlmutter JS. Abnormal cortical responses in patients with writer's cramp. Neurology 1993; 43: 2252–7.
27. Ceballos-Baumann AO, Sheean G, Passingham RE, Marsden CD, Brooks DJ. Botulinum toxin does not reverse the cortical dysfunction associated with writer's cramp. A PET study. Brain 1997; 120: 571–82.

28. Ibanez V, Sadato N, Karp B, Deiber MP, Hallet M. Deficient activation of the motor cortical network in patients with writer's cramp. Neurology 1999; 53: 96–105.
29. Ceballos-Baumann AO, Passingham RE, Warner T et al. Overactive prefrontal and underactive motor cortical areas in idiopathic dystonia. Ann Neurol 1995; 37: 746–57.
30. Odergren T, Stone-Elander S, Ingvar M. Cerebral and cerebellar activation in correlation to the action-induced dystonia in writer's cramp. Mov Disord 1998; 13: 497–508.
31. Pujol J, Roset-Llobet J, Rosinés-Cubells D et al. Brain cortical activation during guitar-induced hand dystonia studied by functional MRI. Neuroimage 2000; 12: 257–67.
32. Tinazzi M, Rosso T, Fiaschi A. Role of the somatosensory system in primary dystonia. Mov Disord 2003; 18: 605–22.
33. Gasser T, Windgassen K, Bereznai B, Kabus C, Ludolph AC. Phenotypic expression of the DYT1 mutation: a family with writer's cramp of juvenile onset. Ann Neurol 1998; 44: 126–8.
34. Kamm C, Naumann M, Mueller J et al. The DYT1 GAG deletion is infrequent in sporadic and familial writer's cramp. Mov Disord 2000; 15(6): 1238–41.
35. Gasser T, Bove CM, Ozelius LJ et al. Haplotype analysis at the DYT1 locus in Ashkenazi Jewish patients with occupational hand dystonia. Mov Disord 1996; 11: 163–6.
36. Bressman SB, Sabatti C, Raymond D et al. The DYT1 phenotype and guidelines for diagnostic testing. Neurology 2000; 54: 1746–52.
37. Poewe W, Lees AJ, Stern GM. Dystonia in Parkinson's disease: clinical and pharmacological features. Ann Neurol 1988; 23: 73–8.
38. Lewitt PA, Burns RS, Newman RP. Dystonia in untreated parkinsonism. Clin Neuropharmacol 1986; 9: 293–7.
39. Zeuner KE, Bara-Jimenez W, Noguchi PS et al. Sensory training for patients with focal hand dystonia. Ann Neurol 2002; 51: 593–8.
40. Byl NN, McKenzie A. Treatment effectiveness for patients with a history of repetitive hand use and focal hand dystonia: a planned, prospective follow-up study. J Hand Ther 2000; 13: 289–301.
41. Lang AE, Sheehy MP, Marsden CD. Anticholinergics in adult-onset focal dystonia. Can J Neurol Sci 1982; 9: 313–19.
42. Brin MF, Fahn S, Moskowitz C et al. Localized injections of botulinum toxin for the treatment of focal dystonia and hemifacial spasm. Mov Disord 1987; 2: 237–54.
43. Jankovic J, Schwartz K, Donovan DT. Botulinum toxin treatment of cranial-cervical dystonia, spasmodic dysphonia, other focal dystonias and hemifacial spasms. J Neurol Neurosurg Psychiatry 1990; 53: 633–9.
44. Poungvarin N. Writer's cramp: the experience with botulinum toxin injections in 25 patients. J Med Assoc Thai 1991; 74: 239–47.
45. Yoshimura DM, Aminoff MJ, Olney RK. Botulinum toxin therapy for limb dystonias. Neurology 1992; 42: 627–30.
46. Cole R, Hallett M, Cohen LG. Double-blind trial of botulinum toxin for treatment of focal hand dystonia. Mov Disord 1995; 10: 466–71.
47. Pullman SL, Greene P, Fahn S, Pedersen SF. Approach to the treatment of limb disorders with botulinum toxin A. Experience with 187 patients. Arch Neurol 1996; 53: 617–24.
48. Ross MH, Charness ME, Sudarsky L, Logigian EL. Treatment of occupational cramp with botulinum toxin: diffusion of toxin to adjacent noninjected muscles. Muscle Nerve 1997; 20: 593–8.
49. Chen R, Karp BI, Goldstein SR et al. Effect of muscle activity immediately after botulinum toxin injection for writer's cramp. Mov Disord 1999; 14: 307–12.
50. Mueller J, Wenning GK, Wissel J, Seppi K, Poewe W. Botulinum toxin treatment in atypical parkinsonian disorders associated with disabling focal dystonia. J Neurol 2002; 249: 300–4.
51. Sheean G. Limb and occupational dystonia. In: Moore P, Naumann M, eds. Handbook of Botulinum Toxin Treatment, 2nd edn. Oxford: Blackwell Science; 2003: 195–218.
52. Marquardt C, Mai N. A computational procedure for movement analysis in handwriting. J Neurosci Methods 1994; 52: 39–45.
53. Pullman SL. Spiral analysis: a new technique for measuring tremor with a digitizing tablet. Mov Disord 1998; 13: 85–9.
54. Goto S, Tsuiki H, Soyama N et al. Stereotactic selective VO-complex thalamotomy in a patient with dystonic writer's cramp. Neurology 1997; 49(4): 1173–4.
55. Taira T, Harashima S, Hori T. Neurosurgical treatment for writer's cramp. Acta Neurochir Suppl 2003; 87: 129–31.
56. Kupsch A, Benecke R, Muller J et al. Pallidal deep-brain stimulation in primary generalized or segmental dystonia. N Engl J Med 2006; 355: 1978–90.
57. Altenmüller E. Causes and cures of focal limb dystonia in musicians. International Society for Study of Tension in Performance 1998; 9: 13–17.
58. Brandfonbrener AG. Musicians with focal dystonia: a report of 58 cases seen during a ten-year period at a performing arts medicine clinic. Med Probl Perform Art 1995: 121–7.
59. Newmark JA, Hochberg FH. Isolated painless manual incoordination in 57 musicians. J Neurol Neurosurg Psychiatry 1987; 50: 291–5.
60. Lim VK, Altenmüller E, Bradshaw JL. Focal dystonia: current theories. Hum Mov Sci 2001; 20: 875–914.
61. Mayer F, Topka H, Boose A, Horstmann T, Dickhuth HH. Bilateral segmental dystonia in a professional tennis player. Med Sci Sports Exerc 1999; 31: 1085–7.
62. McDaniel KD, Cummings JL, Shain S. The "yips": a focal dystonia of golfers. Neurology 1989; 39: 192–5.
63. Kamm C, Naumann M, Mueller J et al. The DYT1 GAG deletion is infrequent in sporadic and familial writer's cramp. Mov Disord 2000; 15(6): 1238–41.
64. Gasser T, Bove CM, Ozelius LJ et al. Haplotype analysis at the DYT1 locus in Ashkenazi Jewish patients with occupational hand dystonia. Mov Disord 1996; 11: 163–6.
65. Cole RA, Cohen LG, Hallett M. Treatment of musician's cramp with botulinum toxin. Med Probl Perform Art 1991; 6: 137–43.
66. Ross MH, Charness ME, Lee D, Logigian EL. Does ulnar neuropathy predispose to focal dystonia? Muscle Nerve 1995; 18: 606–11.
67. Charness ME, Ross MH, Shefner JM. Ulnar neuropathy and dystonia flexion of the fourth and fifth digits: clinical correlation in musicians. Muscle Nerve 1996; 19: 431–7.
68. Lederman RJ. Neuromuscular and musculoskeletal problems in instrumental musicians. Muscle Nerve 2003; 27: 549–61.
69. Elbert T, Candia V, Altenmuller E et al. Alteration of digital representations in somatosensory cortex in focal hand dystonia. Neuroreport 1998; 9: 3571–5.
70. Bara-Jimenez W, Catalan MJ, Hallett M, Gerloff C. Abnormal somatosensory homunculus in dystonia of the hand. Ann Neurol 1998; 44: 828–31.
71. Byl NN, McKenzie A, Nagarajan SS. Differences in somatosensory hand organization in a healthy flutist and a flutist with focal hand dystonia: a case report. J Hand Ther 2000; 13: 302–19.
72. Meunier S, Garnero L, Ducorps A et al. Human brain mapping in dystonia reveals both endophenotypic traits and adaptive reorganization. Ann Neurol 2001; 50: 521–7.
73. Priori A, Pesenti A, Cappellari A, Scarlato G, Barbieri S. Limb immobilization for the treatment of focal occupational dystonia. Neurology 2001; 57: 405–9.
74. Candia V, Elbert T, Altenmüller E et al. Constraint-induced movement therapy for focal hand dystonia in musicians. Lancet 1999; 353: 42.
75. Candia V, Schäfer T, Taub E et al. Sensory motor retuning: a behavioral treatment for focal hand dystonia of pianists and guitarists. Arch Phys Med Rehabil 2002; 83: 1342–8.
76. Candia V, Wienbruch C, Elbert T, Rockstroh B, Ray W. Effective behavioral treatment of focal hand dystonia in musicians alters somatosensory cortical organization. Proc Natl Acad Sci USA 2003; 100: 7942–6.

77. Candia V, Rosset-Liobet J, Elbert T, Pascual-Leone A. Changing the brain through therapy for musicians' hand dystonia. Ann NY Acad Sci 2005; 1060: 335–42.
78. Almasy L, Bressman SB, Raymond D et al. Idiopathic torsion dystonia linked to chromosome 8 in two Mennonite families. Ann Neurol 1997; 42: 670–3.
79. Leube B, Rudnicki D, Ratzlaff T et al. Idiopathic torsion dystonia: assignment of a gene to chromosome 18p in a German family with adult onset, autosomal dominant inheritance and purely focal distribution. Hum Mol Genet 1996; 5: 1673–7.
80. Valente EM, Bentivoglio AR, Cassetta E et al. Identification of a novel primary torsion dystonia locus (DYT 13) on chromosome 1p36 in an Italian family with cranial-cervical or upper limb onset. Neurol Sci 2001; 22: 95–6.
81. Nygaard TG, Trugman JM, de Yebenes JG, Fahn S. Dopa-responsive dystonia: the spectrum of clinical manifestations in a large North American family. Neurology 1990; 40: 66–9.
82. Jankovic J, Demirkiran M. Classification of paroxysmal dyskinesias and ataxias. Adv Neurol 2002; 89: 387–400.
83. Poewe W, Lees AJ. The pharmacology of foot dystonia in parkinsonism. Clin Neuropharmacol 1987; 10(1): 47–56.
84. Katzenschlager R, Costa D, Gacinovic S, Lees AJ. [(123)I]-FP-CIT-SPECT in the early diagnosis of PD presenting exercise-induced dystonia. Neurology 2002; 59: 1974–6.
85. Lücking CB, Durr A, Bonifati V et al. Association between early-onset Parkinson's disease and mutations in the parkin gene. French Parkinson's Disease Genetics Study Group. N Engl J Med 2000; 342: 1560–7.
86. Rinne JO, Lee MS, Thompson PD, Marsden CD. Corticobasal degeneration: a clinical study of 36 cases. Brain 1994; 117: 1183–96.
87. Barclay, CL, Lang AE. Dystonia in progressive supranuclear palsy. J Neurol Neurosurg Psychiatry 1997; 62: 352–6.
88. Boesch SM, Wenning GK, Ransmayr G, Poewe W. Dystonia in multiple system atrophy. J Neurol Neurosurg Psychiatry 2002; 72: 300–3.
89. Rivest J, Quinn N, Marsden CD. Dystonia in Parkinson's disease, multiple system atrophy, and progressive supranuclear palsy. Neurology 1990; 40: 1571–8.
90. Pettigrew LC, Jankovic J. Hemidystonia: a report of 22 patients and a review of the literature. J Neurol Neurosurg Psychiatry 1985; 48: 650–7.
91. Gimenez-Roldan S, Mateo D, Bartolome P. Tardive distonia and severe tardive dyskinesia. Acta Psychiatr Scand 1985; 71: 488–94.
92. Huang CC, Chu NS, Lu CS, Calne DB. Cock gait in manganese intoxication. Mov Disord 1997; 12: 807–8.
93. Owens DG. Dystonia: a potential psychiatric pitfall. Br J Psychiatry 1990; 156: 620–34.
94. Fahn S, Williams DT. Psychogenic dystonia. Adv Neurol 1988; 50: 431–55.
95. Bressman SB, Greene PE. Treatment of hyperkinetic movement disorders. Neurol Clin 1990; 8: 51–75.
96. Coubes P, Roubertie A, Vayssiere N, Hemm S, Echenne B. Treatment of DYT1-generalised dystonia by stimulation of the internal globus pallidus. Lancet 2000; 355: 2220–1.
97. Vidailhet M, Vercueil L, Houeto J-L et al. Bilateral deep-brain stimulation of the globus pallidus in primary generalized dystonia. N Engl J Med 2005; 352: 459–67.
98. Turjanski N, Pirtosek Z, Quirk J et al. Botulinum toxin in the treatment of writer's cramp. Clin Neuropharmacol 1996; 19: 314–20.

11

Laryngeal dystonia

Christy L Ludlow

FORMS OF LARYNGEAL DYSTONIA

The laryngeal dystonias are a subset of laryngeal motor control disorders affecting voice and/or breathing, including adductor and abductor spasmodic dysphonia (SD), voice tremor, and adductor breathing dystonia. A significant proportion, about one-third, of persons with SD also have voice tremor. Diagnosis is symptom based and dependent upon excluding other laryngeal disorders such as those secondary to neurologic diseases/disorders and those laryngeal dysfunction disorders thought to be behavioral in origin (Table 11.1). The laryngeal dystonias are relatively rare, affecting 1 in 100 000 persons.[1]

Among those laryngeal disorders that are secondary to neurologic disease that need to be separated from SD are vocal fold paralysis in the bulbar form of amyotrophic lateral sclerosis causing dysphonia and dysphagia,[2] airway obstruction due to loss of vocal fold opening in multiple system atrophy,[3] hypophonia in Parkinson's disease,[4] and abductor vocal fold paralysis in familial polyneuropathy.[5]

Two poorly understood disorders, muscular tension dysphonia[6] and paradoxical vocal fold function,[7] are thought to have a behavioral component because a large proportion of persons affected respond well to behavioral management.[7,8]

Although previously, the laryngeal dystonias were often misdiagnosed as psychogenic disorders,[9] more recently, these disorders tend to be overdiagnosed. When voice disorder is an early symptom of other underlying neurologic disorders, misdiagnosis can lead to injection of the laryngeal muscles with botulinum toxin in patients who might be not benefit, such as a early-onset bulbar amyotrophic lateral sclensis (ALS).[10] Accurate diagnosis is important, although the symptom complexes among these disorders are not always distinct.[11]

DIAGNOSIS

Spasmodic dysphonia

SD is usually focal to the laryngeal musculature and may involve tone abnormalities in only a few of the laryngeal muscles. As the name implies, spasmodic dysphonia involves intermittent involuntary laryngeal muscle spasms[12] rather than constantly abnormal levels of muscle tone.[13] Adductor spasmodic dysphonia (ADSD) is characterized by intermittent voice stoppages in vowels in the middle of words and difficulty initiating voice on words beginning with vowels.[14] During voice breaks, the vocal folds squeeze together or hyperadduct to such a degree that voicing is stopped.[15] These breaks are due to involuntary spasms in the vocal fold closing muscles, the thyroarytenoid and lateral cricoarytenoid muscles, although spasms can be seen in other muscles such as the cricothyroid in some patients with ADSD.[16,17]

Abductor spasmodic dysphonia (ABSD) occurs in between 10% and 15% of persons with SD.[18] The speech symptoms are breathy breaks due to prolonged voiceless consonants such as 's', 'h', 'p', 't', 'k', and 'f' before a vowel. During the break, the vocal folds have prolonged involuntary opening, preventing rapid voice onset for the following vowel. Vocal fold opening and lengthening muscles, the posterior cricoarytenoid and cricothyroid, respectively, may be involved in ABSD, although some patients have breathy breaks in the middle of vowels as a result of uncontrollable decreases in tone in the thyroarytenoid muscle during a vowel.

Patients with either ADSD or ABSD are symptomatic only during voice for speech, while non-speech tasks such as breathing, sighing, laughter, and crying are unaffected. Singing is usually less affected than speech and most patients can shout better than they can speak.[19] These task-specific differences were previously interpreted as

Table 11.1 Affected and unaffected tasks in the laryngeal dystonias

Disorder	Type	Affected tasks	Unaffected tasks
Spasmodic dysphonias	Adductor	Vowels during speech	Cough, cry, laughter, shout, whisper
	Abductor	Voiceless consonants during speech	Prolonged vowel except in severe cases, cough, cry, laughter, shout, whisper
Voice tremor	Action-induced	Prolonged vowels and voice during speech	Inspiration, cough, cry, laughter
	Essential tremor	Rest, voice, and speech	Cough
Adductor breathing dystonia	Laryngeal obstruction	Inspiration during breathing	Voice and speech, breathing during sleep
	Pharyngeal obstruction	Inspiration during breathing, garbled speech	Breathing during sleep

an indication that the disorder was psychogenic; however, it is now recognized that innate laryngeal gestures may be under separate control in the human brain from learned laryngeal gestures such as those that occur during speech.[20]

The most common complaint of persons with SD is the effort required to speak. Patients also develop fears with speaking on the telephone and in public because of embarrassment caused by their voice problems. Persons with ABSD often also complain of difficulty coordinating breathing with speaking.

Voice tremor

Action-induced voice tremor, only present during speech, often co-occurs with SD.[21,22] In vocal tremor, intermittent hyperadduction of the vocal folds regularly produces breaks in vowels at around 5 Hz.[23] In the abductor form, which is quite rare, breathy modulations or pitch changes are most notable. Because syllables are usually produced at 4 per second in conversational speech, a 5 Hz tremor may not be evident until the patient is asked to produce a prolonged vowel for at least 10 seconds or more.

Adductor breathing dystonia

During breathing, the vocal folds act as a valve in the midline of the upper airway, opening during inspiration[24] and partly closing during exhalation.[25] Patients with a breathing dystonia only have uncontrolled vocal fold closure during inspiration but move their vocal folds normally during speech. Increases in thyroarytenoid muscle during inspiration results in stridor or obstruction.[26] Adductor breathing dystonia is usually continuously present while the patient is awake, reduced during speech, and absent during sleep. Obstruction is exacerbated during forced inspiration when the negative pressure produced by air flow through the glottis sucks the vocal folds together. Adductor breathing dystonia is rare and usually has its onset in middle age. It can be associated with oral–mandibular dystonia. In some patients the obstruction is not at the level of the larynx but rather involves the posterior pharynx. Involuntary tongue retraction and contraction of the superior pharyngeal constrictor can cause the epiglottis to obstruct the hypopharynx. Obstruction occurs as the patient breathes in, producing a negative pressure sucking the walls of the pharynx together.

Adductor breathing dystonia is one form of paradoxical vocal fold dysfunction[27] (PVFD) and differs from other vocal fold breathing dysfunctions, because the dystonic form is continuous while the patient is awake while the other vocal fold dysfunctions are usually episodic, associated with a trigger such as laryngopharyngeal reflux, an airway irritant, asthma, or psychological stressors.[7] PVFD occurring at night may be associated with laryngopharyngeal reflux when gastric juices with a low pH stimulate a glottic closure reflex, or during the day when bending over also causes regurgitation of gastric contents into the larynx.[28] Other patients, often adolescents, develop episodes of PVFD that may be related to psychological triggers or asthma.[7]

ASSESSMENT

Identification of the laryngeal dystonias requires a medical history and physical examination, speech testing, a psychosocial history,[29] and viewing the larynx during breathing, conversational speech, whistling, and phonation using flexible nasolaryngoscopy to visualize the laryngeal movement abnormalities (Table 11.2).

The speech and breathing history can be informative to determine if the disorder is episodic, or constant and chronic for a particular task. Although the severity of SD can wax and wane with 'good days and bad days' if the patient reports that the voice disorder completely abates for days at a time, this is not typical of SD, and may indicate a functional voice disorder, either muscular tension dysphonia or a psychogenic voice disorder.

Complaints of effort are also typical of SD and may include complaints of problems with breathing control while speaking. Patients with psychogenic dysphonia rarely complain of effort, have poor insight into their voice disorder, and discuss it as something occurring independent of themselves, taking little ownership or responsibility for their voice production. On the other hand, patients with SD can often provide a great deal of information on their speaking difficulties and may have considerable insight into their disorder.

The patient's report of the degree of effort on different types of speech sounds is also useful in identifying the type of SD. Sentences or syllable repetitions loaded with glottal stops (words beginning with vowels requiring the vocal folds to close tightly together and then release into vibration) are very difficult for patients with ADSD. Examples are repetition of the vowel 'ee-ee-ee. . . .' and sentences such as 'we eat olives everyday', 'we mow our lawn all year', and 'Sam wants to be in the army' are difficult for patients with ADSD with prolonged voice offsets at the underlined vowels.

In contrast, in ABSD, repetitions of syllables containing voiceless consonants are difficult, such as 'he-he-he. . . ', 'see-see-see. . .' 'pea-pea-pea. . .' or 'key-key-key. . . .' and sentences such as, 'he had half a head of hair', 'a mahogany high boy is heavy', 'the puppy bit the tape', or 'she speaks pleasingly'.

When patients with ADSD and ABSD are asked to repeat different syllables, including those with glottal stops (i-i-i-i-i), voiceless consonants (see-see-see-see-see), and some decoy phrases involving nasal sounds (me-me-me-me-me), they can reliably identify which type is most effortful. Patients with muscular tension

Table 11.2 Assessment of symptoms in the laryngeal dystonias

Disorder	Type	Speech tasks	Nasolaryngoscopy findings
Spasmodic dysphonias	Adductor	e-e-e-e-e-e-e 'we eat eels everyday'	Intermittent lateral–medial hyperadduction, prolonged glottal stops
	Abductor	See-see-see-see-see He-he-he-he-he 'he had half a head of hair', 'a mahogany highboy is heavy'	Prolonged abduction during voiceless consonants prior to vowels
Voice tremor	Action-induced	Tremor on prolonged vowels at speaking pitch, less tremor at high pitch and falsetto	Tremor on voice, less on inspiration
	Essential tremor	Can observe tremor in neck	Tremor at rest involves bobbing of the larynx
Adductor breathing dystonia	Laryngeal obstruction	Stridor on inspiration	Vocal fold medialization on inspiration
	Pharyngeal obstruction	Obstruction on inspiration	Posterior tongue motion moves the epiglottis to the posterior wall of the pharynx

dysphonia or psychogenic dysphonia usually find all syllable types equally difficult.

Nasolaryngoscopy examination

Flexible nasolaryngoscopy is essential for examining patients with laryngeal motor control disorders so that the vocal fold movement abnormalities can be visualized during connected speech when symptoms are most evident. This examination is also necessary to exclude vocal fold paralysis or weakness that may also produce voice and/or breathing abnormalities. On entry into the nasal passages, the superior surface of the velum can be viewed and the degree of closure of the velopharyngeal port during speech tasks can be assessed. The velum should raise to close off the nasopharynx during the vowel 'ee' and a whisper such as 'shhhh' but will lower at rest and during humming and nasal sounds such as 'mama'. Patients with voice tremor may have tremor in the velum during a prolonged vowel such as 'eeeeeeeeeee'. Sentences containing nasal and non-nasal sounds can assess the speed and extent of velar movement, such as 'Mama made some lemon jam' and 'Susie sews socks'. Some patients with ABSD have abnormal movement of the velum during speech, although it is normal for pronged vowels and rises normally during swallowing.

After entering the oropharynx, vocal fold movements can be visualized during both speech and non-speech tasks. During speech, high tongue position vowels ('ee' as in 'tree' and 'oo' as in 'blue') will provide the best view of the larynx. Low back vowels produce posterior tongue positions, which move the epiglottis backwards, obscuring the view of the larynx (e.g. 'ah' as in 'saw').

The vocal folds should be examined for spontaneous movement during quiet respiration to identify tremor or adduction during inspiration for breathing dystonia. Examination of the speed of vocal fold movement for abduction (opening) and adduction (closing) should include speech and non-speech tasks. A rapid 'sniff' followed by an 'ee' at least 3 times in rapid succession allows for examination of the adequacy of opening and closing movements of the vocal folds for speech. Whistling 'Happy Birthday' produces rapid and frequent opening and closing of the vocal folds for non-speech tasks for assessing movement range and symmetry. Most persons will say they can't whistle but the rapid opening and closing of the vocal folds occurs regardless of their skill in whistling a tune.

To examine for symptoms of ADSD, repetitions of vowels, as in 'ee-ee-ee-ee-ee', can assess prolonged vocal fold closing while producing a glottal stop between vowels, resulting in longer voice offsets than normal. Also, sentence production can assess intermittent breaks in all voiced sentences with glottal stops between vowels such as 'we eat eels every day', and counting upwards beginning with 'eighty'.

To examine for symptoms of ABSD, repetition of 'see-see-see-see-see' or 'he-he-he-he-he' will detect prolonged vocal fold opening during voiceless consonants for longer periods than normal. Sentences to examine intermittent spasmodic movements, include 'he had half a head of hair' and 'Peter will keep at the peak' and counting upwards beginning with 'sixty'.

In vocal tremor, the prolonged vowel 'ee' should be produced at different pitches and in glides; usually, tremor is greatest in the low-pitch speaking voice range and reduced at high pitches and in falsetto voice. To determine if tremor is action induced, no tremor will be seen at rest but it may appear during expiration and as soon as the patient goes to speak. In benign essential tremor affecting the larynx, tremor may occur at rest, during both inspiration and expiration, as well as during speaking. If tremor involvement is limited to the vocal folds, then only the intrinsic laryngeal muscles are involved and can be injected with botulinum toxin. On the other hand, if there is a constant superior–inferior (bobbing) motion of the entire larynx, some of the extrinsic laryngeal muscles may also be involved. Finally, if the pharyngeal walls, posterior tongue, and velum are also involved, it will be difficult to manage symptoms using only botulinum toxin injection, and medications may also be needed.

When assessing adductor breathing dystonia, nasolaryngoscopy is important to determine if the range and speed of vocal fold movement are normal during other tasks such as sniffing and whistling, to identify whether stridor is due to abductor vocal fold paralysis or paresis rather than dystonia. Observing vocal fold and pharyngeal movement is important to determine if there is active vocal fold closing during inspiration or whether the obstruction is above the glottis. An otolaryngologist can also examine the laryngeal tissues for signs of laryngopharyngeal reflux to determine if a history of an episodic breathing disorder might be due to gastric reflux stimulating a vocal fold adductory reflex.[28]

Non-dystonic laryngeal movement disorders

Asymmetries in vocal fold movements between the two sides on the whistling task would be indicative of an adductor or abductor paralysis/paresis. Sometimes, asymmetries in movement between the right and left sides are seen during speech in ABSD but are not evident during non-speech tasks such as 'whistling' and 'sniffing', indicating that the disorder is part of the dystonia and not due to vocal fold paralysis.[30] Patients with thinning of the vocal folds or vocal fold bowing can have many different disorders: either Parkinson's disease,[31] a polyneuropathy,[32] or muscle atrophy associated with aging.[33]

A constant harsh quality with an anterior–posterior or a lateral–medial squeeze present during all attempts to speak (termed the isometric larynx[34]), *without intermittent voice breaks*, is more typical of muscular tension dysphonia, considered a 'functional' voice disorder. Differentiating muscular tension dysphonia from ADSD is a frequent dilemma because often patients with ADSD have a constant harshness in addition to their intermittent spasmodic breaks. These SD patients may have an overlaid muscular tension dysphonia as a result of using increased tension in their laryngeal muscles in an attempt to control involuntary movements. Some clinicians have suggested that response to voice therapy is diagnostic in such cases; patients with muscular tension dysphonia often benefit from manual circumlaryngeal therapy, whereas those with SD do not.[8,35]

If a patient has a constant breathy voice without prolonged voiceless consonants which are heard as intermittent breathy breaks, the disorder is more likely a 'functional' voice disorder than ABSD. Patients who are *constantly* aphonic, but have normal vocal fold movements for cough, whistle, throat clear, and swallow, often have psychogenic voice disorders. Total aphonia rarely, if ever, occurs in ABSD. Humming and other task manipulations involving distractions, counting backwards in sevens, along with circumlaryngeal manipulation can sometimes resolve psychogenic voice disorders.[36,37]

PVFD, due to gastric reflux or in association with anxiety and masquerading as asthma, is usually episodic and therefore has very different features from adductor breathing dystonia. Episodes of stridor that occur in the middle of the night or after bending over in the middle of the day suggest gastric reflux. These can be managed by an otolaryngologist using proton pump inhibitors while education by a speech–language pathologist can help the patient understand what is causing the problem and help to reduce the patient's anxiety. If the disorder is exercise-induced, having the patient perform the exercise before the nasolaryngoscopy can be helpful in viewing the laryngeal movement abnormality and can be used to show the patient how to control the symptoms by using short light breaths and avoiding deep inspirations.

TREATMENT OF LARYNGEAL DYSTONIAS

None of the currently available treatments for laryngeal dystonias will reverse the central disorder; all are aimed at only peripheral control of the muscle spasms, either through denervation or muscle excision. The treatments available manage the symptoms for different time windows and with side effects of varying degrees.

Treatments for spasmodic dysphonia

Botulinum toxin injections into the thyroarytenoid muscle or combined with the lateral cricoarytenoid muscle benefit 90% of ADSD patients[38–40] (Table 11.3). Although most patients report significant benefit, even those with a good response do not have a normal voice; the voice is usually 'thin' and reduced in resonance.[41] Small bilateral injections with a starting dose of 1.5–2.5 units on each side[42] were shown effective in a small double-blind trial.[43] Other clinicians have used unilateral injections, producing a unilateral paresis/paralysis.[44] No consistent differences have been found between the two approaches.[45–48] Some clinicians report that unilateral injections can be better controlled to meet patients' needs without producing considerable swallowing and breathiness as side effects.[48] Accurate placement of the toxin in the thyroarytenoid muscle is essential and, usually, placement errors are the basis for a poor result.[49] Continued treatment with botulinum toxin injection is beneficial using outcome measures.[50] However, some patients lose their benefit over time; in such cases, alternating between unilateral and bilateral injections or between injection to the right and then the left can better control symptoms without increasing the dosage.[51] A few patients have developed antibodies to botulinum toxin following laryngeal injections after dosage increases.[52]

Surgical approaches to laryngeal muscle denervation have been used for treatment of SD. The initial success often fades, however, as the central disorder often returns with reinnervation of the laryngeal muscles. Recurrent laryngeal nerve resection was introduced by Dedo[53] in the 1970s but a return of symptoms occurred within a few years in 60% of patients.[54] A recurrent laryngeal nerve avulsion, a more extensive procedure, although used in a smaller number of patients, may have a better long-term rate of symptom control.[55,56] More recently Berke et al developed a denervation–reinnervation procedure, sectioning the branch of the recurrent nerve going to the thyroarytenoid muscle on both sides and then reinnervating with the ansa cervicalis.[57] The procedure initially produces swallowing problems and loss of voice, which then resolve with a resulting voice benefit. The results have recently been replicated in a small series by a second group[58] and a long-term follow-up of patients showed benefit in several patients based on a questionnaire completed by the patients.[59] Isshiki introduced a laryngeal framework approach (midline lateralization thyroplasty type 2) to produce a gap between the vocal folds with a wedge in the anterior commissure. This was reported in six cases, with no postoperative voice evaluation. If such surgical procedures are successful, they might provide patients with longer-term benefits by permanently altering laryngeal structure and function.

Table 11.3 Treatment dosages with botulinum toxin for the laryngeal dystonias

Disorder	Type	Muscle	Dosage
Spasmodic dysphonias	Adductor	Bilateral thyroarytenoid	1.5–2.5 U initial injection 0.5–2.0 U reinjection
		Unilateral thyroarytenoid	7.5–15 U initial injection 5–10 U reinjection
	Abductor	Bilateral posterior cricoarytenoid	Only inject one side at a time, 5 U one side, 5 U, 1–2 weeks later, on opposite side
		Unilateral posterior cricoarytenoid	10 U one side only
Voice tremor	Adductor	Bilateral thyroarytenoid	1.5–2.5 U initial injection 0.5–2.0 U reinjection
		Unilateral thyroarytenoid	7.5–15 U initial injection 5–10 U reinjection
	Abductor	Bilateral posterior cricoarytenoid	Only inject one side at a time, 5 U one side, 5 U, 1–2 weeks later, on opposite side
		Unilateral posterior cricoarytenoid	10 U one side only
Adductor breathing dystonia	Laryngeal obstruction	Bilateral thyroarytenoid	1.5–2.5 U initial injection 0.5–2.0 U reinjection

Treating abductor spasmodic dysphonia

Treatment for ABSD has not been as successful as for ADSD using either botulinum toxin injection or surgery. Most efforts using botulinum toxin have focused on the posterior cricoarytenoid, the only muscle that opens the vocal folds. About 60% of patients benefit[60,61] and their benefit is less and shorter than in ADSD.[47] One reason may be technical: greater skill and experience is needed to inject the posterior cricoarytenoid and few centers see large numbers of these patients. Secondly, great care must be taken to prevent stridor and bilateral airway obstruction, requiring a tracheostomy if both sides are injected. Therefore, most centers inject only one side at a time with 3–5 units and have the patient return in 2 weeks to re-evaluate before deciding to inject the other side. Some centers only inject one side with a dosage of 10 units.

Some patients may not have involuntary spasms of the posterior cricoarytenoid muscles. In one series of patients with spasmodic bursts seen in the cricothyroid muscle during speech, bilateral cricothyroid injections reduced symptoms.[62] An electromyographic study of patients with ABSD not benefited by botulinum toxin found decreases in tone in the thyroarytenoid muscle on one side during speech.[30]

Surgical options have been few. To prevent excessive abduction, one approach combined a myotomy of the posterior cricoarytenoid with a thyroplasty.[63] In a preliminary report, this was performed in three patients with partial success, making the approach experimental.

Voice tremor

A variety of muscles can be affected in vocal tremor[23] and the types of tremor may be either action-induced or continuously present. In addition, the tremor may be focal to just the thyroarytenoid muscle, or involve the muscles of the entire upper airway. This may explain why results have been unreliable when only the thyroarytenoid muscle is injected in the same fashion as in ADSD.[64–66] In general, about 50% of patients are benefited and the degree of benefit has been limited. A combined approach of medication (beta blockers) and botulinum toxin injection is often used. Further research is needed to more carefully categorize patients according to which muscles are affected to produce a more reliable result using botulinum toxin in voice tremor.

Treating adductor breathing dystonia

Patients with an adductor breathing dystonia must be carefully distinguished from those with episodic PVFD, as the treatment regimen differs. Adductor breathing dystonia is rare and only large centers are likely to see enough of these patients for accurate diagnosis. If a patient is shown to have laryngeal obstruction rather than pharyngeal involvement, botulinum toxin injection of the thyroarytenoid muscles, similar to treatment for ADSD, is the best approach to treatment.[26] Injecting the thyroarytenoid muscle bilaterally can reduce the degree of obstruction or stridor; however, there is a trade-off between an improvement in breathing and loss of voice volume and swallowing difficulties.[26,67] Patients with pharyngeal obstruction cannot be managed using botulinum toxin injection, because of the potential for swallowing difficulties. Therefore, the use of medications for management of the dystonia is currently the only approach available for this disorder.

PATHOPHYSIOLOGY AND PATHOGENESIS OF THE LARYNGEAL DYSTONIAS

Very little is understood about these disorders – most research has focused on controlling symptoms through peripheral changes in muscle activation in the larynx. In the 1970s came the first recognition that these were neurologic disorders.[68,69] During the 1980s it was recognized that the symptomatology was similar to other focal dystonias, and the term 'laryngeal dystonia' was first used.[70] Studies on the pathophysiology in the 1990s demonstrated similar abnormalities in central suppression of laryngeal adductor reflexes in both ADSD and ABSD.[71,72] Little attention has been given to the neurologic abnormalities underlying the involuntary muscle spasms. A few studies in the 1990s, using the techniques available at that time, had equivocal findings.[73–75]

With more recent brain imaging techniques, better insight should soon become available on the central abnormalities of these patients. Recently, two neuroimaging studies have been published on SD: both studies compared patients with healthy volunteers before receiving botulinum toxin and then examined changes in the patients' brain activation after receiving botulinum toxin.[76,77] Although the two studies had methodologic differences, one used positron emission tomography and O_2[15] and examined connected speech,[76] while the other used blood oxygen level-dependent changes in functional magnetic romance imaging (fMRI) and examined extended phonation on a vowel.[77] However, both studies had a similar finding of reduced activity in the most lateral M1-S1 regions in the SD patients versus controls, possibly those regions associated with laryngeal sensorimotor control. In one study, however, the hypoactivity in laryngeal sensory regions did not normalize with botulinum toxin injection but was less apparent during whispering.[77] In the other study, the unimodal and heteromodal sensory hypoactivity was reduced in SD but increased with botulinum toxin, and increases in blood flow in the left hemisphere sensory regions were highly correlated with the degree of symptom improvement.[76] These two studies both demonstrate functional neurologic abnormalities that are associated with symptoms of SD in left hemisphere sensorimotor processing for laryngeal control during phonation and whispered speech.

Nothing is known about the etiology of the laryngeal dystonias. Dedo et al first proposed that pathologic changes could be found in the recurrent laryngeal nerve that might indicate a peripheral etiology for the disorder;[68] however, other clinicians could not replicate these findings.[78] More recently, similar studies have yielded conflicting results[79,80] and concluded that the disorder is central in origin.

Only a small percentage of patients have a familial background of either idiopathic torsion dystonia or other focal dystonias;[81] the most frequent condition is writer's cramp, which is found in 11% of patients with SD.[82] The disorder is predominant in females (between 60–80% of those affected)[18,82,83] and develops later than many forms of focal primary dystonia with mean age of onset in one study of 50.7 years.[84] This is in keeping with other adult onset primary cranial dystonias. Events commonly reported preceding the onset of symptoms include a severe upper respiratory infection with an associated voice disorder which does not remit in 30%, with a period of severe stress in 21%.[82] One study found a childhood incidence of measles or mumps in 65% of patients but there was no control group.[82] Onset is usually gradual; the initial voice symptoms may fluctuate over the first 2–6 months before stabilizing and becoming chronic after a year. Improved understanding of the central mechanisms involved in symptom generation in SD is needed to develop new and effective treatment approaches aimed at altering the central abnormality responsible for the generation of spasms. Furthermore, knowledge of risk factors and the mechanisms involved in the pathogenesis might lead to prevention of the disorder. The field has a long way to go to meet these objectives.

REFERENCES

1. Castelon Konkiewitz E, Trender-Gerhard I, Kamm C et al. Service-based survey of dystonia in Munich. Neuroepidemiology 2002; 21(4): 202–6.
2. Watts CR, Vanryckeghem M. Laryngeal dysfunction in amyotrophic lateral sclerosis: a review and case report. BMC Ear Nose Throat Disord 2001; 1(1): 1.
3. Hanson DG, Ludlow CL, Bassich CJ. Vocal fold paresis and Shy–Drager syndrome. Ann Otol Rhinol Laryngol 1983; 92: 85–90.
4. Logemann JA, Fisher HB, Bocshes B. Frequency and cooccurrence of vocal tract dysfunction in the speech of a large sample of Parkinson's patients. J Speech Hear Disord 1978; 434: 47–57.
5. Gacek RR. Hereditary abductor vocal cord paralysis. Ann Otol 1976; 85: 90–3.
6. Morrison MD, Rammage LA, Belisle GM, Pullan CB, Nichol H. Muscular tension dysphonia. J Otolaryngol 1983; 12: 302–6.
7. Christopher KL, Wood R, Eckert RC et al. Vocal-cord dysfunction presenting as asthma. N Engl J Med 1983; 306: 1566–70.
8. Roy N, Bless DM, Heisey D, Ford CN. Manual circumlaryngeal therapy for functional dysphonia: an evaluation of short- and long-term treatment outcomes. J Voice 1997; 11: 321–31.
9. Ginsberg VI, Wallach JJ, Srain JJ, Biller HF. Defining the psychiatric role in spastic dysphonia. General Hospital Psychiatry 1988; 10: 132–7.
10. Roth CR, Glaze LE, Goding GS Jr, David WS. Spasmodic dysphonia symptoms as initial presentation of amyotrophic lateral sclerosis. J Voice 1996; 10(4): 362–7.
11. Leonard R, Kendall K. Differentiation of spasmodic and psychogenic dysphonias with phonoscopic evaluation. Laryngoscope 1999; 109(2 Pt 1): 295–300.
12. Shipp T, Izdebski K, Reed C, Morrissey P. Intrinsic laryngeal muscle activity in a spastic dysphonic patient. Speech Hear Disord 1985; 50: 54–9.
13. Van Pelt F, Ludlow CL, Smith PJ. Comparison of muscle activation patterns in adductor and abductor spasmodic dysphonia. Ann Otol Rhinol Laryngol 1994; 103: 192–200.
14. Barkmeier JM, Case JL, Ludlow CL. Identification of symptoms for spasmodic dysphonia and vocal tremor: a comparison of expert and nonexpert judges. J Commun Disord 2001; 34(1–2): 21–37.
15. Parnes SM, Lavorato AS, Myers EN. Study of spastic dysphonia using videofiberoptic laryngoscopy. Ann Otol 1978; 87: 322–6.
16. Nash EA, Ludlow CL. Laryngeal muscle activity during speech breaks in adductor spasmodic dysphonia. Laryngoscope 1996; 106: 484–9.
17. Bielamowicz S, Ludlow CL. Effects of botulinum toxin on pathophysiology in spasmodic dysphonia. Ann Otol Rhinol Laryngol 2000; 109: 194–203.
18. Blitzer A, Brin MF, Stewart CF. Botulinum toxin management of spasmodic dysphonia (laryngeal dystonia): a 12-year experience in more than 900 patients. Laryngoscope 1998; 108(10): 1435–41.
19. Stewart CF, Allen EL, Tureen P et al. Adductor spasmodic dysphonia: standard evaluation of symptoms and severity. J Voice 1997; 11(1): 95–103.
20. Jurgens U. Neural pathways underlying vocal control. Neurosci Biobehav Rev 2002; 26(2): 235–58.
21. Aronson AE, Hartman DE. Adductor spastic dysphonia as a sign of essential (voice) tremor. Speech Hear Disord 1981; 46: 52–8.
22. Aronson AE, Brown JR, Litin EM, Pearson JS. Spastic dysphonia: II. Comparison with essential (voice) tremor and other neurologic and psychogenic dysphonias. J Speech Hear Disord 1968; 33: 219–31.
23. Koda J, Ludlow CL. An evaluation of laryngeal muscle activation in patients with voice tremor. Otolaryngol Head Neck Surg 1992; 107: 684–96.
24. Horiuchi M, Sasaki CT. Cricothyroid muscle in respiration. Ann Otol Rhinol Laryngol 1978; 87(3 Pt 1): 386–91.
25. Bartlett DJ, Remmers JE, Gautier H. Laryngeal regulation of respiratory airflow. Respir Physiol 1973; 18: 194–204.
26. Marion MH, Klap P, Perrin A, Cohen M. Stridor and focal laryngeal dystonia. Lancet 1992; 339: 457–8.
27. Maschka DA, Bauman NM, McCray PB Jr et al. A classification scheme for paradoxical vocal cord motion. Laryngoscope 1997; 107(11 Pt 1): 1429–35.
28. Loughlin CJ, Koufman JA. Paroxysmal laryngospasm secondary to gastroesophageal reflux. Laryngoscope 1996; 106: 1501–5.
29. Aronson AE. Importance of the psychosocial interview in the diagnosis and treatment of "functional" voice disorders. J Voice 1990; 4: 287–9.
30. Cyrus CB, Bielamowicz S, Evans FJ, Ludlow CL. Adductor muscle activity abnormalities in abductor spasmodic dysphonia. Otolaryngol Head Neck Surg 2001; 124(1): 23–30.
31. Smith ME, Ramig LO, Dromey C, Perez KS, Samandari R. Intensive voice treatment in Parkinson disease: laryngostroboscopic findings. J Voice 1995; 9: 453–9.
32. Dyck PJ, Litchy WJ, Minnerath S et al. Hereditary motor and sensory neuropathy with diaphragm and vocal cord paresis. Ann Neurol 1994; 35: 608–15.
33. Sataloff RT, Rosen DC, Hawkshaw M, Spiegel JR. The aging adult voice. J Voice 1997; 11(2): 156–60.
34. Morrison MD, Rammage LA. Muscle misuse voice disorders: description and classification. Acta Otolaryngol (Stockh) 1993; 113: 428–34.
35. Roy N, Ford CN, Bless DM. Muscle tension dysphonia and spasmodic dysphonia: the role of manual laryngeal tension reduction in diagnosis and management. Ann Otol Rhinol Laryngol 1996; 105: 851–6.
36. Sapir S, Aronson AE. The relationship between psychopathology and speech and language disorders in neurologic patients. J Speech Hear Disord 1990; 55: 503–9.
37. Sapir S. Psychogenic spasmodic dysphonia: a case study with expert opinions. J Voice 1995; 9: 270–81.
38. Gibbs SR, Blitzer A. Botulinum toxin for the treatment of spasmodic dysphonia. Otolaryngol Clin North Am 2000; 33(4): 879–94.
39. Inagi K, Ford CN, Bless DM, Heisey D. Analysis of factors affecting botulinum toxin results in spasmodic dysphonia. J Voice 1996; 10: 306–13.
40. Castellanos PF, Gates GA, Esselman G et al. Anatomic considerations in botulinum toxin type A therapy for spasmodic dysphonia. Laryngoscope 1994; 104: 656–62.
41. Langeveld TPM, van Rossum M, Houtman EH et al. Evaluation of voice quality in adductor spasmodic dysphonia before and after botulinum toxin treatment. Ann Otol Rhinol Laryngol 2001; 110(7): 627–34.
42. Blitzer A, Brin MF. Laryngeal dystonia: a series with botulinum toxin therapy. Ann Otol Rhinol Laryngol 1991; 100: 85–9.
43. Troung DD, Rontal M, Rolnick M, Aronson AE, Mistura K. Double-blind controlled study of botulinum toxin in adductor spasmodic dysphonia. Laryngoscope 1991; 101(6 Pt 1): 630–4.
44. Ludlow CL, Naunton RF, Sedory SE, Schulz GM, Hallett M. Effects of botulinum toxin injections on speech in adductor spasmodic dysphonia. Neurology 1988; 38: 1220–5.
45. Adams SG, Hunt EJ, Charles DA, Lang AE. Unilateral versus bilateral botulinum toxin injections in spasmodic dysphonia: acoustic and perceptual results. J Otolaryngol 1993; 22: 171–5.
46. Langeveld TPM, Drost HA, De Jong RJB. Unilateral versus bilateral botulinum toxin injections in adductor spasmodic dysphonia. Ann Otol Rhinol Laryngol 1998; 107: 280–4.
47. Ludlow CL, Bagley JA, Yin SG, Koda J. A comparison of different injection techniques in the treatment of spasmodic dysphonia with botulinum toxin. J Voice 1992; 6: 380–6.

48. Bielamowicz S, Stager SV, Badillo A, Godlewski A. Unilateral versus bilateral injections of botulinum toxin in patients with adductor spasmodic dysphonia. J Voice 2002; 16(1): 117–23.
49. Galardi G, Guerriero R, Amadio S et al. Sporadic failure of botulinum toxin treatment in usually responsive patients with adductor spasmodic dysphonia. Neurol Sci 2001; 22(4): 303–6.
50. Courey MS, Garrett CG, Billante CR et al. Outcomes assessment following treatment of spasmodic dysphonia with botulinum toxin. Ann Otol Rhinol Laryngol 2000; 109(9): 819–22.
51. Koriwchak MJ, Netterville JL, Snowden T, Courey M, Ossoff RH. Alternating unilateral botulinum toxin type A (BOTOX) injections for spasmodic dysphonia. Laryngoscope 1996; 106(12 Pt 1): 1476–81.
52. Smith ME, Ford CN. Resistance to botulinum toxin injections for spasmodic dysphonia. Arch Otolaryngol Head Neck Surg 2000; 126(4): 533–5.
53. Dedo HH. Recurrent laryngeal nerve section for spastic dysphonia. Ann Otol Rhinol Laryngol 1976; 85: 451–9.
54. Aronson AE, DeSanto LW. Adductor spastic dysphonia: 1 1/2 years after recurrent laryngeal nerve resection. Ann Otol Rhinol Laryngol 1981; 90(1 Pt 1): 2–6.
55. Netterville JL, Stone RE, Rainey C, Zealear DL, Ossoff RH. Recurrent laryngeal nerve avulsion for treatment of spastic dysphonia. Ann Otol Rhinol Laryngol 1991; 100(1): 10–14.
56. Weed DT, Jewett BS, Rainey C et al. Long term follow up of recurrent laryngeal nerve avulsion for the treatment of spastic dysphonia. Ann Otol Rhinol Laryngol 1996; 105(8): 592–601.
57. Berke GS, Blackwell KE, Gerratt BR et al. Selective laryngeal adductor denervation–reinnervation: a new surgical treatment for adductor spasmodic dysphonia. Ann Otol Rhinol Laryngol 1999; 108(3): 227–31.
58. Allegretto M, Morrison M, Rammage L, Lau DP. Selective denervation: reinnervation for the control of adductor spasmodic dysphonia. J Otolaryngol 2003; 32(3): 185–9.
59. Chhetri DK, Mendelsohn AH, Blumin JH, Berke GS. Long-term follow-up results of selective laryngeal adductor denervation–reinnervation surgery for adductor spasmodic dysphonia. Laryngoscope 2006; 116(4): 635–42.
60. Blitzer A, Brin M, Stewart C, Aviv JE, Fahn S. Abductor laryngeal dystonia: a series treated with botulinum toxin. Laryngoscope 1992; 102: 163–7.
61. Bielamowicz S, Squire S, Bidus K, Ludlow CL. Assessment of posterior cricoarytenoid botulinum toxin injections in patients with abductor spasmodic dysphonia. Ann Otol Rhinol Laryngol 2001; 110(5 Pt 1): 406–12.
62. Ludlow CL, Naunton RF, Terada S, Anderson BJ. Successful treatment of selected cases of abductor spasmodic dysphonia using botulinum toxin injection. Otolaryngol Head Neck Surg 1991; 104: 849–55.
63. Shaw GY, Sechtem PR, Rideout B. Posterior cricoarytenoid myoplasty with medialization thyroplasty in the management of refractory abductor spasmodic dysphonia. Ann Otol Rhinol Laryngol 2003; 112(4): 303–6.
64. Hertegard S, Granqvist S, Lindestad PA. Botulinum toxin injections for essential voice tremor. Ann Otol Rhinol Laryngol 2000; 109(2): 204–9.
65. Warrick P, Dromey C, Irish JC et al. Botulinum toxin for essential tremor of the voice with multiple anatomical sites of tremor: a crossover design study of unilateral versus bilateral injection. Laryngoscope 2000; 110(8): 1366–74.
66. Warrick P, Dromey C, Irish J, Durkin L. The treatment of essential voice tremor with botulinum toxin A: a longitudinal case report. J Voice 2000; 14: 410–21.
67. Grillone GA, Blitzer A, Brin MF, Annino DJ, Saint-Hilaire MH. Treatment of adductor laryngeal breathing dystonia with botulinum toxin type A. Laryngoscope 1994; 24: 30.
68. Dedo HH, Townsend JJ, Izdebski K. Current evidence for the organic etiology of spastic dysphonia. Otolaryngology 1978; 86: 875–80.
69. Aminoff MJ, Dedo HH, Izdebski K. Clinical aspects of spasmodic dysphonia. J Neurol Neurosurg Psychiatry 1978; 41: 361–5.
70. Blitzer A, Lovelace RE, Brin MF, Fahn S, Fink ME. Electromyographic findings in focal laryngeal dystonia (spastic dysphonia). Ann Otol Rhinol Laryngol 1985; 94: 591–4.
71. Ludlow CL, Schulz GM, Yamashita T, Deleyiannis FW. Abnormalities in long latency responses to superior laryngeal nerve stimulation in adductor spasmodic dysphonia. Ann Otol Rhinol Laryngol 1995; 104: 928–35.
72. Deleyiannis FW, Gillespie M, Bielamowicz S, Yamashita T, Ludlow CL. Laryngeal long latency response conditioning in abductor spasmodic dysphonia. Ann Otol Rhinol Laryngol 1999; 108(6): 612–19.
73. Schaefer SD, Freeman F, Finitzo T et al. Magnetic resonance imaging findings and correlations in spasmodic dysphonia patients. Ann Otol Rhinol Laryngol 1985; 94: 595–601.
74. Devous MD, Pool KD, Finitzo T et al. Evidence for cortical dysfunction in spasmodic dysphonia: regional cerebral blood flow and quantitative electrophysiology. Brain Lang 1990; 39: 331–44.
75. Pool KD, Freeman FJ, Finitzo T et al. Heterogeneity in spasmodic dysphonia. Arch Neurol 1991; 48: 305–9.
76. Ali SO, Guillemin BA, Thomassen M et al. Alterations in CNS activity induced by botulinum toxin treatment in spasmodic dysphonia: an $H_2{}^{15}O$ PET study. Speech Language Hearing Res 2006; 49: 1127–46.
77. Haslinger B, Erhard P, Dresel C et al. "Silent event-related" fMRI reveals reduced sensorimotor activation in laryngeal dystonia. Neurology 2005; 65(10): 1562–9.
78. Ravits JM, Aronson AE, Desanto LW, Dyck PJ. No morphometric abnormality recurrent laryngeal nerve in spastic dysphonia. Neurology 1979; 29: 1376–82.
79. Kosaki H, Iwamura S, Yamazaki I. Histologic study of the recurrent laryngeal nerve in spasmodic dysphonia. Otolaryngol Head Neck Surg 1999; 120(1): 129–33.
80. Chhetri DK, Blumin JH, Vinters HV, Berke GS. Histology of nerves and muscles in adductor spasmodic dysphonia. Ann Otol Rhinol Laryngol 2003; 112(4): 334–41.
81. Blitzer A, Brin MF, Fahn S, Lovelace RE. Clinical and laboratory characteristics of focal laryngeal dystonia: study of 110 cases. Laryngoscope 1988; 98: 636–40.
82. Schweinfurth JM, Billante M, Courey MS. Risk factors and demographics in patients with spasmodic dysphonia. Laryngoscope 2002; 112(2): 220–3.
83. Adler CH, Edwards BW, Bansberg SF. Female predominance in spasmodic dysphonia. J Neurol Neurosurg Psychiatry 1997; 63(5): 688.
84. Epidemiological Study of Dystonia in Europe (ESDE) Collaborative Group. Sex-related influences on frequency and age of onset of primary dystonia. Neurology 1999; 53: 1871–3

12

Dystonia-plus syndromes

Thomas Gasser, Friedrich Asmus, and Christoph Kamm

INTRODUCTION

In recent classifications of the dystonias, several disorders have been distinguished from 'idiopathic' or 'primary' torsion dystonia based on characteristic clinical features or pharmacologic responses. These diseases have been grouped into a category of 'dystonia-plus syndromes'.[1] This distinction is useful from a nosologic point of view, as dystonia-plus syndromes frequently have distinct genetic etiologies. However, as in most genetically complex disorders, clinical and genetic classifications are not entirely concordant. Not all patients diagnosed according to a given set of clinical criteria prove to have a discernible genetic defect. If they do, the clinical presentation may be highly variable, even within single families, regardless of the underlying genetic cause, and may overlap with other genetic or non-genetic disease entities.

For example, an occasional patient with genetically proven myoclonus-dystonia (M-D, DYT11) may present with pure writer's cramp in his forties[2] and may therefore be misclassified as 'primary dystonia'. Lightning-like myoclonic jerks, which are the clinical hallmark of M-D and which may be found in other members of his family, may only be reported to have prevailed until late adolescence.

On the other hand, myoclonic jerks in affected body parts of patients with primary torsion dystonia (PTD) are quite common. This is reflected in the term 'myoclonic dystonia',[3] which has been coined to draw attention to this fact. To avoid confusion, this term should now only be used to describe this feature of primary dystonia, and not the disease of 'myoclonus-dystonia', which denotes the genetic disorder described in more detail below.

Patients with another dystonia-plus syndrome, dopa-responsive dystonia (DRD, DYT5), may be indistinguishable from those with PTD unless treated with L-dopa. And even then, occasional patients with PTD often show transient or partial therapeutic benefit to L-dopa (although usually not as striking as in DRD), and anticholinergic medication may also be beneficial in both groups.[4] For several of the dystonia-plus syndromes, the respective genetic loci have been mapped, and a few of the genes have been identified. Although the proteins encoded by these genes appear to serve completely distinct cellular functions, the similarities between the different entities exemplified above may point to common molecular pathways in their pathogenesis.

In this chapter, the molecular and genetic basis of three dystonia-plus syndromes is discussed in detail.

- dopa-responsive dystonia, myoclonus-dystonia, and rapid-onset dystonia-parkinsonism.
- Other dystonic syndromes with specific distinguishing clinical features, such as the paroxysmal dystonias, are discussed in other chapters of this book.

DOPA-RESPONSIVE DYSTONIA (DYT5)

The syndrome of DRD was first delineated by Segawa et al in 1976.[5] Since then, the analysis of this syndrome and the underlying molecular biochemical alterations have not only helped to elucidate the molecular pathogenesis of this disease but also provided many valuable insights into the motor function of the basal ganglia.

Clinical presentation

Patients with typical DRD usually present with gait disturbance due to foot dystonia between the ages of 1 and 12 (mean ~6) years. Dystonia often becomes progressively severe during the day (diurnal variation) and is relieved by sleep or rest. The course of the condition is variable, sometimes evolving to severe generalized dystonia that renders the patient wheelchair-bound. Features suggestive of lower extremity spasticity (brisk deep-tendon reflexes, ankle clonus, and/or dystonic extension of the big toe [the striatal toe]) are present in many patients. Parkinsonian symptoms commonly develop later during the disease. In some patients, mild parkinsonism may also be the only manifestation of the disorder (although DRD is certainly a very rare cause in an otherwise-unselected group of patients with adult-onset parkinsonism). Atypical manifestations have been described, such as adult-onset limb, cervical, and craniofacial dystonia,[1,6,7] and some patients may resemble spastic paraplegics.[8] On rare occasions, patients present with myoclonic jerks of the neck accompanying cervical dystonia and the condition could be therefore confused with myoclonus-dystonia.[9] Minimal manifestations, such as stiffness of a leg upon exertion, can also be seen. As in other forms of dystonia, site and age at presentation are interdependent. Onset before the age of 10 years occurs usually in the lower limb, whereas other manifestations, including postural tremor, are commonly seen in cases with later onset.

The most striking clinical feature is the marked and sustained responsiveness to relatively small doses (usually 50–200 mg, but in some cases up to 450 mg may be necessary) of L-dopa/decarboxylase inhibitor.[10] Fluctuations and dyskinesias, often seen as troublesome complications of long-term L-dopa treatment in Parkinson's disease, are rare and, if they occur, only mild in DRD.[11] Treatment should be initiated with slowly increasing doses, and a response is usually seen within days or a few weeks. Rapid dose increases may result in choreic, myoclonic, or tic-like hyperkinesias, which disappear upon dose reduction. Patients have been followed for over 30 years without loss of efficacy. Anticholinergics are also quite effective, although not as completely and consistently as L-dopa. Some patients, particularly those with severe tetrahydrobiopterin (BH_4) deficiency due to compound heterozygous mutations (see below), may require supplementation of 5-hydroxytryptophan (the precursor of serotonin, as phenylalanine hydroxylase also uses BH_4 as a cofactor) and BH_4. Imaging studies using ligands for the pre- and postsynaptic dopaminergic terminals ([^{11}C]-methyphenidate and [^{11}C]-raclopride, respectively) showed that those structures are not compromised in DRD.[12–14] However, a marked increase in the uptake of [^{11}C]-dihydrotetrabenazine (DTBZ), a ligand of the vesicular monoamine transporter (VMAT2), has been interpreted as reflecting the decrease in the intravesicular concentration of dopamine and/or a compensatory up-regulation of VMAT2 expression.[15] Pathologically, a normal number of neurons in the substantia nigra has been found. These neurons, however, are poorly melanized,[16] possibly reflecting the lower rate of dopamine turnover and hence autooxidation.

Recent observations point towards a possibility of discriminating DRD from juvenile-onset parkinsonism by transcranial ultrasound: DRD patients fail to show increased areas of substantia nigra hyperechogenicity.[17]

Genetic and molecular basis

Inheritance of DRD is in most cases autosomal dominant with incomplete penetrance. Apparently sporadic cases with proven mutations occur and may be due to incomplete penetrance in other family members or to new mutational events (which is not uncommon in DRD). Many series showed a higher penetrance (~2.5-fold) in females compared to males. Personal examination of the parents of reportedly sporadic children with DRD often reveals mild parkinsonism of adult onset in a mutation-carrying parent.

The gene for dominant DRD has been mapped to chromosome 14[18] and the causative mutations were identified in the gene for GTP cyclohydrolase I (GCH1).[19] The encoded protein, GTPCH1, catalyzes the first step of BH_4 synthesis, which is in turn a crucial cofactor for tyrosine hydroxylase (TH), the rate-limiting key enzyme in the biosynthesis of dopamine and other amine neurotransmitters.

More than 85 different mutations scattered over all 5 exons of the gene have been found so far,[20] including missense and nonsense mutations, but also mutations affecting splice sites,[21] mutations in the 5′-untranslated region,[22] or large genomic deletions.[23] In as many as 40% of patients with otherwise typical DRD (both familial and sporadic) no mutation can be detected in the coding region, even in some cases with proven linkage to the DRD locus on chromosome 14.[19,22,24] It is assumed that mutations in the introns or regulatory regions of the gene may be responsible in these cases.

Molecular pathogenesis

The molecular pathogenesis of DRD is still not entirely clear. Heterozygous mutations in the *GCH1* gene result in a reduction of enzyme activity beyond what would be expected by a simple loss of function of one allele. Brain levels of total biopterin, neopterin, and dopamine are decreased by more than 80–90% in symptomatic individuals with DRD.[25] Also, activity of GTPCH1 in phytohemagglutinin-stimulated mononuclear blood cells of patients with this type of DRD is decreased to less than 20% of that of normal controls.[19] This phenomenon can probably be explained, at least in part, by a classic 'dominant negative' effect: GTPCH1 normally functions as a homodecameric complex. The integration of abnormal polypeptides derived from the mutant allele into this complex will therefore lead to dysfunction of a large proportion of catalytic units, as only a few will exist entirely of wild-type peptides. Other mechanisms, however, may also play a role. In fact, there is now direct experimental evidence that dominant mutations of *GCH1* may exert their dominant negative effect by also decreasing the level of wild-type protein in the cell: cotransfection of HEK cells with vectors encoding both the mutant and wild-type gene led to accelerated protein degradation.[26]

The deficiency of GTPCH1 activity results in reduced levels of total biopterin (the bulk of which is present as tetrahydrobiopterin (BH_4 in the brain) and neopterin. BH_4 deficiency in turn leads to a reduction of enzymatic activity of TH and other BH_4-dependent enzymes. As a consequence, the concentration of dopamine and its metabolite homovanillic acid (HVA) is reduced in the striatum, which is also measurable in the cerebrospinal fluid (CSF).[27] However, decreased dopamine levels are not only due to low enzymatic activity of TH in the presence of low cofactor concentrations but also to a loss of the TH protein. In fact, a reduction of TH protein content by as much as 97% in the putamen has been found in patients with typical DRD.[27] As levels of TH protein and mRNA in the substantia nigra are normal, it has been hypothesized that the loss of striatal TH is due to increased instability and degradation of the protein in the absence of its cofactor BH_4, within the nigrostriatal processes.

The pattern of striatal dopamine depletion in DRD and idiopathic Parkinson's disease (PD) differs in some respect and its analysis may well provide interesting insights into the function of the basal ganglia. In both DRD and PD, the dopamine deficiency is greater in the putamen than in the caudate nucleus. However, there is evidence that the distribution along the ventrodorsal axis of the striatum may differ between the two disorders, the ventral area being more affected in DRD, while the dorsal portions are more heavily involved in PD. As there is also a differential distribution of relative abundance of D_1 and D_2 receptors in these areas, which in turn are linked to the direct and indirect striatopallidal pathways, respectively, it is possible that the relative difference in dopamine efficiency in D_1 vs D_2 pathways may account, in part, for the different clinical presentation of the two disorders.[28]

Another interesting aspect is the age dependence of clinical symptoms related to dopamine depletion: young-onset cases tend to present with dystonia, whereas later onset is more commonly associated with parkinsonism, both in DRD and in PD. It has been hypothesized that this age effect may be related to differential maturation of dopamine receptors.[29]

Not only TH but also phenylalanine hydroxylase and tryptophan hydroxylase use BH_4 as a cofactor. However, in dominant DRD, only dopamine seems to be deficient to a clinically relevant degree, but not serotonin, the product of tryptophan hydroxylase. The reason for this observation is not entirely clear. It is possible that different expression levels of the respective enzymes in dopaminergic vs serotonergic neurons may play a role. It is also possible that the higher K_m value of TH for BH_4 may contribute to the fact that TH enzymatic activity appears to be much more impaired compared to that of the other two hydroxylases.

Heterozygous, dominant negative mutations in the *GCH1* gene cause a spectrum of clinical manifestations of DRD, as described above. In contrast, patients with homozygous (two identical) or compound heterozygous mutations in the *GCH1* gene *in trans* (a different mutation in each of the two copies of the gene) have a more severe loss of enzyme activity, and suffer from BH_4-deficient hyperphenylalaninemia (HPA), a disorder presenting in infancy with severe neurologic dysfunction (mental retardation, developmental delay, convulsions, truncal hypotonia, and limb hypertonia).[30] Patients with an intermediate phenotype carrying (presumably less deleterious) homozygous or compound heterozygous mutations have been described with a dopa-responsive extrapyramidal syndrome beginning in infancy.[31] The parents, as heterozygous carriers of these recessive mutations, remain clinically asymptomatic.

Diagnosis and differential diagnosis

As more than 85 different mutations have been described that are scattered over the entire gene,[20] the practical role of molecular diagnosis is limited. Fortunately, a suspicion of dopa-responsive dystonia can usually be confirmed by the excellent response to L-dopa treatment, so that molecular analysis is frequently not necessary. A slowly increasing dose up to 300–400 mg/day of L-dopa/decarboxylase inhibitor is given; the effect can usually be seen within days, but may occasionally take weeks. Alternatively, low CSF levels of total biopterin and neopterin,[20] a pathologic phenylalanine loading test,[32] or a reduced activity of GTPCH1 in phytohemagglutinin (PHA)-stimulated peripheral mononuclear cells can be used to substantiate the diagnosis.

Relevant differential diagnoses in childhood-onset DRD include spastic paraplegia and cerebral palsy. A trial of L-dopa/decarboxylase inhibitor (up to 200 mg t.i.d. for 4–6 weeks) should be performed in doubtful cases. Early-onset parkinsonism (EOPD), particularly with *parkin* mutations may present with dystonia at onset and can be clinically very similar to DRD.[33] These patients also show a very good response to L-dopa; however, fluctuations and hyperkinesias appear subsequently during the course of the disease. EOPD can also be distinguished from DRD by abnormal imaging studies using markers of the presynaptic dopaminergic terminals and positron emission tomography (PET) ([^{18}F]-fluorodopa; [^{11}C]-methylphenidate) or single-photon emission computed tomography (SPECT) ([^{123}I]-β-CIT)[13,14] or by transcranial ultrasonography.[17]

DRD due to TH deficiency

A recessive form of dopa-responsive dystonia has been described in patients with a genetic deficiency of TH.[34,35] A complete loss of function of the TH protein appears to be lethal, as judged from knock-out ($TH^{-/-}$) mice. Mutations causing a severe TH deficiency, with enzyme activities <5% of normal lead to a syndrome of developmental motor delay, truncal hypotonia, rigidity, and hypokinesia,[36] a disorder which has been termed 'infantile parkinsonism'. Other mutations have been described, however, with enzymatic activities in the range of 10–20% of normal, with a phenotype more closely resembling DRD.[37]

Dystonia occurring with other defects of pterin synthesis

Homozygous mutations in the genes for 6-pyrovoyltetrahydropterin synthase and sepiapterin reductase, encoding the enzymes catalyzing the subsequent two steps of BH_4-biosynthesis, cause HPA and a severe neurologic syndrome including mental retardation, developmental delay, and seizures. Dystonia is usually not a part of this syndrome, although some patients do show dystonic movements with diurnal fluctuations. Such patients may partially respond to L-dopa therapy, but also need replacement of 5-hydroxytryptophan, the precursor of serotonin, and BH_4.[38]

DRD linked to chromosome 14q31 (DYT14)

In a single family with dopa-responsive dystonia, linkage to a novel locus, termed DYT14, has been located to chromosome 14q13 between D4S283 and D4S70 (maximum lod score of 3.28), clearly distinct from the *GCH1* gene on chromosome 14q22. The clinical picture and pathologic findings closely resemble typical *GCH1*-deficient DRD.[39] To date, linkage to DYT14 has not been confirmed in other families and the gene remains to be discovered.

MYOCLONUS-DYSTONIA

Myoclonus-dystonia is a dystonia-plus syndrome characterized by brief lightning-like myoclonic jerks and dystonia.[40–42]

In its familial form, M-D follows an autosomal dominant inheritance pattern. Families with these clinical features have previously been described under the terms of (familial) essential myoclonus,[43–45] myoclonic dystonia,[46–47] and hereditary dystonia with lightning jerks responsive to alcohol.[48] Affecteds in families from all of these categories have been found to carry mutations in the gene for ϵ-sarcoglycan, the major gene in this disorder.

It is important to distinguish inherited M-D from inherited and sporadic primary dystonia with concomitant myoclonic jerks in the dystonic limb, a condition which has also been called myoclonic dystonia.[3] Occasionally, this distinction may be difficult, and discriminating electrophysiologic criteria have not yet been established.

Gene mapping and cloning

After the initial mapping of a locus in large M-D pedigree to the long arm of chromosome 7 (7q21-31) by Nygaard et al,[49] this finding has been confirmed by several other groups.[50–52] Asmus and coworkers narrowed the critical region to approximately 3 cM. Using a classic positional cloning approach, Zimprich et al then identified five different heterozygous loss-of-function mutations in the gene for ε-sarcoglycan (*SGCE*) in six German families with M-D.[53] Subsequently, many additional mutations were reported.[41,54,55]

The fact that mutations in the ε-sarcoglycan gene are causative in a dystonia-plus syndrome was unexpected, as four other known members of the sarcoglycan family of genes (α-, β-, γ- and δ-sarcoglycan) had already been associated with autosomal recessive limb girdle muscular dystrophies.[56]

By contrast to the other sarcoglycans, which are expressed predominantly or exclusively in muscle, *SGCE* expression is found in a wide variety of embryonic and adult tissues, including several brain regions.[57] In the periphery, the sarcoglycans form a complex, together with other proteins, which links intracellular structural proteins like dystrophin to the extracellular matrix. The function of ε-sarcoglycan in brain is still unknown.

The *SGCE* gene consists of 13 exons (exons 1–11, plus alternatively spliced exons 9b and 11b). Exon 9b contains an Alu-element and can only be detected in traces in mRNA from human leukocytes. The major splice variants either lack exon 2 or exon 8. The use of exon 11b leads to a brain-specific SGCE splice variant with an altered C-terminus.[58,59] The gene encodes a ubiquitously expressed 438-amino acid protein, which has a single transmembrane domain and is 68% homologous to α-sarcoglycan.

Exon deletions, as well as different nonsense and missense mutations of the *SGCE* gene in patients with

M-D, have been published (Figure 12.1).[41,53–55,60–62] From the limited information available to date, there is no indication of a major difference in the phenotype between different types of mutations.

The vast majority of published heterozygous *SGCE* mutations presumably lead to a premature termination of protein translation (nonsense mutations or exon deletions resulting in a premature stop codon, or small deletions or insertions leading to a shift of the reading frame, or splice-site mutations, resulting in aberrant splicing of exons). However, a few mutations have been found to result in single amino acid changes only.[55,58]

Heterozygous loss-of-function mutations are usually associated with autosomal recessive inheritance, as a single allele is usually sufficient to sustain the function of the encoded protein. Exceptions are dominant negative effects, as described above for *GCH1*-deficient DRD. In M-D, the most likely explanation for the dominant pattern of inheritance is the inactivation of the 'healthy' allele in affected individuals by a process called parental genomic imprinting, which is a well-described mechanism of gene regulation in some chromosomal areas, among them the human 7q21 region bearing the *SGCE* gene. There is both genetic and direct experimental evidence for this hypothesis.

The most common mechanism for genomic imprinting is the specific inactivation of one of the parental alleles by methylation of cytosine residues in the promotor region. In the case of *SGCE*, the maternal allele is inactivated; hence, this process is called 'maternal' imprinting. The selective methylation of maternal alleles of the *SGCE* gene could be demonstrated by bisulfite sequencing in cell lines with uniparental disomy of chromosome 7q21, and by analysis of DNA from blood lymphocytes and from brain tissue.[63,64] In addition, sole expression of the paternal allele could be detected in blood lymphocytes by reverse transcription polymerase chain reaction (RT-PCR); (Asmus et al, unpublished observations). Imprinting of the maternal allele explains the marked difference in penetrance of the disease, which depends on the sex of the transmitting parent: less than 5% of mutation carriers manifest the disease if the disease allele is passed on by the mother, while penetrance approaches 95% following paternal transmission. If the mutated allele is inherited from the mother, the intact paternal allele is sufficient to sustain ε-sarcoglycan function (as in most cases of

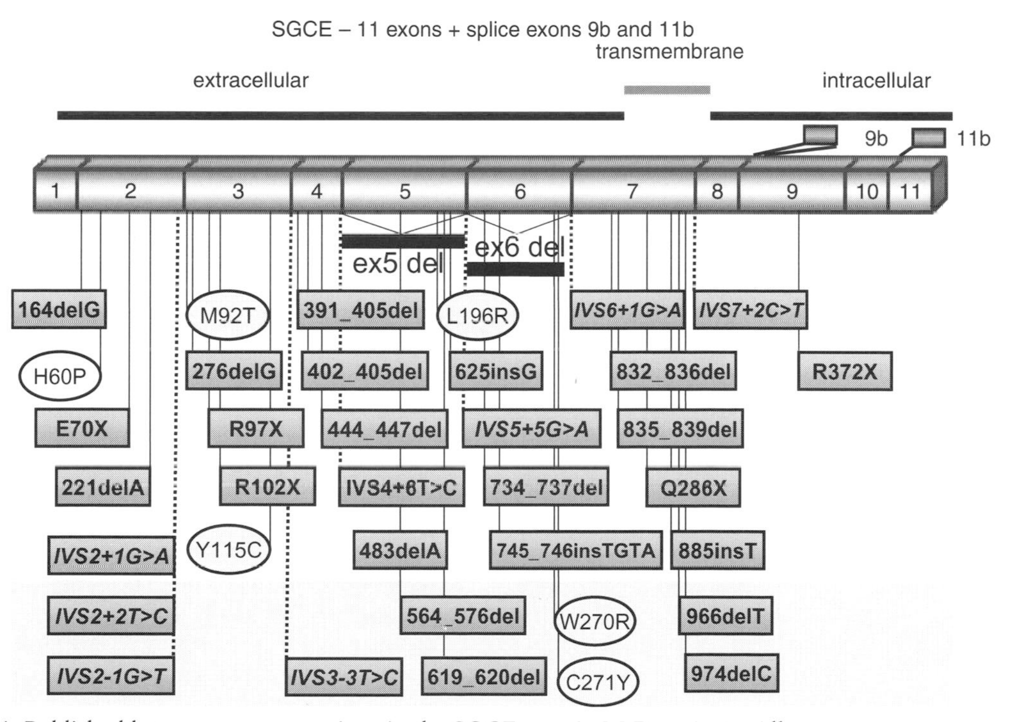

Figure 12.1 Published heterozygous mutations in the *SGCE* gene in M-D patients. All except one mutation (R372X) are located in the extracellular and transmembrane domains of ε-sarcoglycan. Mutations in gray boxes denote nonsense mutations, dashed lines indicate splicing mutations. Missense mutations are given in ovals.

loss-of-function mutations) and the mutation carrier remains healthy. If, on the other hand, the mutated allele is inherited from the father, inactivation of the maternal allele due to imprinting leads to complete ε-sarcoglycan deficiency, and hence to the manifestation of clinical symptoms. Maternal imprinting of the *SGCE* gene has also been demonstrated in the mouse.[65]

Clinical picture

The clinical signs and symptoms of M-D usually develop during childhood or early adolescence and after that take a fluctuating, but usually not progressive course.[40]

The predominant symptom at presentation (mean age at onset 5.4 years, range 0.5–38 years[41]), as well as during the course of the disease in most patients, is myoclonic jerks, affecting predominantly axial muscles (neck and trunk) but also muscles of the upper more than lower extremities, with proximal muscles being more affected than distal ones. Jerks are very brief, 'lightning-like', and are precipitated or aggravated by action and psychological stress, but also occur at rest. More sustained, dystonic movements are observed in about two-thirds of patients, with torticollis and writer's cramp being the most common manifestations. Dystonia of the lower limbs is occasionally seen, leading to dystonic gait disturbances. Usually, dystonia of the extremities accompanies myoclonus and has the characteristics of an action dystonia. Torticollis as the sole manifestation has only been found in a single individual in an M-D pedigree with an otherwise classical phenotype.[41]

Electroencephalographic (EEG) abnormalities and epileptic seizures in several individuals of a single M-D pedigree with an *SGCE* mutation have been reported recently.[61] Additional neurologic manifestations, such as (cerebellar) ataxia, spasticity, or dementia, have not been found so far in M-D patients, unless explained by additional pathology such as perinatal hypoxia.

Most patients experience substantial symptomatic relief by alcohol or benzodiazepines but effective doses may vary considerably and patients can experience a heavy rebound of motor symptoms after single doses of alcohol or benzodiazepines. In contrast to cortical or posthypoxic myoclonus, valproic acid, piracetam, and levetiracetam provide neither significant nor lasting improvement of motor symptoms, although controlled therapeutic trials in M-D have not been performed. In severe cases of M-D, bilateral deep brain stimulation (DBS) to the ventral intermediate (Vim) nucleus of the thalamus or to the internal pallidum have been shown to confer substantial and lasting symptomatic relief.[62,66] In patients with marked limb dystonia accompanying myoclonus, the internal globus pallidus (Gpi) is the preferred target.

Psychiatric features of M-D

Several reports on M-D pedigrees mentioned non-motor features like panic attacks, personality disorders, and alcohol abuse.[41,49,67,68]

In a more systematic investigation of possible psychiatric manifestations, Saunders-Pullman et al assessed three families with linkage to the 7q21 locus.

Symptoms of obsessive-compulsive disorder (OCD) were found to be more common in carriers of the disease-associated haplotype, both with and without motor symptoms, as compared to non-carriers, suggesting that these symptoms may be a primary manifestation of the disease. Recently, this association has been confirmed by the same authors in an extended sample of SGCE mutation carriers (Hess et al., 2007). By contrast, alcohol and benzodiazepine abuse were only detected in patients who experienced motor symptom control by these substances.

Genetic heterogeneity in M-D

Several studies of families and sporadic patients with M-D could only detect *SGCE* mutations in a proportion of the patients tested.[41,60] Whereas in familial cases with a typical phenotype, *SGCE* is certainly the major gene, it seems to play a minor role in sporadic patients. *SGCE* mutations have never been described in patients with an onset of symptoms above 35 years of age.

Prior to the identification of linkage to chromosome 7q21, Klein et al reported a missense change (Val154Ile) in the gene for the dopamine D_2 receptor (DRD2), cosegregating with the phenotype in a single family with M-D.[68] However, in this particular family, a heterozygous *SGCE* mutation was later detected, also cosegregating with the M-D phenotype. As cell culture studies did not show functional effects of the sequence alteration in the D_2 receptor,[69] it is likely that the disease in this family is caused by the *SGCE* mutation, and not by the D2DR variant.

Leung et al identified a novel 18 bp deletion in the *TOR1A* gene (the causative gene in primary torsion dystonia[70] in an M-D sib pair.[71] As both affecteds also carried a heterozygous *SGCE* mutation, the relevance of the 18 bp *TOR1A* deletion for the clinical phenotype remains uncertain.

The mapping of a second locus on chromosome 18p (lod score 3.96) in a family with a typical M-D phenotype and no indication of maternal imprinting was reported by Grimes et al (DYT15).[72] Clinical features in this pedigree are indistinguishable from the classical SGCE phenotype. Interestingly, this genetic region had been implicated in dystonic syndromes before: patients with a deletion of part of chromosome 18p have, among other disturbances, dystonia (18p deletion syndrome,[73]) and one form of adult-onset craniocervical dystonia (DYT7) was mapped to this region,[74] although this finding had not been confirmed in other families.

Occasionally, other conditions such as dopa-responsive dystonia[9] or vitamin E deficiency[75] may mimic M-D.

RAPID-ONSET DYSTONIA-PARKINSONISM (DYT12)

Rapid onset dystonia-parkinsonism (RDP) is a rare, autosomal dominantly inherited movement disorder with incomplete penetrance, characterized by the abrupt or subacute onset of both dystonic symptoms and parkinsonism with prominent bulbar features.[69] To date, 21 families with this condition[95–100] and five possible sporadic cases[96,101–103] have been reported.

Clinical presentation

Most patients experience sudden to subacute onset, over hours to days, of dystonic posturing of the limbs (upper more than lower), bradykinesia with prominent bulbar involvement, postural instability, dysarthria, and dysphagia.[84] In some cases, the acute onset is preceded by stable mild limb dystonia over the course of several years. Onset usually occurs in adolescence or young adulthood, but can also occur in early childhood or late adulthood (as early as 4 and as late as 58 years). Subsequently, symptoms typically remain stable with little or no progression, sometimes even with moderate improvement in some cases. In one family,[78] psychiatric manifestations such as social phobia and depression were noted in five out of eight affected family members and in one obligate gene carrier. In a few cases, seizures and paroxysmal dystonia have also been observed.[76,77] Whereas dystonic features usually predominate, RDP may rarely also present as L-dopa-unresponsive parkinsonism.[83]

In the majority of patients, trigger factors such as emotionally traumatic events, extreme heat or physical exercise, or infection could be identified. Symptoms do not respond significantly to dopaminergic medication. Bilateral pallidal DBS failed to improve symptoms in one sporadic patient.[82]

The differential diagnosis of combined symptoms of generalized dystonia and parkinsonism includes DRD, X-linked dystonia, and parkinsonism (XDP, Lubag),[85] and early-onset autosomal recessive parkinsonism due to mutations in the *parkin* gene.[86]

Biochemical and imaging studies

Although reduced levels of dopamine metabolites in the CSF have been found in some patients, these levels did not correlate with severity of the disease and were also observed in unaffected at-risk individuals and obligate gene carriers.[84] Cranial imaging studies using magnetic reasonance imaging (MRI), computed tomography (CT), and PET imaging of presynaptic dopamine uptake sites[87] were normal, suggesting that RDP is not a neurodegenerative disease, but that symptoms result from neuronal dysfunction. Consistent with this notion, a pathologic study in one patient[78] who had previously undergone unilateral pallidotomy did not reveal evidence of nerve cell loss or gliosis other than that related to surgery.

Genetic studies and molecular pathogenesis

Linkage to an 8 cM region on chromosome 19q13.2 (DYT12) has been established in three families[88] and refined to a 5.9 cM critical interval.[89] Subsequently, six missense mutations in the gene for the Na^+/K^+-ATPase α3 subunit (*ATP1A3*), including de-novo mutations, have been identified in four families and three sporadic patients.[90] The ATP1A3 protein catalyzes the active transport of cations across cell membranes and is responsible for maintaining the electrochemical gradient. All six mutations are located in phylogenetically highly conserved regions of the protein, and five out of six are found in the transmembrane domain. Functional studies and structural predictions suggest that they act as loss-of-function mutations by impairing enzyme activity or stability, presumably leading to a change of cellular Na^+ homeostasis.[91] Differences in protein expression levels of mutant compared to wild-type subunits in transfected cells further suggest that ATP1A3 activity is reduced in RDP patients, with a result equivalent to haploinsufficiency. However, the molecular mechanisms by which these mutations cause an acute non-progressive neuronal phenotype triggered by external factors, followed by continuous specific dysfunction of certain neuronal populations, remain to be determined.

The expression of the *ATP1A3* gene in humans is confined to excitable tissues, i.e. developing and adult brain and heart, and is observed throughout the brain, with the exception of corpus callosum, pituitary gland, and spinal cord.[92] Interestingly, haploinsufficiency due to mutations in the gene encoding the closely related ATP1A2 isoform leads to familial hemiplegic migraine[93] and benign familial infantile convulsions.[94] The fact that mutations in different Na^+/K^+-ATPase isoforms cause clinically distinct neurologic syndromes suggests that expression of these isoforms in the brain is temporally and spatially highly regulated and essential for normal brain function.

Recently, genetic studies in another large RDP family, which ruled out linkage to the DYT12 locus, demonstrated genetic heterogeneity, suggesting at least one additional RDP gene.[79] A comprehensive study of the phenotypic spectrum of RDP in 49 subjects from 21 families (Brashear et al., 2007) provided further evidence for genetic heterogeneity, excluding ATP1A3 mutations in 13 individuals from 11 families, and recommended genetic testing for the ATP1A3 gene when abrupt onset, rostrocaudal gradient and prominent bulbar findings are present.

REFERENCES

1. Schneider SA, Mohire MD, Trender-Gerhard I, Asmus F, et al. Familial dopa-responsive cervical dystonia. Neurology 2006; 66: 599–601.
2. Asmus F, Zimprich A, Tezenas Du Montcel S et al. Myoclonus-dystonia syndrome: epsilon-sarcoglycan mutations and phenotype. Ann Neurol 2002; 52(4): 489–92.
3. Obeso JA, Rothwell JC, Lang AE, Marsden CD. Myoclonic dystonia. Neurology 1983; 33(7): 825–30.
4. Jarman PR, Bandmann O, Marsden CD, Wood NW. GTP cyclohydrolase I mutations in patients with dystonia responsive to anticholinergic drugs. J Neurol Neurosurg Psychiatry 1997; 63(3): 304–8.
5. Segawa M, Hosaka A, Miyagawa F, Nomura Y, Imai H. Hereditary progressive dystonia with marked diurnal fluctuation. Adv Neurol 1976; 14: 215–33.
6. Bandmann O, Marsden CD, Wood NW. Atypical presentations of dopa-responsive dystonia. Adv Neurol 1998; 78: 283–90.
7. Steinberger D, Weber Y, Korinthenberg R et al. High penetrance and pronounced variation in expressivity of GCH1 mutations in five families with dopa-responsive dystonia [published erratum appears in Ann Neurol 1998; 44(1): 147]. Ann Neurol 1998; 43(5): 634–9.
8. Furukawa Y, Graf WD, Wong H, Shimadzu M, Kish SJ. Dopa-responsive dystonia simulating spastic paraplegia due to tyrosine hydroxylase (TH) gene mutations. Neurology 2001; 56(2): 260–3.
9. Leuzzi V, Carducci C, Carducci C et al. Autosomal dominant GTP-CH deficiency presenting as a dopa-responsive myoclonus-dystonia syndrome. Neurology 2002; 59(8): 1241–3.
10. Steinberger D, Korinthenberg R, Topka H et al. Dopa-responsive dystonia: mutation analysis of GCH1 and analysis of therapeutic doses of L-dopa. Neurology 2000; 55(11): 1735–8.
11. Hwang WJ, Calne DB, Tsui JK, Fuente-Fernandez R. The long-term response to levodopa in dopa-responsive dystonia. Parkinsonism Relat Disord 2001; 8(1): 1–5.
12. Kunig G, Leenders KL, Antonini A et al. D_2 receptor binding in dopa-responsive dystonia. Ann Neurol 1998; 44(5): 758–62.
13. Jeon BS, Jeong JM, Park SS et al. Dopamine transporter density measured by [^{123}I]beta-CIT single-photon emission computed tomography is normal in dopa-responsive dystonia. Ann Neurol 1998; 43(6): 792–800.
14. Snow BJ, Nygaard TG, Takahashi H, Calne DB. Positron emission tomographic studies of dopa-responsive dystonia and early-onset idiopathic parkinsonism. Ann Neurol 1993; 34(5): 733–8.
15. Fuente-Fernandez R, Furtado S, Guttman M et al. VMAT2 binding is elevated in dopa-responsive dystonia: visualizing empty vesicles by PET. Synapse 2003; 49(1): 20–8.
16. Rajput AH, Gibb WR, Zhong XH et al. Dopa-responsive dystonia: pathological and biochemical observations in a case. Ann Neurol 1994; 35(4): 396–402.
17. Hagenah JM, Hedrich K, Becker B et al. Distinguishing early-onset PD from dopa-responsive dystonia with transcranial sonography. Neurology 2006; 66(12): 1951–2.
18. Nygaard TG, Wilhelmsen KC, Risch NJ et al. Linkage mapping of dopa-responsive dystonia (DRD) to chromosome 14q. Nat Genet 1993; 5(4): 386–91.
19. Ichinose H, Ohye T, Takahashi E et al. Hereditary progressive dystonia with marked diurnal fluctuation caused by mutations in the GTP cyclohydrolase I gene. Nat Genet 1994; 8(3): 236–42.
20. Furukawa Y. Genetics and biochemistry of dopa-responsive dystonia: significance of striatal tyrosine hydroxylase protein loss. Adv Neurol 2003; 91: 401–10.
21. Weber Y, Steinberger D, Deuschl G, Benecke R, Muller U. Two previously unrecognized splicing mutations of GCH1 in Dopa-responsive dystonia: exon skipping and one base insertion. Neurogenetics 1997; 1(2): 125–7.
22. Bandmann O, Valente EM, Holmans P et al. Dopa-responsive dystonia: a clinical and molecular genetic study. Ann Neurol 1998; 44(4): 649–56.
23. Furukawa Y, Guttman M, Sparagana SP et al. Dopa-responsive dystonia due to a large deletion in the GTP cyclohydrolase I gene. Ann Neurol 2000; 47(4): 517–20.
24. Bandmann O, Nygaard T, Surtees R et al. Dopa-responsive dystonia in British patients: new mutations of the GTP-cyclohydrolase I gene and evidence for genetic heterogeneity. Hum Mol Genet 1996; 5(3): 403–6.
25. Furukawa Y, Nygaard TG, Gutlich M et al. Striatal biopterin and tyrosine hydroxylase protein reduction in dopa-responsive dystonia. Neurology 1999; 53(5): 1032–41.
26. Hwu WL, Chiou YW, Lai SY, Lee YM. Dopa-responsive dystonia is induced by a dominant-negative mechanism. Ann Neurol 2000; 48(4): 609–13.
27. Furukawa Y, Kapatos G, Haycock JW et al. Brain biopterin and tyrosine hydroxylase in asymptomatic dopa-responsive dystonia. Ann Neurol 2002; 51(5): 637–41.
28. Segawa M, Nomura Y, Nishiyama N. Autosomal dominant guanosine triphosphate cyclohydrolase I deficiency (Segawa disease). Ann Neurol 2003; 54 (Suppl 6): S32–S45.
29. Segawa M. Development of the nigrostriatal dopamine neuron and the pathways in the basal ganglia. Brain Dev 2000; 22 (Suppl 1): S1–S4.
30. Blau N, Barnes I, Dhondt JL. International database of tetrahydrobiopterin deficiencies. J Inherit Metab Dis 1996; 19(1): 8–14.
31. Nardocci N, Zorzi G, Blau N et al. Neonatal dopa-responsive extrapyramidal syndrome in twins with recessive GTPCH deficiency. Neurology 2003; 60(2): 335–7.
32. Bandmann O, Goertz M, Zschocke J et al. The phenylalanine loading test in the differential diagnosis of dystonia. Neurology 2003; 60(4): 700–2.
33. Tassin J, Durr A, Bonnet AM et al. Levodopa-responsive dystonia: GTP cyclohydrolase I or parkin mutations? Brain 2000; 123 (Pt 6): 1112–21.
34. Knappskog PM, Flatmark T, Mallet J, Ludecke B, Bartholome K. Recessively inherited L-DOPA-responsive dystonia caused by a point mutation (Q381K) in the tyrosine hydroxylase gene. Hum Mol Genet 1995; 4(7): 1209–12.

35. Ludecke B, Knappskog PM, Clayton PT et al. Recessively inherited L-DOPA-responsive parkinsonism in infancy caused by a point mutation (L205P) in the tyrosine hydroxylase gene. Hum Mol Genet 1996; 5(7): 1023–8.
36. Rijk-Van Andel JF, Gabreels FJ, Geurtz B et al. L-dopa-responsive infantile hypokinetic rigid parkinsonism due to tyrosine hydroxylase deficiency. Neurology 2000; 55(12): 1926–8.
37. Nakashima K, Shimoda M, Sato K et al. Hereditary non-progressive torsion dystonia with intellectual disturbance. Intern Med 1995; 8(4): 310–13.
38. Blau N, Bonafe L, Thony B. Tetrahydrobiopterin deficiencies without hyperphenylalaninemia: diagnosis and genetics of dopa-responsive dystonia and sepiapterin reductase deficiency. Mol Genet Metab 2001; 74(1–2): 172–85.
39. Grotzsch H, Pizzolato GP, Ghika J et al. Neuropathology of a case of dopa-responsive dystonia associated with a new genetic locus, DYT14. Neurology 2002; 58(12): 1839–42.
40. Gasser T. Inherited myoclonus-dystonia syndrome. Adv Neurol 1998; 78: 325–34.
41. Asmus F, Zimprich A, Tezenas Du Montcel S et al. Myoclonus-dystonia syndrome: epsilon-sarcoglycan mutations and phenotype. Ann Neurol 2002; 52(4): 489–92.
42. Saunders-Pullman R, Ozelius L, Bressman SB. Inherited myoclonus-dystonia. Adv Neurol 2002; 89: 185–91.
43. Feldmann H, Wieser S. Klinische Studie zur essentiellen Myoklonie. Arch Psych Z ges Neurol 1964; 205: 555–70.
44. Przuntek H, Muhr H. Essential familial myoclonus. J Neurol 1983; 230(3): 153–62.
45. Fahn S, Sjaastad O. Hereditary essential myoclonus in a large Norwegian family. Mov Disord 1991; 6(3): 237–47.
46. Kyllerman M, Forsgren L, Sanner G et al. Alcohol-responsive myoclonic dystonia in a large family: dominant inheritance and phenotypic variation. Mov Disord 1990; 5(4): 270–9.
47. Gasser T, Bereznai B, Müller B et al. Linkage studies in alcohol-responsive myoclonic dystonia. Mov Disord 1996; 12: 363–70.
48. Quinn NP, Rothwell JC, Thompson PD, Marsden CD. Hereditary myoclonic dystonia, hereditary torsion dystonia and hereditary essential myoclonus: an area of confusion. Adv Neurol 1988; 50: 391–401.
49. Nygaard TG, Raymond D, Chen C et al. Localization of a gene for myoclonus-dystonia to chromosome 7q21-q31. Ann Neurol 1999; 46(5): 794–8.
50. Klein C, Schilling K, Saunders-Pullman RJ et al. A major locus for myoclonus-dystonia maps to chromosome 7q in eight families. Am J Hum Genet 2000; 67(5): 1314–19.
51. Asmus F, Zimprich A, Naumann M et al. Inherited myoclonus-dystonia syndrome: narrowing the 7q21-q31 locus in German families. Ann Neurol 2001; 49: 121–4.
52. Vidailhet M, Tassin J, Durif F et al. A major locus for several phenotypes of myoclonus-dystonia on chromosome 7q. Neurology 2001, 56(9). 1213–16.
53. Zimprich A, Grabowski M, Asmus F et al. Mutations in the gene encoding epsilon-sarcoglycan cause myoclonus-dystonia syndrome. Nat Genet 2001; 29(1): 66–9.
54. Doheny DO, Brin MF, Morrison CE et al. Phenotypic features of myoclonus-dystonia in three kindreds. Neurology 2002; 59(8): 1187–96.
55. Klein C, Liu L, Doheny D et al. Epsilon-sarcoglycan mutations found in combination with other dystonia gene mutations. Ann Neurol 2002; 52(5): 675–9.
56. Lim LE, Campbell KP. The sarcoglycan complex in limb-girdle muscular dystrophy. Curr Opin Neurol 1998; 11(5): 443–52.
57. Ettinger AJ, Feng G, Sanes JR. ε-Sarcoglycan, a broadly expressed homologue of the gene mutated in limb-girdle muscular dystrophy 2D. J Biol Chem 1997; 272(51): 32534–8.
58. Tezenas du Montcel S, Clot F, Vidailhet M et al. Epsilon sarcoglycan mutations and phenotype in French patients with myoclonic syndromes. J Med Genet 2006; 43(5): 394–400.
59. Yokoi F, Dang MT, Mitsui S, Li Y. Exclusive paternal expression and novel alternatively spliced variants of epsilon-sarcoglycan mRNA in mouse brain. FEBS Lett 2005; 579(21): 4822–8.
60. Han F, Lang AE, Racacho L, Bulman DE, Grimes DA. Mutations in the epsilon-sarcoglycan gene found to be uncommon in seven myoclonus-dystonia families. Neurology 2003; 61(2): 244–6.
61. Foncke EM, Klein C, Koelman JH et al. Hereditary myoclonus-dystonia associated with epilepsy. Neurology 2003; 60(12): 1988–90.
62. Asmus F, Salih F, Hjermind LE et al. Myoclonus-dystonia due to genomic deletions in the epsilon-sarcoglycan gene. Ann Neurol 2005; 58(5): 792–7.
63. Muller B, Hedrich K, Kock N et al. Evidence that paternal expression of the epsilon-sarcoglycan gene accounts for reduced penetrance in myoclonus-dystonia. Am J Hum Genet 2002; 71(6): 1303–11.
64. Grabowski M, Zimprich A, Lorenz-Depiereux B et al. The epsilon-sarcoglycan gene (SGCE), mutated in myoclonus-dystonia syndrome, is maternally imprinted. Eur J Hum Genet 2003; 11(2): 138–44.
65. Piras G, El Kharroubi A, Kozlov S et al. Zac1 (Lot1), a potential tumor suppressor gene, and the gene for epsilon-sarcoglycan are maternally imprinted genes: identification by a subtractive screen of novel uniparental fibroblast lines. Mol Cell Biol 2000; 20(9): 3308–15.
66. Trottenberg T, Meissner W, Kabus C et al. Neurostimulation of the ventral intermediate thalamic nucleus in inherited myoclonus-dystonia syndrome. Mov Disord 2001; 16(4): 769–71.
67. Scheidtmann K, Muller F, Hartmann E, Koenig E. [Familial myoclonus-dystonia syndrome associated with panic attacks]. Nervenarzt 2000; 71(10): 839–42. [in German]
68. Klein C, Brin MF, Kramer P et al. Association of a missense change in the D_2 dopamine receptor with myoclonus dystonia. Proc Natl Acad Sci USA 1999; 96(9): 5173–6.
69. Klein C, Gurvich N, Sena-Esteves M et al. Evaluation of the role of the D_2 dopamine receptor in myoclonus dystonia. Ann Neurol 2000; 47(3): 369–73.
70. Ozelius L, Hewett JW, Page CE et al. The early-onset torsion dystonia gene (Dyt1) encodes an ATP-binding protein. Nat Genet 1997; 17: 40–8.
71. Leung JC, Klein C, Friedman J et al. Novel mutation in the TOR1A (DYT1) gene in atypical early onset dystonia and polymorphisms in dystonia and early onset parkinsonism. Neurogenetics 2001; 3(3): 133–43.
72. Grimes DA, Han F, Lang AE et al. A novel locus for inherited myoclonus-dystonia on 18p11. Neurology 2002; 59(8): 1183–6.
73. Klein C, Page CE, LeWitt P et al. Genetic analysis of three patients with an 18p-syndrome and dystonia. Neurology 1999; 52(3): 649–51.
74. Leube B, Rudnicki D, Ratzlaff T et al. Idiopathic torsion dystonia: assignment of a gene to chromosome 18p in a German family with adult onset, autosomal dominant inheritance and purely focal distribution. Hum Mol Genet 1996; 5(10): 1673–7.
75. Angelini L, Erba A, Mariotti C et al. Myoclonic dystonia as unique presentation of isolated vitamin E deficiency in a young patient. Mov Disord 2002; 17(3): 612–14.
76. Dobyns WB, Ozelius LJ, Kramer PL et al. Rapid-onset dystonia-parkinsonism. Neurology 1993; 43(12): 2596–602.
77. Brashear A, deLeon D, Bressman SB et al. Rapid-onset dystonia-parkinsonism in a second family. Neurology 1997; 48(4): 1066–9.
78. Pittock SJ, Joyce C, O'Keane V et al. Rapid-onset dystonia-parkinsonism: a clinical and genetic analysis of a new kindred. Neurology 2000; 55(7): 991–5.

79. Kabakci K, Isbruch K, Schilling K et al. Genetic heterogeneity in rapid onset dystonia-parkinsonism: description of a new family. J Neurol Neurosurg Psychiatry 2005; 76(6): 860–2.
80. Zaremba J, Mierzewska H, Lysiak Z et al. Rapid-onset dystonia-parkinsonism: a fourth family consistent with linkage to chromosome 19q13. Mov Disord 2004; 19(12): 1506–10.
81. Linazasoro G, Indakoetxea B, Ruiz J, Van Blercom N, Lasa A. Possible sporadic rapid-onset dystonia-parkinsonism. Mov Disord 2002; 17(3): 608–9.
82. Deutschlander A, Asmus F, Gasser T, Steude U, Botzel K. Sporadic rapid-onset dystonia-parkinsonism syndrome: failure of bilateral pallidal stimulation. Mov Disord 2005; 20(2): 254–7.
83. Kamphuis DJ, Koelman H, Lees AJ, Tijssen MA. Sporadic rapid-onset dystonia-parkinsonism presenting as Parkinson's disease. Mov Disord 2006; 21(1): 118–19.
84. Brashear A, Butler IJ, Ozelius LJ et al. Rapid-onset dystonia-parkinsonism: a report of clinical, biochemical, and genetic studies in two families. Adv Neurol 1998; 78: 335–9.
85. Nolte D, Niemann S, Muller U. Specific sequence changes in multiple transcript system DYT3 are associated with X-linked dystonia parkinsonism. Proc Natl Acad Sci USA 2003; 100(18): 10347–52.
86. Kitada T, Asakawa S, Hattori N et al. Mutations in the parkin gene cause autosomal recessive juvenile parkinsonism. Nature 1998; 392(6676): 605–8.
87. Brashear A, Mulholland GK, Zheng QH et al. PET imaging of the pre-synaptic dopamine uptake sites in rapid-onset dystonia-parkinsonism (RDP). Mov Disord 1999; 14(1): 132–7.
88. Kramer PL, Mineta M, Klein C et al. Rapid-onset dystonia-parkinsonism: linkage to chromosome 19q13. Ann Neurol 1999; 46(2): 176–82.
89. Kamm C, Leung J, Joseph S et al. Refined linkage to the RDP/DYT12 locus on 19q13.2 and evaluation of GRIK5 as a candidate gene. Mov Disord 2004; 19(7): 845–7.
90. de Carvalho Aguiar P, Sweadner KJ, Penniston JT et al. Mutations in the Na^+/K^+-ATPase alpha3 gene ATP1A3 are associated with rapid-onset dystonia parkinsonism. Neuron 2004; 43(2): 169–75.
91. Rodacker V, Toustrup-Jensen M, Vilsen B. Mutations Phe785Leu and Thr618Met in Na^+,K^+-ATPase, associated with familial rapid-onset dystonia parkinsonism, interfere with Na^+ interaction by distinct mechanisms. J Biol Chem 2006; 281(27): 18539–48.
92. Benfante R, Antonini RA, Vaccari M et al. The expression of the human neuronal alpha3 Na^+,K^+-ATPase subunit gene is regulated by the activity of the Sp1 and NF-Y transcription factors. Biochem J 2005; 386(Pt 1): 63–72.
93. De Fusco M, Marconi R, Silvestri L, Atorino L, Rampoldi L, Morgante L et al. Haploinsufficiency of ATP1A2 encoding the Na+/K+ pump alpha2 subunit associated with familial hemiplegic migraine type 2. Nat Genet 2003; 33: 192–6.
94. Vanmolkot KR, Kors EE, Hottenga JJ, Terwindt GM, Haan J, Hoefnagels WA, et al. Novel mutations in the Na+, K+-ATPase pump gene ATP1A2 associated with familial hemiplegic migraine and benign familial infantile convulsions. Ann Neurol 2003; 54: 360–6.
95. Brashear A, deLeon D, Bressman SB, Thyagarajan D, Farlow MR, Dobyns WB. Rapid-onset dystonia-parkinsonism in a second family. Neurology 1997; 48: 1066–9.
96. Brashear A, Dobyns WB, de Carvalho Aguiar P, Borg M, Frijns CJ, Gollamudi S et al. The phenotypic spectrum of rapid-onset dystonia-parkinsonism (RDP) and mutations in the ATP1A3 gene. Brain 2007; 130: 828–35.
97. Dobyns WB, Ozelius LJ, Kramer PL, Brashear A, Farlow MR, Perry TR et al. Rapid-onset dystonia-parkinsonism. Neurology 1993; 43: 2596–2602.
98. Kabakci K, Isbruch K, Schilling K, Hedrich K, de Carvalho Aguiar P, Ozelius LJ et al. Genetic heterogeneity in rapid onset dystonia-parkinsonism: description of a new family. J Neurol Neurosurg Psychiatry 2005; 76: 860–2.
99. Pittock SJ, Joyce C, O'Keane V, Hugle B, Hardiman MO, Brett F et al. Rapid-onset dystonia-parkinsonism: a clinical and genetic analysis of a new kindred. Neurology 2000; 55: 991–5.
100. Zaremba J, Mierzewska H, Lysiak Z, Kramer P, Ozelius LJ, Brashear A. Rapid-onset dystonia- parkinsonism: a fourth family consistent with linkage to chromosome 19q13. Mov Disord 2004; 19: 1506–10.
101. Deutchlander A, Asmus F, Gasser T, Steude U, Botzel K. Sporadic rapid-onset dystonia-parkinsonism syndrome: failure of bilateral pallidal stimulation. Mov Disord 2005; 20: 254–7.
102. Kamphuis DJ, Koelman H, Lees AJ, Tijssen MA. Sporadic rapid-onset dystonia-parkinsonism presenting as Parkinson's disesase. Mov Disord 2006; 21: 118–9.
103. Linazasoro G, Indakoetxea B, Ruiz J, Van Blercom N, Lasa A. Possible sporadic rapid-onset dystonia-parkinsonism. Mov Disord. 2002; 17: 608–9.

13

Secondary and heredodegenerative dystonia

Yvette M Bordelon and Steven J Frucht

INTRODUCTION

In primary generalized dystonia and idiopathic adult-onset focal dystonia, dystonia occurs in isolation, usually the result of identified or unknown genetic mutations. Dystonia also presents after structural brain injury, exposure to toxins, or in the setting of a progressive neurodegenerative illness. These secondary forms of dystonia form the focus of this chapter. Infarcts, tumors, vascular malformations, and traumatic injuries to the basal ganglia are well-known triggers of dystonia. Exposure to drugs or toxins may cause either acute or chronic dystonia. Dystonia also occurs in a wide range of heredodegenerative illnesses, diseases characterized by progressive neuronal loss with accompanying neurologic symptoms and signs.

The most common causes of secondary dystonia are summarized in Table 13.1: most involve the basal ganglia directly, but secondary dystonia may also occur after injury to cortical or brainstem structures, spinal cord, and even peripheral nerve. Hemidystonia almost always occurs as the result of contralateral basal ganglia injury. Perinatal injury may cause dystonia at the time of brain injury, or with delay. So-called delayed-onset dystonia may begin years after injury, and may progress.[1] Infectious, post-infectious, and inflammatory syndromes associated with dystonia usually present in combination with other movement disorders, including parkinsonism, chorea, athetosis, and tics. Medications such as dopamine receptor antagonists, levodopa, and dopamine agonists may also cause transient dystonia. Toxins such as manganese and carbon monoxide that directly affect the basal ganglia also result in dystonia.

Heredodegenerative causes of dystonia (summarized in Table 13.2) are extremely varied and best classified by etiology: disorders of metabolism, mitochondrial diseases, trinucleotide repeat disorders, parkinsonian disorders, and other degenerative processes without defined cause.

DIAGNOSTIC APPROACH

A brief perusal of Tables 13.1 and 13.2 should convince anyone that arriving at an etiologic diagnosis in a patient with a secondary or heredodegenerative dystonia is a formidable challenge. The differential diagnosis is broad, and there is a natural tendency to adopt a 'shotgun' approach, casting as wide a net as possible with multiple ancillary tests in the hope that one test will secure the diagnosis.

In contrast to this time-consuming and costly approach, we offer an alternative strategy, summarized in Figures 13.1 and 13.2. Age of symptom onset is critically important in guiding the evaluation. The most common causes for dystonia in different age groups are summarized in Table 13.3. Typical age ranges are listed, although there is variability in age of presentation. Brain imaging directs the next step: we routinely rely on magnetic resonance imaging (MRI). Hemidystonia almost always indicates a contralateral structural lesion, and all patients with acute hemidystonia should be promptly imaged to exclude a mass lesion, stroke, or tumor. Characteristic patterns of signal abnormality may aid in the diagnosis, including the 'eye of the tiger' sign in neurodegeneration with brain iron accumulation type I, 'face of the giant panda' in the midbrain of patients with Wilson's disease, and basal ganglia calcification in Fahr's disease.

If radiographic studies are normal, Wilson's disease should be excluded, as this disorder is treatable when diagnosed early and uniformly fatal when missed. Slit-lamp examination by an experienced ophthalmologist, serum ceruloplasmin, and measurement of 24-hour urine

Table 13.1 Causes of secondary dystonia

CNS lesions
Congenital malformations:
- Arteriovenous malformations
- Pachygyria

Brain tumor
Stroke
Hypoxia
Head trauma
Intracranial hemorrhage
Multiple sclerosis
Brainstem lesion, including central pontine myelinolysis
Electrical injury
Cervical cord lesion, including syringomyelia
Spinal stenosis

Peripheral nerve injury

Perinatal cerebral injury
Cerebral palsy
Delayed-onset dystonia
Perinatal hypoxia
Kernicterus

Infectious, post-infectious, and inflammatory
Subacute sclerosing panencephalopathy
Reye's syndrome
Viral encephalitis, including HIV
Creutzfeldt–Jakob disease
Paraneoplastic syndrome-brainstem encephalitis
Systemic lupus erythematosus
Antiphospholipid antibody syndrome
Sjögren's syndrome
Multiple myeloma
Rasmussen's syndrome

Drug-induced
Dopaminomimetic:
- Levodopa
- Dopamine receptor agonists

Dopamine receptor antagonists (primarily D_2 receptors):
- Neuroleptics
- Prochlorperazine, metoclopromide

Antiepileptic medications
Selective serotonin reuptake inhibitors
Ergots

(Continued)

Table 13.1 (Continued)

Buspirone
Cocaine
Monoamine oxidase inhibitors
Flecainide

Toxins
Manganese
Carbon monoxide
Carbon disulfide
Wasp sting
Cyanide
Methanol
Disulfiram
3-Nitropropionic acid

Metabolic disorders
Hypoparathyroidism

Chromosomal abnormality
18q or p deletion

Psychogenic
Conversion disorder
Somatization disorder
Malingering

copper excretion are usually sufficient to exclude the diagnosis. Once Wilson's disease is excluded, the history should be carefully probed for evidence of perinatal hypoxia or exposure to any drug with affinity for the dopamine receptor.

At this point in the work-up, metabolic disorders and heredodegenerative disorders become more likely. Many metabolic disorders can be diagnosed by testing for serum amino acids and organic acids, or documenting specific enzymatic deficiencies in cultures of fibroblasts or leukocytes. These are the most challenging conditions to diagnose, because unique identifying features are absent.

In the remainder of this chapter, we summarize the clinical features and pathogenesis of these disorders, and briefly discuss their treatment.

DISORDERS OF METAL AND MINERAL METABOLISM

Wilson's disease

Wilson's disease, hepatolenticular degeneration, is caused by a mutation in the *ATP7B* gene (13q14) which encodes

Table 13.2 Causes of heredodegenerative dystonia

Metabolic disorders	Defect	Inheritance
Metal and mineral metabolism		
Wilson's disease	Copper metabolism defect *ATP7B* gene Chromosome 13	AR
Neurodegeneration with brain iron accumulation type I (formerly Hallervorden–Spatz disease)	*PANK2* gene Chromosome 20	AR
Neuroferritinopathy	Ferritin light-chain gene Chromosome 19	AD
Idiopathic basal ganglia calcification (Fahr's disease)	*IBGC1* gene Chromosome 14	AD
Lysosomal storage disorders		
Niemann–Pick disease type C	Unesterified cholesterol accumulation *NPC1* and *HE1* genes Chromosomes 18 and 14	AR
GM_1 gangliosidosis	β-Galactosidase gene Chromosome 3	AR
GM_2 gangliosidosis	Hexosaminidase A gene Chromosome 15	AR
Metachromatic leukodystrophy	Arylsulfatase A *ASA/ARSA* gene Chromosome 22	AR
Krabbe's disease	Galactosylceramide β-galactosidase *GALC* gene Chromosome 14	AR
Pelizaeus–Merzbacher disease	Proteolipid protein *PLP* gene	X
Neuronal ceriod-lipofuscinosis (Batten disease)	Intraneuronal accumulation of granular lipopigment 6 gene mutations found	AR
Fucosidosis	Alpha-L-fucosidase *FUCA1* gene Chromosome 1	AR
Inborn errors of metabolism		
Lesch–Nyhan syndrome	HGPRT	X
Aromatic amino acid decarboxylase deficiency	AADC	AR
Triose-phosphate isomerase deficiency	Triose-phosphate isomerase Chromosome 12	AR

(*Continued*)

Table 13.2 (Continued)

Metabolic disorders	**Defect**	**Inheritance**
Guanidinoacetate methyltranferase deficiency	GAMD	AR
Molybdenum cofactor deficiency	MCD and in sulfite oxidase deficiency	AR
Glucose transport defects	*GLUT1* gene Chromosome 1	AD
Amino and organic acidurias		
Glutaric academia type I	Glutaryl-CoA dehydrogenase gene Chromosome 19	AR
Homocystinuria	Cystathionine β-synthase gene Chromosome 21	AR
Priopionic acidemia	Propionyl-CoA carboxylase genes Chromosomes 13 and 3	AR
Methlymalonic aciduria	Methylmalonyl CoA mutase gene Chromosome 6	AR
4-Hydroxybutyric aciduria	Succinic semialdehyde dehydrogenase gene Chromosome 6	AR
3-Methylglutaconic aciduria	3-Methylglutaconyl-CoA hydratase, among other deficiencies	AR
2-Oxoglutaric aciduria	2-Oxoglutarate dehydrogenase	AR
Hartnup disease	Neutral amino acid transporter defect	ND
Mitochondrial disorders		
Leigh disease	Mitochondrial respiratory chain enzyme defects *SURF1* gene	AR, X, maternal
Leber's hereditary optic neuropathy	Mitochonrial respiratory chain complexes I, III, or IV defects	Maternal
Mohr–Tranebjaberg syndrome – dystonia, deafness	Deafness/dystonia peptide (DDP) gene	X
Trinucleotide repeat disorders		
Huntington's disease	*Huntingtin* gene Expanded CAG repeat in *IT15* gene Chromosome 4	AD

(*Continued*)

Table 13.2 (Continued)

Metabolic disorders	Defect	Inheritance
Spinocerebellar ataxia type 3 (Machado–Joseph disease) and other SCAs	Expanded CAG repeat in *ataxin* gene Chromosome 14 (*SCA3*)	AD
Parkinsonian syndromes		
Parkinson's disease	Familial: *parkin*, *synuclein*, and *DJ1* genes	Variable
Progressive supranuclear palsy	Tau	Sporadic
Multiple system atrophy	*synuclein*	Sporadic
Corticobasal ganglionic degeneration	Tau	Sporadic
Juvenile-onset parkinsonism	*parkin* gene	AR
X-linked dystonia-parkinsonism (Lubag)	*DYT3* gene	X
Rapid-onset dystonia-parkinsonism	Chromosome 19	AD
Other degenerative processes		
Ataxia-telangiectasia	*ATM* gene Chromosome 11	AR
Chorea-acanthocytosis	*Chorein* gene Chromosome 9	AR
Rett syndrome	*MECP2* gene	X
Infantile bilateral striatal necrosis	ND	AR, maternal
Neuronal intranuclear inclusion disease	Ubiquinated intranuclear inclusions with polyglutamine tracts	ND
Ataxia with vitamin E deficiency	α-Tocopherol transfer protein gene Chromosome 8	AR
Progressive pallidal degeneration	ND	ND
Sjögren–Larsson syndrome	Fatty alcohol dehydrogenase gene Chromosome 17	AR
Ataxia–amyotrophy–mental retardation–dystonia syndrome	ND	AR

AD = autosomal dominant; AR = autosomal recessive; ND = not determined; X = X-linked.

a copper transporter. It is inherited in autosomal recessive fashion,[2] and numerous point mutations have been described. Certain mutations occur more frequently in particular ethnic groups, such as the H1069Q mutation in those of European descent, R778L found in Asian populations, and H714Q and delC2337 in the Russian population.[2–5] Mutations in the Wilson's disease gene result in abnormal copper metabolism, with accumulation

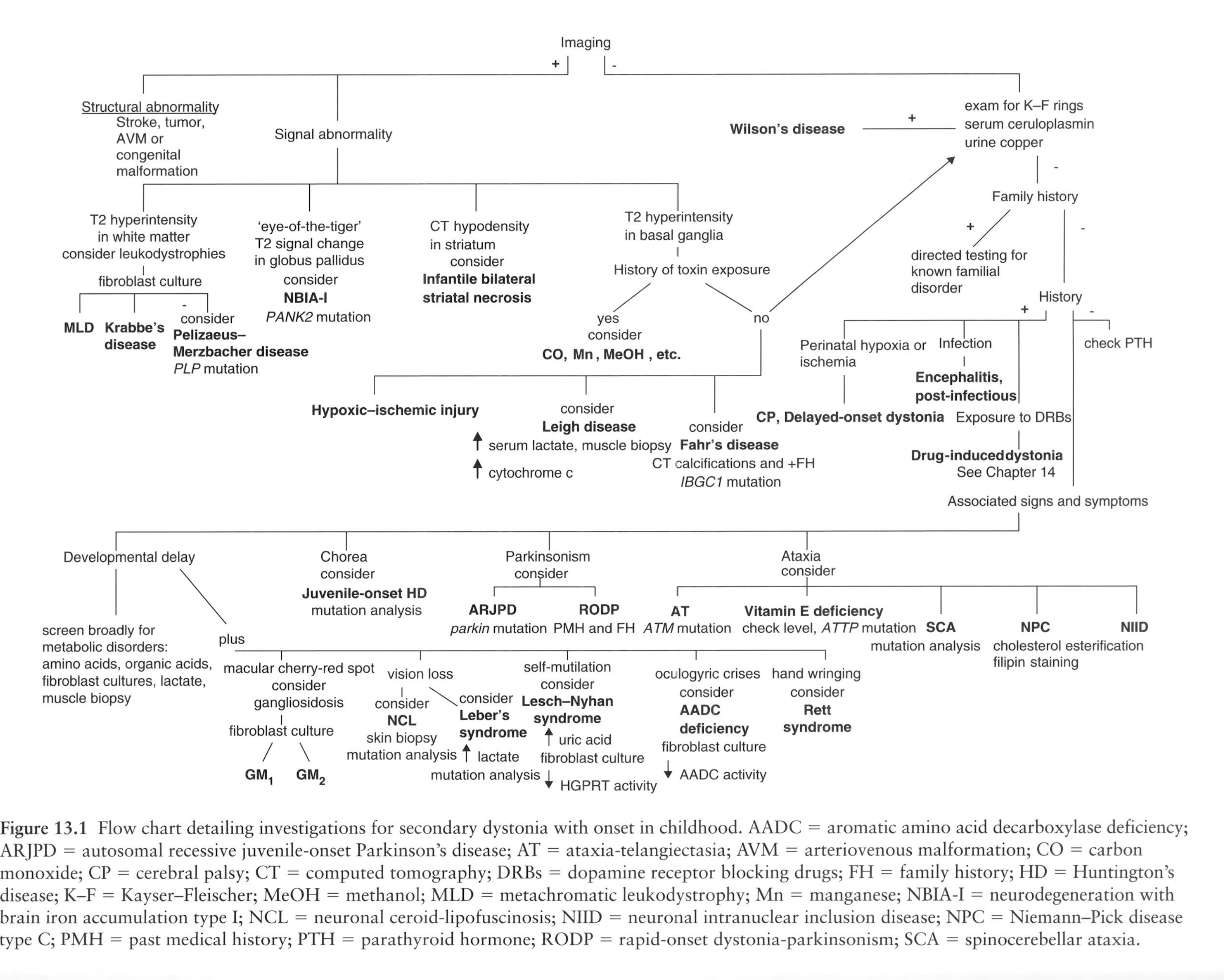

Figure 13.1 Flow chart detailing investigations for secondary dystonia with onset in childhood. AADC = aromatic amino acid decarboxylase deficiency; ARJPD = autosomal recessive juvenile-onset Parkinson's disease; AT = ataxia-telangiectasia; AVM = arteriovenous malformation; CO = carbon monoxide; CP = cerebral palsy; CT = computed tomography; DRBs = dopamine receptor blocking drugs; FH = family history; HD = Huntington's disease; K–F = Kayser–Fleischer; MeOH = methanol; MLD = metachromatic leukodystrophy; Mn = manganese; NBIA-I = neurodegeneration with brain iron accumulation type I; NCL = neuronal ceroid-lipofuscinosis; NIID = neuronal intranuclear inclusion disease; NPC = Niemann–Pick disease type C; PMH = past medical history; PTH = parathyroid hormone; RODP = rapid-onset dystonia-parkinsonism; SCA = spinocerebellar ataxia.

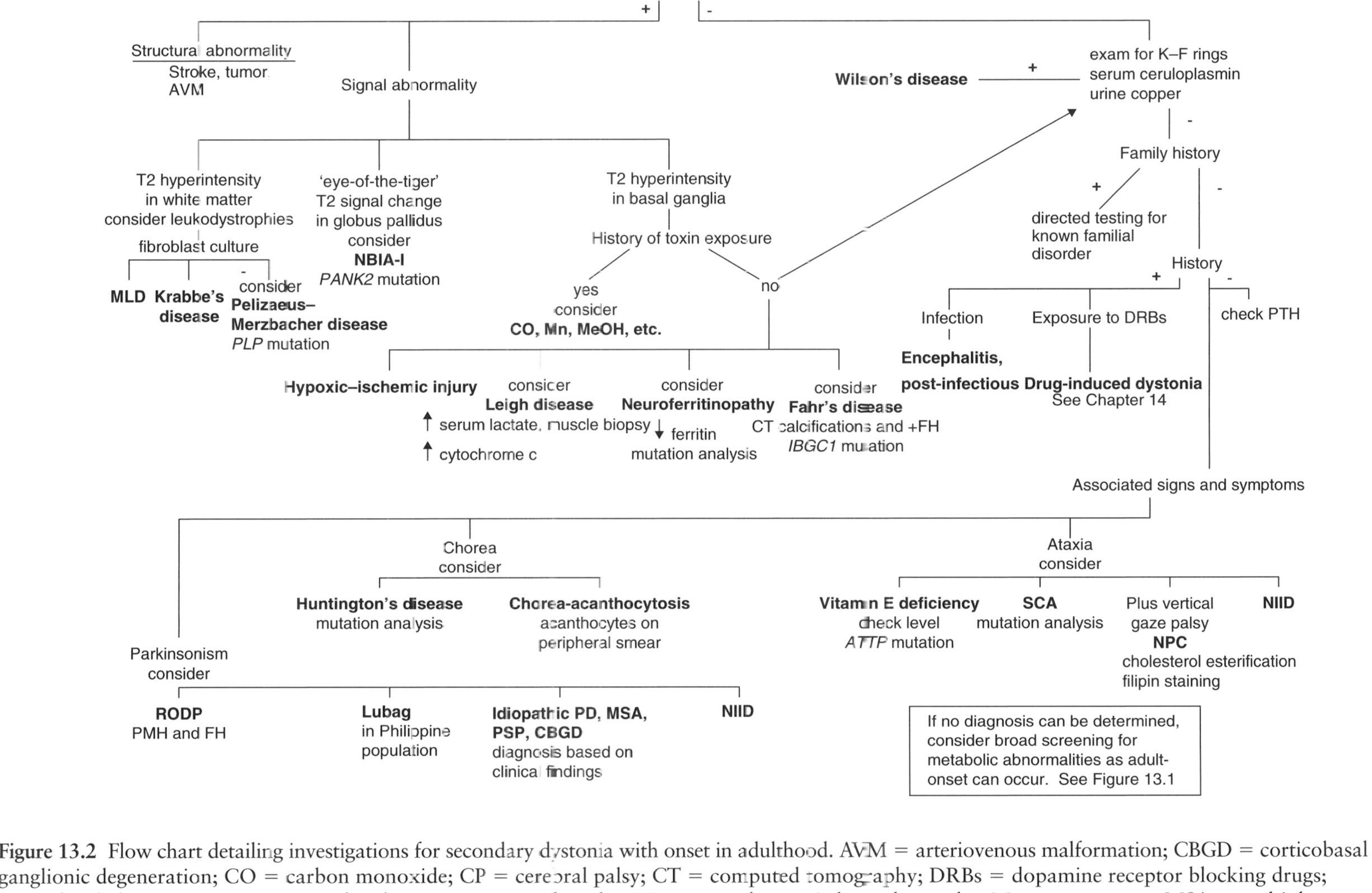

Figure 13.2 Flow chart detailing investigations for secondary dystonia with onset in adulthood. AVM = arteriovenous malformation; CBGD = corticobasal ganglionic degeneration; CO = carbon monoxide; CP = cerebral palsy; CT = computed tomography; DRBs = dopamine receptor blocking drugs; FH = family history; K–F = Kayser–Fleischer; MeOH = methanol; MLD = metachromatic leukodystrophy; Mn = manganese; MSA = multiple system atrophy; NBIA-I = neurodegeneration with brain iron accumulation type I; NCL = neuronal ceroid-lipofuscinosis; NIID = neuronal intranuclear inclusion disease; NPC = Niemann–Pick disease type C; PD = Parkinson's disease; PMH = past medical history; PSP = progressive supranuclear palsy; PTH = parathyroid hormone; RODP = rapid-onset dystonia-parkinsonism; SCA = spinocerebellar ataxia.

Table 13.3 Age at onset of secondary dystonia

Birth	<1 year	1–10 years	10–20 years	Adult
Perinatal injury	Infectious causes	Cerebral palsy	Infectious causes	Stroke, tumor, AVM, hemorrhage
Congenital malformations	GM_1 gangliosidosis	Delayed-onset dystonia	Wilson's disease	Hypoxia, head trauma
Infectious causes	GM_2 gangliosidosis	Infectious causes	Niemann–Pick type C	Infectious, inflammatory causes
Chromosomal deletion	Leukodystrophy	Wilson's disease	GM_2 gangliosidosis	Drug-induced, toxins, psychogenic
	NCL (Batten disease)	NBIA-I	Leukodystrophy	Wilson's disease
	Inborn errors of metabolism	Niemann–Pick type C	NCL (Batten disease)	Neuroferritinopathy
	Amino and organic acidurias	GM_2 gangliosidosis	Leigh disease	Fahr's disease
	Bilateral striatal necrosis	Leukodystrophy	Leber's syndrome	Niemann–Pick type C
		NCL (Batten disease)	Juvenile HD	Leukodystrophy
		Leigh syndrome	ARJPD-parkin mutation	NCL(Batten disease)
		Deafness-dystonia	RODP	Leber syndrome
		Ataxia-telangiectasia	Vitamin E deficiency	HD, SCA3
		Rett syndrome	NIID	PD, PSP, MSA, CBGD
				Lubag, RODP
				Chorea-acanthocytosis

ARJPD = autosomal recessive juvenile-onset Parkinson's disease; AVM = arteriovenous malformation; CBGD = corticobasal ganglionic degeneration; HD = Huntington's disease; MSA = multiple system atrophy; NBIA-I = neurodegeneration with brain iron accumulation type I; NCL = neuronal ceroid-lipofuscinosis; NIID = neuronal intranuclear inclusion disease; PD = Parkinson's disease; PSP = progressive supranuclear palsy; RODP = rapid-onset dystonia-parkinsonism; SCA = spinocerebellar ataxia.

of copper in tissues throughout the body. Clinical manifestations may begin from age 3 to 58 years, typically presenting with hepatic (40%), neurologic (40%), or psychiatric (20%) symptoms and signs.[6–8] Three neurologic presentations have been identified: parkinsonism, generalized dystonia, and a tremor-predominant form. Dystonia is common, often affecting cranial structures, with prominent dysarthria, risus sardonicus or a fixed pseudosmile (see Chapter 9, figure 9.11), and a high-pitched whining on inspiration. Kayser–Fleischer rings are visible in 90–95% of patients with neurologic manifestations of the illness.[7,9] Systemic manifestations of Wilson's disease are common, including hemolytic anemia, renal impairment, pancreatitis, cardiomyopathy, endocrinopathy, osteoarthritis, and osteoporosis.[5]

The diagnosis of Wilson's disease is supported by decreased serum ceruloplasmin (typically less than 20 mg/dl), a 5–10-fold increase in 24-hour urinary copper excretion, and the presence of Kayser–Fleischer rings on slit-lamp examination. Quantification of hepatic copper on liver biopsy is rarely necessary. Mutation analysis is available on a research basis; however, the large number of mutations prevents routine screening.[10,11] Approximately 300 mutations in the *ATP7B* gene have been found to date (http://www.medicalgenetics.med.ualberta.ca/wilson/index.php). A scoring system has been developed based on the clinical signs and symptoms and laboratory testing results. A score of ≥4 suggests that a diagnosis of Wilson's disease is very likely.[10]

Imaging of the brain typically shows T2 hyperintensity in the basal ganglia and thalamus. A characteristic pattern, the 'face of the giant panda', is occasionally visible in the midbrain.[12,13] On pathologic examination, caudate and putamen are often atrophic, with neuronal loss extending to globus pallidus, subthalamic nucleus, thalamus, and brainstem. Alzheimer type II astrocytes are prominent in the cortex, basal ganglia, brainstem nuclei, and cerebellum. Opalski cells may be found in the globus pallidus.[14]

Missing the diagnosis of Wilson's disease is one of the worst errors a neurologist can make. Administration of copper chelators such as penicillamine, trientene, tetrathiomolybdate, or 2,3-dimercaptopropanol, or agents that bind intestinal copper such as zinc sulfate or zinc acetate, is effective in treatment of this disease.[11,15,16] There is debate in the literature whether penicillamine or tetrathiomolybdate should be used as initial treatment, as there is a significant risk of worsening of neurologic symptoms when penicillamine is used.[17] Penicillamine's potential side effects also limit the drug's effectiveness. Patients who do not respond to medical treatment, or in whom hepatic injury is severe, may need liver transplantation, which is curative.

Neurodegeneration with brain iron accumulation type I (formerly Hallervorden–Spatz disease)

This neurodegenerative disorder is transmitted in an autosomal recessive fashion, typically with age of onset between 2 and 10 years. The majority of affected patients possess mutations in a gene on chromosome 20p13 encoding pantothenate kinase 2, a regulatory enzyme important in the biosynthesis of coenzyme A, and the disorder has also been termed pantothenate kinase-associated neurodegeneration (PANK).[18] Dystonia is a prominent presenting sign, present in 87% of patients in one study.[19,20] Cranial and limb dystonia occur early, followed later by axial dystonia. Other neurologic manifestations include chorea, athetosis, rigidity, dysarthria, and dementia. Seizures and retinitis pigmentosa may also occur. The disease is progressive, leading to death in 15–20 years, although atypical forms with later onset and slower progression occur.

Clinical presentation and MRI findings of low T2 signal intensity in the globus pallidus with a central area of increased intensity (the characteristic 'eye of the tiger' sign) should suggest the diagnosis.[21] Recent studies suggest that all cases with a mutation in *PANK2* also possess the 'eye of the tiger' finding on MRI.[20] Pathologic examination reveals iron deposition and cell loss in the pallidum and substantia nigra, associated with axonal spheroids and gliosis.[19,22] Although there are no treatments proven to affect the natural history of the disease, it is reasonable to treat with pantothenate in order to bypass the enzymatic defect.[20]

Neuroferritinopathy

Neuroferritinopathy is a recently described neurodegenerative disorder in which iron accumulates in the brain due to mutations in the gene encoding the ferritin light chain (chromosome 19q13.3).[23] This dominantly inherited disorder typically presents in the fourth to sixth decades of life with dystonia, chorea, and parkinsonism. Dystonic dysarthria is common, and dystonia may also affect the limbs.[24] Laboratory testing reveals a low ferritin level, typically ≤20 mg/dl. Histopathology reveals iron and ferritin deposition extracellularly in the basal ganglia, forebrain, and cerebellum. Cysts may be seen in the globus pallidus. MRI reveals increased T2 signal in the putamen and globus pallidus.[23] Treatment at this time is symptomatic.

Idiopathic basal ganglia calcification (Fahr's disease)

Calcification of the basal ganglia is an incidental finding in 0.3–1% of routine head computed tomography (CT) scans.[25,26] However, in idiopathic basal ganglia calcification (IBGC), also known as Fahr's disease, progressive neurologic and psychiatric dysfunction are caused by calcium deposition within the brain. Parkinsonism, chorea, dystonia, ataxia, dyskinesias, seizures, cognitive impairment, and psychosis have been described.[27–30] The disorder is usually autosomal dominant with an age of onset of 30–50 years.[30] A locus, *IBGC1*, has been identified on chromosome 14q.[31] Calcification is commonly seen in the globus pallidus, putamen, caudate, thalamus, and dentate nucleus. Pathology reveals perivascular iron deposits in the basal ganglia and dentate nucleus.

LYSOSOMAL STORAGE DISORDERS

Niemann–Pick type C

Niemann–Pick type C (NPC) is an autosomal recessive disorder with progressive neurologic and hepatic dysfunction secondary to accumulation of endocytosed unesterified cholesterol.[32] Ninety-five percent of cases are caused by mutations in the *NPC1* gene located on chromosome 18q11, which encodes a protein important for cholesterol trafficking.[33,34] Other cases have been associated with mutations in the *HE1* gene on chromosome 14q24, which encodes a lysosomal protein.[35] Onset is typically in late childhood, and the clinical manifestations include organomegaly, vertical supranuclear gaze palsy, progressive dystonia, ataxia, and dementia. Dystonia is initially focal but often generalizes. Adult-onset cases progress more slowly, whereas infantile onset is characterized by hypotonia and motor delay.[32]

The diagnosis relies on demonstration of abnormal cholesterol esterification and filipin staining in cultured fibroblasts.[36,37] Foamy cells and sea-blue histiocytes are present in bone marrow, spleen, liver, lung, lymph nodes, and tonsils. Cholesterol and other lipids accumulate in the brains of patients with NPC, particularly in the large pyramidal neurons, and ballooned neurons are found in the basal ganglia and thalamus.[32] Axonal spheroids are present in the thalamus, brainstem, and cerebellum.[38] Neurofibrillary tangles are found in the hippocampus, entorhinal cortex, thalamus, and basal ganglia in adults with the disease.[39]

GM_1 gangliosidosis

Mutations in the gene encoding the lysosomal enzyme β-galactosidase result in GM_1 gangliosidosis. This disorder manifests shortly after birth with poor feeding, organomegaly, and failure to thrive.[40] Dystonia may be a prominent feature, or it may be absent.[41] An adult-onset form has been described in which dystonia is more prominent.[42] A macular cherry-red spot is present in 50% of patients. The disorder is autosomal recessive, and the diagnosis can be made enzymatically using cultured fibroblasts, white blood cells, or serum. On pathologic examination, multilamellated neuronal inclusions are found primarily in the basal ganglia.[41]

GM_2 gangliosidoses

GM_2 gangliosides are autosomal recessive lysosomal storage diseases that may present during infancy, childhood, or adulthood.[43] They are caused by mutations in the genes encoding hexosaminidase A (chromosome 15) or B, or the GM_2 activator of hexosaminidase A (both on chromosome 5). There are many forms of GM_2 gangliosidoses, including Tay–Sachs and Sandhoff's diseases. Dystonia is present in many forms of hexosaminidase deficiency and may be prominent in the adult-onset form.[44–47] Motor regression, ataxia, seizures, myoclonus, dementia, and macular cherry-rod spots also occur. Ganglioside GM_2 accumulates in neuronal lysosomes, and 'meganeurites' are observed throughout the cortex.[48]

Leukodystrophies (MLD, Krabbe's disease, and Pelizaeus–Merzbacher disease)

Metachromatic leukodystrophy (MLD) is an autosomal recessive disorder caused by mutations in the *ASA/ARSA* gene (chromosome 22q13), which encodes the lysosomal protein arylsulfatase A.[49] There are three variants of MLD: late-infantile, juvenile, and adult. Dystonia may occur in any form of MLD but typically occurs later in the disease. Ataxia, spasticity, and seizures are frequent concomitant findings. Brain MRI demonstrates diffuse demyelination,[50] and the diagnosis is made by documenting decreased arylsulfatase A activity in leukocytes or cultured fibroblasts. On pathologic examination, there is demyelination and metachromatic granule deposition in oligodendrocytes, macrophages, and neurons.[49]

Krabbe's disease, also known as globoid cell leukodystrophy, is also an autosomal recessively inherited disorder with presentation either in the first year of life, childhood, or adulthood.[51] Mutations have been found in the *GALC* gene on chromosome 14q31 encoding the lysosomal enzyme galactosylceramide β-galactosidase. Typically, psychomotor regression, frequent vomiting, and seizures are the initial manifestation of disease. Progression of disease is rapid, with marked dystonia, optic atrophy, and frequent seizures leading to death within 2 years. In late-onset disease, the clinical features are more variable and the rate of progression may be slower.[52] Brain MRI demonstrates diffuse demyelination. Diagnosis is made by demonstrating the enzyme deficiency in leukocytes or cultured fibroblasts. Pathology reveals extensive demyelination and globoid cells throughout the white matter.[52]

Pelizaeus–Merzbacher disease is a recessive X-linked disorder caused by mutuations in the gene that encodes proteolipid protein (PLP). Demyelination is the cardinal feature,[53] and age of onset and disease progression vary. Disease manifestations include dystonia, ataxia, spasticity, nystagmus, and psychomotor retardation.[54] Brain MRI demonstrates diffuse demyelination. Diagnosis is made by direct mutation analysis. Neuropathology demonstrates central demyelination and axonal loss.

Neuronal ceroid-lipofuscinosis (Batten disease)

Neuronal ceroid-lipofuscinosis (NCL) (Batten disease) is a group of lysosomal storage disorders including eight distinct forms. These disorders are inherited in an autosomal recessive manner and vary in the age of onset. They were originally classified into four groups: infantile NCL or Haltia–Santavuori disease; late-infantile NCL or Janský–Bielschowsky disease; juvenile NCL or Spielmeyer–Vogt–Sjögren disease; and adult NCL or Kufs' disease. Forms of NCL are distinguished by their characteristic neuronal inclusions: granular osmiophilic deposits, curvilinear profiles, fingerprint profiles, and mixed inclusions, respectively.[55] The pathologic hallmark of NCL is accumulation of a granular lipopigment in neurons. Diffuse neuronal loss is also evident.[56] Recent advances have led to the identification of six different gene mutations linked to NCL, termed *CLN1*, *2*, *3*, *5*, *6*, and *8*. The first two genes code for lysosomal enzymes, while *CLN3*, *5*, *6*, and *8* encode transmembrane proteins.[57]

NCLs are characterized by progressive vision loss, cognitive decline, and seizures. Dystonia may occur, and has been described in all forms of the disorder.[58–61] The diagnosis of NCL can be made by the demonstration of lysosomal inclusions on skin biopsy and confirmed by electron microscopy. Biochemical and genetic studies are also available.

Fucosidosis

Fucosidosis is an autosomal recessive disease caused by a deficiency of the lysosomal enzyme α-L-fucosidase. Mutations in the α-fucosidase gene (*FUCA1*) located on chromosome 1 are responsible.[62] The disorder typically manifests during infancy, with progressive psychomotor retardation, dysostosis multiplex, organomegaly, angiokeratoma, seizures, and spasticity.[63] An individual homozygous for a Q422X mutation was reported to have progressive generalized dystonia.[64] The diagnosis is made by demonstrating abnormal enzyme activity in cultured fibroblasts or leukocytes. Electron microscopy reveals the presence of vacuoles in multiple tissues, including brain and liver.[65]

INBORN ERRORS OF METABOLISM

Lesch–Nyhan syndrome

Lesch–Nyhan syndrome is an X-linked disorder resulting from deficiency of hypoxanthine–guanine phosphoribosyltransferase. Clinical manifestations include movement disorders such as dystonia, choreoathetosis, spasticity, self-mutilation, hyperuricemia, and developmental retardation.[66] Symptoms typically begin after 6 months of age. The diagnosis is suggested by elevated levels of uric acid in serum and urine, and secured by absent hypoxanthine guanine phosphoribosyltransferase activity in cultured fibroblasts. No consistent abnormalities have been described on central nervous system (CNS) histopathology.

Aromatic amino acid decarboxylase deficiency

The first patients with aromatic L-amino acid decarboxylase (AADC) deficiency were described by Hyland and Clayton in 1992, and several cases have been subsequently reported.[67–69] Lack of AADC results in reduced levels of the biogenic amines dopamine, serotonin, norepinephrine, and epinephrine. The disorder is inherited in autosomal recessive fashion with typical onset, between 2 and 9 months of age, of characteristic paroxysmal dystonia of the limbs and oculogyric crises. These spells increase in frequency and severity over time. Between spells, bradykinesia, athetosis, myoclonic jerks, tongue thrusting, and flexor spasms may be seen. The diagnosis rests on the demonstration of high levels of plasma levodopa and low levels of plasma dopamine and norepinephrine metabolites. Alternatively, cerebrospinal fluid (CSF) neurotransmitter analysis demonstrates low levels of homovanillic acid and 5-hydroxyindoleacetic acid and elevated 3-O-methyldopa.[70] Direct genetic analysis is available on a research basis to confirm the diagnosis.

Triose-phosphate isomerase deficiency

This autosomal recessive disorder is caused by mutations in triose-phosphate isomerase (TPI) (chromosome 12), a glycolytic enzyme that interchangeably converts glyceraldehyde phosphate and dihydroxyacetone phosphate.[71] Age of onset is typically 2 years, with clinical features of dystonia, tremor, muscular atrophy secondary to anterior horn cell disease, and corticospinal signs.[72] Chronic hemolytic anemia may also occur. The disorder is inherited in an autosomal recessive fashion, and the diagnosis is made by assaying triose-phosphate isomerase levels in red blood cells.

Guanidinoacetate methyltransferase deficiency, molybdenum cofactor deficiency, and glucose transporter protein type 1 deficiency have also been reported to exhibit dystonia as part of their clinical phenotypes.[73–76]

AMINO AND ORGANIC ACIDURIAS

Glutaric acidemia type I

Glutaric acidemia type I is an autosomal recessive disorder caused by mutations in the mitochondrial enzyme glutaryl-coenzyme A dehydrogenase (chromosome 19).[77] Affected patients develop normally during the first months of life, and symptoms may begin acutely or insidiously. Severe generalized dystonia is common, often accompanied by spasticity and seizures.[78] The diagnosis is made by demonstrating elevated glutaric and 3-hydroxyglutaric acids in urine. The enzyme deficiency may also be demonstrated in cultured fibroblasts. Neuronal loss and decreased γ-aminobutyric acid (GABA) levels have been demonstrated in the putamen and caudate.[79,80]

Homocystinuria

Deficiency of cystathionine β-synthase causes homocystinuria, which typically features global developmental delay, cerebral thromboembolism, and anterior dislocation of the optic lens. The disorder is inherited in an autosomal recessive fashion, and many different mutations have been identified in the gene located on chromosome 21.[81] When present, dystonia usually occurs due to infarction of the basal ganglia,[82–84] although this idea has been challenged.[85] Diagnosis is confirmed by documenting the enzyme deficiency in liver or in cultured fibroblasts.

Propionic acidemia

Mutations in the gene encoding propionyl-CoA carboxylase cause propionic acidemia, an autosomal recessive disorder. Symptoms typically begin in infancy, with episodes of ketosis and metabolic acidosis. Infarction of the basal ganglia may be responsible for the movement disorders that occur, which often include dystonia and choreoathetosis.[86–88] Seizures and developmental delay are also common. The diagnosis is made by measurement of organic acids and demonstration of a decrease in propionyl-CoA carboxylase.

Dystonia has been described in various other disorders of amino acid and organic acid metabolism, including methylmalonic aciduria, 4-hydroxybutyric aciduria, 3-methylglutaconic aciduria, 2-oxoglutaric aciduria, and Hartnup disease.[89–94] Measurement of serum and urine amino and organic acids is indicated in children with no other identifiable cause of dystonia.

MITOCHONDRIAL DISORDERS

Leigh disease

Leigh disease, or subacute necrotizing encephalomyelopathy, typically occurs as the result of mutations in the gene encoding SURF1, important for cytochrome coxidase assembly.[95] Other mitochondrial enzymatic abnormalities have been described, including defects in pyruvate dehydrogenase and respiratory complexes I, II, IV, and V.[96] Leigh disease may be inherited in a maternal, X-linked or autosomal recessive fashion. Onset is typically in infancy or childhood, with developmental regression, seizures, brainstem dysfunction, dystonia, ataxia, and optic atrophy. The diagnosis is supported by finding elevated levels of lactate and pyruvate in serum and CSF, abnormal pattern of cytochrome c oxidase expression on muscle biopsy, and abnormal MRI signal and necrosis in the basal ganglia, thalamus, and brainstem.[96]

Leber's hereditary optic neuropathy

Mutations in mitochondrial respiratory chain complexes I, III, or IV may lead to Leber's hereditary optic neuropathy, a disorder characterized by rapid vision loss beginning between 18 and 23 years old.[96] Dystonia, ataxia, or spastic paraplegia may accompany the visual changes.[97,98] Transmission is maternal and the diagnosis is supported by an elevated serum lactate and microangiopathic changes in the optic fundus. Direct DNA mutation analysis is available.

Human deafness-dystonia syndrome (Mohr–Tranebjaerg syndrome)

This unusual disorder results from mutations in the genes encoding DDP1 or DDP2, proteins involved in mitochondrial transport.[99] It is inherited in a recessive X-linked fashion and is characterized by sensorineural deafness, dystonia, cortical blindness, dysphagia, and paranoia.[100,101] Symptoms usually begin in childhood.

TRINUCLEOTIDE REPEAT DISORDERS

Huntington's disease

Huntington's disease (HD) is an autosomal dominant movement disorder caused by an abnormal CAG triplet repeat expansion in the *huntingtin* gene, encoded on chromosome 4.[102] Classically, the disease is characterized by a progressive movement disorder accompanied by cognitive decline and psychiatric abnormalities. Chorea is thought to be related to the early and preferential loss of the enkephalinergic striatal projection neurons to the external segment of the globus pallidus. As the disease progresses and projections to the globus pallidus interna are also affected, rigidity and dystonia predominate. In juvenile-onset cases, dystonia is common early. Striatal and cortical atrophy are prominent, and pathologic examination reveals striatal neuronal loss.[103] Cell loss is also demonstrable in the cortex.

Spinocerebellar ataxia

Machado–Joseph disease or spinocerebellar ataxia type 3 (SCA3) is an autosomal dominant, adult-onset disorder caused by CAG triplet repeat expansions in the gene *ataxin*, encoded on chromosome 14q32.1.[104] Similar to HD, increased repeat length correlates with earlier disease onset and more severe symptoms. Dystonia is a frequent finding in SCA3, particularly in the juvenile-onset form. Progressive ataxia, parkinsonism, and external ophthalmoparesis are the cardinal manifestations.

An updated list of the identified spinocerebellar ataxias is available at http://www.neuro.wustl.edu/neuromuscular/ataxia/domatax.html.

PARKINSONIAN SYNDROMES

Dystonia is not uncommon in parkinsonism. It occurs commonly during 'off' periods in patients with Parkinson's disease (PD) with motor fluctuations, and is also seen in patients with multiple system atrophy. Corticobasal ganglionic degeneration classically features a dystonic hand or foot, and retrocollic dystonia of the neck is common in progressive supranuclear palsy.[105,106]

Approximately 10% of patients with Parkinson's disease have an inherited form of the disease. Mutations identified in families with PD include α-synuclein (chromosome 4q21), *DJ1* (chromosome 1p36), *parkin* (chromosome 6q25–27), *UCH-L1* (ubiquitin C-terminal hydrolase L1, chromosome 4p14), *pink1* (PTEN-induced kinase 1, chromosome 1p35), and *LRRK2* (leucine-rich repeat kinase 2, chromosome 12).[107–113] Dystonia is common in autosomal recessive juvenile Parkinson's disease.[114,115]

X-linked dystonia-parkinsonism (Lubag)

This X-linked disorder was reported in men originating from the island of Panay in the Philippines.[116] Dystonia or parkinsonism may define the clinical presentation. The disorder is linked to the centromere of the X chromosome, and is called DYT3.[117] Female heterozygotes can manifest mild dystonia or chorea. Positron emission tomography (PET) scans reveal decreased striatal glucose metabolism, without decrease in nigrostriatal dopaminergic projection.[118] Neuronal loss and gliosis are observed in a mosaic distribution throughout the striatum, preferentially affecting the lateral putamen.[119]

Rapid-onset dystonia-parkinsonism (see Chapter 12)

This unusual disorder is characterized by the abrupt onset (over hours to weeks) of dystonia, dysarthria, dysphagia, bradykinesia, and postural instability.[120] Symptoms typically begin between the ages of 14 and 45 years, and the disorder often remains stable. It is inherited in an autosomal dominant fashion, linked to chromosome 19q13.[121]

OTHER NEURODEGENERATIVE PROCESSES

Ataxia-telangiectasia

Ataxia-telangiectasia is an autosomal recessive disorder caused by mutations in the *ATM* gene which encodes a member of the phosphoinositol 3-kinase family important for cell cycle regulation and DNA repair.[122] Symptoms typically begin between the ages of 2 and 4 years old, and cerebellar ataxia is the initial and most prominent finding on examination.[123] Telangiectasias are a diagnostic hallmark, found commonly in the conjunctivae, and dystonia is usually seen only in later stages of the disease.[124,125] Cerebellar Purkinje cell loss is characteristic, and degeneration of the posterior and lateral columns of the spinal cord is also seen.[126]

Chorea-acanthocytosis

Chorea-acanthocytosis or neuroacanthocytosis is an autosomal recessive disorder caused by mutations in the gene encoding chorein (chromosome 9), a protein involved in intracellular protein trafficking.[127] Symptoms typically begin in the third to fourth decade of life with prominent and progressive chorea, tics, dystonia, behavioral disinhibition, and cognitive decline.[128] The chorea commonly affects the mouth and tongue, with frequent lip and tongue biting, dysphagia, and dysarthria. Imaging reveals atrophy and signal abnormality of the basal ganglia, particularly the striatum. Neuronal loss is found in the basal ganglia on postmortem examination.[129]

Rett syndrome

Females with Rett syndrome, an X-linked disorder, typically manifest symptoms after the first year of life, with regression of language and motor skills and autistic behavior.[130] Stereotyped wringing of the hands is very characteristic. Spasticity and dystonia may occur.[131,132] Direct mutation analysis of the *Rett* gene is now available.

Infantile bilateral striatal necrosis and familial striatal necrosis

Infantile bilateral striatal necrosis usually occurs acutely and is characterized by chorea, dystonia, rigidity, and ballismus, and a stereotyped cry, grimace, and hyperextension of the neck in response to stimuli.[133] Often, symptoms begin after a respiratory infection. Most cases are sporadic, but some are inherited in an autosomal recessive or maternal pattern. The characteristic findings include spongy degeneration of caudate and putamen, which can be detected on CT or MRI as either hypodensities or T2 hyperintensities, respectively.[134]

Neuronal intranuclear inclusion disease

Clinical manifestations of this disorder typically begin in childhood, but adult onset has been reported. Ataxia, spasticity, parkinsonism, autonomic dysfunction, and cognitive deficits are the core features, but other neurologic deficits occur, including dystonia, chorea, and motor neuropathy.[135–137] Neuronal intranuclear inclusion disease typically occurs sporadically but inherited forms have been described. Intranuclear inclusions composed of eosinophilic, ubiquinated material are found in the central, peripheral, and autonomic nervous systems.[138]

Ataxia with vitamin E deficiency

Approximately 13% of patients with ataxia with vitamin E deficiency exhibit dystonia.[139] This autosomal recessive disorder is caused by mutations in the gene encoding α-tocopherol transfer protein (chromosome 8q).[140] Age of onset is typically under 20 years old, and clinical features include cerebellar ataxia, dysarthria, loss of vibration sense, and deep tendon reflexes. Vitamin E supplementation may retard progression of the disease.

REFERENCES

1. Burke RE, Fahn S, Gold AP. Delayed-onset dystonia in patients with "static" encephalopathy. J Neurol Neurosurg Psychiatry 1980; 43(9): 789–97.
2. Tanzi RE, Petrukhin K, Chernov I et al. The Wilson's disease gene is a copper transporting ATPase with homology to the Menkes disease gene. Nat Genet 1993; 5(4): 344–50.
3. Thomas GR, Forbes JR, Roberts EA, Walshe JM, Cox DW. The Wilson's disease gene: spectrum of mutations and their consequences. Nat Genet 1995; 9(2): 210–17.
4. Shimizu N, Nakazono H, Takeshita Y et al. Molecular analysis and diagnosis in Japanese patients with Wilson's disease. Pediatr Int 1999; 41(4): 409–13.
5. Cox D, Roberts EA. Wilson's disease. www.genetests.org.
6. Dening TR, Berrios GE. Wilson's disease. Psychiatric symptoms in 195 cases. Arch Gen Psychiatry 1989; 46(12): 1126–34.
7. Steindl P, Ferenci P, Dienes HP et al. Wilson's disease in patients presenting with liver disease: a diagnostic challenge. Gastroenterology 1997; 113(1): 212–18.
8. Roberts EA, Cox DW. Wilson's disease. Baillières Clin Gastroenterol 1998; 12(2): 237–56.
9. Demirkiran M, Jankovic J, Lewis RA, Cox DW. Neurologic presentation of Wilson's disease without Kayser–Fleischer rings. Neurology 1996; 46(4): 1040–3.
10. Ferenci P, Caca K, Loudianos G et al. Diagnosis and phenotypic classification of Wilson's disease. Liver 2003; 23(3): 139–42.
11. Roberts EA, Schilsky ML. A practice guideline on Wilson's disease. Hepatology 2003; 37(6): 1475–92.
12. Hitoshi S, Iwata M, Yoshikawa K. Mid-brain pathology of Wilson's disease: MRI analysis of three cases. J Neurol Neurosurg Psychiatry 1991; 54(7): 624–6.
13. van Wassenaer-van Hall HN, van den Heuvel AG, Algra A, Hoogenraad TU, Mali WP. Wilson's disease: findings at MR imaging and CT of the brain with clinical correlation. Radiology 1996; 198(2): 531–6.
14. Bertrand E, Lewandowska E, Szpak GM et al. Neuropathological analysis of pathological forms of astroglia in Wilson's disease. Folia Neuropathol 2001; 39(2): 73–9.
15. LeWitt P. Wilson's disease. In: Noseworthy JH, ed. Neurological Therapeutics: Principles and Practice. London: Martin Dunitz; 2003: 2671–6.
16. Brewer GJ, Askari F, Lorincz MT et al. Treatment of Wilson's disease with ammonium tetrathiomolybdate: IV. Comparison of tetrathiomolybdate and trientine in a double-blind study of treatment of the neurologic presentation of Wilson's disease. Arch Neurol 2006; 63(4): 521–7.
17. Schilsky ML. Treatment of Wilson's disease: what are the relative roles of penicillamine, trientine, and zinc supplementation? Curr Gastroenterol Rep 2001; 3(1): 54–9.
18. Zhou B, Westaway SK, Levinson B et al. A novel pantothenate kinase gene (PANK2) is defective in Hallervorden–Spatz syndrome. Nat Genet 2001; 28(4): 345–9.
19. Dooling EC, Schoene WC, Richardson EP Jr. Hallervorden–Spatz syndrome. Arch Neurol 1974; 30: 70–83.
20. Hayflick SJ, Westaway SK, Levinson B et al. Genetic, clinical, and radiographic delineation of Hallervorden–Spatz syndrome. N Engl J Med 2003; 348(1): 33–40.
21. Sethi KD, Adams RJ, Loring DW, el Gammal T. Hallervorden–Spatz syndrome: clinical and magnetic resonance imaging correlations. Ann Neurol 1988; 24(5): 692–4.
22. Halliday W. The nosology of Hallervorden–Spatz disease. J Neurol Sci 1995; 134(Suppl): 84–91.
23. Curtis AR, Fey C, Morris CM et al. Mutation in the gene encoding ferritin light polypeptide causes dominant adult-onset basal ganglia disease. Nat Genet 2001; 28(4): 350–4.
24. Crompton DE, Chinnery PF, Fey C et al. Neuroferritinopathy: a window on the role of iron in neurodegeneration. Blood Cells Mol Dis 2002; 29(3): 522–31.
25. Koller WC, Cochran JW, Klawans HL. Calcification of the basal ganglia: computerized tomography and clinical correlation. Neurology 1979; 29(3): 328–33.
26. Forstl H, Krumm B, Eden S, Kohlmeyer K. What is the psychiatric significance of bilateral basal ganglia mineralization? Biol Psychiatry 1991; 29(8): 827–33.
27. Flint J, Goldstein LH. Familial calcification of the basal ganglia: a case report and review of the literature. Psychol Med 1992; 22: 581–95.
28. Moskowitz MA, Winickoff RN, Heinz ER. Familial calcification of the basal ganglions: a metabolic and genetic study. N Engl J Med 1971; 285: 72–7.
29. Larsen TA, Dunn HG, Jan JE, Calne DB. Dystonia and calcification of the basal ganglia. Neurology 1985; 35: 533–7.
30. Ellie E, Julien J, Ferrer X. Familial idiopathic striopallidentate calcifications. Neurology 1989; 39: 381–5.
31. Geschwind DH, Loginov M, Stern JM. Identification of a locus on chromosome 14q for idiopathic basal ganglia calcification (Fahr disease). Am J Hum Genet 1999; 65(3): 764–72.
32. Pentchev PG, Vanier MT, Suzuki K, Patterson MC. Niemann–Pick disease type C: a cellular cholesterol lipidosis. In: Scriver CR, Beaudet AL, Sly WS, Valle D, eds. The Metabolic and Molecular Bases of Inherited Disease. New York: McGraw-Hill; 1995: 2625–39.
33. Carstea ED, Morris JA, Coleman KG et al. Niemann–Pick C1 disease gene: homology to mediators of cholesterol homeostasis. Science 1997; 277(5323): 228–31.
34. Morris JA, Zhang D, Coleman KG et al. The genomic organization and polymorphism analysis of the human Niemann–Pick C1 gene. Biochem Biophys Res Commun 1999; 261: 493–8.
35. Naureckiene S, Sleat DE, Lackland H et al. Identification of HE1 as the second gene of Niemann–Pick C disease. Science 2000; 290(5500): 2298–301.
36. Vanier MT, Rodriguez-Lafrasse C, Rousson R et al. Type C Niemann–Pick disease: spectrum of phenotypic variation in

disruption of intracellular LDL-derived cholesterol processing. Biochim Biophys Acta 1991; 1096: 328–37.
37. Roff CF, Goldin E, Comly ME et al. Niemann–Pick type C disease: deficient intracellular transport of exogenously derived cholesterol. Am J Med Genet 1992; 42: 593–8.
38. Elleder M, Jirasek A, Smid F, Ledvinova J, Besley GTN. Niemann–Pick disease type C. Study on the nature of the cerebral storage process. Acta Neuropathol 1985; 66: 325–36.
39. Distl R, Treiber-Held S, Albert F et al. Cholesterol storage and tau pathology in Niemann–Pick type C disease in the brain. J Pathol 2003; 200: 104–11.
40. Stevenson RE, Taylor HA, Parks SE. β-Galactosidase deficiency: prolonged survival in three patients following early central nervous system deterioration. Clin Genet 1978; 13: 305–13.
41. Goldman JE, Katz D, Rapin I, Purpura DP, Suzuki K. Chronic GM1-gangliosidosis presenting as dystonia: I. clinical and pathological features. Ann Neurol 1981; 9: 465–75.
42. Nakano T, Ikeda S, Kondo K, Yanagisawa N, Tsuji S. Adult GM1-gangliosidosis: clinical patterns and rectal biopsy. Neurology 1985; 35: 875–80.
43. Gravel RA, Clarke JTR, Kaback MM et al. The GM2 gangliosidoses. In: Scriver CR, Beaudet AL, Sly WS, Valle D, eds. The Metabolic and Molecular Bases of Inherited Disease. New York: McGraw-Hill; 1995: 2839–79.
44. Meek D, Wolfe LS, Andermann E, Anderman F. Juvenile progressive dystonia: a new phenotype of GM2 gangliosidosis. Ann Neurol 1984; 15: 348–52.
45. Oates CE, Bosch EP, Hart MN. Movement disorders associated with chronic GM2 gangliosidosis. Eur Neurol 1986; 25: 154–9.
46. Hardie RJ, Morgan-Hughes JA. Dystonia in GM2 gangliosidosis. Mov Disord 1992; 7: 390–1.
47. Nardocci N, Bertagnolio B, Rumi V, Angelini L. Progressive dystonia symptomatic of juvenile GM2 gangliosidosis. Mov Disord 1992; 7: 64–7.
48. Purpura DP, Suzuki K. Distortion of neuronal geometry and formation of aberrant synapses in neuronal storage disease. Brain Res 1976; 116: 1–21.
49. Kolodny EH, Fluharty AL. Metachromatic leukodystrophy and multiple sulfatase deficiency: sulfatide lipidosis. In: Scriver CR, Beaudet AL, Sly WS, Valle D, eds. The Metabolic and Molecular Bases of Inherited Disease. New York: McGraw-Hill; 1995: 2693–739.
50. Demaerel P, Faubert C, Wilms G et al. MR findings in leukodystrophy. Neuroradiology 1991; 33: 368–71.
51. Wenger DA, Rafi MA, Luzi R, Datto J, Constantino-Ceccarini E. Krabbe disease: genetic aspects and progress toward therapy. Mol Genet Metab 2000; 70: 1–9.
52. Suzuki K, Suzuki Y, Suzuki K. Galactosylceramide lipidosis: globoid-cell leukodystrophy (Krabbe disease). In: Scriver CR, Beaudet AL, Sly WS, Valle D, eds. The Metabolic and Molecular Bases of Inherited Disease. New York: McGraw-Hill; 1995: 2671–92.
53. Berger J, Moser HW, Forss-Petter S. Leukodystrophies: recent developments in genetics, molecular biology, pathogenesis and treatment. Curr Opin Neurol 2001; 14: 305–12.
54. Koeppen AH, Robitaille Y. Pelizaeus–Merzbacher disease. J Neuropath Exp Neurol 2002; 61: 747–59.
55. Wisniewski KE, Zhong N, Philippart M. Pheno/genotypic correlations of neuronal ceroid lipofuscinoses. Neurology 2001; 57: 576–81.
56. Greenwood RS, Nelson JS. Atypical neuronal ceroid-lipofuscinosis. Neurology 1978; 28: 710–17.
57. Cooper JD. Progress towards understanding the neurobiology of Batten disease or neuronal ceroid lipofuscinosis. Curr Opin Neurol 2003; 16: 121–8.
58. Boustany RM, Alroy J, Kolodny EH. Clinical classification of neuronal ceroid-lipofuscinosis subtypes. Am J Med Genet Suppl 1988; 5: 47–58.
59. Fujita N, Kimura T, Matsubara N, Tabe H, Tanaka K. A case of adult neuronal ceroid lipofuscinosis type A. Rinsho Shinkeigaku 1999; 39: 478–80.
60. Santavouri P, Lauronen L, Kirveskari et al. Neuronal ceroid lipofuscinoses in childhood. Neurol Sci 2000; 21: S35–S41.
61. Simonati A, Santorum E, Tessa A et al. A CLN2 gene nonsense mutation is associated with severe caudate atrophy and dystonia in LINCL. Neuropediatrics 2000; 31: 199–201.
62. Fowler ML, Nakai H, Byers MG et al. Chromosome 1 localization of the human alpha-L-fucosidase structural gene with a homologous site on chromosome 2. Cytogenet Cell Genet 1986; 43: 103–8.
63. Thomas GH, Beaudet AL. Disorders of glycoprotein degradation and structure: alpha-mannosidosis, beta-mannosidosis, fucosidosis, sialidosis, aspartylglucosaminuria, and carbohydrate-deficient glycoprotein syndrome. In: Scriver CR, Beaudet AL, Sly WS, Valle D, eds. The Metabolic and Molecular Bases of Inherited Disease. New York: McGraw-Hill; 1995: 2529–61.
64. Gordon BA, Gordon KE, Seo HC et al. Fucosidosis with dystonia. Neuropediatrics 1995; 26: 325–7.
65. Loeb H, Tondeur M, Jonniaux G, Mockel-Pohl S, Vamos-Hurwitz E. Biochemical and ultrastructural studies in a case of mucopolysaccharidosis "F" (fucosidosis). Helv Pediatr Acta 1969; 24: 519–37.
66. Watts RWE, Spellacy E, Gibbs DA et al. Clinical, post-mortem, biochemical and therapeutic observations on the Lesch–Nyhan syndrome with particular reference to the neurological manifestations. Q J Med 1982; 51: 43–78.
67. Hyland K, Clayton PT. Aromatic L-amino acid decarboxylase deficiency: diagnostic methodology. Clin Chem 1992; 38: 2405–10.
68. Maller A, Hyland K, Milstein S, Biaggioni I, Butler IJ. Aromatic L-amino acid decarboxylase deficiency: clinical features, diagnosis, and treatment of a second family. J Child Neurol 1997; 12: 349–54.
69. Swoboda KJ, Saul JP, McKenna CE, Speller NB, Hyland K. Aromatic L-amino acid decarboxylase deficiency: overview of clinical features and outcomes. Ann Neurol 2003; 54: S49–S55.
70. Swoboda KJ, Hyland K, Goldstein DS et al. Clinical and therapeutic observations in aromatic L-amino acid decarboxylase deficiency. Neurology 1999; 53: 1205–11.
71. Tanaka K, Paglia DE. Pyruvate kinase and other enzymopathies of the erythrocyte. In: Scriver CR, Beaudet AL, Sly WS, Valle D, eds. The Metabolic and Molecular Bases of Inherited Disease. New York: McGraw-Hill; 1995: 3485–511.
72. Poll-The BT, Aicardi J, Girot R, Rosa R. Neurological findings in triosephosphate isomerase deficiency. Ann Neurol 1985; 17: 439–43.
73. Stockler S, Holzbach U, Hanefeld F et al. Creatine deficiency in the brain: a new, treatable inborn error of metabolism. Pediatr Res 1994; 36: 409–13.
74. Schulze A, Hess T, Wevers R et al. Creatine deficiency syndrome caused by guanidinoacetate methyltransferase deficiency: diagnostic tools for a new inborn error of metabolism. J Pediatr 1997; 131: 626–31.
75. Graf WD, Oleinik OE, Jack RM, Weiss AH, Johnson JL. Ahomocysteinemia in molybdenum cofactor deficiency. Neurology 1998; 51: 860–2.
76. Klepper J, Voit T. Facilitated glucose transporter protein type 1 (GLUT1) deficiency syndrome: impaired glucose transport into brain – a review. Eur J Pediatr 2002; 161: 295–304.
77. Zshocke J, Quak E, Guldberg P, Hoffman GF. Mutation analysis in glutaric aciduria type I. J Med Genet 2000; 37: 177–81.

78. Kyllerman M, Skjeldal OH, Lundberg M et al. Dystonia and dyskinesia in glutaric aciduria type I: clinical heterogeneity and therapeutic considerations. Mov Disord 1994; 9: 22–30.
79. Goodman SI, Norenberg MD, Shikes RH, Breslich DJ, Moe PG. Glutaric aciduria: biochemical and morphologic considerations. J Pediatr 1977; 90: 746–50.
80. Leibel RL, Shih VE, Goodman SI et al. Glutaric acidemia: a metabolic disorder causing progressive choreoathetosis. Neurology 1980; 30: 1163–8.
81. Krauss JP, Janosik M, Kozich V et al. Cystathionine beta-synthase mutations in homocystinuria. Hum Mutat 1999; 13: 362–75.
82. Hagberg B, Hambraeus L, Bensch K. A case of homocystinuria with a dystonia neurological syndrome. Neuropadiatrie 1970; 1: 337–43.
83. Davous P, Rondot P. Homocystinuria and dystonia. J Neurol Neurosurg Psychiatry 1983; 46: 283–6.
84. Berardelli A, Thompson PD, Zaccagnini M et al. Two sisters with generalized dystonia associated with homocystinuria. Mov Disord 1991; 6: 163–5.
85. Kempster PA, Brenton DP, Gale AN, Stern GM. Dystonia in homocystinuria. J Neurol Neurosurg Psychiatry 1988; 51: 859–62.
86. Surtees RA, Matthews EE, Leonard JV. Neurologic outcome of propionic acidemia. Pediatr Neurol 1992; 8: 333–7.
87. Nyhan WL, Bay C, Beyer EW, Mazi M. Neurologic nonmetabolic presentation of propionic acidemia. Arch Neurol 1999; 56: 1143–7.
88. Al-Essa M, Bakheet S, Patay Z et al. 18Fluoro-2-deoxyglucose (18FDG) PET scan of the brain in propionic acidemia: clinical and MRI correlations. Brain Dev 1999; 21: 312–17.
89. Kohlschutter A, Behbehani A, Langenbeck U et al. A familial progressive neurodegenerative disease with 2-oxoglutaric aciduria. Eur J Pediatr 1982; 138: 32–7.
90. Darras BT, Ampola MG, Dietz WH, Gilmore HE. Intermittent dystonia in Hartnup disease. Pediatr Neurol 1989; 5: 118–20.
91. Shevell MI, Matiaszuk N, Ledley FD, Rosenblatt DS. Varying neurological phenotypes among muto and mut-patients with methylmalonylCoA mutase deficiency. Am J Med Genet 1993; 45: 619–24.
92. Al Aqeel A, Rashed M, Ozand PT et al. 3-Methylglutaconic aciduria: ten new cases with a possible new phenotype. Brain Dev 1994; 16 (Suppl): 23–32.
93. Rahbeeni Z, Ozand PT, Rashed M et al. 4-Hydroxybutyric aciduria. Brain Dev 1994; 16 (Suppl): 64–71.
94. Stromme P, Stokke O, Jellum E, Skjeldal OH, Baumgartner R. Atypical methylmalonic aciduria with progressive encephalopathy, microcephaly and cataract in two siblings – a new recessive syndrome? Clin Genet 1995; 48: 1–5.
95. Tiranti V, Hoertnagel K, Carrozzo R et al. Mutations of SURF-1 in Leigh disease associated with cytochrome c oxidase deficiency. Am J Hum Genet 1998; 63(6): 1609–21.
96. Schmiedel J, Jackson S, Schafer J, Reichmann H. Mitochondrial cytopathies. J Neurol 2003; 250: 267–77.
97. Novotny EJ Jr, Singh G, Wallace DC et al. Leber's disease and dystonia: a mitochondrial disease. Neurology 1986; 36: 1053–60.
98. Nikoskelainen EK, Marttila RJ, Huoponen K et al. Leber's "plus": neurological abnormalities in patients with Leber's hereditary optic neuropathy. J Neurol Neurosurg Psychiatry 1995; 59: 160–4.
99. Koehler CM, Leuenberger D, Merchant S et al. Human deafness dystonia syndrome is a mitochondrial disease. Proc Natl Acad Sci USA 1999; 96(5): 2141–6.
100. Tranebjaerg L, Schwartz C, Eriksen H et al. A new X linked recessive deafness syndrome with blindness, dystonia, fractures and mental deficiency is linked to Xq22. J Med Genet 1995; 32: 257–63.
101. Jin H, May M, Tranebjaerg L et al. A novel X-linked gene, DDP, shows mutations in families with deafness (DFN-1), dystonia, mental deficiency and blindness. Nat Genet 1996; 14(2): 177–80.
102. Vonsattel JP, DiFiglia M. Huntington disease. J Neuropathol Exp Neurol 1998; 57: 369–84.
103. Vonsattel JP, Myers RH, Stevens TJ et al. Neuropathological classification of Huntington's disease. J Neuropathol Exp Neurol 1985; 44(6): 559–77.
104. Sudarsky L, Coutinho P. Machado–Joseph disease. Clin Neurosci 1995; 3: 17–22.
105. Barclay CL, Lang AE. Dystonia in progressive supranuclear palsy. J Neurol Neurosurg Psychiatry 1997; 62(4): 352–6.
106. Jankovic J, Tintner R. Dystonia and parkinsonism. Parkinsonism Relat Disord 2001; 8(2): 109–21.
107. Polymeropoulos MH, Higgins JJ, Golbe LI et al. Mapping of a gene for Parkinson's disease to chromosome 4q21-q23. Science 1996; 274: 1197–9.
108. Leroy E, Boyer R, Auburger G et al. The ubiquitin pathway in Parkinson's disease. Nature 1998; 395(6701): 451–2.
109. Lucking CB, Durr A, Bonifati V et al. Association between early-onset Parkinson's disease and mutations in the parkin gene. French Parkinson's Disease Genetics Study Group. N Engl J Med 2000; 342(21): 1560–7.
110. Bonifati V, Rizzu P, van Baren MJ et al. Mutations in the DJ-1 gene associated with autosomal recessive early-onset parkinsonism. Science 2003; 299(5604): 256–9.
111. Valente EM, Abou-Sleiman PM, Caputo V et al. Hereditary early-onset Parkinson's disease caused by mutations in PINK1. Science 2004; 304(5674): 1158–60.
112. Hardy J, Cai H, Cookson MR, Gwinn-Hardy K, Singleton A. Genetics of Parkinson's disease and parkinsonism. Ann Neurol 2006; 60(4): 389–98.
113. Paisan-Ruiz C, Jain S, Evans EW et al. Cloning of the gene containing mutations that cause PARK8-linked Parkinson's disease. Neuron 2004; 44(4): 595–600.
114. Ishikawa A, Tsuji S. Clinical analysis of 17 patients in 12 Japanese families with autosomal-recessive type juvenile parkinsonism. Neurology 1996; 47(1): 160–6.
115. Yamamura Y, Kohriyama T, Kawakami H et al. [Autosomal recessive early-onset parkinsonism with diurnal fluctuation (AR-EPDF) – clinical characteristics]. Rinsho Shinkeigaku 1996; 36(8): 944–50. [in Japanese]
116. Evidente VGH, Advincula J, Esteban R et al. Phenomenology of "Lubag" or X-linked dystonia-parkinsonism. Mov Disord 2002; 17: 1271–7.
117. Wilhelmsen KC, Weeks DE, Nygaard T et al. Genetic mapping of "Lubag" (X-linked dystonia-parkinsonism) in a Filipino kindred to the pericentromeric region of the X chromosome. Ann Neurol 1991; 29: 124–31.
118. Eidelberg D, Takikawa S, Wilhelmsen K et al. Positron emission tomographic findings in Filipino X-linked dystonia-parkinsonism. Ann Neurol 1993; 34(2): 185–91.
119. Waters CH, Faust PL, Powers J et al. Neuropathology of lubag (X-linked dystonia parkinsonism). Mov Disord 1993; 8: 387–90.
120. Dobyns WB, Ozelius LJ, Kramer PL et al. Rapid-onset dystonia-parkinsonism. Neurology 1993; 43: 2596–602.
121. Kramer PL, Mineta M, Klein C et al. Rapid-onset dystonia-parkinsonism: linkage to chromosome 19q13. Ann Neurol 1999; 46: 176–82.
122. Gatti RA, Berkel I, Boder E et al. Localization of an ataxia-telangiectasia gene to chromosome 11q22–23. Nature 1988; 336: 577–80.

123. Di Donato S, Gellera C, Mariotti C. The complex clinical and genetic classification of inherited ataxias. II. Autosomal recessive ataxias. Neurol Sci 2001; 22: 219–28.
124. Bodensteiner JB, Goldblum RM, Goldman AS. Progressive dystonia masking ataxia in ataxia-telangiectasia. Arch Neurol 1980; 37: 464–5.
125. Koepp M, Schelosky L, Cordes I, Cordes M, Poewe W. Dystonia in ataxia telangiectasia: report of a case with putaminal lesions and decreased striatal [^{123}I]iodobenzamide binding. Mov Disord 1994; 9: 455–9.
126. Gatti RA, Vinters HV. Cerebellar pathology in ataxia-telangiectasia: the significance of basket cells. Kroc Found Ser 1985; 19: 225–32.
127. Ueno S, Maruki Y, Nakamura M et al. The gene encoding a newly discovered protein, chorein, is mutated in chorea-acanthocytosis. Nat Genet 2001; 28: 121–2.
128. Rampoldi L, Danek A, Monaco AP. Clinical features and molecular bases of neuroacanthocytosis. J Mol Med 2002; 80: 475–91.
129. Hardie RJ, Pullon HW, Harding AE et al. Neuroacanthocytosis. A clinical, haematological and pathological study of 19 cases. Brain 1991; 114: 13–49.
130. Dunn HG, MacLeod PM. Rett syndrome: review of biological abnormalities. Can J Neurol Sci 2001; 28: 16–29.
131. Fitzgerald PM, Jankovic J, Glaze DG, Schultz R, Percy AK. Extrapyramidal involvement in Rett's syndrome. Neurology 1990; 40: 293–5.
132. Fitzgerald PM, Jankovic J, Percy AK. Rett syndrome and associated movement disorders. Mov Disord 1990; 5: 195–202.
133. Mito T, Tanaka T, Becker LE, Takashima S, Tanaka J. Infantile bilateral striatal necrosis. Clinicopathological classification. Arch Neurol 1986; 43(7): 677–80.
134. Roytta M, Olsson I, Sourander P, Svendsen P. Infantile bilateral striatal necrosis. Clinical and morphological report of a case and a review of the literature. Acta Neuropathol (Berl) 1981; 55(2): 97–103.
135. Nangaku M, Motoyoshi Y, Kwak S, Yoshikawa H, Iwata M. [MRI pathology of the globus pallidus in a patient with oculgyric crisis and tremor]. Rinsho Shinkeigaku 1990; 30: 760–4. [in Japanese]
136. O'Sullivan JD, Hanagasi HA, Daniel SE et al. Neuronal intranuclear inclusion disease and juvenile parkinsonism. Mov Disord 2000; 15: 990–5.
137. Zannoli R, Gilman S, Rossi S et al. Hereditary neuronal intranuclear inclusion disease with autonomic failure and cerebellar degeneration. Arch Neurol 2002; 59: 1319–26.
138. Kimber TE, Blumbergs PC, Rice JP et al. Familial neuronal intranuclear inclusion disease with ubiquitin positive inclusions. J Neurol Sci 1998; 160: 33–40.
139. Cavalier L, Ouahchi K, Kayden HJ et al. Ataxia with isolated vitamin E deficiency: heterogeneity of mutations and phenotypic variability in a large number of families. Am J Hum Genet 1998; 62: 301–10.
140. Doerflinger N, Linder C, Ouahchi K et al. Ataxia with vitamin E deficiency: refinement of genetic localization and analysis of linkage disequilibrium by using new markers in 14 families. Am J Hum Genet 1995; 56: 1116–24.

14

Drug-induced and tardive dystonia

Mark J Edwards and Kailash P Bhatia

INTRODUCTION

Soon after the introduction of dopamine receptor blocking drugs (DRBs) in the early 1950s it was observed that dystonia could occur acutely with first exposure. It was later that a dystonic syndrome was recognized in association with the chronic use of DRBs, and later still that acute dystonic reactions were observed to occur with non-DRB prescription drugs and drugs of abuse. Dystonia associated with drug administration is now a common problem encountered in clinical practice. In this chapter we review current knowledge regarding the clinical features, epidemiology, pathophysiology, and treatment of acute dystonic reactions (ADRs) and tardive dystonia (TDT).

ACUTE DRUG-INDUCED DYSTONIA

Definition and clinical features

Acute dystonic reactions occur in the period shortly after the introduction of particular drugs, usually DRBs. Although the time to onset of ADRs following drug exposure is variable, over 50% of patients will develop symptoms within 48 hours of exposure, and over 90% will show symptoms within 5 days.[1]

Clinical features of ADRs are variable, but can be severe and dramatic in nature. Typical presentations are pronounced dystonia of the oromandibular region, often causing mouth-opening spasms. Axial dystonia with hyperextension of the spine, retrocollis, or laryngospasm (which can be life threatening) can also be seen. A sideways twisting of the trunk, Pisa syndrome, is also described as a clinical presentation of ADR.[2] However, this syndrome not only occurs as an ADR but also is seen in Parkinson's disease, progressive supranuclear palsy, and tardive dystonia.[2] Oculogyric crises are characterized by tonic conjugate ocular deviation, which can be associated with psychotic features, including obsessional thoughts and hallucinations.[3] Oculogyric crises are also observed outside the setting of ADRs: e.g. in patients with postencephalitic parkinsonism.[3]

Drugs that cause acute dystonic reactions

DRBs, which are commonly used for the treatment of psychosis, are the drugs most frequently associated with ADRs. As with tardive dystonia (see below), the older DRBs are thought to be the most likely offenders, but it is not entirely certain whether this represents a bias given the longer length of time that such drugs have been available for use in clinical practice compared to the newer 'atypical' antipsychotics. What is clear, however, is that nearly all DRBs are capable of causing ADRs.[4] This also includes DRBs used for treatment of non-psychiatric conditions such as metoclopramide and prochlorperazine in the treatment of nausea and vomiting and also dopamine-depleting and blocking drug such as tetrabenazine.[5]

A growing number of non-DRB drugs have also been associated with ADRs. These include antidepressants (serotonin reuptake inhibitors,[6] monoamine oxidase inhibitors,[7]) calcium antagonists,[8] benzodiazepines,[9] general anesthetic agents,[10] anticonvulsants,[11] and triptans.[12] ADRs also occur with drugs of abuse, including cocaine,[13] crack cocaine,[14] and Ecstasy (3,4-methylenedioxymethamphetamine).[15] A list of the most commonly implicated drugs is given in Table 14.1. Clinically, the ADRs seen with these non-DRB drugs appear to be similar to that seen in association with DRBs.

ADRs can also be seen in patients with parkinsonian disorders when treated with dopaminergic agents.[16] In Parkinson's disease, this typically occurs as the drug level drops ('off-period dystonia'), but is also sometimes seen when the drug level is at its peak ('peak-dose dystonia') or is rising. Alterations in the frequency, dose, and type of dopaminergic drug can be helpful in the

Table 14.1 Drugs commonly associated with ADRs
Dopamine receptor blocking drugs
Antidepressants: serotonin reuptake inhibitors, monoamine oxidase inhibitors
Calcium antagonists
Benzodiazepines
General anesthetic agents
Anticonvulsants (carbamazepine, phenytoin)
Triptans
Ranitidine
Cocaine
Ecstasy

treatment of these symptoms.[16] In the atypical parkinsonian condition multiple system atrophy, levodopa administration can give rise to unusual dystonic spasm of the face, and can be helpful as a differentiating feature of this condition from idiopathic Parkinson's disease.

Risk factors for the development of acute dystonic reactions

Risk factors for the development of ADRs have been mainly studied in psychiatric populations treated with DRBs. In such individuals, male gender, young age (under 30 years old), mental retardation, history of electroconvulsive therapy, dose of DRB, and use of injectable DRBs are all associated with a higher risk of developing ADRs.[17,18] The relative risk associated with male gender and young age may be erroneous, simply reflecting the higher incidence of schizophrenia in young males, and therefore a higher rate of exposure to DRBs.[17,18]

The notion that ADRs occur more frequently in individuals with bipolar disorder as opposed to other psychiatric conditions[19] has been challenged by a prospective study of such patients, where peak DRB dose and age were found to be most predictive of ADRs, as opposed to psychiatric diagnosis.[20] It may be that higher doses of DRBs are more commonly used in those with bipolar disorder (particularly in the manic phase), and that this is responsible for the apparent high prevalence of ADRs in patients with this condition.

Abuse of drugs known to cause ADR (e.g. cocaine) can lead to an increase in the incidence of ADRs when such patients are treated with DRBs.[21] Likewise, patients with HIV (human immunodeficiency virus) or AIDS (acquired immunodeficiency syndrome) have a higher risk of developing ADRs when treated with DRBs,[22] perhaps in some cases due to antiretroviral therapy impairing the normal metabolism of DRBs.[23]

Pathophysiology of acute dystonic reactions

The pathophysiologic mechanism of ADR is unclear. One possibility that has been suggested is that drugs causing ADRs do so by disturbing the balance of dopaminergic and cholinergic neuronal activity in the basal ganglia.[24] Obviously, DRBs are likely to alter this balance due to dopaminergic hypoactivity, but other drugs causing ADR could equally well affect cholinergic neurons. The response of most patients with ADR to anticholinergic drugs supports the hypothesis that relative or actual cholinergic hyperactivity is the mechanism whereby ADRs are produced. A second related hypothesis is that DRBs can cause a paradoxical increase in dopaminergic activity by preferentially blocking presynaptic dopamine receptors.[25] In addition, DRBs may cause an increase in the synthesis and release of dopamine, as well as up-regulation of postsynaptic dopamine receptors.[25] It is informative to note that in patients with Parkinson's disease, ADR can occur at peak or trough dopamine levels. It may therefore be the case that it is the relative balance (or imbalance) of dopaminergic neuronal function that is important in the generation of ADR, rather than the actual level itself.

Sigma receptors, which are widely expressed in motor areas of the brain, have been implicated in the genesis of acute dystonia. The unilateral injection of sigma ligands into the red nucleus of the rat can cause torticollis.[26] Sigma 1 and 2 ligands can both be associated with the production of acute dystonia in animal studies,[27] which can be ameliorated by anticholinergic drugs.[28]

There has been recent interest as to whether dopamine receptor polymorphisms (particularly those of the D_2 receptor) might be important in the pathophysiology of ADR. Although no indication has been found that dopamine receptor polymorphisms are predictive of ADR, an association has been found in one small study between CYP2D6 polymorphisms (a cytochrome P450 enzyme) and ADR.[29] However, this finding was not confirmed by a separate study.[30]

Treatment of acute dystonic reactions

Treatment of ADRs can be clinically urgent, not only as symptoms can be very distressing to the patient but also as serious consequences can occur, including respiratory arrest[31] and rhabdomyolysis.[32] Fortunately, the majority of ADRs can be successfully treated with injectable anticholinergic drugs. Typically, 1–2 mg of benztropine is injected intravenously, and will terminate the attack. Injectable antihistamines such as chlorpheniramine have also been used either in addition or as sole treatment. Benzodiazapines can sometimes be helpful as adjunctive treatment: e.g. 1–2 mg of clonazepam. For those with severe dystonia, relevant management of any systemic complications, particularly compromise of the airway, is essential.

There is evidence to suggest that pretreatment with anticholinergic drugs can reduce the incidence of ADR.[33] This strategy should therefore be considered when DRBs are prescribed to those at particular risk of ADRs, such as cocaine users and those with HIV/AIDS.

TARDIVE DYSTONIA

Introduction and definition

Following the introduction of DRBs in 1952 for the treatment of psychosis, it soon emerged that abnormal involuntary movements could occur in association with chronic DRB administration.[34,35] Initial reports were of rather rapid involuntary movements that tended to involve the mouth and face, leading to the use of the term tardive dyskinesia (TDK) to describe them.

At around the same time as these early reports of TDK were appearing in the medical literature, there were others which reported dystonia related to the long-term use of DRBs.[36,37] It was Keegan and Rajput,[38] however, who first coined the term 'dystonia tarda' in 1973 when reporting a series of patients with torticollis and axial dystonia secondary to the use of DRBs. Other 'tardive' syndromes have been reported in association with DRB use, including tics[39] and tremor.[40]

There has been some confusion generated by the parallel development of the two terms tardive dystonia (TDT) and tardive dyskinesia (TDK). Although both can be caused by DRBs, there has been a tendency to call all DRB-associated movement disorders TDK. Many reports of movement disorders associated with DRBs have therefore mixed cases of TDT and TDK, making it difficult to separate out risk factors and epidemiologic features specifically related to TDT. This may explain why there have been so few case series of patients specifically with TDT. To date, only three large series to have been published (Burke et al,[41] Kang et al,[42] and Kiriakakis et al,[43]) with a combined total of just over 200 patients.

In this regard, criteria have been suggested to aid the clinical definition of TDT. Burke et al[41] defined TDT as:

> an involuntary movement disorder predominated by dystonia and associated with the use of dopamine receptor antagonists. The dystonia must have been present for more than a month and occur either during treatment with DRBs or within 3 months of its discontinuation.

This definition allowed for the presence of choreiform movements, but dystonia had to be the dominant movement disorder. A family history of dystonia was an exclusion criterion, as was the presence of other possible causes for dystonia. A more recent clinical classification of TDT by Adityanjee and colleagues[44] has attempted to stratify patients with TDT based on the dominance of dystonia over any other movement disorder. Under this system, patients are classified as:

- type I – pure TDT in the absence of any other movement disorder
- type II – dystonia coexists with dyskinetic movements of the same body part, but dystonia is predominant
- type III – dystonia coexists with dyskinetic movements in the same or different body parts, but dystonia is less prominent than dyskinesias
- type IV – dystonia coexists with a variety of movement disorders.

It may be useful in a research setting, as the authors of these criteria suggest, to use these criteria to separate out those patients with pure (type I) TDT from those with TDT associated with TDK, in order to aid research into risk factors and pathophysiologic features that are specific for TDT. In clinical practice, however, we would suggest that it is probably most useful to identify TDT (and therefore plan its treatment) by the observation of predominant dystonia in a patient with a history of DRB use when all other relevant causes have been excluded.

Clinical features

Onset of dystonia in TDT typically occurs in one body part, most commonly the neck or face, but spread to a contiguous body part may follow to cause segmental dystonia, or further to produce generalized dystonia. Onset in the arms, trunk, or legs is reported, but is less common. It is rare for TDT to remain as focal dystonia – only 16% of one series remained with focal involvement.[43] There appears to be a relationship between age of onset and distribution of dystonia, mirroring the pattern observed in idiopathic primary dystonia (ID): thus, patients with young-onset disease typically have limb-onset disease, which can spread to become generalized; patients who present in mid-life have segmental dystonia; and patients with an older age of onset tend to have craniocervical involvement. Progression of dystonia typically occurs over months to years: the largest clinical study of patients with TDT found a mean progression of 1.8 years, but with a wide range from 1 month to 14 years.[43] The most rapid onset tends to be seen in younger patients.

Although, clinically, patients with TDT can look very similar to those with ID, there are some features that can be useful in distinguishing the two conditions. Retrocollis and axial extension dystonia causing marked hyperextension of the neck and trunk are quite characteristic of TDT. The extensor neck spasms can be so severe that they often lead to loss of hair, causing a bald patch at the back of the head due to constant friction of the head with the back rest. In contrast, simple torticollis, laterocollis, muscle hypertrophy, head tremor, and a positive family history are more commonly observed in ID.[41,43,45,46] A sensory geste is less commonly observed in TDT but can be present.

Interestingly, typical writer's cramp or other task-specific dystonias do not appear to occur as a manifestation of TDT. Leg and trunk involvement were seen, respectively, in 26% and 44% of patients with TDT in the large series of Kiriakakis et al.[43] Adult onset of leg and axial dystonia is unusual in ID. Bruxism as the sole feature of TDT has been described.

Other movement disorders may be associated with TDT. Most common is the association with the typical stereotyped orofacial dyskinesias of TDK, and it appears that older patients have a greater propensity to develop this pattern of movement disorder. Parkinsonism, tremor, and akathisia can also occur with TDT.[43]

Differential diagnosis

One should bear in mind that there are conditions other than TDT where psychiatric disturbance and dystonia (which may affect the craniocervical region in the main) are encountered together. Most important amongst these (as the condition is treatable) is Wilson's disease, a disorder in which psychiatric disturbance, various movement disorders including dystonia, and sometimes systemic complications can occur. Serum copper and ceruloplasmin, urinary copper excretion, slit-lamp examination for Kayser–Fleischer rings, and sometimes liver biopsy are necessary to make the diagnosis. Other conditions that can present with dystonia and psychiatric disturbance include Huntington's disease, dentatorubral-pallidoluysian atrophy (DRPLA), and pantothenate kinase-associated neurodegeneration (PKAN) for which genetic tests are available, as well as a positive family history in some cases and imaging abnormalities (particularly in PKAN). Delayed-onset dystonia following birth injury and metachromatic leukodystrophy can be excluded by a careful history and cerebral imaging.

As mentioned above, coincidental idiopathic primary dystonia and psychiatric disturbance may be the cause of the clinical presentation rather than TDT, even given exposure to DRB. Although the clinical features outlined above provide a guide to distinguishing the two conditions, such a distinction can be difficult to make with certainty. In younger patients, particularly those with generalized dystonia, it can therefore be useful to perform a *DYT1* gene test. This genetic abnormality is the commonest cause of early-onset primary generalized dystonia,[47] and can therefore be a useful test in the differential diagnosis of certain patients with suspected TDT. The *DYT1* gene has been found to be negative in a series of patients with TDT.[48]

In the majority of patients with suspected TDT where clear exposure to DRB has occurred prior to the onset of the dystonia and the clinical phenotype is typical, testing for Wilson's disease and cerebral imaging with computed tomography (CT) or magnetic resonance imaging (MRI) are sufficient as screening tests for alternative diagnoses.

How common is tardive dystonia

It is difficult to be accurate regarding the true prevalence of TDT, because, as mentioned earlier, many epidemiologic studies have included patients with TDK and other DRB-associated movement disorders rather than pure TDT. Most studies have been retrospective and have taken place in a variety of settings, including in- and outpatient psychiatric services. However, a broad impression of the prevalence of TDT can be gained by examining data from the 10 cross-sectional studies into the prevalence of movement disorders in patients with psychiatric disease treated with DRB that have been performed.[49–59] The prevalence of TDT in these studies ranges from 0.5% to 21%, with a mean of 3%. The figure of 21% is from a study by Sethi and collegues,[52] who explained the high prevalence of TDT they discovered by their systematic examination of patients in the study by neurologists specializing in movement disorders. This might indicate that other studies not employing this type of approach may have underestimated the prevalence of TDT within DRB-treated populations. When patients with all types of drug-induced movement disorders are studied, TDT is a relatively common phenotype: for example, it accounts for 24% of a sample of 125 patients with drug-induced movement disorders reported by Miller and Jankovic.[60]

Risk factors for the development of tardive dystonia

Type of drug

Despite the impression that the older generation of DRBs might be more likely to produce TDT, it is clear that there are no 'safe' DRBs. Even the newer 'atypical' DRBs are capable of producing TDT, including olanzapine,[61] risperidone,[62] quetiapine,[63] aripiprazole,[64] ziprasidone,[65] and even clozapine.[66] Chlorpromazine, thioridazine, and haloperidol are most commonly reported as associated with TDT, but this may simply reflect the length of time they have been in use in clinical practice, and the way in which they have been used (average dose, average length of treatment). It remains to be seen whether the modern trend towards the use of atypical DRBs for the treatment of psychosis will lead to a reduction in the incidence of DRB-induced movement disorders including TDT.

DRBs are not only prescribed for the treatment of psychosis. Such drugs are used for the treatment of other psychiatric conditions, including depression, anxiety, and acute confusional states. DRBs such as metoclopramide and prochlorperazine are commonly prescribed for the treatment of nausea and vertigo. In populations of patients with TDT, over 20% may have been prescribed DRBs for conditions such as these where alternative treatment might have been appropriate.[43]

There is no evidence to suggest that the concurrent use of non-DRB drugs (such as anticholinergics) in patients taking DRBs increases (or decreases) their risk of developing TDT.

Duration of exposure

There is no clear relationship between duration of exposure to DRB and the subsequent occurrence or severity of TDT. Although mean exposure time prior to the onset of TDT is in the region of 6 years,[43] there is clearly no 'safe' exposure time to DRB, and patients have been reported who have developed TDT after exposures as short as 4 days (Figure 14.1).[43] Likewise, those on very long-term treatment cannot be considered to be safe from developing TDT: exposure times as long as 23 years have been reported before the onset of TDT.[43] In this regard, there is some evidence that the onset of TDT can be triggered in patients on long-term stable DRB therapy by either a change in DRB, the addition of another DRB, or even a change in a stable dose of DRB.

Diagnosis

It is not surprising that the majority of those with TDT have psychiatric disorders, or that the majority of these patients have a diagnosis of schizophrenia, given that psychiatric disease, and schizophrenia in particular, are the major indications for DRB. There is no evidence that there is a particular psychiatric diagnosis that puts patients at an increased or decreased risk of developing TDT during treatment with DRB. Although there is less evidence available, patients without psychiatric disorders are clearly capable of developing TDT when exposed to DRB, and there is no reason to suspect that their risk of developing TDT with DRB exposure is any greater or less than those with psychiatric disorders.

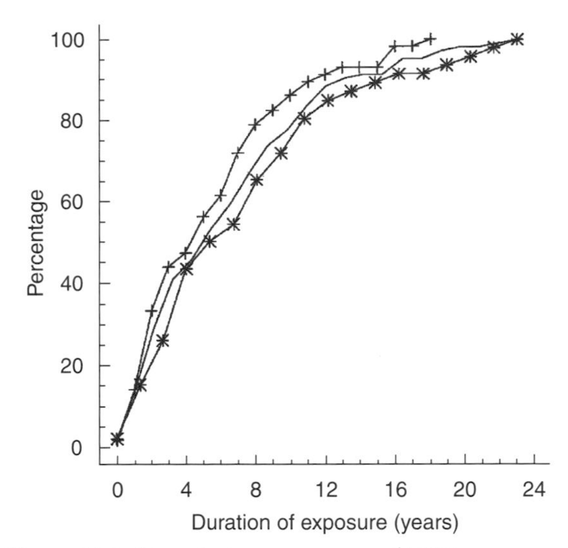

Figure 14.1 Cumulative percentage of TDT as a function of duration of exposure to DRB. Males (+); females (*); all patients (−). (Reproduced from Kiriakakis et al,[43] with permission.)

Age and gender

There does appear to be an association between the age at onset of the DRB-associated movement disorder and the type of tardive movement disorder produced. An older age of onset is associated with the production of TDK rather than TDT,[67] and if TDT does occur in older patients, lower limb involvement and generalized dystonia are less likely.[41] There is a male predominance observed in studies of TDT (approximately 2: 1), and men also tend to have a lower age at onset of TDT compared with women.[43] This may simply reflect the differences between men and women regarding the prevalence and age at onset of schizophrenia, which is both more common in men than women, and also tends to occur at a younger age in men. It is likely, therefore, that men are more frequently prescribed DRB, and at a younger age than women. Indeed, the age at first exposure to DRB was found to be 27 years for males and 36 years for females in one case series.[43]

Natural history of tardive dystonia – outcome and remission

Unfortunately, spontaneous remission of TDT is rare. Summarizing the six published case series (a total patient group of 231 patients),[41–43,68–70] remission was only seen in 10% of cases, after a mean follow-up of 7 years (Table 14.2). The chance of remission occurring is not influenced by age at onset, type of DRB, gender, or the distribution and extent of dystonia. The two factors that do appear to be related to the chance of remission are the discontinuation of DRB therapy and the total duration of DRB exposure. Patients with TDT in whom DRBs have been discontinued are more likely to experience a remission of their TDT (12/54 patients vs 3/52 patients in one series[43]). Patients with TDT with an exposure to DRB of greater than 10 years are five times less likely to experience a remission than those with an exposure to DRB of less than 1 year.[43]

Pathophysiology of tardive dystonia

The majority of research into the pathophysiology of tardive syndromes has focused on TDK, rather than TDT. The clinical classification of subjects in such studies is not always clear, and it is therefore likely that a number of patients with TDT are included. The data presented below must therefore be considered with this in mind, as TDT and TDK may have different underlying mechanisms.

Dopamine receptor hypersensitivity is the leading pathophysiologic theory behind the origins of both TDK and TDT.[25,71] It is suggested that enhanced D_1 receptor stimulation by endogenous dopamine in the presence of D_2 receptor blockade by DRBs might lead to a critical imbalance between direct and indirect pathway activity in the basal ganglia.[71] A slowly developing sensitization of D_1-mediated striatal output is consistent with the delayed onset of dystonia, and its persistence after DRB withdrawal. In addition, blockade of D_1 receptors and stimulation of D_2 receptors (by the D_1 antagonist and D_2 agonist bromocriptine) has been found to be beneficial in some patients with TDK.[72] Conversely, up-regulation of D_2 receptors due to dopamine receptor blockade has been identified in patients on long-term DRB therapy. Using [^{11}C]-raclopride positron emission tomography (PET), Silvestri and colleagues[73] have demonstrated a decrease in [^{11}C]-raclopride binding (consistent with an up-regulation of D_2 receptors), in patients on long-term DRB treatment, although none of these patients had TDT/TDK.

It has been proposed that γ-aminobutyric acid (GABA) may play a role in the pathogenesis of TDT/TDK.[74] Abnormalities in glutamic acid decarboxylase (GAD) – an enzyme involved in the synthesis of GABA – have been found in experimental animals treated with DRBs[75] and in humans with TDK.[76] Other clinicians have failed to replicate these findings, however.[77] In keeping with a possible role for abnormalities in GABA in the pathogenesis of TDT/TDK, there is some clinical evidence to support the efficacy of GABA agonists in the treatment of TDT/TDK.[78] However, a recent Cochrane review has concluded that insufficient evidence currently exists to truly determine the usefulness of such drugs.[79]

Table 14.2 Details of remission rates in patients with tardive dystonia reported in six case series

Study	Patients (*n*)	Follow-up from onset (years)	Follow-up from DRB withdrawal (years)	Remitting patients (*n*)
Burke et al, 1982[41]	42	3.1	1.5	5
Gimenez-Roldan et al, 1985[67]	9	4.7	n.s.	0
Kang et al, 1986[42]	67	4.8	2.8	5
Gardos et al, 1987,[69]	10	5.2	n.s.	0
Wojcik et al, 1991[68]	29	7.3	n.s.	0
Kiriakakis et al, 1998[43]	107	8.3	3.9	15

DRB = dopamine receptor blocking drug; n.s = not stated.

As with ADRs, recent interest has focused on the possible role of genetic polymorphisms in the genesis of TDT. Polymorphisms in a number of genes have been studied, including estrogen, opioid, and dopamine receptor genes, and genes involved in oxidative phosporylation. The most promising finding is of an association between a ser/gly polymorphism in the dopamine D_3 receptor and TDK:[80] not only has this polymorphism been identified in patients with TDK[80] but also it has been found in a primate model of TDK which has a high susceptibility to DRB-induced side effects.[81] The functional relevance of this polymorphism is unclear at the present time. This finding has not been confirmed by all investigators. For example, Mihara and colleagues found no association between TDT and polymorphisms in the D_2 and D_3 receptor genes, but numbers were small in this study, with only nine TDT patients.[82]

Recent research has also proposed a possible role for oxidative stress in the pathogenesis of TDT. It is hypothesized that DRBs are a cause of oxidative stress in the basal ganglia. Evidence in support of this hypothesis comes from cerebrospinal fluid (CSF) studies in patients taking DRB in whom lipid peroxidation was higher than control subjects,[83] and also from studies in animal models and humans showing that vitamin E administration may reduce DRB induced changes in monoamine metabolism, protect against DRB-induced cell death, and perhaps even reduce TDK symptoms in some patients.[84–86] Controlled studies of vitamin E in TDK have not, however, been able to demonstrate a benefit.[87] It is possible that DRBs may cause excitotoxicity in the basal ganglia. There is evidence that DRBs can increase the striatal release of glutamate,[88] and this could, in turn, increase the chance of excitotoxic damage. These hypotheses open the way for further studies of neuroprotective and antioxidant agents, both in patients with TDT and in those at risk of developing TDT.

Treatment of tardive dystonia

Treatments available for TDT are symptomatic, and there is no evidence that any particular treatment can increase the chance of a remission occurring. The most important 'treatment' therefore is that of prevention, by ensuring that DRBs are only used when absolutely necessary, and then for the shortest time possible.

For those with focal or segmental TDT, or in patients with more widespread dystonia, but with specific problems associated with a body part, botulinum toxin (BT) injections are often the most effective treatment. In one study of the use of BT in 34 patients with TDT, moderate to marked improvement was noted in 29 of 38 body parts injected.[89] All of the patients in this study had failed to respond to standard drug treatment.

In those in whom botulinum toxin is unhelpful or not appropriate, a variety of drugs can be tried, including anticholinergics, baclofen, benzodiazepines, tetrabenazine, reserpine, and levodopa. There is no clear way of predicting individual response to such drugs, and often a combination of two or more agents is necessary. Unfortunately, all of these drugs can cause psychiatric side effects, particularly at high doses. It is common practice to use anticholinergic drugs first, which should be introduced slowly and cautiously. Using such an approach, it is sometimes possible to reach high doses, particularly in younger patients, without the emergence of side effects and with a beneficial effect on the dystonia. Tetrabenazine and reserpine can be used in addition to anticholinergics, or alone if anticholinergics are not tolerated, but depression is a notable side effect. Oral baclofen can be helpful, but can be associated with sedation and depression. Intrathecal baclofen is sometimes used for patients with axial dystonia with good results in some case reports. However, long-term problems with catheter displacement, infection, and pump failure can occur. Benzodiazepines (in particular clonazepam) are sometimes useful as adjunctive agents, but are associated with side effects, including sedation, mood disturbance, and dependence. Levodopa is rarely helpful, but at least can be trialed without a major risk of side effects.

There is increasing evidence that patients with TDT may paradoxically benefit from the reintroduction of a particular DRB. Clozapine is the drug most studied in this respect, and a number of open-label and double-blinded trials have demonstrated some moderate benefit, although not all trials have reached this conclusion (for a review see Reference 90). There are reports of other atypical DRBs being beneficial in the treatment of TDT, including risperidone,[91,92] olanzapine,[93] and quetiapine.[94–96] It must be noted that treatment with clozapine requires strict monitoring of blood counts due to the risk of neutropenia. There is clearly a risk that the reintroduction of DRBs may worsen TDT, and therefore the treatment of TDT with atypical DRBs should be considered only after other treatment strategies have failed. As a caveat to this, some patients with TDT will clearly require ongoing DRB treatment for psychosis and, in such patients, trials of clozapine and perhaps other atypical DRBs are indicated.

Although recent studies in the pathophysiology of TDT have suggested that oxidative stress induced by DRB may play a role, a controlled study of vitamin E supplementation failed to produce a benefit.[88] Additional treatments for which benefit has been claimed in open studies of small numbers of patients include morphine[97] and electroconvulsive therapy.[98,99] Dietary supplementation with branched-chain amino acids has been found to significantly decrease TDK symptoms in one uncontrolled study,[100] and encouragingly also in a recent placebo-controlled trial,[101] but results of the use of such treatment has not been published in patients with TDT.

The recent interest and notable success of pallidal deep brain stimulation for patients with idiopathic primary dystonia has led to the use of this technique in a small number of patients with TDT. One patient with TDT reported by Trottenberg and colleagues was implanted with bilateral internal globus pallidus (GPi) and ventral intermediate thalamic (VIM) stimulators.[102] Dystonic symptoms were improved by stimulation through the GPi electrodes, but stimulation via the VIM stimulators alone produced no benefit, and simultaneous stimulation via GPi and VIM electrodes produced no additional benefit over GPi stimulation alone. This group has more recently published a small series of five patients with TDT treated with GPi stimulation. They reported an average improvement of 87% in the Burke Fahn Marsden dystonia rating scale in these patients. Thalamotomy has also been applied to patients with TDT, with apparent benefit.[103]

A small number of patients with TDT (usually those with generalized dystonia) develop sudden severe exacerbations of their dystonia, sometimes triggered by intercurrent illness. This not only occurs in patients with TDT but also has been reported in patients with other forms of dystonia. This syndrome of 'status dystonicus' or 'dystonic storm' is a medical emergency, as the severity of the dystonia can compromise bulbar function, and can result in myoglobinuria and renal failure.[104] Such patients should be managed in an intensive care setting, but despite the severity of the symptoms, episodes are usually self-limiting.

CONCLUSIONS

1. ADRs can be associated with a variety of drugs, not just DRBs, and although, typically, symptoms are readily treated with injectable anticholinergic drugs, they can be severe, and even life threatening.
2. TDT is a disabling, chronic condition associated with DRB use.
3. There is no 'safe' DRB and no 'safe' exposure time.
4. Remission from TDT is rare, and symptomatic treatment is difficult. DRBs should therefore only be used in situations where no other therapeutic options are available.
5. Treatment of focal dystonia due to TDT is most often treated with botulinum toxin. A range of medications are available for those in whom botulinum toxin is not appropriate, but responses to such drugs vary widely between patients. In those with refractory, severe TDT, atypical DRB or deep brain stimulation are viable treatment strategies.

REFERENCES

1. Keepers GA, Casey DE. Predictors of neuroleptic-induced dystonia. J Clin Psychopharmacol 1987; 7: 342–5.
2. Suzuki T, Koizumi J, Moroji T et al. Clinical characteristics of the Pisa syndrome. Acta Psych Scand 1990; 82: 454–7.
3. Sachdev P. Tardive and chronically recurrent oculogyric crises. Mov Disord 1993; 8(1): 93–7.
4. Raja M, Azzoni A. Novel antipsychotics and acute dystonic reactions. Pharmacol Biochem Behav 2000; 67(3): 497–500.
5. Bateman DN, Darling WM, Boys R, Rawlins MD. Extrapyramidal reactions to metoclopramide and prochlorperazine. Q J Med 1989; 71(264): 307–11.
6. Arnone D, Hansen L, Kerr JS. Acute dystonic reaction in an elderly patient with mood disorder after titration of paroxetine: possible mechanisms and implications for clinical care. J Psychopharmacol 2002 ; 16(4): 395–7.
7. Jarecke CR, Reid PJ. Acute dystonic reaction induced by a monoamine oxidase inhibitor. J Clin Psychopharmacol 1990; 10(2): 144–5.
8. Micheli F, Pardal MF, Gatto M et al. Flunarizine- and cinnarizine-induced extrapyramidal reactions. Neurology 1987; 37(5): 881–4.
9. Hooker EA, Danzl DF. Acute dystonic reaction due to diazepam. J Emerg Med 1988; 6(6): 491–3.
10. Hariharan V. Acute dystonic reaction following general anaesthesia. Acta Anaesthesiol Scand 2001; 45(4): 520.
11. Kerrick JM, Kelley BJ, Maister BH, Graves NM, Leppik IE. Involuntary movement disorders associated with felbamate. Neurology 1995 ; 45(1): 185–7.
12. Garcia G, Kaufman MB, Colucci RD. Dystonic reaction associated with sumatriptan. Ann Pharmacother 1994; 28(10): 1199.
13. Fines RE, Brady WJ, DeBehnke DJ. Cocaine-associated dystonic reaction. Am J Emerg Med 1997; 15(5): 513–15.
14. Catalano G, Catalano MC, Rodriguez R. Dystonia associated with crack cocaine use. South Med J 1997; 90(10): 1050–2.
15. Priori A, Bertolasi L, Berardelli A, Manfredi M. Acute dystonic reaction to ecstasy. Mov Disord 1995; 10(3): 353.
16. Cubo E, Gracies JM, Benabou R et al. Early morning off-medication dyskinesias, dystonia, and choreic subtypes. Arch Neurol 2001; 58(9): 1379–82.
17. Keepers GA, Casey DE. Predictors of neuroleptic-induced dystonia. J Clin Psychopharmacol 1987; 7: 342–5.
18. Priori A, Bertolasi L, Berardelli A, Manfredi M. Predictors of acute dystonia in first-episode psychotic patients. Am J Psychiatry 1994; 151(12): 1819–21.
19. Nasrallah HA, Churchill CM, Hamdan-Allan GA. Higher frequency of neuroleptic-induced dystonia in mania than in schizophrenia. Am J Psychiatry 1988; 145(11): 1455–6.
20. Khanna R, Das A, Damodaran SS. Prospective study of neuroleptic-induced dystonia in mania and schizophrenia. Am J Psychiatry 1992; 149(4): 511–13.
21. van Harten PN, van Trier JC, Horwitz EH, Matroos GE, Hoek HW. Cocaine as a risk factor for neuroleptic-induced acute dystonia. J Clin Psychiatry 1998; 59(3): 128–30.
22. van Der Kleij FG, de Vries PA, Stassen PM, Sprenger HG, Gans RO. Acute dystonia due to metoclopramide: increased risk in AIDS. Arch Intern Med 2002; 162(3): 358–9.
23. Kelly DV, Beique LC, Bowmer MI. Extrapyramidal symptoms with ritonavir/indinavir plus risperidone. Ann Pharmacother 2002; 36(5): 827–30.

24. Neale R, Gerhardt S, Liebman JM. Effects of dopamine agonists, catecholamine depletors, and cholinergic and GABAergic drugs on acute dyskinesias in squirrel monkeys. Psychopharmacology (Berl) 1984; 82(1–2): 20–6.
25. Marsden CD, Jenner P. The pathophysiology of extrapyramidal side-effects of neuroleptic drugs. Psychol Med 1980; 10(1): 55–72.
26. Matsumoto RR, Hemstreet MK, Lai NL et al. Drug specificity of pharmacological dystonia. Pharmacol Biochem Behav 1990; 36(1): 151–5.
27. Matsumoto RR, Pouw B. Correlation between neuroleptic binding to sigma(1) and sigma(2) receptors and acute dystonic reactions. Eur J Pharmacol 2000; 401(2): 155–60.
28. Yoshida K, Takahashi H, Sato K, Higuchi H, Shimizu T. Biperiden hydrochlorate ameliorates dystonia of rats produced by microinjection of sigma ligands into the red nucleus. Pharmacol Biochem Behav 2000; 67(3): 497–500.
29. Scordo MG, Spina E, Romeo P et al. CYP2D6 genotype and antipsychotic-induced extrapyramidal side effects in schizophrenic patients. Eur J Clin Pharmacol 2000; 56(9–10): 679–83.
30. Armstrong M, Daly AK, Blennerhassett R, Ferrier N, Idle JR. Antipsychotic drug-induced movement disorders in schizophrenics in relation to CYP2D6 genotype. Br J Psychiatry 1997; 170: 23–6.
31. Stevens CB. Acute laryngeal dystonic reactions. Psychosomatics 1990; 31(2): 236–7.
32. Cavanaugh JJ, Finlayson RE. Rhabdomyolysis due to acute dystonic reaction to antipsychotic drugs. J Clin Psychiatry 1984; 45(8): 356–7.
33. Spina E, Sturiale V, Valvo S et al. Prevalence of acute dystonic reactions associated with neuroleptic treatment with and without anticholinergic prophylaxis. Int Clin Psychopharmacol 1993; 8(1): 21–4.
34. Faurbye A, Rasch PJ, Petersen PB, Brandborg G, Pakkenberg H. Neurological symptoms in pharmacotherapy of psychoses. Acta Psychiatr Scand 1964; 40: 10–27.
35. Crane GE. Persistent dyskinesia. Br J Psychiatry 1973; 122: 395–405.
36. Druckman R, Seelinger D, Thulin B. Chronic involuntary movements induced by phenothiazines. J Nerv Ment Dis 1962; 135: 69–76.
37. Angle CR, McIntire MS. Persistent dystonia in a brain-damaged child after ingestion of phenothiazine. Pediatr Pharmacol Ther 1968; 73: 124–6.
38. Keegan DL, Rajput AH. Drug induced dystonia tarda: treatment with L-dopa. Dis Nerv Syst 1973; 34: 167–9.
39. Bharucha KJ, Sethi KD. Tardive tourettism after exposure to neuroleptic therapy. Mov Disord 1995; 10(6): 791–3.
40. Tarsy D, Indorf G. Tardive tremor due to metoclopramide. Mov Disord 2002; 17(3): 620–1.
41. Burke RE, Fahn S, Jankovic J et al. Tardive dystonia: late-onset and persistent dystonia caused by antipsychotic drugs. Neurology 1982; 32: 1335–46.
42. Kang UJ, Burke RE, Fahn S. Natural history and treatment of tardive dystonia. Mov Disord 1986; 1: 193–208.
43. Kiriakakis V, Bhatia KP, Quinn NP, Marsden CD. The natural history of tardive dystonia. A long-term follow-up study of 107 cases. Brain 1998; 121: 2053–66.
44. Adityanjee, Aderibigbe YA, Jampala VC, Mathews T. The current status of tardive dystonia. Biol Psychiatry 1999; 45(6): 715–30.
45. Molho ES, Feustel PJ, Factor SA. Clinical comparison of tardive and idiopathic cervical dystonia. Mov Disord 1998; 13: 486–9.
46. Bhatia KP, Quinn NP, Marsden CD. Clinical features and natural history of axial predominant adult onset primary dystonia. J Neurol Neurosurg Psychiatry 1997; 63: 788–91.
47. Bressman SB, Sabatti C, Raymond D et al. The DYT1 phenotype and guidelines for diagnostic testing. Neurology 2000; 54(9): 1746–52.
48. Bressman SB, de Leon D, Raymond D et al. Secondary dystonia and the DYTI gene. Neurology 1997; 48(6): 1571–7.
49. Friedman JH, Kucharski LT, Wagner RL. Tardive dystonia in a psychiatric hospital. J Neurol Neurosurg Psychiatry 1987; 50: 801–3.
50. Yassa R, Nair V, Dimitry R. Prevalence of tardive dsytonia. Acta Psychiatr Scand 1986; 73: 629–33.
51. Gureje O. The significance of subtyping tardive dyskinesia: a study of prevalence and associated factors. Psychol Med 1989; 19: 121–8.
52. Sethi KD, Hess DC, Harp RJ, Prevalence of dystonia in veterans on chronic antipsychotic therapy. Mov Disord 1990; 5: 319–21.
53. Sachdev P. The prevalence of tardive dystonia in patients with chronic schizophrenia (letter). Aust N Z J Psychiatry 1991; 25: 446–8.
54. Inada T, Yagi G, Kaijima K et al. Clinical variants of tardive dyskinesia in Japan. Jpn J Psychiatry Neurol 1991; 45: 67–71.
55. Chiu H, Shum P, Lau J, Lam L, Lee S. Prevalence of tardive dyskinesia, tardive dystonia, and respiratory dyskinesia among Chinese psychiatric patients in Hong Kong. Am J Psychiatry 1992; 149; 1081–5.
56. Micheli F, Fernandez Pardal M, Gatto M et al. Bruxism secondary to chronic antidopaminergic drug exposure. Clin Neuropharmacol 1993; 16: 315–23.
57. Pourcher E, Baruch P, Bouchard RH, Filteau MJ, Bergeron D. Neuroleptic associated tardive dyskinesias in young people with psychoses [see comments]. Bradykinesia J Psychiatry 1995; 166: 768–72. Comment in Br J Psychiatry 1995; 167: 410–11.
58. Raja M. Tardive dystonia: prevalence, risk factors, and comparison with tardive dyskinesia in a population of 299 acute psychiatric inpatients. Eur Arch Psychiatry Clin Neurosci 1995; 245: 145–51.
59. Van Harten PN, Matroos GE, Hoek HW, Kahn RS. The prevalence of tardive dystonia, tardive dyskinesia, parkinsonism and akathisia. The Curacao Extrapyramidal Syndromes Study: 1. Schizophr Res 1996; 19: 195–203.
60. Miller LG, Jankovic J. Neurologic approach to drug-induced movement disorders: a study of 125 patients. South Med J 1990; 83(5): 525–32.
61. Dunayevich E, Strakowski SM. Olanzapine-induced tardive dystonia. Am J Psychiatry 1999; 156(10): 1662.
62. Vercueil L, Foucher J. Risperidone-induced tardive dystonia and psychosis. Lancet 1999; 353(9157): 981.
63. Ghelber D, Belmaker RH. Tardive dyskinesia with quetiapine. Am J Psychiatry 1999; 156(5): 796–7.
64. Pinniti NR, Mago, Adityangi A. Tardive dystonia – associated prescription of aripiprazole. J Neuropsychiatry Clin Neurosci 2006; 18(3): 426–7.
65. Papapetropoulos S, Wheeler S, Singer C. Tardive dystonia associated with ziprasidone. Am J Psychiatry 2005; 162(11): 2191.
66. Bruneau MA, Stip E. Metronome or alternating Pisa syndrome: a form of tardive dystonia under clozapine treatment. Int Clin Psychopharmacol 1998; 13(5): 229–32.
67. Gimenez-Roldan S, Mateo D, Bartolome P. Tardive dystonia and severe tardive dyskinesia. A comparison of risk factors and prognosis. Acta Psychiatr Scand 1985; 71: 488–94.
68. Wojcik JD, Falk WE, Fink JS, Cole JO, Gelenberg AJ. A review of 32 cases of tardive dystonia. Am J Psychiatry 1991; 148: 1055–9.
69. Gardos G, Cole JO, Salomon M, Schniebolk S. Clinical forms of severe tardive dyskinesia. Am J Psychiatry 1987; 144: 895–902.
70. Klawans HL, Tanner CM, Goetz CG. Epidemiology and pathophysiology of tardive dyskinesias. Adv Neurol 1988; 49: 185–97.

71. Trugman JM, Leadbetter R, Zalis ME, Burgdorf RO, Wooten GF. Treatment of severe axial tardive dystonia with clozapine: case report and hypothesis. Mov Disord 1994; 9(4): 441–6.
72. Lieberman JA, Alvir J, Mukherjee S, Kane JM. Treatment of tardive dyskinesia with bromocriptine. A test of the receptor modification strategy. Arch Gen Psychiatry 1989; 46(10): 908–13.
73. Silvestri S, Seeman MV, Negrete JC et al. Increased dopamine D_2 receptor binding after long-term treatment with antipsychotics in humans: a clinical PET study. Psychopharmacology (Berl) 2000; 152(2): 174–80.
74. Gunne LM, Haggstrom JE. Pathophysiology of tardive dyskinesia. Psychopharmacology Suppl 1985; 2: 191–3.
75. Gunne LM, Haggstrom JE, Sjoquist B. Association with persistent neuroleptic-induced dyskinesia of regional changes in brain GABA synthesis. Nature 1984; 309: 347–9.
76. Andersson U, Haggstrom JE, Levin ED. Reduced glutamic acid decarboxylase activity in the subthalamic nucleus in patients with tardive dyskinesia. Mov Disord 1989; 4: 37–46.
77. Mithani S, Atmadja S, Baimbridge KG, Fibiger HC. Neuroleptic-induced oral dyskinesias: effects of progabide and lack of correlation with regional changes in glutamic acid decarboxylase and choline acetyltransferase activities. Psychopharmacology (Berl) 1987; 93(1): 94–100.
78. Thaker GK, Nguyen JA, Strauss ME et al. Clonazepam treatment of tardive dyskinesia: a practical GABAmimetic strategy. Am J Psychiatry 1990; 147: 445–51.
79. Soares KV, McGrath JJ, Deeks JJ. Gamma-aminobutyric acid agonists for neuroleptic-induced tardive dyskinesia. Cochrane Database Syst Rev 2001; (2): CD000203.
80. Lohmann PL, Bagli M, Krauss H et al. CYP2D6 polymorphism and tardive dyskinesia in schizophrenic patients. Pharmacopsychiatry 2003; 36(2): 73–8.
81. Werge T, Elbaek Z, Andersen MB, Lundbaek JA, Rasmussen HB. Cebus apella, a nonhuman primate highly susceptible to neuroleptic side effects, carries the GLY9 dopamine receptor D_3 associated with tardive dyskinesia in humans. Pharmacogenomics J 2003; 3(2): 97–100.
82. Mihara K, Kondo T, Higuchi H et al. Tardive dystonia and genetic polymorphisms of cytochrome P4502D6 and dopamine D2 and D3 receptors: a preliminary finding. Am J Med Genet 2002; 114(6): 693–5.
83. Pall HS, Williams AC, Blake DR, Lunec J. Evidence of enhanced lipid perioxidation in the cerebrospinal fluid of patients taking phenothiazines. Lancet 1987; 2: 596–9.
84. Abilio VC, Araujo CC, Bergamo M et al. Vitamin E attenuates reserpine-induced oral dyskinesia and striatal oxidized glutathione/reduced glutathione ratio (GSSG/GSH) enhancement in rats. Prog Neuropsychopharmacol Biol Psychiatry 2003; 27(1): 109–14.
85. Behl C, Rupprecht R, Skutella T, Holsboer F. Haloperidol-induced cell death – mechanism and protection with vitamin E in vitro. Neuroreport 1995; 7(1): 360–4.
86. Michael N, Sourgens H, Arolt V, Erfurth A. Severe tardive dyskinesia in affective disorders: treatment with vitamin E and C. Neuropsychobiology 2002; 46(Suppl 1): 28–30.
87. Adler LA, Rotrosen J, Edson R et al. Vitamin E treatment for tardive dyskinesia. Veterans Affairs Cooperative Study #394 Study Group. Arch Gen Psychiatry 1999; 56(9): 836–41.
88. See RE, Lynch AM. Chronic haloperidol potentiates stimulated glutamate release in caudate putamen, but not prefrontal cortex. Neuroreport 1995; 6(13): 1795–8.
89. Tarsy D, Kaufman D, Sethi KD et al. An open-label study of botulinum toxin A for treatment of tardive dystonia. Clin Neuropharmacol 1997; 20(1): 90–3.
90. Fernandez HH, Friedman JH. Classification and treatment of tardive syndromes. Neurologist 2003; 9(1): 16–27.
91. Chen JY, Bai YM, Pyng LY, Lin CC. Risperidone for tardive dyskinesia. Am J Psychiatry 2001; 158(11): 1931–2.
92. Bai YM, Yu SC, Chen JY et al. Risperidone for pre-existing severe tardive dyskinesia: a 48-week prospective follow-up study. Int Clin Psychopharmacol 2005; 20(2): 79–85.
93. Lucetti C, Bellini G, Nuti A et al. Treatment of patients with tardive dystonia with olanzapine. Clin Neuropharmacol 2002; 25(2): 71–4.
94. Bouckaert F, Herman G, Peuskens J. Rapid remission of severe tardive dyskinesia and tardive dystonia with quetiapine. Int J Geriatr Psychiatry 2005; 20(3): 287–8.
95. Gourzis P, Polychronopoulos P, Papapetropoulos S et al. Quetiapine in the treatment of focal tardive dystonia induced by other atypical antipsychotics: a report of 2 cases. Clin Neuropharmacol 2005; 28(4): 195–6.
96. Alptekin K, Kivircik BB. Quetiapine-induced improvement of tardive dyskinesia in three patients with schizophrenia. Int Clin Psychopharmacol 2002; 17(5): 263–4.
97. Berg D, Becker G, Naumann M, Reiners K. Morphine in tardive and idiopathic dystonia. J Neural Transm 2001; 108: 1035–41.
98. Kaplan Z, Benjamin J, Zohar J. Remission of tardive dystonia with ECT. Convuls Ther 1991; 7(4): 280–3.
99. Sienaert P, Peuskens J. Remission of tardive dystonia (blepharospasm) after electroconvulsive therapy in a patient with treatment-refractory schizophrenia. J ECT 2005; 21(2): 132–4.
100. Richardson MA, Bevans ML, Weber JB et al. Branched chain amino acids decrease tardive dyskinesia symptoms. Psychopharmacology (Berl) 1999; 143(4): 358–64.
101. Richardson MA, Bevans ML, Read LL et al. Efficacy of the branched-chain amino acids in the treatment of tardive dyskinesia in men. Am J Psychiatry 2003; 160: 1117–24.
102. Trottenberg T, Paul G, Meissner W et al. Pallidal and thalamic neurostimulation in severe tardive dystonia. J Neurol Neurosurg Psychiatry 2001; 70(4): 557–9.
103. Trottenberg T, Volkmann J, Deuschl G et al. Treatment of severe tardive dystonia with pallidal deep brain stimulation. Neurology 2005; 64(2): 344–6.
104. Hillier CE, Wiles CM, Simpson BA. Thalamotomy for severe antipsychotic induced tardive dyskinesia and dystonia [letter]. J Neurol Neurosurg Psychiatry 1999; 66: 250–1.
105. Manji H, Howard RS, Miller DH et al. Status dystonicus: the syndrome and its management. Brain 1998; 121(Pt 2): 243–52.

15

Paroxysmal dyskinesias

Pablo Mir, Susanne A Schneider, and Kailash P Bhatia

DEFINITION, HISTORICAL ASPECTS, AND CLASSIFICATION

Paroxysmal dyskinesias are a rare heterogeneous group of conditions manifesting as abnormal involuntary movements that recur episodically and last only a brief duration.[1,2] The abnormal movements may be choreic, dystonic, ballistic, or other, or a mixture of these. The conditions can be inherited or acquired. Between episodes, the patient is generally normal. Hence, conditions such as tic disorders, where there may be paroxysmal worsening, or task- or action-induced dystonias such as musicians or writing dystonia, are traditionally not considered as forms of paroxysmal dyskinesias.

Gower probably gave the first description of paroxysmal movement disorders but called it epilepsy. The term paroxysmal choreoathetosis entered the literature in 1940, when Mount and Reback gave the first clear descriptions of an episodic hyperkinetic condition describing a 23-year-old man who had episodes of "choreo-dystonia" which could last several hours.[3] There were more than 20 other family members also affected, with a clear autosomal dominant pattern of inheritance. As more families with a similar disorder were described,[4–6] it became clear that these episodes of paroxysmal choreoathetosis seemed to be precipitated by drinking alcohol, coffee or tea, and by fatigue and smoking. Phenytoin and phenobarbitone were not found helpful. Richards and Barnett,[6] noting the torsion spasms and increased tone in the limbs added 'dystonia' to the description of Mount and Reback, and this disorder thus came to be known as paroxysmal dystonic choreoathetosis (PDC).

In 1967 Kertesz described an episodic disorder termed paroxysmal kinesigenic choreoathetosis (PKC).[7] It was noted that attacks in those affected were induced by sudden movement, i.e. kinesigenic. However, Kertesz probably did not recognize this as a new disorder but felt that this may represent an entity within the previously described condition of PDC, as suggested by the title of the paper. As more cases and families were described, it became clear that this disorder was different from PDC as the attacks were relatively brief and the conditon responded well to antiepileptic drugs.[8]

A third form of episodic dyskinesia was described by Lance in 1977, reporting a family who had attacks lasting between 5 and 30 minutes provoked by prolonged exercise and not by sudden movement.[8] Lance referred to this paroxysmal exercise-induced dyskinesia (PED) as the 'intermediate type' because the attack duration seemed longer than PKC but less than typical PDC. In the same paper, Lance also suggested a classification of the paroxysmal dyskinesias based primarily upon the duration of attacks, dividing them into three types:

- PKC, in which there were brief attacks of up to 5 minutes induced by sudden movement;
- PDC, in which attacks were not induced by sudden movement and were of long duration, up to 4–6 hours;
- PED, which was induced by exercise and the attack duration was between PKC and PDC.

These terms have been used widely in the literature over the years.

In 1995, Demirkiran and Jankovic[1] pointed out that the attacks in these disorders were not necessarily choreic or dystonic and could be any form of dyskinesia. Hence, they suggested classifying these disorders broadly into two main groups: paroxysmal kinesigenic dyskinesia (PKD), if the attacks were induced by sudden movement; or paroxysmal non-kinesigenic dyskinesia (PKND), if they were not. These two groups broadly correspond to PKC and PDC of the earlier classification of Lance 1977.[8] Apart from these two main forms, PED continued as a separate entity (Table 15.1). Each type was to be further classified as either idiopathic or secondary ('symptomatic'), depending on

Table 15.1 Summary of clinical and genetic characteristics of the three main forms of paroxysmal dyskinesia

	PKD	PED	PKND
Duration	Very brief	2 minutes to 2 hours	30 minutes to 1 hour
Triggering factors	Sudden movements, increase in speed, amplitude, force, strength	Prolonged or sustained exercise	Alcohol, coffee, coke, tobacco, emotions, hunger, fatigue
Age at onset	7–15 years (6 months to 33 years)	2–30 years	2–79 years
Treatment	Carbamazepine	Gabapentin L-Dopa	Benzodiazepines Anticonvulsants Acetazolamide L-Dopa
Gene	Chromosome 16p11 (RE-PED-WC)	Chromosome 16p11 (RE-PED-WC)	Chromosome 2q33-q35 (MR-1)

PKD = paroxysmal kinesigenic dyskinesia; PED = paroxysmal exercise-induced dyskinesia; PNKD = paroxysmal non-kinesigenic dyskinesia.

the etiology. In the idiopathic form, which is often familial, imaging and other investigations are unremarkable and there are no other signs to suggest a neurodegenerative or symptomatic cause.

A fourth form of paroxysmal disorder, referred to as paroxysmal hypnogenic dyskinesia (PHD), in which dyskinetic episodes occurred only at night during sleep has also been recognized and added to the main three.[1,2] In addition, we propose that the term 'paroxysmal dyskinesias plus' could be applied (in the same way as it is used for idiopathic primary dystonia) to describe some rare families in the recent literature where those affected are said to have additional interictal neurologic features such as spasticity.[9] These features are not the norm in the four typical forms mentioned above. Apart from the idiopathic forms, secondary ('symptomatic') paroxysmal dyskinesias would be those caused by environmental insults. A whole host of different etiologies can cause the secondary paroxysmal dyskinesias.[1,10] Lastly, it must be recognized that certain cases may not fall easily into the current classification of the main four subtypes.[11]

CLINICAL ASPECTS

Paroxysmal kinesigenic dyskinesia (paroxysmal kinesigenic choreoathetosis)

As was noted in the original description of 10 cases by Kertesz,[7] those affected have brief dyskinetic episodes precipitated by sudden movement. The kinesigenic form usually occurs from early childhood and is more common in males. In one report of a series of 26 idiopathic cases, the mean age of onset was 13 years (range 1–39).[12] In the same series, there was a notable predominance of males (7:1), which has also been mentioned by earlier authors.[2] A preceding 'aura'-like sensation in the limb which gets involved in an attack has been reported in 63% of cases with PKD.[12] The attacks frequently manifest as dystonia or choreodystonia induced by a sudden change in position, classically from a sitting to standing position, or by a sudden change in velocity while walking or running. However startle, hyperventilation, and even continuous exercise can also trigger them. Rarely, episodes occur at rest and occasionally in sleep. Attacks commonly involve the hemi-body, which can either be the same side or alternating sides.[1,2,12] Rarely, the episodes become generalized. Speech can be affected but consciousness is not lost. Typically, PKD attacks are very brief and frequently last for seconds. Although Demirkiran and Jankovic have mentioned that PKD attacks can last up to 5 minutes,[1] in our experience the attacks in the idiopathic form are very brief and in the majority of cases do not exceed more than 1 minute.[12] There can be dozens of attacks per day. Most cases are idiopathic and apparently sporadic. Family history is clearly present in about 25% of cases and usually follows an autosomal dominant pattern of inheritance.[12] These findings have also been replicated in a large series by Bruno et al,[13] who suggested the specific criteria for PKD (Table 15.2).

Overall, prognosis for the idiopathic form is good and in our experience the condition may often abate in adult life, as the attack frequency tends to decrease with age.

Table 15.2 Clinical criteria for paroxysmal kinesigenic dyskinesia (PKD) as proposed by Bruno et al[13]
• Identified kinesigenic trigger for the attacks • Short duration of attacks (<1 minute) • No loss of consciousness or pain during attacks • Exclusion of other organic diseases and normal neurologic examination • Control of attacks with phenytoin or carbamazepine, if tried • Age at onset between 1 and 20 years, if no family history of PKD

The association of PKC/PKD with epilepsy

Recently, epilepsy has been recognized to be an associated feature in both sporadic and familial cases with PKC. There have also been a few reports describing families with 'benign' infantile convulsions and later onset of episodes of paroxysmal choreoathetosis (called the infantile convulsions and choreoathetosis – ICCA syndrome).[14–19] The first description was by Szepetowski et al[17] of four French families said to have the ICCA syndrome, as those affected had afebrile infantile seizures and paroxysmal involuntary movements. Lee et al soon followed, with a report of a Chinese family who had a similar condition.[20] Although clinical details were somewhat sparse (in retrospect), the attacks of paroxysmal choreoathetosis in the ICCA syndrome resembled PKC in being very brief, frequent and induced by sudden exertion and, interestingly, also by ongoing exercise.[17,20] Other families with epilepsy and PKD have also been recently recognized. Hattori et al described seven Japanese families and two sporadic cases with benign infantile convulsions and paroxysmal dyskinesias.[15,20] Seventeen individuals developed afebrile complex partial infantile convulsions between 12 months and 3 years of age, followed later by brief paroxysmal dyskinesia resembling PKC. Most families were autosomal dominant, but in some only siblings were affected, suggesting a possible recessive inheritance and genetic heterogeneity. Another family with PKC and epilepsy has been described recently.[21] In this autosomal dominant family from India, individuals with PKC did not have infantile convulsions. However, some had sporadic episodes of generalized tonic-clonic seizures in teenage years with spontaneous remission of their epilepsy a few years later, although the PKC attacks continued.[22] PKD has also been associated with interictal myoclonus.[23]

Paroxysmal exercise-induced dyskinesia

In this condition, episodes of involuntary movements occur after exercise such as walking or swimming. The dystonic episodes usually cease in 10–15 minutes after stopping the exercise. In the initial family described by Lance in 1977,[8] affected members had attacks lasting between 5 and 30 minutes, provoked usually by walking. The inheritance pattern was autosomal dominant. Plant et al reported a mother and daughter with similar exercise-induced attacks, although attacks could also be initiated by repetitive passive movement of the limbs and by vibration. Munchau et al[24] reported an autosomal dominant family with PED who also had associated migraine. In this, some members could have jaw dystonia due to chewing gum. Exposure to cold has also been reported to bring on attacks in affected individuals.[25]

Sporadic examples of exercise-induced dystonia of the intermediate type of PDC are rare and only a few cases have been reported in the literature.[25] Although, traditionally, PED was thought to be distinct from the kinesigenic form (as usually, the attacks come on after 10 or 15 minutes of continuing exercise rather than at the initiation of movement), recently there have been some familial cases with infantile convulsions and paroxysmal dyskinesias resembling PKD (the so-called ICCA syndrome) in whom the episodes were induced by sudden movements or ongoing exercise.[14–19]

PED plus syndrome

Recently, a family with an apparently recessive disorder characterized by rolandic epilepsy, paroxysmal exercise-induced dystonia, and writers' cramp (RE-PED-WC syndrome) affecting three members of the same generation, has been linked to chromosome 16p 12-11.2[26] in the same region as the families with the ICCA syndrome[17,20] and PKD (see Genetics section), suggesting an overlap between these disorders. There is also a syndrome of exercise-induced dystonia associated with atypical absences, alternating hemiplegia, and ataxia that was improved by corticosteroid treatment.[27]

Paroxysmal non-kinesigenic dyskinesia (paroxysmal dystonic choreoathetosis)

Since the initial description by Mount and Reback,[3] a number of families have been reported with an autosomal dominant inheritance with a fairly similar clinical description between families.[6,28,29] PNKD is characterized by attacks of dyskinesia which are frequently precipitated by alcohol, caffeine, stress, or fatigue.

Patients with PNKD have longer (10 minutes to 6 hours) and less frequent attacks (1–3/day) than patients with PKD/PKC, followed by long attack-free intervals. The dyskinesia may be of any form, but often tends to be more dystonic or choreic in nature. More males than females are affected (1.4:1),[2] and onset is usually in childhood, with a tendency for the attacks to diminish with age.[29]

Details of typical clinical features of a large English family with 18 affected members were described by Jarman et al.[29] In all cases the onset of symptoms was very early in life, in the second year in seven individuals and as early as age 6 months and 2 months in two other individuals. Witnessed attacks consisted of generalized choreoathetosis in two individuals. In one case there was associated dysarthria in the attack. Attacks started in one limb or one side and progressed to become generalized. The attack duration varied from 10 minutes to 12 hours; however, the majority of attacks were between 30 and 180 minutes. All adults reported a decline in attack duration and frequency with age. One individual who was 85 years old had only 1 attack a year and that was very mild. Coffee, alcohol, anger and excitement, hunger and sleep deprivation were general precipitants, as well as cold and exercise in two individuals. All affected individuals reported a remarkable response to sleep, with 5–10 minutes of sleep being sufficient to abort an attack while some found drinking cold fluids or vigorous exercise while the attack was still mild could abort it. There was some diurnal fluctuation, with a tendency to attacks in the afternoon or evening but not in the morning.[29] Recently, Bruno et al[30] have confirmed these findings in 14 kindreds with classic PNKD.

There has been speculation as to why alcohol and coffee precipitate attacks in PNKD.[28] Fink et al postulated a surge of dopamine release induced by alcohol, for example, followed by relative dopamine deficiency could cause the dystonia. This notion is supported by the fact that some patients with PNKD respond to l-dopa with sleep benefit.[28,29] A surge in cerebrospinal (CSF) dopamine metabolites has been noted, supporting the theory of Fink et al in another family with PNKD.[29]

Generally, PNKD cases have no detectable abnormalities between attacks, although there has been one report of a patient with PNKD who also had some interictal dystonia.[31] There has also been a family with PNKD with additional myokymia.[32]

With regard to investigations, routine tests as well as electroencephalograms (EEGs) and brain imaging in the idiopathic cases are normal. Pathologic examination at autopsy in two cases also revealed no abnormalities.[8]

PNKD associated with spasticity

A large German family in whom affected members had choreo-dystonic attacks induced by alcohol, fatigue, and exercise (and thus similar to PNKD) was reported by Auburger et al.[9] However, some affected individuals also had marked spastic paraparesis and other clinical features, including perioral paresthesias, double vision, headache, and generalized myoclonic jerks, and seizures were also present. This condition is therefore different from typical PNKD and can be considered as a PNKD plus syndrome.

Paroxysmal hypnogenic dyskinesia

In PHD, the attacks of paroxysmal dyskinesia occur at night in sleep (hence, hypnogenic), and this disorder is often erroneously suspected to represent night terrors or some other sleep disorder.[33] In a typical PHD attack, the patient awakens with a cry followed by involuntary dystonic and ballistic limb movements that are very brief, lasting seconds and rarely over 1 minute. The movements often involve the legs. There is no loss of consciousness. Usually there are no detectable concurrent EEG abnormalities. Several attacks (sometimes even 20–25) can occur each night.

Lugaresi and Cirignotta[34] gave one of the first clear descriptions of this condition in five patients who had attacks in sleep almost every night. Lee et al[35] and others also described similar familial cases with a clear autosomal dominant inheritance pattern. It has now become clear that in a large proportion of these cases, especially the familial variety, these nocturnal dyskinesias are due to mesial frontal lobe seizures which are difficult to pick up on surface EEG recordings.[36] Describing the salient features in six families from Canada, Australia, and the UK, Scheffer et al suggested the eponym autosomal dominant nocturnal frontal lobe epilepsy (ADNFLE) to describe this disorder.[36] The gene responsible for ADNFLE has been discovered in a few families (see Genetics section).

Benign paroxysmal torticollis in infancy

BPT is a relatively rare disorder with onset in infancy and episodes of torticollis with or without tortipelvis.[37] The duration is hours, rarely up to a few days. The episodes are infrequent, with 1–2 occurring in a day at times. There have been some suggestions of a relationship to migraine (basilar variety) and kinestosis.[37] This is because, with time, episodes of head tilt become less prominent, and are replaced by vertigo, vomiting, lassitude, and migraine-like headaches. Recently, two cases with BPT were described from families with familial hemiplegic migraine linked with calcium channel gene (CACLNA1).[38] This is interesting, given the hypothesis (see Pathophysiology section) that the paroxysmal dyskinesias may be caused by ion channel abnormalities.

Secondary ('symptomatic') paroxysmal dyskinesias

Secondary paroxysmal dyskinesias are probably more common than initially thought. In a series by Blakeley and Jankovic, 17 of 76 patients with paroxysmal dyskinesias (22%) had an identifiable cause.[10] Secondary cases are notable for their variability in age of onset, the presence of both kinesigenic and non-kinesigenic symptoms in some patients, the prevalence of sensory precipitants, and most importantly, the reversal of symptoms when the underlying etiology is treated in some patients.[22] The association of PKC/PDC with multiple sclerosis is the most common.[39–43] Other causes include stroke,[10,44–49] transient cerebral ischemia,[50–55] antiphospholipid syndrome,[56] central and peripheral trauma,[10,57–62] hypoglycemia,[63–65] hyperglycemia,[66–68] hypoparathyroidism,[69,70] pseudohypoparathyroidism,[71] thyrotoxicosis,[72] basal ganglia calcifications,[73] kernicterus,[10] meningovascular syphilis,[10] HIV (human immunodeficiency virus) infection,[74] and cytomegalovirus encephalitis.[10] Clinically, there may be some clues about the cause; for instance, in multiple sclerosis the attacks are often precipitated by hyperventilation. On examination, we can find some signs such as spasticity which would suggest multiple sclerosis or phalangeal shortening suggesting pseudohypoparathyroidism. Since there are multiple possible causes of secondary paroxysmal dyskinesias, most individuals with this movement disorder would therefore required basic investigation, including brain imaging, preferably magnetic resonance imaging (MRI) scan, and appropriate blood tests or other investigations.

GENETICS OF PAROXYSMAL DYSKINESIAS

Paroxysmal non-kinesigenic dyskinesia

Two groups separately linked families with PNKD to chromosome 2q.[28,75] Fink and co-workers performed a genome-wide search in a large American kindred of Polish descent with 28 affected members and mapped PNKD on chromosome 2q33-q35.[28] Fouad et al also showed tight linkage between PNKD and microsatellite markers on distal 2q (2q31-q36) in a five-generation Italian family with 20 affected members.[28,75] The smallest region of overlap of the candidate intervals identified by these two groups placed the PNKD locus in a 6-cM interval. In a six-generation British family, Jarman and co-workers confirmed linkage to distal chromosome 2q and narrowed the candidate region to a 4-cM interval.[76] Linkage to the same genetic location, designated FPD1 (familial paroxysmal dyskinesia type 1), was also confirmed by Hofele et al[77] in a German family, originally described by Przuntek and Monninger[78] as classical Mount and Reback type of PNKD, and other typical PNKD families, including one from North America of German descent[79] as well as a Japanese family.[80] These studies suggest a level of genetic homogeneity for classical familial PNKD/PDC.

After a number of candidate genes were excluded,[79–81] the gene for responsible for PNKD was discovered to be the myofibrillogenesis regulator 1 (MR-1) gene.[82] Mutations in this gene cause paroxysmal dystonic choreoathetosis.[82] This gene encodes an enzyme in a stress response pathway.[83] Lee et al[83] found that the mutations cause changes (Ala to Val) in the N-terminal region of two MR-1 isoforms. The MR-1L isoform is specifically expressed in brain and is localized to the cell membrane, whereas the MR-1S isoform is ubiquitously expressed and shows diffuse cytoplasmic and nuclear localization. Bioinformatic analysis reveals that the MR-1 gene is homologous to the hydroxyacylglutathione hydrolase (HAGH) gene. HAGH functions in a pathway to detoxify methylglyoxal, a compound present in coffee and alcoholic beverages and produced as a by-product of oxidative stress, thus suggesting a possible mechanism (Figure 15.1) whereby alcohol, coffee, and stress precipitate attacks in PNKD. Mutations in the MR-1 gene have been confirmed to be the cause of PNKD in numerous families all over the world[84] and as far apart as Oman and Serbia.[85,86]

PKD/PKC, the ICCA syndrome, and PED (RE-PED-WC syndrome)

These three disorders have to be considered together as they are all linked to the small arm of the pericentromic region of chromosome 16. Szepetowski et al[17] linked four French families with infantile convulsions and paroxysmal choreoathetosis (the ICCA syndrome) called to a 10-cM interval around the pericentromeric region of chromosome 16. Linkage to the same locus was confirmed in a Chinese ICCA family.[20] Since the clinical characteristics of the paroxysmal dyskinetic episodes in the ICCA syndrome were very similar to those described for PKD, it was not surprising that eight Japanese families,[87] as well as an African-American kindred[88] with typical PKC, were mapped by linkage

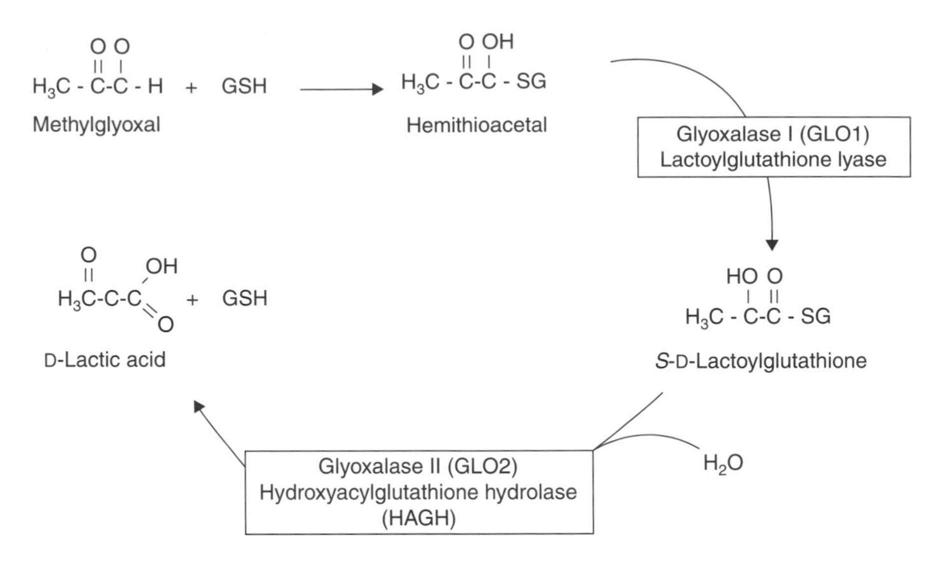

Figure 15.1 PNKD is caused by mutations in the myofibrillogenesis regulator 1 (MR-1) gene, a homologue to the hydroxyacylglutathione hydrolase (HAGH) gene, which pays a role in detoxification of methylglyoxal. The glyoxylase process is depicted here. Methylglyoxal and glutathione non-enzymatically form a hemithioacetal intermediate. Glyoxylase I catalyzes the formation of *S*-D-lactoylglutathione. HAGH then catalyzes the hydrolysis of *S*-D-lactoylglutathione to D-lactate and reduced glutathione (GSH). (Adopted from Lee et al.[13,83])

analysis to the same pericentromeric region of chromosome 16. The PKC region in the Japanese families spanned 12.4 cM and overlapped by 6.0 cM the ICCA region. The fact that there was an increased prevalence of afebrile infantile convulsions in the Japanese families with PKC[87] suggested the possibility that the same one gene may be responsible for both PKC and ICCA. However, the PKC interval identified in the African-American family in which individuals have PKC alone (and no infantile seizures) overlaps by 3.4 cM with the ICCA region and by 9.8 cM with the PKC region identified in Japanese families. Thus, it was unclear whether there were two (or more) genes giving rise to both ICCA and PKC in these families or a single gene in this interval. Furthermore, the autosomal recessive family with RE-PED-WC syndrome described by Guerrini et al[26] (see above in Clinical aspects) was also linked to chromosome 16 within the ICCA region but outside the 3.4 cM overlap between ICCA and PKC. Thus, it appears that the RE-PED-WC syndrome might also be allelic to ICCA but is probably not allelic to PKC. In addition, as epilepsy is the most striking feature of both the ICCA and RE-PED-WC syndromes and some of the ICCA attacks were induced by exercise, it has been suggested that there are common underlying genes for these two conditions which may be different from that giving rise to isolated PKC.

Swoboda et al[19] highlighted a role for locus heterogeneity when reporting linkage data on 11 families with PKD, with infantile convulsions also present in nine families. Ethnic background was diverse, including two Afro-American, Taiwanese, Ashkenazi Jewish, Dutch, Mexican, and mixed European ancestry. Linkage was confirmed to chromosome 16 and overlapped the ICCA region, which the authors narrowed down to 3.2 cm. However, one family with classic PKC and infantile convulsions failed to share a common haplotype, thus suggesting heterogeneity. It is also interesting to note the paper by Valente et al[21] in this context. They identified a family with PKC from India and linked it to a second locus on the long arm of chromosome 16, distinct from the locus of the Japanese families with PKC, hence this is referred to as episodic kinesigenic dyskinesia 2 locus (*EKD2*). The localization of PKC in the African-American family overlaps with both these regions.[88] The African-American PKC locus may thus be allelic with either the Japanese or Indian PKC locus or represent yet another gene altogether. In addition, there are also families with PKD not linked to chromosome 16 at all, suggesting evidence of yet another locus.[89]

The gene(s) causing these disorders are as yet unknown but there are a group of ion channel genes which lie in this pericentromeric region of chromosome

16, within the ICCA and PKC intervals, which are good candidates and are being currently investigated.

Finally, it is also interesting to note that a recent paper described linkage of seven families with benign neonatal infantile convulsions (without paroxysmal dyskinesias) to the same region as ICCA on 16p12-q12,[14] thus suggesting that there may be a family of genes causing different paroxysmal disorders on the pericentromeric region of chromosome 16.

Paroxysmal hypnogenic dyskinesia

One ADNFLE locus was first mapped by Phillips et al[90] on chromosome 20q13.2 in an Australian family. The obvious candidate was the α4 subunit of the neuronal acetylcholine receptor, a ligand gated channel gene. Two different mutations in two families in the α_4 subunit of the neuronal acetylcholine receptor (*CHRNA4*) on 20q13.2 were found. The mutations observed were missense mutations in an Australian family and a Japanese family and a three base pair insertion in the case of a Norwegian family.[91–93] However, a British family with ADNFLE was not found to be linked to *CHRNA4* on chromosome 20q but to a locus on chromosome 15q24 close to a *CHRNA3/CNRNA5/CHRNB4* nicotinic acetylcholine receptor gene cluster.[94] Also, seven other families with ADNFLE and seven sporadic cases were unlinked to these loci on chromosomes 20q13.2 and 15q24, thereby suggesting the existence of at least a third ADNFLE locus and genetic heterogeneity of this disorder. This has been confirmed by the finding of mutations of a β subunit of the nicotinic acetylcholine receptor gene causing nocturnal frontal lobe epilepsy.[95,96]

Paroxysmal dyskinesias plus

The genetics of the PED plus syndrome (RE-PED-WC syndrome) have been discussed above together with PKD/PKC and the ICCA syndrome.

The German family with PNKD associated with spasticity was linked to a locus different to typical PNKD on chromosome 1p which has been designated CSE (choreoathetosis/spasticity episodic).[9] Linkage analysis in this family placed the disease locus in a 12-cM interval on chromosome 1p21 between flanking markers. The gene is yet to be determined, but several potassium channel genes have been mapped to this region and lie in a cluster. Further investigations are needed to determine the gene for this disorder. No other similar families have been reported so far.

PATHOPHYSIOLOGY

Over the years, the pathophysiology of these disorders has been debated. The main arguments have been whether these conditions are a form of epilepsy or whether they represent a basal ganglia disorder. It has been suggested by some that the primary pathophysiologic process may be of epilepsy, perhaps at a subcortical level, given the paroxysmal character of attacks, prodromic aura-like symptoms in many, the short duration of the attacks, and the response to antiepileptic drugs.[97,98] In support of this hypothesis are several reports of families in which some individuals presented with either or both paroxysmal dyskinesias and epilepsy, with different age-related expressions.[26,99] On the other hand, the occurrence of dystonia in 70–80% of paroxysmal dyskinesia episodes might indicate a pathophysiologic process similar to primary dystonia, where deficits in cortical, brainstem, and spinal inhibitory circuits, due to disordered basal ganglia modulation of cortical motor output, have been detected. Evidence to support the role of the basal ganglia in the pathophysiology of paroxysmal dyskinesias is based on the observation of secondary paroxysmal dyskinesias in association with focal basal ganglia lesions.[10]

Few studies to date have investigated the pathophysiology of paroxysmal dyskinesias. Franssen et al investigated the contingent negative variation (CNV) in one patient with PKD.[99] The slow negative wave component of the CNV was more pronounced compared to control subjects (the opposite to the pattern observed in primary dystonia), but this was normalized after phenytoin treatment. Lee et al studied forearm reciprocal inhibition in 10 patients with PKD and found a paradoxical facilitation of H reflex size in the first phase of reciprocal inhibition (a pattern not routinely observed in primary dystonia).[100] More recently, Mir et al[101] assessed a number of electrophysiologic parameters in 11 patients with PKD, a proportion of them on and off treatment. A reduced short intracortical inhibition, a reduced early phase of transcallosal inhibition, and a reduced first phase of spinal reciprocal inhibition (RI) in subjects with PKD were identified. Cortical silent period, the startle response, and the second and third phases of RI were normal. Treatment with carbamazepine normalized the abnormalities in transcallosal inhibition, but had no effect on other parameters.

Invasive long-term electrode monitoring of a patient with secondary PKD was reported to show consistent ictal discharge recorded from the ipsilateral caudate nucleus with a concomitant discharge recorded from the supplementary sensory motor cortex, without significant spread to other areas.[102] Invasive monitoring has also been performed in a child with severe PNKD, which recorded an ictal discharge from the caudate nuclei with no cortical correlate. ^{18}F-dopa and ^{11}C-raclopride PET (positron emission tomography) scans in the same patient revealed a marked reduction in the density of presynaptic dopa decarboxylase activity in the striatum, together with an increased density of postsynaptic dopamine D_2 receptors. Ictal and postictal SPECT (single-photon emission computed tomography) studies have shown basal ganglia hyperactivity associated with dyskinetic attacks in PKD.[103,104] However, a study with ^{99m}Tc-HMPAO (hexamethyl propyleneamine oxime) SPECT has found the opposite pattern, with a decrease in cerebral blood flow in the basal ganglia on the contralateral side of choreoathetotic movements.[105] Increase in cerebral blood flow in the left medial thalamus during a PKD attack has been observed in a study using ^{123}I-IMP SPECT.[106]

It is possible that a common, genetically determined, pathophysiologic abnormality is variably expressed in the cerebral cortex and in basal ganglia.[107] It has been hypothesized that this abnormality might be in ion channels. The paroxysmal dyskinesias have many similarities to other episodic disorders of the nervous system such as episodic ataxias and periodic paralysis.[108] Many of these paroxysmal neurologic disorders are now known to be 'channelopathies' due to mutations of genes regulating ion channels.[109–115] In this regard it is interesting to note the many similarities between PKD and episodic ataxia type 1 (EA1). Like PKD, the episodes of ataxia in EA1 are often provoked by kinesigenic stimuli, are brief (lasting seconds to a few minutes), and can occur several times a day.[116] Both conditions have a early age of onset and there is tendency for both to abate in adulthood. EA1 typically responds to acetazolamide and also to anticonvulsants.[116,117] Interestingly, PKD also has similarities to hereditary hyperekplexia, an inherited disorder of the glycine receptor gene (GLRA1), characterized clinically by continuous muscle stiffness in the first year of life, and later an exaggerated startle response.[118] Discrete abnormalities in the first phase of RI in PKD that resemble the pattern observed in patients with hereditary hyperekplexia have been shown.[104,119,120] There are also reports of families with multiple episodic disorders: for example, paroxysmal dyskinesia in a family with episodic ataxia, and association of episodic problems like migraine and epilepsy in families with paroxysmal ataxia or dyskinesias.[21,24,121,122] Furthermore, paroxysmal dyskinesias are observed in the tottering mouse, which inherits a mutation in the P/Q-type calcium channel.[123] Thus, the familial paroxysmal dyskinesias are also believed to be due to defects in genes regulating ion channels. However, as mentioned earlier, so far the only identified mutations in channel genes are in ADFNLE, where there is a mutation of a ligand gated ion channel gene, and BPT, where some cases with mutation in a calcium channel gene have been reported. Surprisingly, the gene for PNKD did not turn out to be an ion channel gene and this condition is caused by mutations in the MR-1 gene, which encodes an enzyme in a stress response pathway.[83] However, the exact mechanism of how intermittent attacks of dyskinesias occur in PNKD remains unclear and it is possible that there is some associated interaction with ion channels. The genes for PKD and PED are still unknown.

TREATMENT OF PAROXYSMAL DYSKINESIAS

PKD responds dramatically to different antiepileptic drugs, but there appears to be a particularly good response to carbamazepine, even with relatively low doses.[12,29,124,125] More recently, it has been reported that PKC patients have a good response to the newer antiepileptics, including gabapentin,[126] lamotrigine,[127,128] levetiracetam,[129] and topiramate,[130] but our own experience is that carbamazepine is the drug of choice. PNKD is thus more difficult to treat than PKD with drugs; however, over the years, many patients learn to avoid precipitants and thus either avoid or even abort attacks. Most patients with PNKD generally do not benefit from antiepileptic drugs. However, clonazepam can be helpful in some and clobazam was reportedly beneficial in one case. Anticonvulsants may be useful in some but not all cases of PED.[25] Other drugs which may be helpful in some cases include l-dopa, acetazolamide, and trihexiphenidyl, which can be tried in turn. Generally, PED is more difficult to treat than PKC. In drug refractory cases, stereotactic surgery may be considered, particularly if attacks are predominantly one-sided. There has been a report of unilateral pallidotomy being useful in a case with PED.[25] Regarding the treatment of PHD, antiepileptics, particularly carbamazepine, are very effective in most cases.[36] In secondary, as in idiopathic paroxysmal dyskinesias, it is more difficult to control symptoms in PNKD and mixed disease than in PKD.[131] The treatments that have been used have not been uniformly effective, but anticonvulsant drugs and clonazepam have been the most beneficial.[10] Treatment of the underlying etiology has been reported to improve the symptoms in some cases. Botulinum toxin injections into the agonist muscle have been found effective in some patients with focal paroxysmal dystonia.[22] It is interesting to note that acetazolamide is helpful for some patients with paroxysmal dyskinesias,[29] as it also is in patients with known channelopathies such as periodic paralysis[132] and episodic ataxias.

FUTURE DIRECTIONS

The discovery of the genes will also lead to the possibility of developing animal models and functional cellular studies. This has already become possible for ADNFLE, which is known to be caused by mutations of the brain nicotinic acetylcholine receptor gene, a ligand gated channel. How these mutations cause epileptogenesis is not clearly understood, but functional studies have been performed expressing the mutant gene in cell lines, and undertaking single cell recordings using patch-clamp techniques to compare with the wild type. By this method, several different effects for different mutations of the α_4 or β_2 subunits of the nicotinic acetylcholine receptor gene have been observed, which include a decrease in maximal current amplitude[133] or increase,[134] decreases in acetylcholine affinity[133] and reduction in calcium entry into cells.[92,134] The pathophysiologic mechanisms of PNKD related to dysfunction of the MR-1 gene product have been speculated on (see Figure 15.1)[83] but further work is needed.

REFERENCES

1. Demirkiran M, Jankovic J. Paroxysmal dyskinesias: clinical features and classification. Ann Neurol 1995; 38(4): 571–9.
2. Fahn S. The paroxysmal dyskinesias. In: Marsden CD, Fahn S, eds. Movement Disorders. Oxford: Butterworth Heinmann, 1994: 310–45.
3. Mount LA, Reback S. Familial paroxysmal choreoathetosis. Arch Neurol Psychiatry 1940; 44: 841–7.
4. Forsman H. Hereditary disorder characterized by attacks of muscular contractions, induced by alcohol amongst other factors. Acta Med Scand 1961; 170: 517–33.
5. Lance JW. Sporadic and familial varieties of tonic seizures. J Neurol Neurosurg Psychiatry 1963, 26: 51–9.
6. Richards RN, Barnett HJ. Paroxysmal dystonic choreoathetosis. A family study and review of the literature. Neurology 1968; 18(5): 461–9.
7. Kertesz A. Paroxysmal kinesigenic choreoathetosis. An entity within the paroxysmal choreoathetosis syndrome. Description of 10 cases, including 1 autopsied. Neurology 1967; 17(7): 680–90.
8. Lance JW. Familial paroxysmal dystonic choreoathetosis and its differentiation from related syndromes. Ann Neurol 1977; 2(4): 285–93.
9. Auburger G, Ratzlaff T, Lunkes A et al. A gene for autosomal dominant paroxysmal choreoathetosis/spasticity (CSE) maps to the vicinity of a potassium channel gene cluster on chromosome 1p, probably within 2 cM between D1S443 and D1S197. Genomics 1996; 31(1): 90–4.
10. Blakeley J, Jankovic J. Secondary paroxysmal dyskinesias. Mov Disord 2002; 17(4): 726–34.
11. Pourfar MH, Guerrini R, Parain D et al. Classification conundrums in paroxysmal dyskinesias: a new subtype or variations on classic themes? Mov Disord 2005; 20(8): 1047–51.
12. Houser MK, Soland VL, Bhatia KP et al. Paroxysmal kinesigenic choreoathetosis: a report of 26 patients. J Neurol 1999; 246(2): 120–6.
13. Bruno MK, Hallett M, Gwinn-Hardy K et al. Clinical evaluation of idiopathic paroxysmal kinesigenic dyskinesia: new diagnostic criteria. Neurology 2004; 63(12): 2280–7.
14. Caraballo R, Pavek S, Lemainque A et al. Linkage of benign familial infantile convulsions to chromosome 16p12-q12 suggests allelism to the infantile convulsions and choreoathetosis syndrome. Am J Hum Genet 2001; 68(3): 788–94.
15. Hattori H, Fujii T, Nigami H et al. Co-segregation of benign infantile convulsions and paroxysmal kinesigenic choreoathetosis. Brain Dev 2000; 22(7): 432–5.
16. Sadamatsu M, Masui A, Sakai T et al. Familial paroxysmal kinesigenic choreoathetosis: an electrophysiologic and genotypic analysis. Epilepsia 1999; 40(7): 942–9.
17. Szepetowski P, Rochette J, Berquin P et al. Familial infantile convulsions and paroxysmal choreoathetosis: a new neurological syndrome linked to the pericentromeric region of human chromosome 16. Am J Hum Genet 1997; 61(4): 889–98.
18. Thiriaux A, de St Martin A, Vercueil L et al. Co-occurrence of infantile epileptic seizures and childhood paroxysmal choreoathetosis in one family: clinical, EEG, and SPECT characterization of episodic events. Mov Disord 2002; 17(1): 98–104.
19. Swoboda KJ, Soong B, McKenna C et al. Paroxysmal kinesigenic dyskinesia and infantile convulsions: clinical and linkage studies. Neurology 2000; 55(2): 224–30.
20. Lee WL, Tay A, Ong HT et al. Association of infantile convulsions with paroxysmal dyskinesias (ICCA syndrome): confirmation of linkage to human chromosome 16p12-q12 in a Chinese family. Hum Genet 1998; 103(5): 608–12.
21. Valente EM, Spacey SD, Wali GM et al. A second paroxysmal kinesigenic choreoathetosis locus (EKD2) mapping on 16q13-q22.1 indicates a family of genes which give rise to paroxysmal disorders on human chromosome 16. Brain 2000; 123(Pt 10): 2040–5.
22. Blakeley J, Jankovic J. Secondary causes of paroxysmal dyskinesia. Adv Neurol 2002; 89: 401–20.
23. Cochen DC, V, Bourdain F, Apartis E et al. Interictal myoclonus with paroxysmal kinesigenic dyskinesia. Mov Disord 2006; 21(9): 1533–5.
24. Munchau A, Valente EM, Shahidi GA et al. A new family with paroxysmal exercise induced dystonia and migraine: a clinical and genetic study. J Neurol Neurosurg Psychiatry 2000; 68(5): 609–14.
25. Bhatia KP, Soland VL, Bhatt MH et al. Paroxysmal exercise-induced dystonia: eight new sporadic cases and a review of the literature. Mov Disord 1997; 12(6): 1007–12.
26. Guerrini R, Bonanni P, Nardocci N et al. Autosomal recessive rolandic epilepsy with paroxysmal exercise-induced dystonia and writer's cramp: delineation of the syndrome and gene mapping to chromosome 16p12-11.2. Ann Neurol 1999; 45(3): 344–52.
27. Neville BG, Besag FM, Marsden CD. Exercise induced steroid dependent dystonia, ataxia, and alternating hemiplegia associated with epilepsy. J Neurol Neurosurg Psychiatry 1998; 65(2): 241–4.
28. Fink JK, Hedera P, Mathay JG et al. Paroxysmal dystonic choreoathetosis linked to chromosome 2q: clinical analysis and proposed pathophysiology. Neurology 1997; 49(1): 177–83.
29. Jarman PR, Bhatia KP, Davie C et al. Paroxysmal dystonic choreoathetosis: clinical features and investigation of pathophysiology in a large family. Mov Disord 2000; 15(4): 648–57.
30. Bruno MK, Lee HY, Auburger GW et al. Genotype–phenotype correlation of paroxysmal nonkinesigenic dyskinesia. Neurology 2007; 68(21): 1782–9.
31. Bressman SB, Fahn S, Burke RE. Paroxysmal non-kinesigenic dystonia. Adv Neurol 1988; 50: 403–13.

32. Byrne E, White O, Cook M. Familial dystonic choreoathetosis with myokymia; a sleep responsive disorder. J Neurol Neurosurg Psychiatry 1991; 54(12): 1090–2.
33. Scheffer IE, Bhatia KP, Lopes-Cendes I et al. Autosomal dominant frontal epilepsy misdiagnosed as sleep disorder. Lancet 1994; 343(8896): 515–7.
34. Lugaresi E, Cirignotta F. Hypnogenic paroxysmal dystonia: epileptic seizure or a new syndrome? Sleep 1981; 4(2): 129–38.
35. Lee BI, Lesser RP, Pippenger CE et al. Familial paroxysmal hypnogenic dystonia. Neurology 1985; 35(9): 1357–60.
36. Scheffer IE, Bhatia KP, Lopes-Cendes I et al. Autosomal dominant nocturnal frontal lobe epilepsy. A distinctive clinical disorder. Brain 1995; 118(Pt 1): 61–73.
37. Drigo P, Carli G, Laverda AM. Benign paroxysmal torticollis of infancy. Brain Dev 2000; 22(3): 169–72.
38. Giffin NJ, Benton S, Goadsby PJ. Benign paroxysmal torticollis of infancy: four new cases and linkage to CACNA1A mutation. Dev Med Child Neurol 2002; 44(7): 490–3.
39. Berger JR, Sheremata WA, Melamed E. Paroxysmal dystonia as the initial manifestation of multiple sclerosis. Arch Neurol 1984; 41(7): 747–50.
40. de Seze J, Stojkovic T, Destee M et al. Paroxysmal kinesigenic choreoathetosis as a presenting symptom of multiple sclerosis. J Neurol 2000; 247(6): 478–80.
41. Ostermann PO, Westerberg CE. Paroxysmal attacks in multiple sclerosis. Brain 1975; 98(2): 189–202.
42. Shibasaki H, Kuroiwa Y. Painful tonic seizure in multiple sclerosis. Arch Neurol 1974; 30(1): 47–51.
43. Tranchant C, Bhatia KP, Marsden CD. Movement disorders in multiple sclerosis. Mov Disord 1995; 10(4): 418–23.
44. Camac A, Greene P, Khandji A. Paroxysmal kinesigenic dystonic choreoathetosis associated with a thalamic infarct. Mov Disord 1990; 5(3): 235–8.
45. Lee MS, Marsden CD. Movement disorders following lesions of the thalamus or subthalamic region. Mov Disord 1994; 9(5): 493–507.
46. Merchut MP, Brumlik J. Painful tonic spasms caused by putaminal infarction. Stroke 1986; 17(6): 1319–21.
47. Nijssen PC, Tijssen CC. Stimulus-sensitive paroxysmal dyskinesias associated with a thalamic infarct. Mov Disord 1992; 7(4): 364–6.
48. Riley DE. Paroxysmal kinesigenic dystonia associated with a medullary lesion. Mov Disord 1996; 11(6): 738–40.
49. Sunohara N, Mukoyama M, Mano Y et al. Action-induced rhythmic dystonia: an autopsy case. Neurology 1984; 34(3): 321–7.
50. Baquis GD, Pessin MS, Scott RM. Limb shaking – a carotid TIA. Stroke 1985; 16(3): 444–8.
51. Bennett DA, Fox JH. Paroxysmal dyskinesias secondary to cerebral vascular disease – reversal with aspirin. Clin Neuropharmacol 1989; 12(3): 215–6.
52. Galvez-Jimenez N, Hanson MR, Hargreave MJ et al. Transient ischemic attacks and paroxysmal dyskinesias: an under-recognized association. Adv Neurol 2002; 89: 421–32.
53. Margolin DI, Marsden CD. Episodic dyskinesias and transient cerebral ischemia. Neurology 1982; 32(12): 1379–80.
54. Yanagihara T, Piepgras DG, Klass DW. Repetitive involuntary movement associated with episodic cerebral ischemia. Ann Neurol 1985; 18(2): 244–50.
55. Zaidat OO, Werz MA, Landis DM et al. Orthostatic limb shaking from carotid hypoperfusion. Neurology 1999; 53(3): 650–1.
56. Engelen M, Tijssen MA. Paroxysmal non-kinesigenic dyskinesia in antiphospholipid syndrome. Mov Disord 2005; 20(1): 111–3.
57. Biary N, Singh B, Bahou Y et al. Posttraumatic paroxysmal nocturnal hemidystonia. Mov Disord 1994; 9(1): 98–9.
58. Drake ME Jr, Jackson RD, Miller CA. Paroxysmal choreoathetosis after head injury. J Neurol Neurosurg Psychiatry 1986; 49(7): 837–8.
59. George MS, Pickett JB, Kohli H et al. Paroxysmal dystonic reflex choreoathetosis after minor closed head injury. Lancet 1990; 336(8723): 1134–5.
60. Perlmutter JS, Raichle ME. Pure hemidystonia with basal ganglion abnormalities on positron emission tomography. Ann Neurol 1984; 15(3): 228–33.
61. Richardson JC, Howes JL, Celinski MJ et al. Kinesigenic choreoathetosis due to brain injury. Can J Neurol Sci 1987; 14(4): 626–8.
62. Robin JJ. Paroxysmal choreoathetosis following head injury. Ann Neurol 1977; 2(5): 447–8.
63. Newman RP, Kinkel WR. Paroxysmal choreoathetosis due to hypoglycemia. Arch Neurol 1984; 41(3): 341–2.
64. Schmidt BJ, Pillay N. Paroxysmal dyskinesia associated with hypoglycemia. Can J Neurol Sci 1993; 20(2): 151–3.
65. Shaw C, Haas L, Miller D et al. A case report of paroxysmal dystonic choreoathetosis due to hypoglycaemia induced by an insulinoma. J Neurol Neurosurg Psychiatry 1996; 61(2): 194–5.
66. Haan J, Kremer HP, Padberg GW. Paroxysmal choreoathetosis as presenting symptom of diabetes mellitus. J Neurol Neurosurg Psychiatry 1989; 52(1): 133.
67. Clark JD, Pahwa R, Koller C et al. Diabetes mellitus presenting as paroxysmal kinesigenic dystonic choreoathetosis. Mov Disord 1995; 10(3): 353–5.
68. Morres CA, Dire DJ. Movement disorders as a manifestation of nonketotic hyperglycemia. J Emerg Med 1989; 7(4): 359–64.
69. Barabas G, Tucker SM. Idiopathic hypoparathyroidism and paroxysmal dystonic choreoathetosis. Ann Neurol 1988; 24(4): 585.
70. Soffer D, Licht A, Yaar I et al. Paroxysmal choreoathetosis as a presenting symptom in idiopathic hypoparathyroidism. J Neurol Neurosurg Psychiatry 1977; 40(7): 692–4.
71. Yamamoto K, Kawazawa S. Basal ganglion calcification in paroxysmal dystonic choreoathetosis. Ann Neurol 1987; 22(4): 556.
72. Fischbeck KH, Layzer RB. Paroxysmal choreoathetosis associated with thyrotosicosis. Ann Neurol 1979; 6(5): 453–4.
73. Micheli F, Fernandez Pardal MM, Casas P et al. Sporadic paroxysmal dystonic choreoathetosis associated with basal ganglia calcifications. Ann Neurol 1986; 20(6): 750.
74. Mirsattari SM, Berry ME, Holden JK et al. Paroxysmal dyskinesias in patients with HIV infection. Neurology 1999; 52(1): 109–14.
75. Fouad GT, Servidei S, Durcan S et al. A gene for familial paroxysmal dyskinesia (FPD1) maps to chromosome 2q. Am J Hum Genet 1996; 59(1): 135–9.
76. Jarman PR, Davis MB, Hodgson SV et al. Paroxysmal dystonic choreoathetosis. Genetic linkage studies in a British family. Brain 1997; 120(Pt 12): 2125–30.
77. Hofele K, Benecke R, Auburger G. Gene locus FPD1 of the dystonic Mount–Reback type of autosomal-dominant paroxysmal choreoathetosis. Neurology 1997; 49(5): 1252–7.
78. Przuntek H, Monninger P. Therapeutic aspects of kinesiogenic paroxysmal choreoathetosis and familial paroxysmal choreoathetosis of the Mount and Reback type. J Neurol 1983; 230(3): 163–9.
79. Raskind WH, Bolin T, Wolff J et al. Further localization of a gene for paroxysmal dystonic choreoathetosis to a 5-cM region on chromosome 2q34. Hum Genet 1998; 102(1): 93–7.
80. Matsuo H, Kamakura K, Saito M et al. Familial paroxysmal dystonic choreoathetosis: clinical findings in a large Japanese family and genetic linkage to 2q. Arch Neurol 1999; 56(6): 721–6.

81. Grunder S, Geisler HS, Rainier S et al. Acid-sensing ion channel (ASIC) 4 gene: physical mapping, genomic organisation, and evaluation as a candidate for paroxysmal dystonia. Eur J Hum Genet 2001; 9(9): 672–6.
82. Rainier S, Thomas D, Tokarz D et al. Myofibrillogenesis regulator 1 gene mutations cause paroxysmal dystonic choreoathetosis. Arch Neurol 2004; 61(7): 1025–9.
83. Lee HY, Xu Y, Huang Y et al. The gene for paroxysmal non-kinesigenic dyskinesia encodes an enzyme in a stress response pathway. Hum Mol Genet 2004; 13(24): 3161–70.
84. Chen DH, Matsushita M, Rainier S et al. Presence of alanine-to-valine substitutions in myofibrillogenesis regulator 1 in paroxysmal nonkinesigenic dyskinesia: confirmation in 2 kindreds. Arch Neurol 2005; 62(4): 597–600.
85. Hempelmann A, Kumar S, Muralitharan S et al. Myofibrillogenesis regulator 1 gene (MR-1) mutation in an Omani family with paroxysmal nonkinesigenic dyskinesia. Neurosci Lett 2006; 402(1–2): 118–20.
86. Stefanova E, Djarmati A, Momcilovic D et al. Clinical characteristics of paroxysmal nonkinesigenic dyskinesia in Serbian family with Myofibrillogenesis regulator 1 gene mutation. Mov Disord 2006; 21(11): 2010–5.
87. Tomita H, Nagamitsu S, Wakui K et al. Paroxysmal kinesigenic choreoathetosis locus maps to chromosome 16p11.2-q12.1. Am J Hum Genet 1999; 65(6): 1688–97.
88. Bennett LB, Roach ES, Bowcock AM. A locus for paroxysmal kinesigenic dyskinesia maps to human chromosome 16. Neurology 2000; 54(1): 125–30
89. Spacey SD, Valente EM, Wali GM et al. Genetic and clinical heterogeneity in paroxysmal kinesigenic dyskinesia: evidence for a third EKD gene. Mov Disord 2002; 17(4): 717–25.
90. Phillips HA, Scheffer IE, Berkovic SF et al. Localization of a gene for autosomal dominant nocturnal frontal lobe epilepsy to chromosome 20q 13.2. Nat Genet 1995; 10(1): 117–8.
91. Hirose S, Iwata H, Akiyoshi H et al. A novel mutation of CHRNA4 responsible for autosomal dominant nocturnal frontal lobe epilepsy. Neurology 1999; 53(8): 1749–53.
92. Steinlein OK, Magnusson A, Stoodt J et al. An insertion mutation of the CHRNA4 gene in a family with autosomal dominant nocturnal frontal lobe epilepsy. Hum Mol Genet 1997; 6(6): 943–7.
93. Weiland S, Witzemann V, Villarroel A et al. An amino acid exchange in the second transmembrane segment of a neuronal nicotinic receptor causes partial epilepsy by altering its desensitization kinetics. FEBS Lett 1996; 398(1): 91–6.
94. Phillips HA, Scheffer IE, Crossland KM et al. Autosomal dominant nocturnal frontal-lobe epilepsy: genetic heterogeneity and evidence for a second locus at 15q24. Am J Hum Genet 1998; 63(4): 1108–16.
95. De Fusco M, Becchetti A, Patrignani A et al. The nicotinic receptor beta 2 subunit is mutant in nocturnal frontal lobe epilepsy. Nat Genet 2000; 26(3): 275–6.
96. Phillips HA, Favre I, Kirkpatrick M et al. CHRNB2 is the second acetylcholine receptor subunit associated with autosomal dominant nocturnal frontal lobe epilepsy. Am J Hum Genet 2001; 68(1): 225–31.
97. Singh R, Macdonell RA, Scheffer IE et al. Epilepsy and paroxysmal movement disorders in families: evidence for shared mechanisms. Epileptic Disord 1999; 1(2): 93–9.
98. Stevens H. Paroxysmal choreo-athetosis. A form of reflex epilepsy. Arch Neurol 1966; 14(4): 415–20.
99. Franssen H, Fortgens C, Wattendorff AR et al. Paroxysmal kinesigenic choreoathetosis and abnormal contingent negative variation. A case report. Arch Neurol 1983; 40(6): 381–5.
100. Lee MS, Kim WC, Lyoo CH et al. Reciprocal inhibition between the forearm muscles in patients with paroxysmal kinesigenic dyskinesia. J Neurol Sci 1999; 168(1): 57–61.
101. Mir P, Huang YZ, Gilio F et al. Abnormal cortical and spinal inhibition in paroxysmal kinesigenic dyskinesia. Brain 2005; 128(Pt 2): 291–9.
102. Lombroso CT. Paroxysmal choreoathetosis: an epileptic or non-epileptic disorder? Ital J Neurol Sci 1995; 16(5): 271–7.
103. Hayashi R, Hanyu N, Yahikozawa H et al. Ictal muscle discharge pattern and SPECT in paroxysmal kinesigenic choreoathetosis. Electromyogr Clin Neurophysiol 1997; 37(2): 89–94.
104. Ko CH, Kong CK, Ngai WT et al. Ictal ^{99m}Tc ECD SPECT in paroxysmal kinesigenic choreoathetosis. Pediatr Neurol 2001; 24(3): 225–7.
105. Kitagawa N, Hayashi M, Akiguchi I et al. [Ictal ^{99m}TC-HMPAO-SPECT in a case of paroxysmal kinesigenic choreoathetosis]. Rinsho Shinkeigaku 1998; 38(8): 767–70. [in Japanese]
106. Shirane S, Sasaki M, Kogure D et al. Increased ictal perfusion of the thalamus in paroxysmal kinesigenic dyskinesia. J Neurol Neurosurg Psychiatry 2001; 71(3): 408–10.
107. Guerrini R, Parmeggiani L, Casari G. Epilepsy and paroxysmal dyskinesia: co-occurrence and differential diagnosis. Adv Neurol 2002; 89: 433–41.
108. Bhatia KP, Griggs RC, Ptacek LJ. Episodic movement disorders as channelopathies. Mov Disord 2000; 15(3): 429–33.
109. Browne DL, Gancher ST, Nutt JG et al. Episodic ataxia/myokymia syndrome is associated with point mutations in the human potassium channel gene, KCNA1. Nat Genet 1994; 8(2): 136–40.
110. de Carvalho AP, Sweadner KJ, Penniston JT et al. Mutations in the Na^+/K^+-ATPase alpha3 gene ATP1A3 are associated with rapid-onset dystonia parkinsonism. Neuron 2004; 43(2): 169–75.
111. Jurkat-Rott K, Lehmann-Horn F, Elbaz A et al. A calcium channel mutation causing hypokalemic periodic paralysis. Hum Mol Genet 1994; 3(8): 1415–9.
112. Litt M, Kramer P, Browne D et al. A gene for episodic ataxia/myokymia maps to chromosome 12p13. Am J Hum Genet 1994; 55(4): 702–9.
113. Ophoff RA, Terwindt GM, Vergouwe MN et al. Familial hemiplegic migraine and episodic ataxia type-2 are caused by mutations in the Ca^{2+} channel gene CACNL1A4. Cell 1996; 87(3): 543–52.
114. Ptacek LJ, Tawil R, Griggs RC et al. Sodium channel mutations in acetazolamide-responsive myotonia congenita, paramyotonia congenita, and hyperkalemic periodic paralysis. Neurology 1994; 44(8): 1500–3.
115. Vahedi K, Joutel A, Van Bogaert P et al. A gene for hereditary paroxysmal cerebellar ataxia maps to chromosome 19p. Ann Neurol 1995; 37(3): 289–93.
116. Brunt ER, van Weerden TW. Familial paroxysmal kinesigenic ataxia and continuous myokymia. Brain 1990; 113(Pt 5): 1361–82.
117. Griggs RC, Moxley RT III, Lafrance RA et al. Hereditary paroxysmal ataxia: response to acetazolamide. Neurology 1978; 28(12): 1259–64.
118. Shiang R, Ryan SG, Zhu YZ et al. Mutations in the alpha 1 subunit of the inhibitory glycine receptor cause the dominant neurologic disorder, hyperekplexia. Nat Genet 1993; 5(4): 351–8.
119. Brown P. Neurophysiology of the startle syndrome and hyperekplexia. Adv Neurol 2002; 89: 153–9.
120. Floeter MK, Andermann F, Andermann E et al. Physiological studies of spinal inhibitory pathways in patients with hereditary hyperekplexia. Neurology 1996; 46(3): 766–72.
121. Zuberi SM, Eunson LH, Spauschus A et al. A novel mutation in the human voltage-gated potassium channel gene (Kv1.1) associates with episodic ataxia type 1 and sometimes with partial epilepsy. Brain 1999; 122(Pt 5): 817–25.
122. Eunson LH, Rea R, Zuberi SM et al. Clinical, genetic, and expression studies of mutations in the potassium channel gene

KCNA1 reveal new phenotypic variability. Ann Neurol 2000; 48(4): 647–56.

123. Fureman BE, Jinnah HA, Hess EJ. Triggers of paroxysmal dyskinesia in the calcium channel mouse mutant tottering. Pharmacol Biochem Behav 2002; 73(3): 631–7.
124. Kato M, Araki S. Paroxysmal kinesignenic choreoathetosis. Report of a case relieved by carbamazepine. Arch Neurol 1969; 20(5): 508–13.
125. Wein T, Andermann F, Silver K et al. Exquisite sensitivity of paroxysmal kinesigenic choreoathetosis to carbamazepine. Neurology 1996; 47(4): 1104–6.
126. Chudnow RS, Mimbela RA, Owen DB et al. Gabapentin for familial paroxysmal dystonic choreoathetosis. Neurology 1997; 49(5): 1441–2.
127. Pereira AC, Loo WJ, Bamford M et al. Use of lamotrigine to treat paroxysmal kinesigenic choreoathetosis. J Neurol Neurosurg Psychiatry 2000; 68(6): 796–7.
128. Uberall MA, Wenzel D. Effectiveness of lamotrigine in children with paroxysmal kinesigenic choreoathetosis. Dev Med Child Neurol 2000; 42(10): 699–700.
129. Chatterjee A, Louis ED, Frucht S. Levetiracetam in the treatment of paroxysmal kinesiogenic choreoathetosis. Mov Disord 2002; 17(3): 614–5.
130. Huang YG, Chen YC, Du F et al. Topiramate therapy for paroxysmal kinesigenic choreoathetosis. Mov Disord 2005; 20(1): 75–7.
131. Blakeley J, Jankovic J. Secondary causes of paroxysmal dyskinesia. Adv Neurol 2002; 89: 401–20.
132. Ptacek LJ. Channelopathies: ion channel disorders of muscle as a paradigm for paroxysmal disorders of the nervous system. Neuromuscul Disord 1997; 7(4): 250–5.
133. Bertrand S, Weiland S, Berkovic SF et al. Properties of neuronal nicotinic acetylcholine receptor mutants from humans suffering from autosomal dominant nocturnal frontal lobe epilepsy. Br J Pharmacol 1998; 125(4): 751–60.
134. Kuryatov A, Gerzanich V, Nelson M et al. Mutation causing autosomal dominant nocturnal frontal lobe epilepsy alters Ca^{2+} permeability, conductance, and gating of human $\alpha_4\beta_2$ nicotinic acetylcholine receptors. J Neurosci 1997; 17(23): 9035–47.

16

Psychogenic dystonia

Martin Cloutier, Tamara Pringsheim, and Anthony E Lang

BACKGROUND

The history of dystonia is marked by a swinging pendulum of thought: from psychogenic to organic, and there and back again. The controversy surrounding the history of dystonia has made clinicians approach the diagnosis of psychogenic dystonia with understandable caution.

Early descriptions of idiopathic torsion dystonia date back to the beginning of the 20th century. Although originally described as a manifestation of psychiatric disease, several turn of the century neurologists recognized the organic nature of dystonia.[1–3] Attitudes toward dystonia changed in the 1940s and 1950s, perhaps as a result of the puzzling nature of the syndrome, and failure to understand its underlying pathology.[4] Commonly, physicians once more thought of dystonia as a psychiatric disorder, and patients with dystonia were sent for psychiatric evaluation and management. Over the next 20 years, clinicians became increasingly convinced that a true disorder of neurologic function was responsible for dystonia, and discouraged the notion of psychogenic causes. A hard line, denying the occurrence of dystonia secondary to psychological dysfunction, was taken in large part as a reaction to the recognition of the harm that had been done to patients with 'organic' dystonia who had been previously diagnosed and treated as having a psychiatric disorder. However, the pendulum has moved away from this extreme, with the recognition that in a small but definite proportion of patients with dystonia primary psychological factors are causative.

In order to better understand why theories of dystonia have swung so dramatically from organic to psychogenic, one must closely consider some aspects of the disease and its manifestations. Idiopathic torsion dystonia typically begins as a highly focal, action-specific movement disorder. For example, patients describe plantar flexion and inversion of the foot while walking forward, but not while running or walking backward, or writing is impaired in the absence of interference with other manual tasks. Symptoms may later progress to affect other tasks and other body segments. The appearance of dystonia is often quite bizarre. For example, dystonia involving the trunk, pelvis, and legs can cause a very peculiar gait that is often mistaken as hysterical. Focal and segmental dystonias also have interesting features such as amelioration by unusual sensory tricks ('gestes antagonistes') which could suggest psychogenicity to the inexperienced clinician. Cranial dystonias such as blepharospasm may be aggravated by trying to read or watch television, whereas manifestations of oromandibular dystonia may be minimal until the person attempts to eat or speak. These symptoms, especially blepharospasm, are often markedly diminished by the stress or alerting effect of a visit to the physician's office, resulting in suspicion of psychogenic disease in a patient who claims to be functionally blind at home. Some patients, especially those with cervical dystonia, may give a history of full spontaneous remission of symptoms in the past with later recurrence, sometimes precipitated by emotional upset. It is the variable nature of the dystonia that has made it most puzzling to clinicians, and has led to debate regarding the etiology of the symptoms. Experience and observation have proven that this is indeed an organic syndrome and often 'unusual' but characteristic features such as task specificity and the ameliorative effect of sensory tricks are used in support of the diagnosis. That said, psychogenic dystonia does exist, and must be recognized. Much of this chapter is reproduced with approval by the editor from a previous review on the topic.[5]

EPIDEMIOLOGY

Although psychogenic dystonia makes up a significant percentage of psychogenic movement disorders seen at subspecialty clinics, it accounts for a small minority of patients with idiopathic or symptomatic dystonia. Combined data on psychogenic movement disorders seen at Columbia-Presbyterian Medical Center,[6] the Toronto Western Hospital (unpublished data), Cleveland Clinic Florida (unpublished data), and Albany Medical Center[7] are presented in Table 16.1 Dystonia makes up the largest subgroup, accounting for 33% of psychogenic movement disorders seen at these clinics. This is mostly due to the large number of psychogenic dystonia cases seen at Columbia-Presbyterian Medical Center, which during the time of this data collection, served as a Dystonia Medical Research Foundation center of excellence and therefore probably had a strong referral bias. In the other groups, tremor was the most common psychogenic movement disorder, followed by dystonia. In our recent evaluation of 279 patients with psychogenic movement disorders, 89 (32%) had dystonia, while 91 (33%) had tremor, 51 (18%) had myoclonus, and the remainder had a variety of less common phenotypes.[8]

Looking at the percentage of patients with dystonia who had a psychogenic origin of their symptoms, Marsden quotes a figure of 1% at the National Hospital for Neurology and Neurosurgery in London (21 of 2221 patients with idiopathic or symptomatic dystonia),[4] while Fahn's group at the Dystonia Clinical Research Center had a figure of 2.6% (21 of 814 patients).[6] Factor et al reported that 2.9% of all the patients with dystonia seen at their clinic were diagnosed as psychogenic.[7] These numbers are all from tertiary-care movement disorders clinics and are probably higher than the true prevalence of psychogenic dystonia. Clearly, the vast majority of patients with dystonia have an organic basis for their symptoms.

CLINICAL FEATURES AND DIAGNOSIS

Overall, a psychogenic movement disorder is not a diagnosis of exclusion. Several important historical and particularly clinical features are required in support of this consideration. Of all the psychogenic movement disorders, psychogenic dystonia is probably the most difficult to diagnose. This is based on skillful observation and examination of the patient by an experienced clinician, which will reveal inconsistencies suggestive of a psychogenic origin of the patient's symptoms. Expertise in the evaluation of movement disorders is necessary to make a diagnosis of psychogenic dystonia since there is no biologic marker for the condition. Currently, neuroimaging and electrophysiologic testing are of limited use in the diagnosis of psychogenic dystonia, although that role is evolving.

Table 16.2 provides a list of important historical and clinical clues to the diagnosis of psychogenic movement

Table 16.1 Combined data on psychogenic movement disorders seen at Columbia-Presbyterian Medical Center, Toronto Western Hospital, Cleveland Clinic Florida, and Albany Medical Center

Psychogenic movement disorder	Columbia-Presbyterian Medical Center (%)	Toronto Western Hospital (%)	Cleveland Clinic Florida (%)	Albany Medical Center (%)	Total (%)
Dystonia	82 (53)	34 (20)	14 (25)	6 (21)	136 (33)
Tremor	21 (13)	52 (30)	18 (32)	15 (54)	106 (26)
Myoclonus	11 (7)	34 (20)	4 (14)	4 (14)	53 (13)
Parkinsonism	3 (2)	14 (8)	2 (7)	2 (7)	19 (5)
Gait disorder	14 (9)	7 (4)	1 (2)	0	22 (5)
Blepharospasm facial movements	4 (2)	0	4 (7)	1 (4)	9 (2)
Tics	2 (1.3)	0	2 (3.6)	0	4 (1)
Stiff person	1 (0.6)	0	0	0	1 (0.2)
Other	14 (9)	30 (18)	13 (23)	1 (4)	58 (14)
Total	152	171	56	28	407

Columbia-Presbyterian Medical Center data includes all types of psychogenic movement disorders.[6]
Toronto Western Hospital (AE Lang, unpublished data) and Cleveland Clinic Florida (N Galvez Jiminez, pers comm) data listed only predominant psychogenic movement disorders.
Albany Clinic.[7]

Table 16.2 Important clues suggesting a psychogenic movement disorder

Historical clues
Abrupt onset
Minor trauma (litigation or compensation often present)
Static course
Purely paroxysmal or paroxysmal worsening (exclude other paroxysmal dyskinesias)
Spontaneous cures/remissions
Multiple somatizations/undiagnosed conditions
Other psychiatric illness
Employed in allied health professions
Clear secondary gain

Clues on physical examination
Movements incongruous with organic movement disorders:
- Mixed (often bizarre) movement disorders:
- Paroxysmal attacks (including pseudoseizures)
- Precipitated paroxysms (often suggestible/startle)

Movement inconsistent:
- Over time-variability
- Selective disabilities (exclude task-specific movement disorders)
- Distractibility (exclude tics, akathisia)
- Suggestibility
- Entrainment by complex repetitive motor tasks (especially tremor)

Response to placebo with suggestion:
- Worsening or improving

Refuses videotaping (infrequent; might suggest malingering)

disorders in general. Importantly, none of these are definitive and many of these features may also be seen in organic movement disorders. For example, abrupt onset or rapid progression to maximum severity is a common feature of psychogenic dystonia (and other psychogenic movement disorders) but it can be seen in some heredodegenerative dystonias such as Wilson's disease or rapid-onset dystonia-parkinsonism. Paroxysmal movement disorders are commonly psychogenic, but idiopathic and secondary paroxysmal dyskinesias and dystonias – kinesigenic or non-kinesigenic – must be ruled out before the definitive diagnosis is made.

Fahn and Williams developed a classification system for psychogenic dystonia which is now used to classify psychogenic movement disorders of all types.[6] This classification system allows the neurologist to categorize the degree of diagnostic certainty as documented, clinically established, probable, or possible. Table 16.3 outlines the features of each diagnostic category. Williams and colleagues have subsequently combined the categories of documented and clinically established to form a category of clinically definite dystonia, as both categories imply a definite diagnosis.[9]

Psychogenic dystonia can be extremely difficult to diagnose given the unusual clinical features of organic dystonia, as previously mentioned. This diagnosis requires considerable experience in the assessment of various organic dystonic syndromes, since it is based on the presence of clinical inconsistencies and incongruities with organic dystonia. Incongruous features include:

- rapid onset and progression with fixed postures followed by static course
- paroxysms (often triggered)
- marked ('active') resistance to passive movement, often with the inability to activate the same muscles on command
- elaborate, bizarre, or complex abnormal movements
- extreme slowness of voluntary movements, clinically different from true bradykinsesia, since there is often preserved amplitude of movement and a lack of fatiguing
- extreme pain with the dystonic spasms
- variable direction of 'dystonic' posturing
- foot dystonia (especially fixed), beginning in the adult.

Features that are generally inconsistent with organic dystonia include:

- being witnessed free of dystonia on surreptitious observation
- dystonia subsides on distraction
- dystonia changes or is precipitated with suggestion.

Although organic dystonia often does fluctuate over time, it usually behaves in a stereotyped pattern, whereas psychogenic dystonia can show inconsistent variation over time. Table 16.4 lists features which help distinguish psychogenic from organic dystonia. Once again, it is important to emphasize that these features are simply 'suggestive' clues and no more. Organic dystonias may also manifest any or all of these features, and the incongruities and inconsistencies listed above are critical in support of the diagnosis.

Fahn and Williams reported on the largest series of patients with psychogenic dystonia.[6] Among a total of 39 cases of psychogenic dystonia, diagnosed with various degrees of certainty, 17 met the criteria for documented

Table 16.3 Classification system for psychogenic movement disorders by Fahn and Williams[6]

Category	Criteria
Documented[a]	• Movement disorder is persistently relieved by psychotherapy, psychological suggestion, or administration of placebo • Absence of symptoms when unaware of being observed
Clinically established[a]	• Movement disorder is inconsistent over time or is incongruent with the clinical presentation of an organic movement disorder • Supportive evidence is provided by the presence of other physical signs that are definitely psychogenic (e.g. false weakness, non-anatomic sensory loss), multiple somatizations, or an obvious psychiatric disturbance
Probable	Three categories of patients: 1. Movements are inconsistent or incongruent with an organic disorder but no other features exist to support a psychogenic origin 2. Abnormal movements are consistent and congruent with an organic disorder, but physical signs are present that are definitely psychogenic[b] 3. Movements are consistent and congruent with an organic disorder, but multiple somatizations are present[b]
Possible	• Obvious psychiatric disturbance present in a patient with abnormal movements that are consistent and congruent with an organic movement disorder • Supportive evidence includes inappropriate affect, discrepancy between the movement disorder and the reported disability, and the presence of secondary gain

[a]Documented and clinically established groups could be combined as clinically definite.
[b]These features are not uncommon in patients with organic movement disorders. We would not support using these criteria to give a diagnosis of a probable psychogenic movement disorder.

psychogenic dystonia and 4 were considered clinically established. The authors reported on these 21 patients in detail.

There were 19 females and 2 males. Age of onset was between 8 and 58 years. They differentiated between the 14 patients with continual dystonia and 7 having only paroxysmal dystonia. The former group had a mean age of onset of 23 years and the latter 33 years. Many of the patients had clinical features that were considered suspicious of a non-organic etiology. Dystonia was considered incongruent or inconsistent in 19 of the 21 patients. Nine patients reported prominent pain; 14 patients had false weakness and 5 had false sensory signs; 8 had multiple somatizations; 11 had dystonia at rest from the onset, another atypical feature of organic dystonia; 5 had superimposed paroxysmal episodes that were vaguely similar to seizures; 7 had other movement disorders that were also considered psychogenic; 5 patients had excessive non-organic slowness of movements.

Onset was in lower limbs in 14 patients, including 7 of the 11 patients who were 25 years of age or older. It frequently evolved to generalized dystonia – again, even in adult-onset cases.

Before the authors' assessment, none of the patients were diagnosed as having a pure psychogenic disorder, although some were believed to have a mixture of organic dystonia with superimposed psychogenic features. Some patients had invasive procedures before the correct diagnosis was made: 1 patient had a previous right thalamotomy, 1 patient had carotid arteriography, 1 patient underwent a tendon transplantation, and 1 patient had received intrathecal baclofen.

The duration of symptoms from onset to their assessment was between 1 month and 15 years. The 5 patients who had symptoms for less than 2 months before the diagnosis was made had a complete remission. Among all 21 patients, 9 had a complete and permanent remission and another 4 had a moderate or considerable relief of their symptoms. The duration of follow-up was not specified.

Lang reviewed 18 patients with a diagnosis of clinically definite psychogenic dystonia.[10] According to the Fahn and Williams classification, 4 of these met the definition of documented psychogenic dystonia and 14 were clinically established. Thirteen of the 18 patients were female. The mean age of onset was 35.5 ± 12.7

Table 16.4 Features suggestive of psychogenic dystonia[9a]

Onset with resting dystonia
Adult onset with leg involvement
Fixed spasm
Rapid progression
Spread to maximum disability early in the course
Dystonic movements inconsistent over time
No sensory trick
Selective disabilities
Abilities inconsistent with fixed spasms
Pain or tenderness to touch and exaggeration with passive movement
Lack of improvement after sleep
Attempted voluntary movement to command in the opposite direction of the dystonic posturing may activate antagonist muscles with little apparent action in agonist muscles
Paroxysmal dystonia (isolated or combined with persistent dystonia)
Other paroxysmal movements
Other psychogenic movement disorders
Other non-organic neurologic signs
Precipitants
Remissions, spontaneous or with placebo
Absence of family history

[a]Any or all of these features can also be seen present in organic dystonias. See text for details.

years, with a range between 17 and 59 years. The mean duration of symptoms before the first assessment was 3.8 ± 6.9 years, but one patient had symptoms for 30 years before the diagnosis was made. Fourteen patients had a known precipitant before the onset of dystonia; in 6 patients, this was a local injury and in 5 a motor vehicle accident, usually with a whiplash injury, was reported.

The onset of dystonia was sudden in 9 patients, progressed over days in 6 patients, whereas the temporal evolution of the symptoms remained uncertain in 3 patients. In most patients, the maximum severity was reached rapidly, either immediately or over days, certainly an atypical course for organic dystonia. Onset was in the lower limbs in 7 patients, and generalized dystonia from onset was present in 3 patients. Again, these features are very rare in adults with organic dystonia. After the onset, there was a progression to generalized dystonia in 5 other patients.

At first assessment, 12 of the patients had dystonia at rest. Ten patients reported superimposed paroxysmal changes in their dystonia, and in 4 patients these paroxysmal events were triggered by non-physiologic means during examination.

Prominent pain was a common feature, reported by 14 patients. There was pronounced tenderness of the muscles involved and exaggeration of pain with attempted passive manipulation; 10 patients had other psychogenic movement disorders and 15 had non-organic neurologic abnormalities on examination, usually give-way weakness or false sensory signs; 8 patients had multiple somatizations. Six patients were receiving financial benefits for their disabilities and 2 patients had pending litigation. Thirteen patients went through multiple investigations before their assessment, and 6 patients had therapeutic trials with at least three medications. One patient had two right-sided thalamotomies.

Follow-up was available for only 8 patients. One patient had a complete remission and 2 patients showed marked improvement. Another patient who had obvious generalized dystonia when first evaluated was seen later at a lay symposium on dystonia and appeared normal. One other patient had a moderate improvement and in 3 patients the dystonia persisted unchanged.

Factor and colleagues reported 28 patients with various psychogenic movement disorders, including 5 patients with dystonia.[7] These 5 patients were aged between 22 and 50 years old, and 4 were female; 2 patients had left foot dystonia, 2 patients had blepharospasm, and 1 patient had paroxysmal generalized dystonia. As a group, they shared many of the features of the patients reported by Fahn and Williams and Lang, such as additional non-organic neurologic signs and potential secondary gains. Interestingly, 7 of the 28 patients with a psychogenic movement disorder also had a distinct organic movement disorder.[7]

Another not uncommon presentation of psychogenic dystonia is facial dystonia. Patients will typically present with unilateral eye closure, and contralateral mouth deviation. This presentation in considered incongruent with organic dystonia and cannot be explained by neuroanatomic pathways.

Bentivoglio and colleagues reported a patient with psychogenic dystonia who was also a carrier of the *DYT1* mutation.[11] Four other family members, over three generations, were affected with organic primary torsion dystonia. The adult-onset inconsistent episodes of severe dystonia, leading to a temporary wheelchair-bound state, followed by complete spontaneous remission, with the additional non-organic neurologic signs led the authors to the correct diagnosis. The sense of guilt of having transmitted a severe movement disorder to her son was believed to be the source of her conversion disorder.

The concept of *post-traumatic movement disorders* warrants separate discussion. Of note, is the occurrence of movement disorders, particularly dystonia, accompanying the complex regional pain syndrome (CRPS), which is characterized by a combination of sensory, autonomic, and other motor disturbances following trauma to a limb. This is now divided into CRPS type I (clinical syndrome not limited to the distribution of a single peripheral nerve, previously referred to as reflex sympathetic dystrophy [RSD]) and CRPS type II after partial injury of a nerve or one of its branches, often referred to previously as causalgia. Motor manifestations described in these patients include dystonic posturing, weakness, tremor, and myoclonic jerks. Despite the attention given to these motor manifestations in recent times, the pathophysiologic mechanisms remain obscure.

Van Hilten and colleagues, among others, champion the concept of *multifocal or generalized tonic dystonia of complex regional pain syndrome,* which they feel has an unequivocal organic basis, is associated with a particular HLA-type predisposition (HLA-DR13), and responds to intrathecal baclofen.[12–14] However, many of the features reported to be typical of this disorder are also characteristic of psychogenic dystonia, including precipitation by minor injury, rapid onset with fixed postures, unusual distributions, spontaneous remissions, atypical pain and tenderness, non-anatomic sensory changes, and weakness. Verdugo and Ochoa studied 58 CRPS patients with a movement disorder seen at their clinic in an effort to understand the essence of positive motor phenomena seen in patients with CRPS.[15] Of the 58 patients, 47 had sustained a minor physical injury at work. Patients exhibited various combinations of dystonic spasms, coarse postural or action tremor, and irregular jerks. Patients underwent rigorous clinical and laboratory evaluation aimed at characterizing their neurologic disturbance. Only patients with CRPS I or RSD displayed abnormal movements, and all patients exhibited pseudoneurologic signs, suggesting that the abnormal movements were also non-organic in nature. Features of the abnormal movements experienced by patients, such as paroxysmal worsening of dystonic postures, and the clenched fist syndrome were characteristic of psychogenic abnormal movements. Video surveillance tapes were forwarded to the clinic for 4 patients, confirming a diagnosis of malingering. The authors conclude that the abnormal movements of CRPS I are of somatoform or malingering origin. In contrast to these findings, Birklein and colleagues reported that 'irregular myoclonic jerks and dystonic muscle contractions' were present in 33 of 122 CRPS I patients but also in 11 of 23 CRPS II cases.[16] This remains a controversial area. As more definitive diagnostic tools become available for psychogenic dystonia, further studies of patients with unusual forms of dystonia following minor peripheral injury will be necessary. The study of Schrag and her colleagues sheds important light on this difficult group of patients. These authors reviewed 103 patients with fixed dystonia, 41 of whom were evaluated intensively.[17] Fifteen (36%) had clinically definite psychogenic dystonia and in only 4 (10%) was there no suggestion of a psychogenic movement disorder. Twenty-six of the 41 patients had developed dystonia following some form of peripheral injury; of these, 23 had evidence for a psychogenic cause (5 documented, 3 clinically established, and 15 probable). Fifteen of these 26 cases had evidence of CRPS, 13 of whom were diagnosed as psychogenic dystonia (3 documented, and 10, probable). Forty-one percent (7/17) of those in whom general practice notes could be obtained and evaluated had evidence for a somatization disorder and in most of these the diagnosis was only evident after review of past records was possible, raising concerns about the accuracy of the past history provided by patients with neurologically unexplained symptoms.[18]

A similar disorder has been termed post-traumatic cervical dystonia.[19–21] Our groups at the Toronto Western Hospital Movement Disorders Unit and Comprehensive Pain Program have recently evaluated 16 patients with what we prefer to designate as *post-traumatic painful torticollis*.[22] These patients developed a characteristic, exceedingly painful fixed head tilt and shoulder elevation after a motor vehicle accident or work-related accident. The onset of the abnormal posturing is very often within the first week after the accident. Additional abnormalities on physical examination were common, including non-dermatomal sensory loss, give-way limb weakness, psychogenic dystonia of the limb or jaw, and psychogenic tremor. Litigation or compensation was present in all 16 patients. Oral medications commonly used for dystonia and even botulinum toxin were generally ineffective or worsened pain, although 1 patient had excellent response to both active and placebo botulinum toxin injections. Sodium amytal interview resulted in improvement in posture, pain, or both, in all 13 patients undergoing this procedure, and marked improvement or normalization of sensory deficit occurred in 7 of the 13 patients. These patients met the accepted criteria for the diagnosis of peripheral trauma-induced dystonia.[23] However, our clinical and psychological evaluations strongly support the importance of contributing psychological factors to the etiology of this condition. As outlined in the following section, we have argued that this is a disorder occurring in psychologically vulnerable individuals following minor physical injuries.

PSYCHOPATHOLOGY

Patients with psychogenic dystonia are considered in the *Diagnostic and Statistical Manual of Mental Disorders* to suffer from conversion disorder, motor subtype. Conversion disorder falls into the category of somatoform disorders. Conversion theory holds that primary or secondary gain or both underlie symptom production. Primary gain refers to the conversion of psychological distress into physical symptoms. Secondary gain refers to external factors that may be influenced by the symptom development, such as the sympathy and attention of family members.[24] Morris et al have recently proposed the concept of 'deceptive signaling' to account for psychogenic movement disorders.[25]

Studies of patients with motor conversion disorder have revealed a number of trends. Comorbidity between motor conversion and both Axis I (clinical disorders) and Axis II (personality disorders) is significant. In fact, the majority of patients with motor conversion have at least one comorbid Axis I diagnosis, with rates of depression ranging from 26% to 71%, and anxiety disorder present in 7–38%.[9,26–28] Personality disorders were diagnosed in 42–67% of patients, and included a variety of personality subtypes, with dependent and borderline personalities being most common.

In the study of *post-traumatic painful torticollis* from our center described above, psychological evaluations suggested that psychological conflicts and/or stress were being expressed via somatic channels in 11 of 12 tested patients. The onset of physical trauma in these patients, in the context of critical psychological factors, might result in ongoing contraction and guarding of the neck and shoulder musculature associated with pain and non-dermatomal sensory deficits, a process which is primarily unconscious. It was postulated that injury may trigger poorly defined central mechanisms in psychologically vulnerable individuals who are at risk of developing these features.[22] Indeed, other psychogenic movement disorders may also result from the triggering of such processes in vulnerable individuals, leading to motor dysfunction. Further studies are required to establish the importance of this dynamic interplay. It is critical that these include similar assessments in patients with established organic movement disorders.

NEUROIMAGING

There have been no neuroimaging studies evaluating psychogenic dystonia. One major stumbling block is the non-specific but critical confounding effect of the ongoing motor activity on widespread sensory and motor brain regions, particularly since the vast majority of patients with psychogenic dystonia maintain the abnormal postures at rest, and even in the lighter stages of sleep. The work of Eidelberg and colleagues in their studies using [18F]-fluorodeoxyglucose positron emission tomography (FDG PET) in patients with idiopathic torsion dystonia and essential blepharospasm might suggest novel approaches to the study of psychogenic dystonia.[29] Studying clinically affected *DYT1* carriers in a sleep state, when involuntary movements were suppressed by sleep, allowed observation of the primary functional abnormality in brain metabolism in these patients without the secondary effects of movement (this abnormal neural network was similar to that found in asymptomatic *DYT1* carriers). FDG PET in awake and sleeping patients with essential blepharospasm also allowed the distinction to be made between the functional substrate of the disorder and the brain activity resulting from the clinical manifestations.[30] Such a technique could be applied to patients with psychogenic dystonia. It will be important to compare these patients with the organic counterparts as well as normal controls feigning the same type of movements.

Interesting studies in patients with psychogenic paralysis may provide further insights or ideas of how to pursue these issues in psychogenic dystonia. For example, Marshall and colleagues measured changes in regional cerebral blood flow in a woman with long-standing left-sided paralysis due to motor conversion disorder.[31] When the patient moved her right leg the areas activated included the dorsolateral prefrontal cortex bilaterally, and left lateral premotor areas, left primary sensorimotor cortex, bilateral secondary somatosensory areas (inferior parietal cortex), and the vermis and cerebellar hemispheres bilaterally. Preparation to move the right leg activated a subset of these areas, including the dorsolateral prefrontal cortex bilaterally, right lateral premotor and bilateral inferior parietal cortex, and the vermis and cerebellar hemispheres, but not the left primary sensorimotor cortex. Preparation to move the (paralyzed) left leg activated the left lateral premotor cortex and the cerebellar hemispheres bilaterally, indicating the patient's readiness to move the paralyzed leg. Attempting to move the paralyzed leg led to activation of movement-related areas, including the left dorsolateral prefrontal cortex and the cerebellar hemispheres bilaterally, but no activation of the right premotor areas or of right primary sensorimotor cortex was seen. Instead, the right anterior cingulate and orbitofrontal cortices were significantly activated during this condition (when compared with preparing to move the left leg). The authors proposed that these areas actively inhibited movement of the left leg despite dorsolateral prefrontal cortex activation and downstream activation of the cerebellum. They proposed that the orbitofrontal cortex may be the distal source of unconscious inhibition while the anterior cingulate, which mediates emotion and action, is the proximal site that disconnects premotor/prefrontal areas from primary motor cortex. The authors speculated that in the absence of functional or structural pathology, it is a disturbance of the will to move that triggers the hemiparalysis via pathologic activation of orbitofrontal and cingulate cortex. Supporting suggestions that hypnosis and conversion disorders are pathogenetically linked, the same researchers found that hypnotically induced paralysis of the left leg activated similar brain areas to those of motor conversion disorder.[32]

Other clinicians have found reversible alterations in regional cerebral blood flow in the thalamus and basal ganglia contralateral to hysterical 'sensorimotor' loss, with lower activation in the contralateral caudate nucleus predicting poorer recovery at follow-up.[33] Functional magnetic resonance imaging (FMRI) has also been used to evaluate patients with hysterical sensory loss and functional pain syndromes.[34] Similar studies in psychogenic dystonia are awaited with interest; however, as mentioned, there are important confounding factors, particularly the effects of the ongoing persistent muscle activity, which will need to be addressed if these are to provide useful pathophysiologic insights.

NEUROPHYSIOLOGIC STUDIES

Electrophysiologic studies are extremely useful in defining the psychogenic nature of some movement disorders, most notably myoclonus and tremor.[35] Unfortunately, to date, the utility of neurophysiologic assessment in psychogenic dystonia has not been established. Comparison of electromyographic (EMG) activity in the sternocleidomastoid and splenius capitis muscles of patients with idiopathic torticollis with that of controls matching the head posture or imitating tremulous torticollis has provided information regarding the pattern of rhythmic drive to the muscles of the neck which could be useful in differentiating organic from psychogenic torticollis.[36] Control subjects showed a significant peak in the autospectrum of the splenius capitis EMG at 10–12 Hz, which was absent in all patients with organic torticollis. Patients with torticollis had evidence of a 4–7 Hz drive to the splenius capitis and sternocleidomastoid that was absent in coherence spectra from controls. The activity in the sternocleidomastoid and splenius capitis was in phase in patients but not in controls. These EMG features might prove useful in differentiating organic from psychogenic dystonia, although the extent to which the findings in controls can be applied to patients with psychogenic dystonia is not known.

A variety of electrophysiologic features have been defined in patients with organic forms of dystonia. However, it is unclear whether many of the electrophysiologic features decribed in dystonia are a primary feature of the disorder or simply secondary to the abnormal postures, in which case they would be of little help in differentiating psychogenic from non-psychogenic dystonias. For example, abnormalities of recurrent spinal inhibition are widely described in patients with dystonia.[31] However, similar findings may be evident in normal individuals purposely maintaining those limbs in a dystonic-like posture (K Bhatia, pers comm). Similar concerns might apply to changes in cortical sensory maps of dystonic limbs. However, Meunier and colleagues have found disorganization of finger representation in the somatosensory cortex of the non-dystonic hand in patients with unilateral task-specific dystonia using magnetoencephelography, suggesting that this may very well be a primary phenomenon rather than secondarily induced by the abnormal posture.[37] An important example of the potential influence of prolonged dystonic postures on neuronal function with neuroplastic adaptive responses comes from the unpublished anecdotal experience with psychogenic dystonia patients undergoing thalamotomy. Lenz and colleagues described careful electrophysiologic studies of dystonia patients performed at the time of thalamic surgery. They demonstrated increased receptive fields and an increased thalamic representation of dystonic body parts which was believed to be a hallmark of the dystonic state.[38] However, we are aware of 2 patients with psychogenic dystonia who were treated by thalamotomy who had similar electrophysiologic studies with identical expanded sensory receptive fields, supporting the possibility that this is a consequence of the dystonic movement itself, rather than part of the underlying pathogenesis. This is further supported by the recent study of Espay et al[39] who found that measures of cortical inhibition, resting short- and long-interval intracortical inhibition, and the cortical silent period were reduced in patients with psychogenic dystonia as well as in those with organic dystonia, suggesting that these electrophysiologic abnormalities may in fact be a consequence rather than a cause of dystonia.

There is a great need for further electrophysiologic and imaging studies in psychogenic dystonia. However, considerable care will have to be taken to address the important confounding secondary or compensatory changes that occur as a consequence of the abnormal movements.

TREATMENT AND PROGNOSIS

Patients with psychogenic dystonia can experience profound disability due to their condition, making proper diagnosis and treatment essential. Patients with lower limb symptoms may become wheelchair-bound. Psychogenic dystonia patients may reach the point of requiring assistance for self-care tasks, lose their ability to work, and be unable to participate in activities they formally enjoyed.[6]

Studies of patients with psychogenic movement disorders in general, including psychogenic dystonia, show that prognosis is better in patients with a shorter duration of symptoms prior to diagnosis. In one study of 30 patients admitted to hospital with motor conversion symptoms of less than 3 months' duration prior to diagnosis and treatment, 63% of patients had complete remission of their symptoms, 27% were improved, and only 10% were unchanged or worse after 2–5 years. The majority of patients were symptom-free within 6 months of receiving the diagnosis of conversion.[40]

In studies where the majority of the cases have had a long duration between initial presentation and diagnosis, remission rates have not been nearly as favorable. Rates of complete resolution of symptoms range from 10% to 28%, with the average length of time between presentation and diagnosis of 18 months to 2 years.[9,27,28] However, these numbers may not represent the prognosis in unselected psychogenic dystonia since they come from movement disorders clinics, with a clear referral bias toward more severe and long-lasting cases. In collaboration with our group, Feinstein et al found a significant correlation between the mode of onset and the course of symptoms, with a more sudden onset predicting a better outcome, as well as a significant correlation between the extent of psychiatric comorbidity and the course of symptoms.[27] Crimlisk and colleagues found that a new psychiatric diagnosis coinciding with the unexplained motor symptoms was associated with a favorable prognosis at long-term follow-up, whereas receipt of financial benefits and pending litigation at the time of admission to hospital predicted a poor prognosis.[28]

In dealing with these patients, appropriate investigation should be undertaken to exclude organic dystonia and reassure the patient and clinician that no organic basis for the symptoms has been overlooked. This should be completed before the diagnosis of psychogenic dystonia is raised with the patient. Fahn and Williams recommended that patients suspected of having psychogenic dystonia be admitted to hospital.[6,9] This is due to the reluctance of most patients to accept a psychological explanation for their symptoms, and concern regarding proper follow-up and treatment once this diagnosis is made. It will also expedite the completion of any necessary investigation and allow more intensive observation and evaluation. Certainly, we would agree that this is necessary for complex cases where the diagnosis is uncertain or for the more entrenched and long-standing symptoms, especially when profound disability is present. On the other hand, this approach is not mandatory in all patients and the benefit of such intensive care to long-term outcome has not been proven. Placebo and suggestion can be used to exacerbate movements or relieve them, and may provide further diagnostic information. Utilization of placebo is controversial, and there are legal and ethical concerns. The deception that it implies can endanger the physician–patient relationship. Furthermore, the response to placebo is typically not lasting, and further treatment will be necessary. Psychiatric consultation should be obtained to identify coexisting psychopathology or psychosocial issues which can be treated accordingly. The collaboration between the neurologist and the psychiatrist is of great importance. It would be counterproductive and detrimental to the patient if the psychiatrist expresses doubt regarding the psychological basis of the disorder and insists on further investigation for an organic etiology. It is also important, as emphasized earlier in the chapter, that underlying psychiatric disturbances in a patient with dystonia not be accepted as causative of the movement disorder, especially when the clinical features are compatible with idiopathic or symptomatic forms of dystonia.

Cases of unequivocal malingering and rare examples of Munchausen syndrome are dealt with quite differently than those with conversion disorder. Individuals with the former two conditions are consciously and purposefully causing their symptoms for financial or psychological gain. We will not discuss these further.

In patients with conversion disorder, the diagnosis of psychogenic dystonia should be presented in an assertive but supportive fashion only after the diagnosis is certain and planned investigations are complete. The absence of a severe neurologic disorder should be stated clearly. This should be emphasized in a very positive light, underscoring the potential for recovery in view of the absence of an underlying 'brain disease'. The unconscious nature of symptom production should be explained (i.e. emphasizing that it is not believed that the patient is feigning or purposefully causing the symptoms), as well as the ability of psychological conflicts to express themselves via somatic channels. Preferably, both neurologist and psychiatrist should participate in this exercise. Providing analogies of physical symptoms commonly accepted (correctly or not) as caused by stress by the lay public such as high blood pressure, duodenal ulcer, chest or abdominal pains, dermatitis, etc. helps the patient and family to understand the potential for psychological factors to induce dystonia. We often emphasize the interactions or 'connections' of the large parts of the brain involved in emotional or psychological function with those that control movement and posture. Treatment employing psychotherapy, physical therapy, and psychopharmacologic therapy may be necessary and, when appropriate, should be started in hospital. Intensive follow-up is required for the best outcome, although considerable research is required to evaluate the impact of various possible treatment strategies. Outcomes are generally poor when patients are simply given the diagnosis and returned to their referring physician for ongoing management or it is left to the referring physician to discuss the diagnosis and arrange further care.

CONCLUSION

Psychogenic dystonia is a rare cause of dystonia, but does occur and often results in profound disability. It is difficult to diagnose with certainty, and this should only be undertaken by a neurologist with considerable experience with organic dystonias. A great deal of controversy surrounds the primary role of psychological factors in the pathogenesis of dystonia following minor injury. The pathophysiology of psychogenic dystonia is poorly understood, but may improve with novel neuroimaging techniques or the development of new electrophysiologic strategies. Prompt diagnosis and treatment is necessary, given the poor prognosis of conversion disorders when considerable delays occur between symptom onset and diagnosis. There is a major need for research evaluating various treatment options, given the overall poor prognosis experienced by these patients.

REFERENCES

1. Schwalbe W. Eine eigentumliche tonische Krampfform mit hysterischen symptomene. Inaug Diss. Berlin: G. Schade; 1908.
2. Oppenheim H. Uber eine eigenartige Krampfkrankheit des kindlichen und jugendlichen Alters (Dysbasia lordotica progressive, Dystonia musculorum deformans). Neurol Centrabl 1911; 30: 1090–107.
3. Flatau E, Sterling W. Progressiver Torsionspasms bie Kindern. Z gesamte Neurol Psychiatr 1911; 7: 586–612.
4. Marsden CD. Psychogenic problems associated with dystonia. Adv Neurol 1995; 65: 319–26.
5. Pringsheim T, Lang A. Psychogenic dystonia. Rev Neurol (Paris) 2003; 159: 885–91.
6. Fahn S, Williams D. Psychogenic dystonia. Adv Neurol 1988; 50: 431–55.
7. Factor SA, Podskalny GD, Mohlo ES. Psychogenic movement disorders: frequency, clinical profile and characteristics. J Neurol Neurosurg Psychiatry 1995; 59: 406–12.
8. Baik JS, Lang AE. Gait abnormalities in psychogenic movement disorders. Mov Disord 2007; 22: 395–9.
9. Williams DT, Ford B, Fahn S. Phenomenology and psychopathology related to psychogenic movement disorders. Adv Neurol 1995; 65: 231–57.
10. Lang AE. Psychogenic dystonia: a review of 18 cases. Can J Neurol Sci 1995; 22: 136–43.
11. Bentivoglio AR, Loi M, Valente EM et al. Phenotypic variability of DYT1-PTD: does the clinical spectrum include psychogenic dystonia? Mov Disord 2002; 17: 1058–63.
12. van Hilten JJ, Van de Beek WJ, Hoff JI, Voormolen JH, Delhaas EM. Intrathecal baclofen for the treatment of dystonia in patients with reflex sympathetic dystrophy. N Engl J Med 2000; 343: 625–30.
13. van Hilten JJ, Van de Beek WJT, Vein AA, Van Dijk JG, Middelkoop HAM. Clinical aspects of multifocal or generalized tonic dystonia in reflex sympathetic dystrophy. Neurology 2001; 56: 1762–5.
14. van Hilten JJ, Van de Beek WJT, Roep BO. Multifocal or generalized tonic dystonia of complex regional pain syndrome: a distinct clinical entity associated with HLA-DR13. Ann Neurol 2000; 48: 113–16.
15. Verdugo RJ, Ochoa JF. Abnormal movements in complex regional pain syndrome: assessment of their nature. Muscle Nerve 2000; 23: 198–205.
16. Birklein F, Riedl B, Sieweke N, Weber M, Neundorfer B. Neurological findings in complex regional pain syndromes – analysis of 145 cases. Acta Neurol Scand 2000; 101: 262–9.
17. Schrag A, Trimble M, Quinn N, Bhatia K. The syndrome of fixed dystonia: an evaluation of 103 patients. Brain 2004; 127: 2360–72.
18. Schrag A, Brown RJ, Trimble MR. Reliability of self-reported diagnoses in patients with neurologically unexplained symptoms. J Neurol Neurosurg Psychiatry 2004; 75: 608–11.
19. Goldman S, Ahlskog JE. Posttraumatic cervical dystonia. Mayo Clin Proc 1993; 68: 443–8.
20. Tarsy D. Comparison of acute- and delayed-onset posttraumatic cervical dystonia. Mov Disord 1998; 13: 481–5.
21. Samii A, Pal PK, Schulzer M, Mak E, Tsui JKC. Post-traumatic cervical dystonia: a distinct entity? Can J Neurol Sci 2000; 27: 55–9.
22. Sa DS, Mailis A, Nicholson K, Lang AE. Posttraumatic painful torticollis. Mov Disord 2003; 18: 1482–91.
23. Jankovic J. Can peripheral trauma induce dystonia and other movement disorders? Yes! Mov Disord 2001; 16: 7–12.
24. American Psychiatric Association. Diagnostic and Statistical Manual of Mental Disorders, 4th edn. Washington, DC: American Psychiatric Association; 1994.
25. Morris JG, de Moore GM, Herberstein M. Psychogenic gait: an example of deceptive signaling. In: Hallett M, Fahn S, Jankovic J et al, eds. Psychogenic Movement Disorders: Neurology and Neuropsychiatry. Philadelphia: Lippincott Williams and Wilkins; 2006: 69–75.
26. Binzer M, Eisemann M. Childhood experiences and personality traits in patients with motor conversion symptoms. Acta Psychiatr Scand 1998; 98: 288–95.
27. Feinstein A, Stergiopoulos V, Fine J, Lang AE. Psychiatric outcome in patients with a psychogenic movement disorder. Neuropsychiatry Neuropsychol Behav Neurol 2001; 14: 169–76.
28. Crimlisk HL, Bhatia K, Cope H et al. Slater revisited: 6 year follow-up study of patients with medically unexplained motor symptoms. BMJ 1998; 316: 582–6.
29. Eidelberg D, Moeller J, Antonini A et al. Functional brain networks in DYT1 dystonia. Ann Neurol 1998; 44: 303–12.
30. Hutchison M, Nakamura T, Moeller JR et al. The metabolic topography of essential blepharospasm. Neurology 2000; 55: 673–7.

31. Marshall JC, Halligan PW, Fink GR, Wade DT, Frackowiak RSJ. The functional anatomy of hysterical paralysis. Cognition 1997; 64: B1–8.
32. Halligan PW, Athwal BS, Oakley DA, Frackiowiak RSJ. Imaging hypnotic paralysis: implications for conversion hysteria. Lancet 2000; 355: 986–7.
33. Vuilleumier P, Chicherio C, Assal F et al. Functional neuroanatomical correlates of hysterical sensorimotor loss. Brain 2001; 124: 1077–90.
34. Mailis-Gagnon A, Giannoylis I, Downar J et al. Altered central somatosensory processing in chronic pain patients with "hysterical" anesthesia. Neurology 2003; 60: 1501–7.
35. Brown P, Thompson PD. Electrophysiological aids to the diagnosis of psychogenic jerks, spasms and tremor. Mov Disord 2001; 16: 595–9.
36. Tijssen MAJ, Marsden JF, Brown P. Frequency analysis of EMG activity in patients with idiopathic torticollis. Brain 2000; 123: 677–86.
37. Meunier S, Garnero L, Ducorps A. Human brain mapping in dystonia reveals both endophenotypic traits and adaptive reorganization. Ann Neurol 2001; 50: 521–7.
38. Lenz FA, Jaeger CJ, Seike MS et al. Thalamic single neuron activity in patients with dystonia: dystonia-related activity and somatic sensory reorganization. J Neurophysiol 1999; 82: 2372–92.
39. Espay AJ, Morgante F, Purzner J et al. Cortical and spinal abnormalities in psychogenic dystonia. Ann Neurol 2006; 59: 825–34.
40. Binzer M, Kullgren G. Motor conversion disorder. A prospective 2 to 5 year follow-up study. Psychosomatics 1998; 39: 519–27.

17

Drug therapy of torsion dystonia

Paul Greene

INTRODUCTION

The last decade has seen an increase in the treatment options for many forms of dystonia, primarily due to the dramatic expansion in the use of botulinum toxin (BTX) and the more recent application of deep brain stimulation to both childhood and adult dystonia. During this period, despite the discovery of the *DYT1* gene, there have been few new developments in the pharmacologic treatment of dystonia. Nonetheless, there still is an important role for drug therapy of both idiopathic and some symptomatic forms of dystonia:

- Patients with dopa-responsive dystonia (DRD) have dramatic, sustained improvement taking small doses of levodopa.[1] Unless an alternative diagnosis is certain (e.g. a gene for an alternative form of dystonia has been found in the family), a trial of levodopa as initial therapy should be strongly considered. This applies primarily to childhood-onset dystonia, but patients with adult-onset dystonia and a history of a relative with childhood-onset dystonia might also be candidates for a trial of levodopa.
- Many children with dystonia have disabling symptoms in multiple regions of the body, so that the use of BTX injections as sole therapy is impractical. Despite the reassuring safety record of BTX to date, the consequences of chronic BTX injections over multiple decades are unknown. It is, therefore, preferable to treat children with medication when possible.
- Most patients with adult-onset dystonia have symptoms primarily in one region of the body (usually involving neck, upper face, vocal cords, upper extremity, or oromandibular muscles). Some patients, however, require treatment of muscles that are not limited to a single segment and it may not be practical to inject BTX into a sufficient number of contracting muscles. These patients may be candidates for medication trials.
- Some patients with focal or segmental dystonia will fail to improve significantly after BTX treatment or develop resistance to the injections.[2] Until there is more data about the role of deep brain stimulation in focal, adult-onset dystonia, these patients may benefit from medications.

I will discuss the most common medications used to treat dystonia, considering the evidence for efficacy, indications, and adverse effects. In uncontrolled studies, small response rates may suggest placebo effect. However, it is well to keep in mind that even well-designed prospective, placebo-controlled trials may fail to detect significant benefit that occurs in only a small percentage of patients.

DOPAMINERGIC AGENTS

Patients with Segawa variant dystonia or DRD usually develop symptoms in the lower extremities before puberty and may have parkinsonism, corticospinal tract signs, improvement after sleep, and a family history of levodopa-responsive dystonia.[3] Patients with DRD improve dramatically with small doses of levodopa – ranging from 50 mg/day to 900 mg/day of levodopa with decarboxylase inhibitor (mean = 250 mg/day).[3] It is necessary to initiate therapy with very small doses of levodopa (usually 50 mg/day) because higher doses may produce unpleasant dyskinesias. Supplemental carbidopa may be necessary at these low doses to prevent nausea. Symptoms in these patients may also improve with dopamine agonists or anticholinergic medications.[3] If there is any chance that a patient has DRD, a trial of Sinemet (carbidopa + levodopa) should be performed.

The results of controlled, oral studies of dopaminergic agents in dystonia have been contradictory. Several small controlled studies found benefit from bromocriptine or lisuride.[4–8] Other studies failed to find such benefit from bromocriptine, amantadine, or levodopa.[9–13] An early review of studies up to 1985 concluded that improvement from dopaminergic agents was rarely dramatic, and that these agents worsened symptoms in almost 20% of patients.[14] Later open-label reports came to similar conclusions.[15,16] Despite these disappointing results, an occasional patient with non-DRD does seem to improve, suggesting more than a placebo response.[17]

Most patients with dystonia tolerate dopaminergic agents well. Nausea, orthostatic hypotension, confusion or hallucinations and dopa dyskinesias have been reported in patients with dystonia, but are uncommon. However, a substantial minority will experience worsening of symptoms or the development of superimposed levodopa dyskinesias.

ANTICHOLINERGICS

A prospective, placebo-controlled, study documented the efficacy of high-dose trihexyphenidyl in alleviating the symptoms of dystonia in children and young adults.[18] Thirty-one childhood-onset patients were studied, with a mean age at time of treatment of 18.6 years: 67% of patients treated with trihexyphenidyl improved, which was significantly better than those treated with placebo; 68% continued to benefit from trihexyphenidyl after a mean 2.4 years at a mean dose of 40 mg/day. There has not been another prospective controlled study in children, although uncontrolled reports have found similar benefit in children.[12,19,20] One retrospective study found only modest benefit in patients with DYT1 dystonia, but the age at therapy was not specified.[21] Several case reports and small series have suggested that anticholinergics may be effective for children and young adults with dystonia after cerebral infarct,[22] cerebral hemorrhage,[23] delayed-onset dystonia after birth injury,[24] and other causes.[25]

It has been more difficult to determine the effectiveness of oral anticholinergic agents in treating adults with focal dystonia. There have been several small prospective studies of the acute administration of anticholinergic agents (usually by the intravenous or intramuscular route) in adult-onset dystonia.[4,13,26–28] These older studies had varying degrees of control and blinding and concluded that acute administration of anticholinergics is effective in dystonia and predicts long-term improvement with oral anticholinergic agents. However, a somewhat larger study found no statistically significant benefit and attributed the modest benefit to sedation.[29] None of three published prospective studies of oral anticholinergics in adult-onset dystonia meet modern criteria for well-designed studies.[12,30,31] One open-label study of 38 patients using blinded ratings found benefit in 45% of patients with a mean dose of 23 mg/day of trihexyphenidyl.[31] Anticholinergics were not well tolerated, and many patients stopped medication due to forgetfulness, constipation, dry mouth, blurred vision, etc.

In addition to the studies cited above, there are open-label reports of the use of anticholinergics in adults with dystonia, some finding benefit[15,19,32–34] and others finding minimal if any benefit.[16,29,35]

In both children and adults, the dose of anticholinergic medications must be increased gradually if side effects are to be avoided. Benefit may not appear for many weeks on a constant dose, and so lengthy trials are more likely to be productive.[18] Most patients require high doses of anticholinergic agents before improvement is seen. The effective dose varies from patient to patient and from agent to agent. For example, the published effective doses of trihexyphenidyl vary from 5 mg/day to 120 mg/day,[18] and of ethopropazine from 50 mg/day to 800 mg/day.[15] Many anticholinergics have been used to treat dystonia, including trihexyphenidyl, benztropine, biperiden, ethopropazine, atropine, procyclidine, orphenadrine, scopolamine, and trans-derm scopolamine. Side effects may vary from agent to agent, so that switching anticholinergic medications is sometimes helpful. Peripheral side effects such as blurred vision, constipation, dry mouth, and urinary retention can usually be treated with pilocarpine eye drops for blurred vision and with pyridostigmine for the other side effects. Central nervous system side effects such as short-term memory loss, confusion, or psychosis are frequently dose-limiting, especially in adults. Other central side effects occasionally occur, such as restlessness, chorea, or exacerbation of a pre-existing tic disorder.[18] Abrupt withdrawal of anticholinergics may not only precipitate cholinergic crisis but may also cause dramatic increase in dystonia.[36]

BACLOFEN

Baclofen is a derivative of γ-aminobutyric acid (GABA) that reduces spinal cord interneuron and motor neuron excitability, possibly via activation of the presynaptic $GABA_B$ receptor by the L isomer.[37] There have been no controlled studies of baclofen in the treatment of dystonia, but in retrospective studies at the Movement Disorder Center at Columbia Medical Center, we found baclofen to be of marked benefit in a significant minority of children and of some benefit in a small minority of adults with dystonia.[15,38–40] Baclofen was the medication most often used in one study of patients with DYT1 dystonia, but age at therapy was not specified.[21]

In other small series, there was no significant benefit from baclofen.[41,42] There have been several reports of improvement in dystonia in a handful of patients with various focal dystonias using a combination of baclofen and valproate.[43–46]

Side effects are a major limiting factor in treating adults with baclofen. Even with gradual increase in dosage, lethargy, upset stomach, dizziness, 'floppiness', dry mouth, or urinary urgency or hesitation prevent treatment with high doses of baclofen in many patients. Confusion, hallucinosis, and paranoia have been reported, but are rare. Rapid decrease in the dose of baclofen may precipitate psychosis or seizures, so all patients should be warned not to discontinue baclofen abruptly. Baclofen is better tolerated in children, although the same kinds of side effects can be seen.

BENZODIAZEPINES

Benzodiazepines are frequently used in the treatment of dystonia, but documentation of benefit in well-designed controlled studies is lacking. There have been many uncontrolled reports of benefit from benzodiazepines, including clonazepam, diazepam, and others.[15,32–34,47–50] Benzodiazepines were the medications most often successful in one series of patients with symptomatic hemidystonia.[25] Sedation and ataxia are the limiting side effects for most patients taking benzodiazepines. Patients with dystonia can sometimes tolerate very large doses of benzodiazepines if the doses are increased gradually. Some patients taking high doses of clonazepam become irritable. Nocturnal drooling and depression are possible side effects of benzodiazepines, but seem to be rare. There is always concern that patients taking benzodiazepines may develop withdrawal on stopping the medication, or develop tachyphylaxis. Patients with dystonia do get withdrawal symptoms if benzodiazepine doses are lowered rapidly, and it may be difficult to determine if the resulting worsening of dystonia represents evidence that the medication produced unsuspected benefit. We have rarely seen tachyphylaxis in patients with dystonia.

ANTIDOPAMINERGIC AGENTS

Paradoxically, occasional patients with dystonia seem to improve with a variety of antidopaminergic agents. Some controlled studies with pimozide and the investigational dopamine depleter/dopamine receptor blocker tetrabenazine found benefit.[26,51–53] Other controlled studies found no benefit.[12,13] Open-label studies with pimozide, haloperidol, α-methylparatyrosine, or tetrabenazine have also produced mixed results: some studies reported benefit,[15,16,32,54–57] whereas other studies found improvement in only 9–11% of patients.[4,27,35,48,58,59] Some patients seemed to improve with the combination of tetrabenazine and lithium.[57] Patients with severe dystonia, or acute exacerbation of dystonia ('dystonic storm') sometimes improve with the combination of a dopamine receptor blocker, a dopamine depleter, and an anticholinergic agent.[20,60] In the case of tardive dystonia, dopamine depleters such as reserpine and tetrabenazine are especially useful.[61]

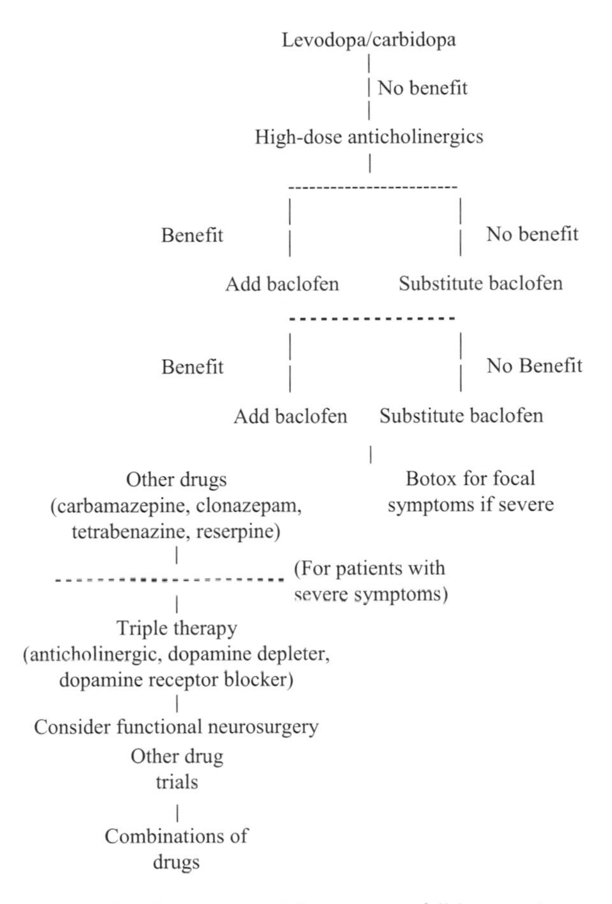

Figure 17.1 Treatment of dystonia in children and adolescents.

With the exception of reserpine, tetrabenazine and the atypical neuroleptic clozapine, dopamine receptor blockers can produce tardive symptoms (akathisia, dyskinesias, or even dystonia) in patients with dystonia, and these may become more disabling than the original symptoms. At this time, clozapine is the only atypical neuroleptic that does not produce tardive syndromes, although there are very few reports of tardive syndromes from the atypical neuroleptic quetiapine. Clozapine[62–66] and quetiapine[67,68] have both been reported to help some patients with tardive dystonia affecting various parts of the body. Clozapine was effective in some patients with idiopathic dystonia[69,70] but not in others.[71] One single-blinded, uncontrolled study found clozapine to benefit the jerky movements in spasmodic torticollis but not the head deviation.[72] In addition to the risk of tardive syndromes, patients with dystonia often tolerate antidopaminergic agents poorly. Sedation, apathy, nausea, orthostatic hypotension, insomnia, acute dystonic reactions, acute akathisia, worsening of dystonic symptoms, and confusion have all been seen with these agents, but usually can be reversed with reduction in dose or discontinuation of the medication. Depression, especially with dopamine depleters, is uncommon, but can be severe and can be life threatening if not recognized and treated, usually with reduction in dose. Drug-induced parkinsonism is often the limiting factor in treating patients who seem to benefit from dopamine depleters. The parkinsonism is reversible and dose dependent and can be controlled with reduction in dose. Unfortunately, dystonia does not improve in some patients until parkinsonism appears. In these patients, parkinson symptoms may be reduced by the addition of anticholinergic agents, amantadine, or levodopa. This is not always effective, however, and addition of dopaminergic agents may also reverse improvement in dystonic symptoms induced by the antidopaminergic treatment.

CARBAMAZEPINE

Carbamazepine occasionally produces dystonia as a toxic effect in patients treated for seizures.[73] Paradoxically, it has been reported to treat dystonia in some uncontrolled series.[15,74,75] Some carbamazepine successes may have been patients with DRD, since these patients improve with carbamazepine, although not to the same degree as with levodopa.[3] However, some patients who improved with carbamazepine did not have DRD, as they did not improve with levodopa.[74,75] Patients with paroxysmal kinesigenic dystonia improve dramatically with carbamazepine, phenytoin, and other anticonvulsants.[76]

OTHER AGENTS

Many other medications have been used to treat dystonia in isolated cases. Tricyclic antidepressants,[15,47,49] dantrolene,[47] propranolol,[31] phenytoin,[49] clonidine,[15,26] monoamine oxidase (MAO) inhibitors,[77] barbiturates,[77] and L-tryptophan[78] have generally not been noted to produce improvement in the small number of cases tried. Sporadic reports of improvement with amphetamines[79] have not been vigorously pursued. Tetrahydrobiopterin has been reported to benefit some patients with dystonia,[80] but most of these patients probably had DRD. Double-blind studies of the GABAergic agent γ-vinyl GABA[81] and the muscle relaxant tizanidine[82] did not document benefit in dystonia. A subsequent open trial of tizanidine (with an initial placebo wash-in) in 9 patients with cranial dystonia found that 22% (2/9) improved at tolerated doses, and benefit was transient in both of these.[83] Antihistamines have occasionally been reported to produce benefit, and it has been suggested that the effect may not be entirely due to their anticholinergic properties.[84,85] Cyproheptadine, which has serotonin antagonist properties, has been reported to help dystonia in two reports by the same group.[86,87] 5-Hydroxytryptophan, a serotonin precursor, was reported to benefit some patients with torticollis,[88] but not patients with Meige syndrome.[77] Individual reports claimed benefit from salmon calcitonin[89] and cannibidiol.[90] Lasting benefit using lithium was reported in 26% (9/34) of patients with torticollis and cranial dystonia, but only 4 of these improved on lithium alone.[33] Mexiletine, an oral antiarrhythmic related to lidocaine, was found to be of benefit in uncontrolled studies in small numbers of patients with torticollis, blepharospasm, and generalized dystonia.[91–93] Riluzole was described to benefit some patients with torticollis in an uncontrolled study with blinded video ratings.[94] Despite some anecdotal reports of benefit in focal and generalized dystonia with levetiracetam,[95,96] a prospective, uncontrolled study in 10 patients found no benefit in any of the 7 patients that tolerated the planned dose target of 1000 mg twice a day.[97]

SUMMARY

Treating dystonia requires patience and persistence on the part of the patient, family, and physician. Medications are often successful in children and adolescents and a large minority of patients improve dramatically. Unless surgery becomes a first-line treatment for dystonia in children, medications will remain the mainstay of therapy. A L-dopa trial is often the first maneuver. Anticholinergics remain the medication most likely to produce benefit in most children, but baclofen and benzodiazepines remain reasonable options. Treatment with the other medications listed above may be appropriate where surgery is inappropriate or ineffective. While dopamine receptor blocking agents may help a small percentage of patients, the risk of tardive syndromes makes the use of these agents undesirable except for the most severely affected patients. Medications are much less effective in adults, and many adults can benefit from botulinum toxin or surgical procedures. Medications remain an option for selected adults, as outlined above. With the exception of dopaminergic agents, which are much less likely to benefit adults, medication trials in adults proceed in the same order as trials in children.

REFERENCES

1. Segawa M, Hosaka A, Miyagawa F et al. Hereditary progressive dystonia with marked diurnal fluctuation. Adv Neurol 1976; 14: 215–33.
2. Greene PE, Fahn S, Diamond B. Development of resistance to botulinum toxin type A in patients with torticollis treated with injections of botulinum toxin type A. Mov Disord 1994; 9: 213–17.
3. Nygaard TG, Marsden CD, Fahn S. Dopa-responsive dystonia: long-term treatment response and prognosis. Neurology 1991; 41: 174–81.
4. Stahl SM, Berger PA. Bromocriptine, physostigmine, and neurotransmitter mechanisms in the dystonias. Neurology 1982; 32: 889–92.
5. Bassi S, Ferrarese C, Frattola L et al. Lisuride in generalized dystonia and spasmodic torticollis. Lancet 1982; i: 514–15.
6. Obeso JA, Luquin MR. Bromocriptine and lisuride in dystonias. Neurology 1984; 34: 135.
7. Quinn NP, Lang AE, Sheehy MP et al. Lisuride treatment of dystonia. Neurology 1984; 34(Suppl 1): 223. [abstract]
8. Nutt JG, Hammerstad JP, Carter J et al. Lisuride treatment of cranial dystonia. Neurology 1984; 34(Suppl 1): 223. [abstract]
9. Lees A, Shaw KM, Stern GM. Bromocriptine and spasmodic torticollis. BMJ 1976; 1: 1343.
10. West HH. Treatment of spasmodic torticollis with amantadine: a double-blind study. Neurology 1977; 27: 198–9.
11. Juntunen J, Kaste M, Iivanainen M et al. Bromocriptine treatment of spasmodic torticollis. Arch Neurol 1979; 36: 449–50.
12. Girotti F, Scigliano G, Nardocci N et al. Idiopathic dystonia: neuropharmacological study. J Neurol 1982; 227: 239–47.
13. Giménez-Roldán S, Mateo D, Orbe M et al. Acute pharmacologic tests in cranial dystonia. Adv Neurol 1988; 49: 451–66.
14. Lang AE. Dopamine agonists in the treatment of dystonia. Clin Neuropharmacol 1985; 8: 38–57.
15. Greene P, Shale H, Fahn S. Analysis of open-label trials in torsion dystonia using high dosages of anticholinergics and other drugs. Mov Disord 1988; 3: 46–60.
16. Defazio G, Lamberti P, Lepore V et al. Facial dystonia: clinical features, prognosis and pharmacology in 31 patients. Ital J Neurol Sci 1989; 10: 553–60.
17. Van Gerpen JA. Dopa-responsive dystonic camptocormia. Neurology 2006; 66: 1779.
18. Burke RE, Fahn S, Marsden CD. Torsion dystonia: a double-blind, prospective trial of high-dosage trihexyphenidyl. Neurology 1986; 36: 160–4.
19. Fahn S. High dosage anticholinergic therapy in dystonia. Neurology 1983; 33: 1255–61.
20. Marsden CD, Marion MH, Quinn N. The treatment of severe dystonia in children and adults. J Neurol Neurosurg Psychiatry 1984; 47: 1166–73.
21. Anca MH, Zaccai TF, Badarna S et al. Natural history of Oppenheim's dystonia (DYT1) in Israel. J Child Neurol 2003; 18: 325–30.
22. Vogels OJM, Maassen B, Rotteveel JJ et al. Focal dystonia and speech impairment responding to anticholinergic therapy. Pediatr Neurol 1994; 11: 346–8.
23. Pidcock FS, Hoon AH Jr, Johnston MV. Trihexyphenidyl in post-hemorrhagic dystonia: motor and language effects. Pediatr Neurol 1999; 20: 219–22.
24. Hoon AH Jr, Freese PO, Reinhardt EM et al. Age dependent effects of trihexyphenidyl in extrapyramidal cerebral palsy. Pediatr Neurol 2001; 25: 55–8.
25. Chuang C, Fahn S, Frucht SJ. The natural history and treatment of acquired hemidystonia: report of 33 cases and review of the literature. J Neurol Neurosurg Psychiatry 2002; 72: 59–67.
26. Lal S, Hoyte K, Kiely ME et al. Neuropharmacological investigations and treatment of spasmodic torticollis. Adv Neurol 1979; 24: 335–51.
27. Tanner CM, Glantz RH, Klawans HL. Meige disease: acute and chronic cholinergic effects. Neurology 1982; 32: 783–5.
28. Povlsen UJ, Pakkenberg H. Effect of intravenous injection of biperiden and clonazepam in dystonia. Mov Disord 1990; 5: 27–31.
29. Lang AE, Sheehy MP, Marsden CD. Anthicholinergics in adult-onset focal dystonia. Can J Neurol Sci 1982; 9: 313–19.
30. Nutt JG, Hammerstad JP, deGarmo P et al. Cranial dystonia: double-blind crossover study of anticholinergics. Neurology 1984; 34: 215–17.
31. Jabbari B, Scherokman B, Gunderson CH et al. Treatment of movement disorders with trihexyphenidyl. Mov Disord 1989; 4: 202–12.
32. Gollomp SM, Fahn S, Burke RE et al. Therapeutic trials in Meige syndrome. Adv Neurol 1983; 37: 207–13.
33. Jankovic J, Ford J. Blepharospasm and orofacial-cervical dystonia: clinical and pharmacological fingings in 100 patients. Ann Neurol 1983; 13: 402–11.
34. Rondot P, Marchand MP, Dellatolas G. Spasmodic torticollis – review of 220 patients. Can J Neurol Sci 1991; 18: 143–51.
35. Marsden CD, Lang AE, Sheehy MP. Pharmacology of cranial dystonia. Neurology 1983; 33: 1100–1.
36. Gimenez-Roldan S, Mateo D, Martin M. Life-threatening cranial dystonia following trihexyphenidyl withdrawal. Mov Disord 1989; 4: 349–53.
37. Davidoff RA. Antispasticity drugs: mechanisms of action. Ann Neurol 1985; 17: 107–16.
38. Greene P, Fahn S. Baclofen in the treatment of idiopathic dystonia in children. Mov Disord 1992; 7: 48–52.
39. Greene P. Baclofen in the treatment of dystonia. Clin Neuropharmacol 1992; 15: 276–88.
40. Fahn S, Hening WA, Bressman S et al. Long-term usefulness of baclofen in the treatment of essential blepharospasm. Adv Ophthalmol Plast Reconstr Surg 1985; 4: 219–26.
41. Marsden CD. The focal dystonias. Semin Neurol 1982; 2: 324–33.
42. Arthurs B, Flanders M, Codère F et al. Treatment of blepharospasm with medication, surgery and type A botulinum toxin. Can J Ophthalmol 1987; 22: 24–8.
43. Sandyk R. Blepharospasm-successful treatment with baclofen and sodium valproate. S Afr Med J 1983; 64: 955–6.
44. Sandyk R. Treatment of writer's cramp with sodium valproate and baclofen. A case report. S Afr Med J 1983; 63: 702–3.
45. Sandyk R. Beneficial effect of sodium valproate and baclofen in spasmodic torticollis. S Afr Med J 1984; 65: 62–3.
46. Brennan MJ, Ruff P, Sandyk R. Efficacy of a combination of sodium valproate and baclofen in Meige's disease (idiopathic orofacial dystonia). Br Med J (Clin Res Ed) 1982; 285: 853.
47. Ortiz A. Neuropharmacological profile of Meige's disease: overview and a case report. Clin Neuropharmacol 1983; 6: 297–304.
48. Altrocchi PH. Spontaneous oral-facial dyskinesia. Arch Neurol 1972; 26: 506–12.

49. Paulson GW. Meige's syndrome: dyskinesia of the eyelids and facial muscles. Geriatrics 1972; 27: 69–73.
50. Keats S. Dystonia musculorum deformans progressiva: experience with diazepam. Dis Nerv Syst 1963; 24: 624–9.
51. Asher SW, Aminoff MJ. Tetrabenazine and movement disorders. Neurology 1981; 31: 1051–4.
52. Jankovic J. Treatment of hyperkinetic movement disorders with tetrabenazine: a double-blind, placebo-controlled study. Ann Neurol 1982; 11: 41–7.
53. Kakigi R, Shibasaki H, Kuroda Y et al. Meige's syndrome associated with spasmodic dysphagia. J Neurol Neurosurg Psychiatry 1983; 46: 589–90.
54. Mandell S. The treatment of dystonia with L-dopa and haloperidol. Neurology 1970; 20: 103–6.
55. Gilbert GJ. The medical treatment of spasmodic torticollis. Arch Neurol 1972; 27: 503–6.
56. Tolosa ES, Lai C. Meige disease: striatal dopaminergic preponderance. Neurology 1979; 29: 1126–30.
57. Jankovic J, Orman J. Tetrabenazine therapy of dystonia, chorea, tics and other dyskinesias. Neurology 1988; 38: 391–4.
58. Bigwood GF. Treatment of spasmodic torticollis. N Engl J Med 1972; 286: 1161–2.
59. Lang AE, Marsden CD. Alphamethylparatyrosine and tetrabenazine in movement disorders. Clin Neuropharacol 1982; 5: 375–87.
60. Manji H, Howard RS, Miller DH et al. Status dystonicus: the syndrome and its management. Brain 1998; 121: 243–52.
61. Kang UJ, Burke RE, Fahn S. Natural history and treatment of tardive dystonia. Mov Disord 1986; 1: 193–208.
62. Lieberman JA, Saltz BL, Johns CA et al. The effects of clozapine on tardive dyskinesia. Br J Psychiatry 1991; 158: 503–10.
63. van Harten PN, Kamphuis DJ, Matroos GE. Use of clozapine in tardive dystonia. Prog Neuropsychopharmacol Biol Psychiatry 1996; 20: 263–74.
64. Friedman JH. Clozapine treatment of psychosis in patients with tardive dystonia: report of three cases. Mov Disord 1994; 9: 321–4.
65. Trugman JM, Leadbetter R, Zalis ME et al. Treatment of severe axial tardive dystonia with clozapine: case report and hypothesis. Mov Disord 1994; 9: 441–6.
66. Raja M, Maisto G, Altavista MC et al. Tardive lingual dystonia treated with clozapine. Mov Disord 1996; 11: 585–6.
67. Bouckaert F, Herman G, Peuskens J. Rapid remission of severe tardive dyskinesia and tardive dystonia with quetiapine. Int J Geriatr Psychiatry 2005; 20: 287–8.
68. Gourzis P, Polychronopoulos P, Papapetropoulos S et al. Quetiapine in the treatment of focal tardive dystonia induced by other atypical antipsychotics: a report of 2 cases. Clin Neuropharmacol 2005; 28: 195–6.
69. Hanagasi HA, Bilgic B, Gurvit H et al. Clozapine treatment in oromandibular dystonia. Clin Neuropharmacol 2004; 27: 84–6.
70. Karp BI, Goldstein SR, Chen R et al. An open trial of clozapine for dystonia. Mov Disord 1999; 14: 652–7.
71. Theil A, Dressler D, Kistel C et al. Clozapine treatment of spasmodic torticollis. Neurology 1994; 44: 957–8.
72. Burbaud P, Guehl D, Lagueny A et al. A pilot trial of clozapine in the treatment of cervical dystonia. J Neurol 1998; 245: 329–31.
73. Bimpong-Buta K, Froescher W. Carbamazepine-induced choreoathetoid dyskinesias. J Neurol Neurosurg Psychiatry 1982; 45: 560.
74. Garg BP. Dystonia musculorum deformans: implications of therapeutic response to levodopa and carbamazepine. Arch Neurol 1982; 39: 376–7.
75. Geller M, Kaplan B, Christoff N. Dystonic symptoms in children: treatment with carbamazepine. JAMA 1974; 229: 1755–7.
76. Goodenough DJ, Fariello RG, Annis Bl et al. Familial and acquired paroxysmal dyskinesias. A proposed classification with delineation of clinical features. Arch Neurol 1978; 35: 827–31.
77. Marsden CD. Blepharospasm-oromandibular dystonia syndrome (Brueghel's syndrome). J Neurol Neurosurg Psychiatry 1976; 39: 1204–9.
78. Lal S, Young SN, Kiely ME et al. Effect of L-tryptophan on spasmodic torticollis. Can J Neurol Sci 1981; 3: 305–8.
79. Myerson A, Loman J. Amphetamine sulfate in treatment of spasmodic torticollis. Arch Neurol Psychiatry 1942; 48: 823–8.
80. LeWitt PA, Miller LP, Levine RA et al. Tetrahydrobiopterin in dystonia: identification of abnormal metabolism and therapeutic trial. Neurology 1986; 36: 760–4.
81. Carella F, Girotti F, Scigliano G et al. Double-blind study of oral gamma-vinyl GABA in the treatment of dystonia. Neurology 1986; 36: 98–100.
82. ten Houten R, Lakke JPWF, de Jong P et al. Spasmodic torticollis: treatment with tizanidine. Acta Neurol Scand 1984; 70: 373–6.
83. Lang AE, Riley DE. Tizanidine in cranial dystonia. Clin Neuropharmacol 1992; 15: 142–7.
84. Granana N, Ferrea M, Scorticati MC et al. Beneficial effects of diphenhydramine in dystonia. Medicina 1999; 59: 38–42.
85. van't Groenewout JL, Stone MR, Vo VN et al. Evidence for the involvement of histamine in the antidystonic effects of diphenhydramine. Exp Neurol 1995; 134: 253–60.
86. Fasanella RM, Aghajanian GK. Treatment of benign essential blepharospasm with cyproheptadine. N Engl J Med 1990; 322: 778.
87. Fasanella RM. Relief of benign essential blepharospasm and ? memory loss by cyproheptadine. Conn Med 1993; 57: 565–6.
88. Mori K, Fujita Y, Shimabukuro H, Ito M, Handa H. Some considerations for treatment of spasmodic torticollis. Clinical and experimental studies. Confin Neurol 1975; 37: 265–9.
89. Patti F, Marano P, Nicoletti F et al. Generalized and focal dystonic syndromes: possible therapy with salmon calcitonin. Eur Neurol 1985; 24: 386–91.
90. Snider SR, Consroe P. Treatment of Meige syndrome with cannabidiol. Neurology 1984; 34(Suppl 1): 147.
91. Ohara S, Hayashi R, Momoi H et al. Mexiletine in the treatment of spasmodic torticollis. Mov Disord 1998; 13: 934–40.
92. Ohara S, Tsuyuzaki J, Hayashi R. Mexiletine in the treatment of blepharospasm: experience with the first three patients. Mov Disord 1999; 14: 173–5.
93. Lucetti C, Nuti A, Gambaccini G et al. Mexiletine in the treatment of torticollis and generalized dystonia. Clin Neuropharmacol 2000; 23: 186–9.
94. Muller J, Wenning GK, Wissel J et al. Riluzole therapy in cervical dystonia. Mov Disord 2002; 17: 198–9.
95. Sullivan KL, Hauser RA, Louis ED et al. Levetiracetam for the treatment of generalized dystonia. Parkinsonism Relat Disord 2005; 11: 469–71.
96. Yardimci N, Karatas M, Kilinc M et al. Levetiracetam in Meige's syndrome. Acta Neurol Scand 2006; 114: 63–6.
97. Tarsy D, Ryan RK, Ro SI. An open-label trial of levetiracetam for treatment of cervical dystonia. Mov Disord 2006; 21: 734–5.

18

Botulinum toxin

Ronald Tintner and Joseph Jankovic

INTRODUCTION

Dystonia is a neurologic disorder characterized by sustained, repetitive, and patterned muscle contractions that produce twisting and repetitive movements or abnormal postures.[1] Dystonia can be generalized and affect many regions of the body, including the trunk and legs, or it can be relatively focal or segmental. Focal dystonia affects a single body part and includes cervical dystonia (CD; also known as spasmodic torticollis), blepharospasm (bilateral, involuntary, synchronous, forceful eye closure), oromandibular dystonia (OMD; forceful involuntary jaw opening or closing), laryngeal dystonia (LD; spasmodic dysphonia – strained or breathy voice), and limb dystonias (task-specific focal dystonia such as writer's cramp or other occupational cramps). Generalized dystonia is usually treated with orally administered medications, intrathecal baclofen infusions, or surgery such as ablation or high-frequency stimulation of the globus pallidus or thalamus.[2]

Because of its local action, restricted to or near the site of intramuscular injection, and thus limiting side effects, botulinum toxin (BTX) has become the predominant mode of therapy for focal and segmental dystonias. The use of BTX in different forms of dystonias is covered in the respective chapters and, therefore, we concentrate here on the overlapping BTX-related issues common to all the dystonic disorders.

HISTORY

Justinus Kerner first described the clinical symptoms of food-borne botulism between 1817 and 1822 and also suggested a possible therapeutic use of BTX, which he called 'sausage poison'.[3] The symptoms associated with BTX poisoning can be categorized as generalized (fatigue, dizziness), oculomotor (double and blurred vision), oral (dysphagia, dry mouth, dysarthria, sore throat), gastrointestinal (GI) (constipation, nausea, vomiting, abdominal cramps, diarrhea), and somatic (bulbar, arm, leg, and diaphragmatic and chest muscle weakness, and paresthesias).[4,5] Botulism can be incurred not from only GI intake but also through the skin. This was initially seen after traumatic or surgical wounds, described in 1943, and after drug abuse in the mid-1980s. In 1895, Emile Van Ermengem first isolated the bacterium *Clostridium botulinum*; in 1944, Edward Schantz cultured *C. botulinum* and isolated the toxin; and in 1949, Burgen et al discovered that BTX blocks neuromuscular transmission. The first medical use for botulinum toxin was conceived and implemented by Alan Scott in 1973 for strabismus.

BTX consists of a naturally occurring group of seven peptides, produced by *C. botulinum* (CB). These are immunologically distinct neurotoxin serotypes produced by different strains of the bacterium. In addition, this bacterium also produces tetanus toxin, which acts in a similar manner.

Botulinum toxin type A (BTX-A) is the serotype used most extensively in clinical practice. A formulation of BTX-A approved for clinical use in the USA in December 1989, Botox (Allergan), was based largely on the results of two double-blind, placebo-controlled studies.[6,7] Many different botulinum toxins are now available on the market in one or more countries (Table 18.1). Four of them contain BTX-A (Botox, Dysport, Xeomin, and CBTXA), as well as a new preparation, free of complexing proteins (NT 201),[8] and the other contains BTX type B (BTX-B; Myobloc/NeuroBloc).[9,10]

Initially approved under the Orphan Drug Act, for the treatment of blepharospasm and hemifacial spasm (HFS) and strabismus, Botox was approved in December 2000 for the treatment of CD. At the same time, BTX-B (Myobloc in the USA, NeuroBloc in Europe; Elan

Table 18.1 Commercially available formulations of botulinum toxin and some characteristics

	Botox	Dysport	Xeomin	Chinese type A botulinum toxin (CBTX-A)	Neuronox	Myobloc/ NeuroBloc
Manufacturer	Allergan, Inc., Irvine, CA, USA	Ipsen Ltd, Slough, Berks, UK	Merz Pharmaceuticals, Frankfurt, Germany	Lanzhou Institute of Biological Products, Lanzhou, China	CJ Corp/Medy-Tox, Inc., South Korea	Elan plc, Dublin, Ireland
BTX serotype	A	A	A	A	A	B
Strain	Hall A	Ipsen strain	Hall A	?	?	Bean B
Site of SNARE hydrolysis	SNAP-25	SNAP-25	SNAP-25	SNAP-25	SNAP-25[b]	VAMP
Conversion factor (from Botox)	1[a]	3[a]	1[a]	1.08[c]	1[a]	40[a]
Reconstituted pH Specific biological potency, mouse units/ng BNT	Lyophilized 7.4 60	Lyophilized 7.4 100	Lyophilized 7.4 167	Lyophilized 6.0 ?	Lyophilized 6.8 ?	Solubilized 5.6 5
Other constituents (per vial)	HAS 500 μg NaCl 900 μg	HSA 125 μg Lactose 2500 μg	HSA 1 mg Sucrose 5 mg	Gelatin 5mg Dextran 25 mg Sucrose 25 mg	HSA 500 μg NaCl 900 μg	?
Stability (months)	24	15	36	?	?	24
Product-specific units/vial	100	500	100	100	100	$1.0/2.5/10.0 \times 10^3$

BTN = botulinum neurotoxin; HSA = human serum albumin.
[a]From Dressler.[169]
[b]From manufacturer PDF.
[c]From Tang and Wan.[170]

Pharmaceuticals) was approved for treatment of CD. Botulinum toxins are now used for a large number of disorders of hyperactive muscles or glands, although official approval is for a much smaller number of indications.[11–18] In the USA, both Botox and Myobloc are approved for cervical dystonia. In addition, Botox has been approved in the USA, for axillary hyperhydrosis and moderate to severe glabellar lines associated with corrugator and/or procerus muscle activity (frown lines) in adult patients less than 65 years of age.

BOTULINUM TOXIN – BASIC SCIENCE

Preparation of botulinum toxin

Current preparations of BTX are harvested and purified from the medium of cultured CB, as opposed to in-vitro synthesis. BTX-A is the serotype used most extensively in clinical practice. The material used from 1989 until 1998 (specifically for Botox) was a single batch prepared from the Hall strain of CB and consisted of a protein complex containing the neurotoxin as well as non-neurotoxic proteins. A new batch of Botox, used since 1998, has higher neurotoxic activity per mg of protein and, therefore, seems to be less antigenic (see below). While Botox is a freeze-dried preparation, Myobloc is marketed in a solubilized form.

Chemistry

Several excellent reviews of the pharmacology of BTX have been published and the reader is referred to these publications for additional information.[19–29] The botulinum neurotoxins act enzymatically at the neuromuscular junction to cleave a number of nerve terminal proteins critical to normal neurotransmitter release.[28,30] Three proteins form the so-called SNARE complex:[30] vesicle-associated membrane protein (VAMP), syntaxin, and SNAP-25 (synaptosomal protein with a molecular weight of 25 kDa). VAMP, also known as synaptobrevin, is attached to the membrane of transmitter-containing vesicles. Syntaxin and SNAP-25 are located on the inner plasma membrane of the nerve terminal. Soluble NSF (N-ethylmaleimide sensitive factor) attachment protein binds tightly to this preformed complex, which permits the association of NSF, from which is derived the term SNARE (soluble N-ethylmaleimide sensitive factor attachment protein receptor). The SNARE complex serves an essential role in synaptic transmission by bringing the synaptic vesicle membrane into close proximity to the plasma membrane to allow exocytosis of acetylcholine (ACh) or other transmitters into the synaptic cleft. This complex forms a multimeric array around the vesicle attachment site, although the exact stoichiometry of this is not known at the moment.

The BTX molecule is synthesized as a single chain and then cleaved to form a two-chain molecule with a disulfide bond joining a heavy chain and a light chain. The proposed mechanism of action involves three steps (Figure 18.1).

First, the toxin binds to a membrane receptor via the heavy chain. This imparts specificity to the site of action of BTX, as BTX introduced intracellularly can impair exocytosis in any cell. The nature of this receptor is complicated and has been the subject of years of speculation and inquiry. Current evidence suggests that the receptors are composed of gangliosides and proteins that cooperate to form high-affinity toxin-binding sites. Gangliosides seem to constitute relatively low-affinity toxin-binding sites that serve to capture *Clostridium* neurotoxins to facilitate interactions with cell surface receptor proteins. Gangliosides are ubiquitous glycosphingolipids in the outer leaflet of plasma membranes. They are classified according to the number and position of sialic acids present. Polysialiogangliosides, which are present almost exclusively in neurons and neuroendocrine cells, bind to *Clostridium* neurotoxins with the greatest affinity.[31] The protein components have recently been identified. SV2 and synaptotagmin (specifically synaptotagmin I and II), also known as Syt I and Syt II, are two proteins that span the membrane of synaptic vesicles and have domains that lie within the lumen of the vesicle. These luminal domains are exposed during cycles of exo-endocytosis. BTX-A binds to the intraluminal domain of SV2, which acts as a high-affinity binding component of the BTX-A receptor complex.[32,33] SV2 is involved in regulating the presynaptic interactions with calcium that drive vesicular exocytosis. BTX-B binds to synaptotagmins I and II. This interaction is stoichiometric, highly specific, facilitated by gangliosides, and is mediated by a region of Syt that is transiently exposed outside of cells during exocytosis.[34] Cholinergic neurons at the neuromuscular junction express Syt II and are the major physiologic target of BTX-B. Using motor neurons that innervate the diaphragm, binding and uptake of BTX-B is activity-dependent and can be blocked by synaptotagmin fragments in conjunction with gangliosides at the neuromuscular junction.[34] Synaptotagmin I (Syt I) is a less effective receptor, but at high local ganglioside concentrations, Syt I may also mediate entry of BTX-B into neurons that lack Syt II. Therefore, the sensitivity of a particular neuron terminal to BTX-B might depend on the local levels of gangliosides and whether it expresses Syt I or Syt II. Exposure of these receptors at the surface of nerve terminals also increases when a synapse

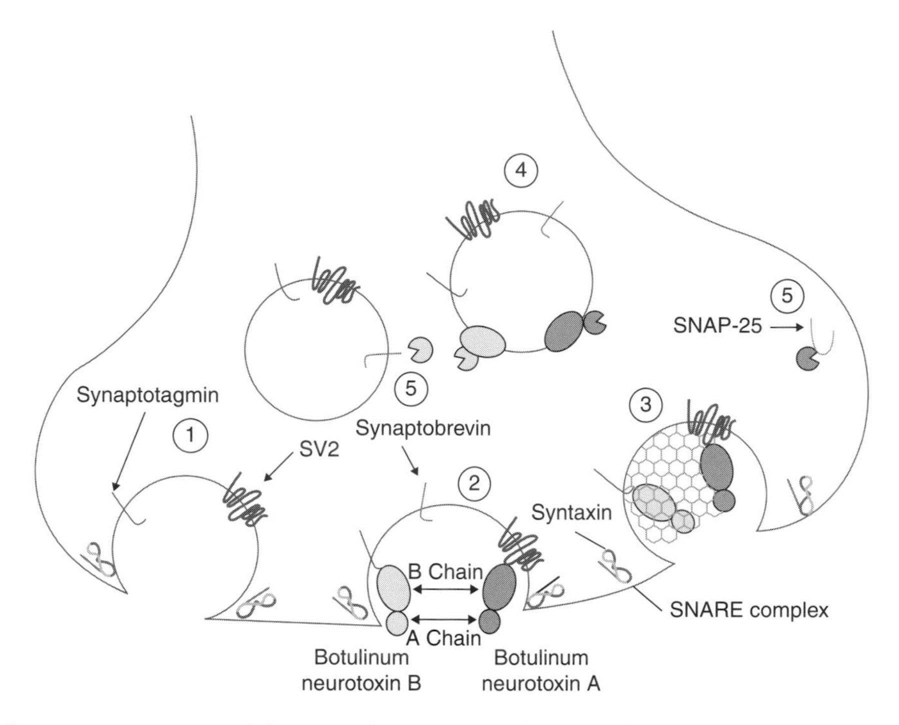

Figure 18.1 The presynaptic terminal depicting the proteins and site involved in the mechanism of action of botulinum toxins A and B. (1) The synaptic vesicle approaches and fuses with the plasma membrane. This is mediated by a multimeric complex of SNARE complexes. As this occurs, the lumen of the vesicle becomes exposed to the extracellular environment and the intraluminal domains of SV2 (for BTX-A) and synaptotagmin (for BTX-B) become exposed to the cytoplasm. (2) The two chain dimer of botulinum toxin becomes available to the intrinsic luminal domains of their receptors and their appropriate proteins. Binding is accomplished. (3) The botulinum toxin is internalized in the endocytotic membrane, within a clathrin cage, and brought within the cell. (4) Once within the cell, the toxin experiences a pH change. This results in hydrolysis of the botulinum toxin into two separate chains. The light chains become activated to act as a peptidase. (5) Cleavage of their appropriate SNARE protein (SNAP-25 for BTX-A, BTX-C, and BTX-E and synaptobrevin for BTX-B, BTX-D, BTX-F and BTX-G), disruption of the SNARE complex, and loss of exocytotic ability.

releases more ACh (i.e. actively exocytosing), thus giving the toxins an additional advantage of preferably attacking active nerve terminals. The identification of two structurally unrelated receptors for BTX-A and BTX-B sheds new light on a remarkable evolutionary adaptation. Although the toxins originated from a common ancestral precursor protein, both the A and the B chains have evolved to interact with structurally very different proteins. Syt-II also acts as receptor for BTX-G.[33–35]

It is important to remember that even if cholinergic receptors are required for BTX entry into an intact neuron, that does not mean that there is specificity for inhibition of ACh release. First, there are a variety of co-transmitters with ACh in 'cholinergic' neurons[36] and vesicular release of those co-transmitters is impaired as much as ACh, once the toxin is in the cell.

Secondly, the heavy and light chains are internalized (endocytosis). As the pH inside the endocytosome decreases, the disulfide bond that joins the heavy and light chain is enzymatically cleaved and the light chain then dissociates and is exocytosed into the cytoplasm of the presynaptic terminal.

The third step is proteolysis. Once the light chain is cleaved free, it is able to act as a zinc endopeptidase that lyses its target protein, thus preventing proper docking of the presynaptic ACh vesicle with the presynaptic membrane, and blocking the release of the neurotransmitter into the neuromuscular junction. Toxin serotypes A, C, and E hydrolyze SNAP-25, whereas serotypes B, D, F, and G cleave VAMP. BTX type C additionally cleaves syntaxin.[37] Besides lysing and inactivating the cleaved protein, the product of this hydrolysis is a truncated peptide. It has been shown that these truncated peptides can further interfere with normal organelle trafficking at the synaptic ending and the longer these abnormal truncated peptides persist, the longer the physiologic dysfunction.[38,39] The different toxins create different and differentially acting truncated peptides. In addition, the protease activity associated with the different serotypes persists for different lengths of time. Although the actual duration of the effect of different BTX serotypes varies in different species and preparations, the rank ordering does not. In an interesting biochemical study performed in rat cerebellar neurons[40] (since these experiments are not practical at motor nerve endings), the authors quantified the half-life of the effect of each toxin, the speed of replenishment of their substrates, and the degradation of the cleaved products. The half-lives of inhibition for BTX-A, BTX-C, BTX-B, BTX-F, and BTX-E were approximately 31, 25, 10, 2, and 0.8 days, respectively. This is equivalent to the neuromuscular paralysis times found in mice, and the recovery of neurotransmitter release coincided with the reappearance of the intact SNAREs. A limiting factor for the short in-vivo durations of action of BTX-F and BTX-E is the replenishment of synaptobrevin or SNAP-25, whereas the longer action of BTX-A, BTX-B, or BTX-C results from the persistence of protease activity. Hydrolysis of the intracellular docking proteins causes a functional denervation at the neuromuscular junction. When BTX-A was injected into human extensor digitorum brevis (EDB),[41] all EDB motor action potentials decreased within 48 hours, with peak decline at day 21, whereas atrophy peaked at day 42. With time (>28 days in rats) there is associated sprouting;[42] however, a second, distinct phase of the recovery process followed, with a return of vesicle turnover to the original terminals, accompanied by an elimination of the by then superfluous sprouts. It is not clear what happens with multiple injection cycles over long periods of time, but after true denervation (e.g. after peripheral nerve transaction) there is a limited period of time in which reinnervation remains possible. It is not known if this happens with chronic BTX therapy.

How does botulinum toxin work in dystonia?

Although it seems that the mechanism of BTX action is via denervation of motor endplates, other potential mechanisms of action have been proposed.[43] For example, one of the most striking and important features of BTX treatment is its ability to decrease associated sensory symptoms. The potential analgesic effect of BTX was first suggested by the observation that a higher-than-expected percentage of patients with CD experienced decreased pain and burning than could be attributed to an observable decrease in the intensity and severity of dystonic movements. BTX is extremely potent in inhibition of release, and possibly enzymatic hydrolysis of, substance P, which may be important in myopathic pain.[44,45] As a result, BTX is now being intensely studied as a potential analgesic.[46–50] Using a randomized, double-blind, paired study design, Sycha et al[51] compared the effects of 100 mouse units of BTX vs pure saline and found no direct effect on acute, non-inflammatory pain and failed to observe any anti-inflammatory effects of BTX. The strong placebo effect should always be considered when designing and interpreting studies of BTX treatment of pain disorders.[52] Thus, studies examining the effect of BTX on sensory (primarily pain) thresholds have generally not found an effect,[53] although they may show alterations in secondary effector-mediated responses such as neurogenic flare.[54,55] It is likely that sensory processes are involved at some point, as there is evidence that BTX treatment can result in changes in the central nervous system (CNS). Blood et al[56] used diffusion tensor imaging to examine six patients with primary focal dystonias. They found that all patients exhibited an abnormal white matter hemispheric asymmetry in a focal region between the pallidum and the thalamus. This asymmetry was absent 4 weeks after the same patients were treated with intramuscular botulinum toxin injections. Secondary alteration of central sensorimotor physiology and an additional primary effect on muscle spindle function may be critical in the long-term efficacy of BTX in dystonia.[57] One study demonstrated differential suppression of the tonic vibration reflex (TVR) by BTX-A treatment.[58] Specifically, 10 patients with writer's cramp were evaluated electrophysiologically before and 3 weeks after treatment. The ratio between pre- and postinjection values of maximal M-wave (M-max), maximal voluntary contraction (MVC), and TVR were measured in the injected wrist muscles. In all the subjects, BTX-A injection reduced the TVR more than the M-max and MVC. Long-term evaluation of 2 patients disclosed that, after 7 months, when some clinical benefits persisted, M-max and MVC had fully recovered, whereas the TVR was still depressed. The authors suggest that 'this special sensitivity of the TVR to suppression by BTX-A injection could be mediated by the chemodenervation of intrafusal muscle fibers, leading to a reduction in spindle inflow to the central nervous system during vibration'. This alteration in spindle afferent activity might form the basis for the treatment of dystonia with muscle afferent block[59] as well as providing a mechanism for BTX to alter sensory input to the CNS.

Dose equivalence and comparative actions of BTX preparations

Dose equivalence between formulations of BTX, even of the same serotype, remains problematic. All BTX preparations are standardized to the same type of bioassay, but the units are not therapeutically equivalent, although the reason is not clear. The two initial manufacturers of BTX-A use somewhat different bioassay methodologies, including different dilution media, which differentially activate the enzyme. The activity of the preparations has been expressed as mouse units, where 1 unit (U) is the median lethal intraperitoneal dose in mice. This assay measures the potency of the toxin–protein complex to traverse the journey from peritoneum to site of lethality (probably the respiratory and laryngeal musculature); thus, factors protective in the systemic milieu that increase potency in this assay, such as the non-neurotoxic proteins that are part of the BTX complex, may be irrelevant in the milieu of the muscle itself. In one direct comparison study using the same mouse lethality assay system, Botox was 2.86 times as potent as Dysport,[60] which is close to other estimates of Dysport:Botox ratio.[61,62] In another study of CD, Dysport at 3:1 was a little more effective than Botox, with a few more side effects, suggesting an equivalency ratio less than 3:1,[63] whereas a study on writer's cramp found that 1 unit of Botox was roughly equivalent to about 3.5 units of Dysport.[64] A bioassay that assesses local effects of regional denervation in muscle may be an appropriate method to assess relative potency of BTX,[65] but in-vitro assays have been also proposed.[66,67] It has been suggested that each BTX product can be considered as a unique drug and the idea of standard assay can be abandoned.[68]

Calculating equivalent doses of BTX-A and BTX-B is even more uncertain. Sloop et al[69] compared the dose–response (DR) curves, maximal paralysis, and post-exercise M-wave facilitation of BTX-A and BTX-B by injecting in EDB. They demonstrated that human muscle paralysis resulting from BTX-B injection is not as complete or long-lasting as that resulting from BTX-A. Whether M-wave amplitude is a reliable measure of clinical response and whether the doses of BTX-A and BTX-B, with B/A ratio of about 45:1, are comparable is, however, debatable. There is some evidence in patients who receive BTX for cosmesis that BTX-B has a quicker onset of action and BTX-A has longer benefit for glabellar wrinkles,[70] but this has not been confirmed by well-designed, controlled studies. One controlled, but not blinded, study of 30 consecutive patients treated with BTX-B, of which 5 patients also received BTX-A, suggested that BTX-B may have more autonomic side effects than BTX-A, an observation consistent with descriptions of clinical botulism.[71] In patients with CD, side effects consisted of dryness of mouth (total 21/24, duration 4.4 ± 2.0 SD weeks, 10 severe, 7 moderate, 4 mild), accommodation difficulties (7), conjunctival irritation (5), reduced sweating (4), swallowing difficulties (3), heartburn (3), constipation (3), bladder voiding difficulties (2), head instability (1), dryness of nasal mucosa (1), and thrush (1). In 6 patients with focal hyperhidrosis, side effects consisted of accommodation difficulties (4), dryness of mouth (2), and conjunctival irritation (1). The authors concluded that autonomic side effects occur far more often after BTX-B than after BTX-A, suggesting systemic spread of BTX-B. There is a report on three individual patients who received BTX-B and who subsequently developed parasympathetic dysfunction of the visual system after injections of BTX-B at remote sites.[72] In a prospective study, however, using both quantitative physiologic measurements as well as questionnaires, patients with CD were randomized to receive either BTX-A or BTX-B in a double-blind manner. Efficacy and physiologic questionnaire measures of autonomic function were assessed at baseline and 2 weeks after injection. Patients treated with BTX-B had significantly less saliva production and greater severity of constipation than those treated with BTX-A, but did not differ in other tests of autonomic functions.[73]

In a study by the Dystonia Study Group, subjects with CD who had a previous response from BTX-A were randomly assigned to BTX-A or BTX-B at 1:40 U dose ratio, and evaluated in a blinded fashion at baseline, 4 weeks, 8 weeks, and 2-week intervals thereafter until loss of 80% of clinical effect or completion of 20 weeks of observation. Of a total of 139 subjects (BTX-A, n = 74; BTX-B, n = 65), dysphagia and dry mouth were significantly more frequent with BTX-B (dysphagia, BTX-A 19% vs BTX-B 48%; dry mouth, BTX-A 41% vs BTX-B 80%).[74] This finding of increased autonomic nervous system (ANS) adverse effects, may be partially a factor of initial exposure, since in a multiple injection study: 'Dry mouth frequency decreased with each session despite increasing doses whereas flu-like syndrome and weakness increased'.[75]

THERAPEUTIC TRIALS

Blepharospasm and hemifacial spasm

Blepharospasm is a focal cranial dystonia characterized by sustained, involuntary spasms of the orbicularis oculi muscle, resulting in eyelid closure. HFS is another disorder associated with, usually unilateral, eyelid spasms with additional involvement of other facial nerve innervated muscles. HFS, however, is not a dystonia but rather a peripherally induced movement disorder due to hyperexcitability of the facial nerve (usually due to compression of the facial nerve by a vascular loop).

BTX injections in the orbicularis oculi have become the primary therapeutic modality for both blepharospasm and HFS. In the first published double-blind placebo-controlled trial of BTX-A, all 12 patients with blepharospasm improved by 72% in the severity score and by 61% in the self-assessment score.[7] There have been several open trials since. In a long-term follow up of 90 treated patients there was moderate or marked improvement in 94% with 12.4 weeks duration of maximum, but longer duration of any, effect. In all, 41% of patients reported some adverse effects (ptosis, blurred vision, diplopia, tearing); in all but 2% of affected patients, the side effects generally spontaneously resolved within 2 weeks.[76] In another report of long term clinical experience with BTX-A for blepharospasm,[77] of 178 cases followed between 1980 and 2001, 10 were lost to follow-up; of the remaining patients, 93% reported improvement after treatments. The mean duration of improvement was 3.6 months. Twelve patients (76%) who underwent more than 14 treatments maintained stable relief. Three patients (1.7%) had a total remission of spasms. Side effects were exclusively local. In yet another 10-year experience, it was shown that over the long term, there is neither loss of efficacy nor increased dose requirement and the frequency of complications tends to decline with repeat injections.[78] More recently, NT 201 has been studied in 300 patients with blepharospasm, 256 of whom completed the study, and found no difference in efficacy or adverse effects between NT 201 and Botox. The adjusted mean change in the Jankovic Rating Scale was −2.90 for the NT 201 and −2.67 for the Botox group; the frequency of ptosis, the most common adverse effect, was 6.08% and 4.52%, respectively.[79]

A 2005 Cochrane Database Review[80] concluded that:

> There are no high quality, randomised, controlled efficacy data to support the use of BTX for blepharospasm. Despite this, other studies suggest that BTX is highly effective and safe for treating blepharospasm and support its use. The effect size (90% of patients benefit) seen in open studies makes it very difficult and probably unethical to perform new placebo-controlled trials of efficacy of BTX for blepharospasm.

An open trial with BTX-B[81] in patients non-responsive to BTX-A (that were AB positive) found generally disappointing results in patients with blepharospasm and HFS.

There is an ongoing debate surrounding the optimal injection sites. The orbicularis oculi consists of three portions:

- an orbital portion, surrounding the orbital margin, including the brow
- a palpebral (tarsal or septal) portion consisting of thin bundles of fibers that concentrically cross the eyelids in front of the orbital septum
- at the lid margin (pretarsal portion of the orbicularis oculi), a small group of fine muscle fibers known as the ciliary (or Riolan's) muscle.

Price et al[82] compared four different treatment site applications in a prospective trial of 92 patients with blepharospasm and HFS. Patients were assigned randomly to one of four different treatment groups: standard (medial and lateral aspects of upper eyelid, and lateral and central portion of lower eyelid), brow (medial and lateral aspects of upper eyebrow and lateral and central portion of lower eyelid), inner orbital (medial to the lateral orbital margin), or outer orbital (just lateral to the lateral orbital margin). In the patients with blepharospasm, those assigned to the standard group had a significantly longer duration of effect than for those in the other groups, whereas of the patients with HFS, those in the outer orbital group had significantly shorter duration of effect than those in the other groups. The inner orbital treatment produced significantly more episodes of ptosis (13% of treatments). However, the standard treatment produced the most epiphora and ocular irritation (18% of treatments). Thus, the standard treatment produces the longest duration of effect in the blepharospasm group but with the most transient ocular irritation and epiphora. In the HFS group, the brow treatment had an equally long duration of effect as that of the standard treatment, with fewer side effects. It is not clear from the methods section exactly where in the eyelids the injections were made: i.e. relative to the inferior margin of the upper eyelid. Another controlled study showed that an injection in the most inferior aspect (pretarsal) rather than septal portions of the orbicularis oculi is associated with significantly less ptosis.[83] In 10 patients with blepharospasm treated unsuccessfully with bilateral periorbital injections, injecting BTX into the pretarsal region of the orbicularis oculi proved to be highly efficacious; in addition, 26/30 of the patients with hemifacial spasm preferred these ciliary injections.[84] Other studies have confirmed the superior efficacy of pretarsal injection in patients with blepharospasm.[85,86]

Oromandibular dystonia (see Chapter 9)

Oromandibular dystonia consists of involuntary spasms of masticatory, lingual, and pharyngeal muscles, resulting in jaw closing dystonia (JCD), jaw opening dystonia (JOD), jaw deviation dystonia (JDD), or a combination of these abnormal movements, and its management represents a formidable challenge. For JCD, the masseters, temporalis, or internal pterygoids may be injected; for JOD, the submentalis complex or external pterygoids, and for JDD, various combinations may be needed. We have reviewed the use of BTX in these conditions at greater length recently.[87] Tan and Jankovic[88] reported their long-term experience with BTX for OMD in 162 patients over a period of 10 years (mean follow-up period = 4.4 years). More than half the patients had JCD. BTX treatments were administered into the masseter muscles, submentalis complex, or both. The mean doses (± SD) of BTX (per side) were 54 ± 15 U for the masseters and 29 ± 17 U for the submentalis complex. The mean total duration of response was 16 ± 7 weeks. The mean global effect of BTX was 3.1 (range 0–4, where 4 equals the complete abolition of the dystonia). A score >3, was seen in 80% of the JCD patients, but in only 40% of the JOD, 33% of the JDD and 52% of the mixed dystonia patients. Adverse effects were reported in at least one visit in 31.5% of patients with BTX and complications such as dysphagia and dysarthria were reported in 11% of all treatment visits. Using a broader range of muscles and electromyographic (EMG) localization, Brin et al[89] also found that patients with JOD and JDD may not respond as well as those with JCD.

Bruxism is a diurnal or nocturnal jaw activity manifested by clenching, grinding, bracing, and gnashing of the teeth. Possibly a manifestation of dystonia, bruxism is a common occurrence in otherwise normal individuals. However, it does seem to appear more frequently in patients with dystonia and was present in 79% of 79 patients with cranial-CD.[90] In an open trial of 18 subjects with severe bruxism, BTX-A injections of the masseter muscles (mean dose 62 U per side, range 25–100 U) were an effective treatment.[91] The mean peak effect on a scale of 0–4 (4 is equal to total abolishment of grinding) was 3.4; mean total duration of response was 19 weeks. Only one subject reported dysphagia.

Laryngeal dystonia (spasmodic dysphonia) (see Chapter 11)

Laryngeal dystonia may produce strained or breathy voice, referred to as spasmodic dysphonia (SD), which has been categorized primarily into adductor spasmodic dysphonia (strain-strangled voice interrupted by voiceless pauses), which accounts for the vast majority of cases of LD, and abductor spasmodic dysphonia (whispering, breathy voice). Prior to the introduction of BTX, treatment consisted of speech therapy or unilateral nerve resections, neither of which was completely satisfactory. The use of BTX in SD has been reviewed elsewhere.[92,93] In contrast to the adductor form of SD, which is easily managed with BTX, the abductor form of SD is more difficult to treat. Blitzer et al[94] performed a retrospective analysis of a 12-year experience in which more than 900 patients with SD were treated with BTX. While the adductor patients, injected into the thyroarytenoid muscle, had an average benefit of 90% of normal function (lasting an average of 15 weeks), the abductor patients, usually injected into the posterior cricoarytenoid muscle, had an average benefit of 67% of normal function (lasting an average of 11 weeks). Adverse effects included mild breathiness and coughing on fluids in the adductor patients, and mild stridor in a few of the abductor patients.

The primary controversy involving the use of BTX in SD involves technique. The main approaches now used are percutaneous injection through the cricothyroid membrane under EMG guidance, either unilaterally or bilaterally, or transorally under visual laryngoscopic control. The main side effect is prolonged breathy hypophonia, which is seen more with large bilateral injections. Langeveld et al[95] compared unilateral (5 U in the left thyroarytenoid muscle) and bilateral (2.5 U in both sides) percutaneous BTX-A injections in a prospective, crossover study in 27 patients with adductor spasmodic dysphonia. Voice quality, duration of effect, and side effects were assessed. There was no difference between the procedures in duration of voice improvement or in the occurrence of breathy dysphonia. Although more patients preferred the bilateral injection, this approach was associated with more and longer-lasting side effects, particularly dysphagia. A large Australian clinical experience has also been reported;[96] a consecutive series of 169 patients with SD were studied prospectively, of whom 144 were treated with BTX injections between 1983 and 1999. Adductor SD (89.4%) was more frequent than abductor SD (1.8%) or mixed SD (4.7%). The median treatment outcome score was excellent in 63.2%, very good in 18.5%, satisfactory in 14.7% and unsatisfactory in 3.5% of patients. Poorer treatment outcome was associated with abductor SD (odds ratio [OR] = 4.69, confidence interval [CI] = 1.23–17.92 and age >65 years old (OR = 2.83, CI = 0.95–8.42). Mild post-injection paralytic dysphonia was associated with longer-lasting treatment and superior treatment outcome rating. The authors hypothesize that mild post-injection paralytic dysphonia may be a marker for more effective and lasting treatment in adductor SD. BTX-B has been reported in cases to also be effective for SD.[97]

Warrick et al[98] examined the efficacy of BTX-A for the closely related entity of voice tremor using either a bilateral 2.5 U or a unilateral 15 U EMG-guided injection, followed by the other injection type 16–18 weeks later. A minority of patients demonstrated objective reduction of tremor; however, 8 of 10 patients wished to be reinjected at the conclusion of the study. A reduction in vocal effort appeared to be coincident with reduction in laryngeal airway resistance after BTX injection.

In another study unilateral and bilateral injections were compared.[99] Sixteen patients received unilateral injections (72 injections total) and 33 patients bilateral injections (133 injections total). Individual assignments to injection type were based on treatment previously received and dose was adjusted according to the patient's previous treatment response rather than on any kind of randomized basis. Compared to patients receiving bilateral injections, those patients receiving unilateral injections more frequently noted a statistically significant benefit of ≥3 months, side effects of ≤2 weeks duration, as well as simultaneous 3-month benefit. Injection type had no effect on optimal BTX dosing with repeat injections. These authors concluded that unilateral injections provided a more optimal and consistent efficacy/side-effect profile.

Treatment with BTX for SD results in improved quality of life. In 5 patients with OMD and 18 with SD, BTX-A injections were effective on the basis of quality-of-life criteria.[100] The mean total benefit score on the Glasgow Benefit Inventory, which was used to quantify the health benefit of treatment, was +38.04 (possible range = −100 to +100). Also in a study of 27 consecutive new patients presenting with SD, voice-related quality of life (V-RQOL) was low and botulinum toxin injections improved it significantly for each injection cycle studied.[101]

Cervical dystonia (see Chapter 8)

Cervical dystonia is the most common form of focal dystonia seen in movement disorders clinics. It consists of jerky or sustained, but nearly always patterned (same muscles involved), movements of the head and neck. The goal of treatment of CD is not only to treat the abnormal postures and associated neck pain but also to prevent secondary complications such as contractures, cervical radiculopathy, and myelopathy.[102] This topic has been reviewed in recent articles.[103–105]

Muscle selection

Several muscles are involved in neck movement, particularly the sternocleidomastoid (SCM), splenius capitus, scalenus complex, levator scapulae, and semispinalis capitis. One of the challenges in BTX treatment of CD has been to determine which muscles to inject. This difficulty is compounded by the fact that multiple muscle combinations can produce the same movements, the particular pattern of abnormal muscle activity is highly individualized, and that antagonist muscles may contract more intensely and may be more hypertrophic than the agonist muscles. Only the latter group of muscles should be targeted for BTX injection. Although some investigators have suggested that after injection of BTX, the pattern of muscle activity may change,[106] this is quite rare in our experience. Some investigators have also shown that although there are no further changes in the EMG activity of the injected SCM subsequent to the first dose of BTX-A, there may be a progressive change in the contralateral (i.e. antagonist) muscle.[107]

Selection of methods used to target and inject muscles remains controversial: i.e. it should be determined solely by clinical inspection or with the addition of EMG analysis. Even the specifics of 'EMG guidance' can vary. EMG can be used to confirm localization of the needle to a muscle or confirm and possibly quantify the occurrence of specific muscular activity during ongoing dystonic movements.[108–111] In comparison to an EMG mapping study, the clinical predictions of individual muscle involvement by four movement disorder specialists were only 59% sensitive and 75% specific. Muscle hypertrophy, shoulder elevation, and dominant head vector did not bolster clinical accuracy.[112] One study showed that patients did better with EMG-guided than strictly clinically guided injections.[113] The difference in the overall magnitude of this effect was, however, small and there was no difference between groups in the number of patients returning for booster injections. Although patients with retrocollis, head tilt, and shoulder elevation in particular demonstrated additional benefit with EMG-guided Botox injection, the patients that did not have EMG assistance got higher doses of Botox, suggesting more severe disease. In the Dystonia Study Group Botulinum Toxin A vs B in cervical dystonia trial, there was no benefit shown for patients that received EMG guidance, although the study was not designed to answer this question.[114] We reserve EMG for non-responding patients or those in whom proper identification of the target muscle by palpation is difficult. This issue is discussed at length in a position paper by one of the authors (JJ).[115] Frequency of individual muscle involvement and typical BTX doses in CD are given in the Table 18.2.

Other localization techniques may become useful in the future and may include anatomically based methods such as ultrasonography.[59] An excellent mode of visualizing exactly which muscles were being injected was

Table 18.2 Cervical muscles frequently injected with botulinum toxin (BTX): functions, relative involvement in cervical dystonia, and typical botulinum toxin doses

Muscle	Action	BTX (U)[a]
Sternocleidomastoid	Contralateral rotation; anterior flexion	40–70
Trapezius	Elevation of scapula and shoulder, extension of neck	25–100
Splenius capitis	Ipsilateral rotation; extension of neck	60–100
Levator scapulae	Elevate scapulae and shoulder	25–60
Scalene complex	Ipsilateral turn with neck flexion (anterocollis)	15–50
Deep post-vertebrals:	Ipsilateral tilt, neck extension	
Longissimus capitis		55–90
Semispinalis capitis		30–60
Hyoid muscles	Head flexion (anterocollis)	10–30

From Dressler.[171]
Movements refer to the neck; maximal involvement = 1.
[a]Botox units.

described in a paper using BTX to denervate the scalene muscles in apparent neurogenic thoracic outlet syndrome.[116] The muscles were first localized with EMG, then BTX-A was co-administered with radiopaque dye under fluoroscopy. The degree of confirmation with this technique is far greater than with EMG, but as yet there are no proponents for widespread use of this technique. Computed tomography (CT) has also been used.[117]

Efficacy

The efficacy of BTX in CD has been demonstrated in both controlled and open-label trials[118, 119] and in an evidence-based medicine criteria analysis.[120, 121] In one double-blind placebo-controlled trial, 61% of patients injected with BTX-A improved; 74% of patients subsequently improved during a later open phase at a higher dose of Botox.[122] In general, improvement rates run from as low as 65%, but no complete improvement, to as high as 92%, and near-complete improvement in 83%, with further improvement after repeated treatments being seen up to 5 years. A recent large-scale retrospective analysis (616 patients) with BTX-A showed sustained significant benefit, as measured by a disease severity score, independent of the type of CD. Pronounced individual differences were found in response to this treatment, even in patients with similar initial clinical scores and doses of BTX-A. Whereas secondary non-response was seen in about 5% of patients, antibody tests revealed neutralizing serum antibodies in only 2%.[123] Lew et al[124] have reviewed the prior studies with BTX-B, which taken together, showed about a 25% reduction in the TWSTRS (Toronto Western Spasmodic Torticollis Rating Scale) score and duration of action of 12–16 weeks.[125–127] The two pivotal studies, one using BTX-A (Botox) and the other BTX-B (Myobloc), that led to the approval of BTX by the Food and Drug Administration (FDA) in CD, have not been published, but have been recently reviewed.[119]

CD may also cause pain outside the neck per se. BTX-A safely improved headache associated with craniocervical dystonia when administered for the primary condition of craniocervical dystonia, measured with headache diaries, Headache Impact Test (HIT-6), and Migraine Disability Assessment Scale (MIDAS).[128]

Complications

The most common complication of BTX for CD is pharyngeal weakness manifested by dysphagia. Although usually mild and rarely disabling, it may require a change to a soft diet to prevent aspiration.[129] In one study, 33% of patients receiving their first dose of BTX experienced dysphagia and a greater number displayed radiographic swallowing abnormalities.[113] Dysphagia has been reported to occur on average 9.7 days after injection and last on average 3.5 weeks.[123] Dysphagia most commonly occurs with bilateral injections of the SCM or scalenus muscles, presumably because of local spread of the toxin from these muscles to posterior pharyngeal muscles. This complication may occur less frequently if the biologic activity of the toxin is contained within the target muscle by using multiple small injections rather than a single large bolus.[130] Neck weakness is the second most common local complication following BTX treatment of CD. In addition, BTX-B has a relatively high incidence of injection site pain and dry mouth.[124–127] It is not clear whether the dry mouth noted with BTX-B was present but interpreted as dysphagia in a subset of the patients in the earlier trials with BTX-A.

Although BTX has been considered the treatment of choice for CD, it has been formally compared to medical therapy in only one study. Brans et al[131] compared the effectiveness of BTX-A with that of trihexyphenidyl in a prospective, randomized, double-blind design. Sixty-six consecutive patients with idiopathic CD were randomized to treatment with trihexyphenidyl tablets plus placebo injection or placebo tablets plus BTX-A injections. Dysport or saline was injected under EMG guidance at study entry and again after 8 weeks. Patients were assessed for efficacy at baseline and after 12 weeks by different clinical rating scales. Sixty-four patients completed the study, 32 in each group. Mean dose of BTX-A was 292 U (first session) and 262 U (second session). Mean dose of trihexyphenidyl was 16.2 mg. The changes on the Disability section of the TWSTRS (TWSTRS-Disability) (primary outcome), Tsui Scale, and the General Health Perception Subscale were significantly improved in favor of BTX-A. Furthermore, adverse effects were significantly less frequent in the BTX-A group.

Dosing

Several studies have attempted to determine optimum dosing in patients with CD. Poewe et al[132] performed a prospective multicenter placebo-controlled double-blind dose ranging study in a homogeneous group of previously untreated patients with rotational torticollis to obtain objective data on DR relations. Seventy-five patients were randomly assigned to receive treatment with placebo or total doses of 250, 500, and 1000 Dysport U divided between one splenius capitis and the contralateral SCM. Seventy nine percent reported subjective improvement at one or more follow-up visits. Decreases in the modified Tsui scale score were significant at week 4 for the 500 and 1000 U groups vs placebo. There was a positive relation between dose injected and the duration of clinical benefit. Ninety-four percent of patients treated with placebo and about 50% of patients receiving 200 and 500 U requested reinjection by 8 weeks, whereas only 39% of those having received 1000 U asked for a second treatment by this time. A dose relation was also established for the number of adverse events overall and for the incidence of neck muscle weakness and voice changes. They concluded that although magnitude and duration of improvement was greatest after injections of 1000 U of Dysport, it was at the cost of significantly more adverse events. They suggested a starting dose of 500 U Dysport, with upward titration if clinically necessary.

Another double-blind, randomized study, involving 31 patients with CD (patients had received at least two previous Dysport injections), examined low-dose therapy.[133] The patients received either a mean total target dose of 547 ± 113 mouse units (MU) at a concentration of 500 MU Dysport/ml or a 4-times-diluted preparation of 130 ± 32 MU at a concentration of 125 MU Dysport/ml). TWSTRS and self-rating before and after injection revealed comparable clinical improvement in both groups; however, 3 patients in the low-dose group received reinjections due to insufficient effects from the previous injection. These findings again suggest that low-dose treatment of CD with Dysport may be clinically effective during maintenance therapy, at least for a limited period of time. The authors suggest that the low-dose Dysport effects may have been potentiated by the long-lasting effects of previous Dysport treatments at conventional doses.

Resistance and other clinical factors

Several factors can influence failure to respond to BTX. Primary non-response results from contractures (long-standing disease), insufficient dosage of BTX, injection of the incorrect muscles, or some other technical factor (e.g. failure to properly prepare the BTX). In CD, about half of these patients will subsequently benefit from BTX injections.[134] More recently, in a long-term study (median 5.5 years, range 1.5–10 years)[135] in 78 patients with idiopathic CD, treatment with BTX-A was assessed using patient and treating neurologist scores as well as 'Global Burden of Disease', as expressed on Visual Analog Scales (VAS, 0–10). By combining these outcome measures, 67% of the patients were characterized as having a good effect, and 33% an unsatisfactory effect. This outcome (good or unsatisfactory effect) was independent of the severity of head deviation or complexity pattern of CD prior to treatment, the delay from onset to start of BTX treatment, or the number of treatments. The complexity pattern remained stable during treatment in 64% of the patients, became less complex in 19%, whereas 17% of the patients developed more complex patterns.

EMG may be required to properly localize the muscles primarily responsible for the dystonic posture in the patients that do not respond well.[134] However, even after these factors are considered, some patients will still fail to benefit. This is believed to result from the involvement of inaccessible deep neck musculature, but no studies have specifically analyzed these patients.

Cervical dystonia is due to a number of different etiologies, including genetic predisposition, local trauma, and certain drugs, which may affect the responsiveness to BTX. In one study, the response of patients with tardive CD was similar to that of idiopathic CD, although the tardive patients required higher BTX-A doses by about 30%, partly because of greater pain, larger muscles, and more complicated movements.[136] Acute-onset CD (occurring within 4 weeks of trauma) is characterized by markedly reduced cervical mobility, prominent shoulder elevation with trapezius hypertrophy, isometric contraction of the affected muscles without involuntary movements, lack of effect of sensory tricks, or activation maneuvers. Although patients with post-traumatic CD do not generally respond to BTX injections as well as patients with idiopathic dystonia, this is usually the most effective treatment, particularly for pain relief. By contrast, delayed-onset CD (between 3 months and 1 year after trauma) is clinically indistinguishable from non-traumatic idiopathic CD with respect to response to BTX.[137]

In a multicenter study of 100 patients with cervical dystonia, we examined the immunogenicity of BTX-B and correlated the clinical response with the presence of blocking antibodies using a novel mouse protection assay. A third of the patients who were negative for BTX-B antibodies at baseline became positive for BTX-B antibodies at last visit. Thus, the high antigenicity of BTX-B limits its long-term efficacy.[138]

Writer's cramp and other limb dystonias and tremors (see Chapter 10)

Most limb dystonias consist of position- or task-specific dystonias such as writer's and musician's cramp, but also include foot dystonias. The latter is typically present in children with generalized dystonia, such as DYT1 dystonia, or adults with Parkinson's disease. Prior to BTX, treatment with systemic agents or local surgery rarely provided satisfactory results.

Muscle selection

Large groups of muscles can be localized clinically. Although writer's cramp and other hand and distal arm dystonias can affect both flexor and extensor muscles, success can usually be achieved by injecting the forearm flexor compartment exclusively, with little significant morbidity, whereas wrist drop after injection of extensors is not uncommon. When more precise determination of muscles is needed, especially if there are relatively high risks of clinically significant morbidity, EMG guidance is needed for correct localization of desired limb muscles.[64] In one study, the accuracy of muscle localization in 38 muscles in patients with focal hand dystonia without EMG guidance was examined.[139] Only 37% of needle placement attempts reached the target muscles or muscle fascicles.

Clinical efficacy

Jankovic and Schwartz[137] injected forearm muscles with BTX-A in 130 treatment sessions for writer's cramp without EMG guidance – 116 into wrist flexors and 52 into wrist extensors. The average peak response was 2.3 (0 = none to 4 = maximum), average latency to onset was 5.6 days, and average duration of response was 9.2 weeks. Temporary hand weakness occurred in 54% of all patients. However, the frequency of adverse effects has, dramatically increased since the initial report, as a result of using lower doses in specific, targeted muscles most involved in the production of the abnormal movement or posture. In an open-label prospective analysis, Pullman et al[140] injected BTX-A into selected upper and lower limb muscles under EMG guidance in 187 patients with limb disorders, including 136 with dystonia, during an 8-year period. Average BTX efficacy (calculated as an arithmetic combination of changes in the three clinical ratings before and after administration of BTX) was 65% overall and 83.5% for focal hand dystonia. BTX-A injections relieved pain, independent of motor function, in 82.7% of patients with painful muscle spasms. The only notable adverse effect of BTX injection in limbs was transient weakness in injected or neighboring muscles. Over a 5-year period, Ross et al[141] treated 40 patients with hand dystonias with BTX-A using either standard EMG recording of voluntary potentials or muscle twitch stimulation guide injection. Moderate to complete improvement in dystonia occurred in 28 patients (70%) after the first injection and in 34 patients (85%) after the second. Of note, weakness of uninjected muscles, immediately adjacent to those injected, was found in 25/40 patients (63%). Spread to, and weakness of, adjacent uninjected muscles was a major factor contributing to suboptimal outcome in 6/39 (15%) such patients.[141] A randomized, placebo-controlled trial of BTX-A for writer's cramp has also been performed.[142] Forty participants were randomized to treatment with either BTX-A or placebo injections in two sessions; the trial duration was 12 weeks. The primary outcome measure was the patient's decision to continue the particular treatment. In addition, clinical rating scales of impairment and disability were used as secondary outcome measures. Assessments were made at baseline and 2 months (secondary outcomes) and 3 months (primary outcome), but patients were followed for a total of 1 year. Fourteen of 20 patients (70%) receiving BTX-A vs 6 of 19 patients (31.6%) in the placebo group ($p = 0.03$) chose to continue treatment. The changes on most of the clinical rating scales were also significantly in favor of BTX-A. Side effects reported were hand weakness, which was mostly mild and always transient, and pain at the injection site. After 1 year, 20 of 39 patients were still under treatment with perceived benefit.

The observation that some patients treated for focal dystonia with BTX noted improvement in their tremor led to studies examining the effects of BTX specifically on tremor. In a placebo-controlled study,[143] 25 patients with hand tremor of 2+ (moderate) to 4+ (severe) on the tremor severity rating scale were randomized to receive either 50 U of BTX or placebo injections into the wrist flexors and extensors of the dominant limb. If patients failed to respond to the initial injection, they were eligible to receive another injection of 100 U 4 weeks later. Rest, postural, and kinetic tremors were evaluated at 2–4-week intervals over a 16-week study period, using tremor severity rating scales, accelerometry, and assessments of improvement and disability. Four weeks after injection, 75% of BTX-treated patients vs 27% of placebo-treated patients ($p < 0.05$) reported mild to moderate improvement (peak effect rating >2) and this effect was maintained for the duration of the study. There were no significant improvements in functional rating scales, although trends were observed for some items. Postural accelerometry measurements showed a greater than 30% reduction in amplitude in 9 of 12 BTX-treated subjects and in 1 of 9 placebo-treated subjects ($p < 0.05$). Although all patients treated with BTX reported some degree of finger weakness, no severe, irreversible, or unexpected adverse events occurred. This and other studies[144] have demonstrated that chemodenervation with BTX may significantly ameliorate essential tremor in patients who fail to improve with conventional pharmacologic therapy. As a result of long-term experience with hundreds of patients treated with BTX for various tremors, we have modified our protocol and have markedly decreased the dosage in the forearm extensor muscles (to <15 U) with little or no finger extensor weakness.

Although BTX is clearly a useful treatment in some patients with hand tremor, it has been found particularly effective in patients with head tremor.[145]

RESISTANCE TO BOTULINUM TOXIN – ANTIBODY DEVELOPMENT

Secondary failure to respond to BTX usually indicates the development of immunoresistance due to neutralizing antibodies. Antibody development relates to the inverse of the specific biologic activity, and this has been determined for the different preparations of BTX.[146] For Botox, the specific biologic activity is 60 MU-EV/ng neurotoxin, for Dysport 100 MU-EV/ng neurotoxin, and for Myobloc/NeuroBloc 5 MU-EV/ng neurotoxin. For Myobloc/NeuroBloc this has been calculated by these authors to translate into an antibody-induced therapy failure rate of 44% in patients treated for cervical dystonia, whereas for BTX-A preparations this figure is approximately 5%. Although neutralizing antibodies have been thought to develop in less than 10% of treated patients,[147] more recent studies of BTX-A and BTX-B in patients treated for CD suggest a frequency as high as 18%, according to yet unpublished data.[119]

We analyzed longitudinal follow-up data on 45 patients (32 women; mean age, 68.8 years) currently followed in the Baylor College of Medicine Movement Disorders Clinic, who have received BTX treatments continuously for at least 12 years (mean 15.8 ± 1.5 years).[148] Antibody (Ab) testing was carried out in 22 patients due to non-responsiveness; blocking Abs were confirmed by the mouse protection assay in 4 of 22 (18%) patients. Of the Ab-negative patients, 16 resumed responsiveness after dose adjustments and 2 persisted as non-respondents.

The development of neutralizing antibodies is a serious problem because it essentially eliminates future response to that type of BTX, but the patient may respond to an alternative serotype of BTX.[126] However, the high antigenicity of BTX-B limits its long-term efficacy.[138] Four of nine patients (44%) with cervical dystonia receiving BT-B (NeuroBloc/Myobloc, Elan Pharmaceuticals) experienced complete therapy failure with BT-B-AB titers in excess of 10 mU/ml on the mouse diaphragm assay.[149] This pilot result was confirmed in a multicenter study of 100 patients with cervical dystonia; one-third of the patients who were negative for BTX-B Abs at baseline became positive for BTX-B antibodies at the last visit.[138]

A new batch of Botox has been used since 1997. It has a higher activity per mg protein, but comparable unit efficacy[150] and, because of the lower protein load, it promised to have a lower risk of antibody production. A double-blind, multicenter study crossover design of 133 patients compared the efficacy and safety of BTX-A (Botox) produced from both original and current bulk toxin sources for the treatment of CD.[151] Adverse events were assessed at each visit. Efficacy was assessed at 2 and 6 weeks post-injection using the severity and pain-disability subscales of the TWSTRS. Efficacy and adverse effects and dosing were virtually identical after treatment with either batch of BTX-A. In our experience, this new preparation decreased the risk of antibody formation by a factor of six.[152] In a retrospective comparison of 130 patients treated for CD with original Botox, 42 of whom were exposed only to the original BTX-A used before 1998 (25 ng protein/100 U), and 119 treated only with the current BTX type A (5 ng of protein/100 U), blocking antibodies were detected in 4 of 42 (9.5%) patients treated only with original BTX-A but in none of the 119 patients treated exclusively with current BTX type A ($p < 0.004$). However, a patient with craniocervical dystonia injected with the new, lower-protein formulation of BTX-A who developed secondary resistance has been reported,[153] with subsequent reduction of blepharospasm with BTX-B.

Detection of blocking antibodies

There are several methods for detecting blocking antibodies in patients who lose responsiveness to BTX. The gold standard is the highly specific, but relatively insensitive and cumbersome assay, the mouse protection assay (MPA), which evaluates the ability of increasing dilutions of a patient's serum to protect mice from lethal doses of BTX-A. Another bioassay involves a unilateral brow injection (UBI) in which a test dose (20 U of Botox) is administered and, if the brow is paralyzed and the patient is unable to frown on the injected side this indicates that the patient is BTX responsive and, therefore, does not have blocking antibodies.[154] Ever more sophisticated and quantitative bioassays have been developed using quantitative EMG and reduction of evoked or maximal motor unit amplitude,[155,156] and reduction of sudomotor activity.[157] One of these – the so-called EDB Test[158] – involves injection of BTX-A into an indicator muscle, the EDB, combined with amplitude measurements of compound muscle action potentials (CMAPs) elicited by electrical nerve stimulation of the peroneal nerve before and after the injection. A recent study[159] concludes that:

> the EDB test correlates better with the clinical response than the antibody assays and that EDB decrement does not always correlate quantitatively with the BTXA antibody titers. In patients with secondary nonresponsiveness, it is recommended that an EDB test is the initial investigation of choice. In those patients where the EDB test does not demonstrate resistance to BTXA, a reexamination of the patients and carefully placed injections under EMG guidance may improve results.

Antibodies can be assayed directly in vitro; however, in-vitro antibody assays, including the Western blot assay (WBA), do not correlate well with clinical responses because they do not detect specific blocking antibodies. More recently, an assay using immunoprecipitation of ^{125}I-labeled BTX has been developed.[160] Hanna et al[161] compared the WBA to the immunoprecipitation (IPA) and bioassays. Both in-vitro assays had high specificity, although the sensitivity of the IPA was higher than the MPA. In addition, the IPA seems to display positivity earlier than the MPA, and as such, it may prognosticate future non-responsiveness. Eyebrow (and frontalis) test injections correlated well with clinical and immunologic results and are useful in the assessment of BTX non-responders and in an algorithm for management of BTX non-responders.[154] In addition, several risk factors have been identified for the development of BTX antibodies, including short (<3 month) interval between treatments and 'booster' injections, high cumulative doses, duration of treatment, and possibly young age. Resistance with antibody formation has very rarely been reported in conditions other than CD, although rare cases of resistance (although not well documented by appropriate antibody assays) have been noted in patients with laryngeal dystonia.[162,163] In order to evaluate the feasibility of low-dose treatments, Rollnik et al[164] demonstrated that low-doses of Dysport, diluted with albumin, were effective without the development of antibodies in 115 patients suffering CD, blepharospasm, and HFS over a period of 2 years in an open-label, non-controlled pilot study.

Antibody levels can decline after cessation of therapy, although they may not regain responsiveness (usually temporary) to the same type of BTX for at least 18 months.[165] Thirteen patients with various dystonic syndromes and complete secondary therapy failure underwent monitoring period of at least 750 days after loss of response; two or more BTX-A antibody tests using the quantitative mouse diaphragm assay were performed.[166] Eight of 13 BTX-A antibody titers decreased. The onset of decrease could be detected after between approximately 500 and 1750 days. After 1250–2250 days, they had dropped below a level of 0.002 U/ml, where it is felt that secondary unresponsiveness is unlikely. However, 5 of 13 BT-A-AB titers did not decrease. The authors expressed their hopes that these patients might again become responsive to BTX-A, but there may well be an anamnestic response. Unfortunately, once patients develop blocking antibodies, even if the titer subsequently decreases, a rechallenge with the same type of BTX usually again stimulates the production of antibodies. Even when these patients are reinjected with an alternate type of BTX, they are at a high risk of developing blocking antibodies to the second BTX, presumably because of cross-reactivity.[167,168]

SUMMARY

Botulinum toxin provides a tool to perform selective chemical denervation. This has been shown to be effective in a variety of forms of dystonia. Although the dystonia can be generalized or multifocal, even the more widespread forms may display the most troublesome features for individual patients in a limited anatomic area. In general, BTX is very safe and primary toxicity is due to local spread. Systemic spread is very rare. Two different serologic subtypes of the toxin are available clinically, providing an alternative mode of therapy for patients that develop immunoresistance to one or the other. Various preclinical studies suggest that BTX-A is more potent and long-lasting than BTX-B, but this remains to be demonstrated in a clinical trial. Therapy has been limited by the development of blocking antibodies. This appears to be far less likely when using the newer preparation of BTX-A, which is more pure: i.e. has a greater neurotoxic activity per mg of total protein. Besides blocking neuromuscular activity by inhibition of ACh release, botulinum toxin appears to have effects on pain that may occur by different mechanisms, such as inhibition of peptide release.

REFERENCES

1. Jankovic J, Fahn S. Dystonic Disorders. In: Jankovic J, Tolosa E, eds. Parkinson's Disease and Movement Disorders. Baltimore: Williams and Wilkins; 1998: 513–51.
2. Jankovic J. Treatment of dystonia. Lancet Neurol 2006; 5(10): 864–72.
3. Erbguth FJ, Naumann M. Historical aspects of botulinum toxin: Justinus Kerner (1786–1862) and the 'sausage poison'. Neurology 1999; 53(8): 1850–3.
4. Arnon SS, Schechter R, Inglesby TV et al. Botulinum toxin as a biological weapon: medical and public health management. JAMA 2001; 285(8): 1059–70.
5. Cherington M. Clinical spectrum of botulism. Muscle Nerve 1998; 21(6): 701–10.
6. Tsui JK, Eisen A, Stoessl AJ, Calne S, Calne DB. Double-blind study of botulinum toxin in spasmodic torticollis. Lancet 1986; 2(8501): 245–7.
7. Jankovic J, Orman J. Botulinum A toxin for cranial–cervical dystonia: a double-blind, placebo-controlled study. Neurology 1987; 37(4): 616–23.
8. Benecke R, Jost WH, Karnovsky P et al. A new botulinum toxin type A free of complexing proteins for treatment of cervical dystonia. Neurology 2005; 64(11): 1949–51.
9. Eleopra R, Tugnoli V, Quatrale R et al. Clinical use of non-A botulinum toxins: botulinum toxin type C and botulinum toxin type F. Neurotox Res 2006; 9(2–3): 127–31.
10. Dressler D, Eleopra R. Clinical use of non-A botulinum toxins: botulinum toxin type B. Neurotox Res 2006; 9(2–3): 121–5.
11. Truong DD, Jost WH. Botulinum toxin: clinical use. Parkinsonism Relat Disord 2006; 12(6): 331–55.
12. Schurch B. Botulinum toxin for the management of bladder dysfunction. Drugs 2006; 66(10): 1301–18.
13. Ramachandran M, Eastwood DM. Botulinum toxin and its orthopaedic applications. J Bone Joint Surg Br 2006; 88(8): 981–7.
14. Cheng CM, Chen JS, Patel RP. Unlabeled uses of botulinum toxins: a review, part 2. Am J Health Syst Pharm 2006; 63(3): 225–32.
15. Cheng CM, Chen JS, Patel RP. Unlabeled uses of botulinum toxins: a review, part 1. Am J Health Syst Pharm 2006; 63(2): 145–52.
16. Pullman SL. The myriad uses of botulinum toxin. Ann Intern Med 2005; 143(11): 838–9.
17. Comella CL, Pullman SL. Botulinum toxins in neurological disease. Muscle Nerve 2004; 29(5): 628–44.
18. Jankovic J. Botulinum toxin in clinical practice. J Neurol Neurosurg Psychiatry 2004; 75(7): 951–7.
19. Dressler D, Adib Saberi F. Botulinum toxin: mechanisms of action. Eur Neurol 2005; 53(1): 3–9.
20. Thakker MM, Rubin PA. Pharmacology and clinical applications of botulinum toxins A and B. Int Ophthalmol Clin 2004; 44(3): 147–63.
21. Simpson LL. Identification of the major steps in botulinum toxin action. Annu Rev Pharmacol Toxicol 2004; 44: 167–93.
22. Rossetto O, Morbiato L, Caccin P, Rigoni M, Montecucco C. Presynaptic enzymatic neurotoxins. J Neurochem 2006; 97(6): 1534–45.
23. Foster KA, Bigalke H, Aoki KR. Botulinum neurotoxin – from laboratory to bedside. Neurotox Res 2006; 9(2–3): 133–40.
24. Huang W, Foster JA, Rogachefsky AS. Pharmacology of botulinum toxin. J Am Acad Dermatol 2000; 43(2 Pt 1): 249–59.
25. Humeau Y, Doussau F, Grant NJ, Poulain B. How botulinum and tetanus neurotoxins block neurotransmitter release. Biochimie 2000; 82(5): 427–46.
26. Schiavo G, Matteoli M, Montecucco C. Neurotoxins affecting neuroexocytosis. Physiol Rev 2000; 80(No. 2): 718–66.
27. Turton K, Chaddock JA, Acharya KR. Botulinum and tetanus neurotoxins: structure, function and therapeutic utility. Trends Biochem Sci 2002; 27(11): 552–8.
28. Dolly O. Synaptic transmission: inhibition of neurotransmitter release by botulinum toxins. Headache 2003; 43 (Suppl 1): 16–24.
29. Aoki KR. Physiology and pharmacology of therapeutic botulinum neurotoxins. Curr Probl Dermatol 2002; 30: 107–16.
30. Montecucco C, Schiavo G, Pantano S. SNARE complexes and neuroexocytosis: how many, how close? Trends Biochem Sci 2005; 30(7): 367–72.
31. Halpern JL, Neale EA. Neurospecific binding, internalization, and retrograde axonal transport. Curr Top Microbiol Immunol 1995; 195: 221–41.
32. Dong M, Yeh F, Tepp WH et al. SV2 is the protein receptor for botulinum neurotoxin A. Science 2006; 312(5773): 592–6.
33. Mahrhold S, Rummel A, Bigalke H, Davletov B, Binz T. The synaptic vesicle protein 2C mediates the uptake of botulinum neurotoxin A into phrenic nerves. FEBS Lett 2006; 580(8): 2011–14.
34. Dong M, Richards PA, Goodnough MC et al. Synaptotagmins I and II mediate entry of botulinum neurotoxin B into cells. J Cell Biol 2003; 162(7): 1293–303.
35. Figgitt DP, Noble S. Botulinum toxin B: a review of its therapeutic potential in the management of cervical dystonia. Drugs 2002; 62(4): 705–22.

36. Anderson RL, Gibbins IL, Morris JL. Five inhibitory transmitters coexist in pelvic autonomic vasodilator neurons. Neuroreport 1997; 8(14): 3023–8.
37. Jahn R. Neuroscience. A neuronal receptor for botulinum toxin. Science 2006; 312(5773): 540–1.
38. Meunier FA, Lisk G, Sesardic D, Dolly JO. Dynamics of motor nerve terminal remodeling unveiled using SNARE-cleaving botulinum toxins: the extent and duration are dictated by the sites of SNAP-25 truncation. Mol Cell Neurosci 2003; 22(4): 454–66.
39. Dolly JO, Lisk G, Foran PG et al. Insights into the extended duration of neuroparalysis by botulinum neurotoxin A relative to the other shorter-acting serotypes: differences between motor nerve terminals and cultured neurons. In: Brin M, Hallett M, Jankovic J, eds. Scientific and Therapeutic Aspects of Botulinum Toxins. Philadelphia: Lippincott, Williams and Wilkins; 2002: 91–102.
40. Foran PG, Mohammed N, Lisk G et al. Evaluation of the therapeutic usefulness of botulinum neurotoxin B, C1, E, and F compared with the long lasting type A. Basis for distinct durations of inhibition of exocytosis in central neurons. J Biol Chem 2003; 278(2): 1363–71.
41. Hamjian JA, Walker FO. Serial neurophysiological studies of intramuscular botulinum-A toxin in humans. Muscle Nerve 1994; 17(12): 1385–92.
42. de Paiva A, Meunier FA, Molgo J, Aoki KR, Jolly JO. Functional repair of motor endplates after botulinum neurotoxin type A poisoning: biphasic switch of synaptic activity between nerve sprouts and their parent terminals. Proc Natl Acad Sci USA 1999; 96(6): 3200–5.
43. Giladi N. The mechanism of action of botulinum toxin type A in focal dystonia is most probably through its dual effect on efferent (motor) and afferent pathways at the injected site. J Neurol Sci 1997; 152(2): 132–5.
44. Barwood S, Baillieu C, Boyd R et al. Analgesic effects of botulinum toxin A: a randomized, placebo-controlled clinical trial. Dev Med Child Neurol 2000; 42(2): 116–21.
45. Purkiss J, Welch M, Doward S, Foster K. Capsaicin-stimulated release of substance P from cultured dorsal root ganglion neurons: involvement of two distinct mechanisms. Biochem Pharmacol 2000; 59(11): 1403–6.
46. Aoki KR. Evidence for antinociceptive activity of botulinum toxin type A in pain management. Headache 2003; 43 (Suppl 1): 9–15.
47. Foster KA. A new wrinkle on pain relief: re-engineering clostridial neurotoxins for analgesics. Drug Discov Today 2005; 10(8): 563–9.
48. Reisner L. Biologic poisons for pain. Curr Pain Headache Rep 2004; 8(6): 427–34.
49. Mense S. Neurobiological basis for the use of botulinum toxin in pain therapy. J Neurol 2004; 251 (Suppl 1): I1–7.
50. Raj PP. Botulinum toxin therapy in pain management. Anesthesiol Clin North America 2003; 21(4): 715–31.
51. Sycha T, Samal D, Chizh B et al. A lack of antinociceptive or antiinflammatory effect of botulinum toxin A in an inflammatory human pain model. Anesth Analg 2006; 102: 509–16.
52. Breuer B, Sperber K, Wallenstein S et al. Clinically significant placebo analgesic response in a pilot trial of botulinum B in patients with hand pain and carpal tunnel syndrome. Pain Med 2006; 7(1): 16–24.
53. Blersch W, Schulte-Matter WJ, Przywara S et al. Botulinum toxin A and the cutaneous nociception in humans: a prospective, double-blind, placebo-controlled, randomized study. J Neurol Sci 2002; 205(1): 59–63.
54. Kramer HH, Angerer C, Erbguth F, Schmelz M, Birklein F. Botulinum Toxin A reduces neurogenic flare but has almost no effect on pain and hyperalgesia in human skin. J Neurol 2003; 250(2): 188–93.
55. Voller B, Sycha T, Gustorff B et al. A randomized, double-blind, placebo controlled study on analgesic effects of botulinum toxin A. Neurology 2003; 61(7): 940–4.
56. Blood AJ, Tuch DS, Makris N et al. White matter abnormalities in dystonia normalize after botulinum toxin treatment. Neuroreport 2006; 17(12): 1251–5.
57. Hallett M. How does botulinum toxin work? Ann Neurol 2000; 48(1): 7–8.
58. Trompetto C, Curra A, Buccolieri A et al. Botulinum toxin changes intrafusal feedback in dystonia: a study with the tonic vibration reflex. Mov Disord 2006; 21(6): 777–82.
59. Mezaki T, Matsumoto S, Sakamoto T, Mizutani K, Kaji R. [Cervical echomyography in cervical dystonia and its application to the monitoring for muscle afferent block (MAB)]. Rinsho Shinkeigaku 2000; 40(7): 689–93. [in Japanese]
60. Van den Bergh PY, Lison DF. Dose standardization of botulinum toxin. Adv Neurol 1998; 78: 231–5.
61. Odergren T, Hjaltason H, Kaakkola S et al. A double blind, randomised, parallel group study to investigate the dose equivalence of Dysport and Botox in the treatment of cervical dystonia. J Neurol Neurosurg Psychiatry 1998; 64(1): 6–12.
62. Sampaio C, Ferreira J, Simoes F et al. DYSBOT: a single-blind, randomized parallel study to determine whether any differences can be detected in the efficacy and tolerability of two formulations of botulinum toxin type A – Dysport and Botox – assuming a ratio of 4:1. Mov Disord 1997; 12(6): 1013–18.
63. Ranoux D, Gury C, Fondarai J, Mas JL, Zuber M. Respective potencies of Botox and Dysport: a double blind, randomised, crossover study in cervical dystonia. J Neurol Neurosurg Psychiatry 2002; 72(4): 459–62.
64. Das CP, Dressler D, Hallett M. Botulinum toxin therapy of writer's cramp. Eur J Neurol 2006; 13(Suppl): 55–9.
65. Pearce LB, Borodic GE, Johnson EA, First ER, MacCallum R. The median paralysis unit: a more pharmacologically relevant unit of biologic activity for botulinum toxin. Toxicon 1995; 33(2): 217–27.
66. Pellizzari R, Rossetto O, Washbourne P et al. In vitro biological activity and toxicity of tetanus and botulinum neurotoxins. Toxicol Lett 1998; 102–103: 191–7.
67. Sheridan RE, Deshpande SS, Smith T. Comparison of in vivo and in vitro mouse bioassays for botulinum toxin antagonists. J Appl Toxicol 1999; 19(Suppl 1): S29–33.
68. Guyer BM. Some unresolved issues with botulinum toxin. J Neurol 2001; 248 (Suppl 1): 11–13.
69. Sloop RR, Cole BA, Escutin RO. Reconstituted botulinum toxin type A does not lose potency in humans if it is refrozen or refrigerated for 2 weeks before use. Neurology 1997; 48(1): 249–53.
70. Lowe NJ, Yamauchi PS, Lask GP, Patnaik R, Moore D. Botulinum toxins types A and B for brow furrows: preliminary experiences with type B toxin dosing. J Cosmet Laser Ther 2002; 4(1): 15–18.
71. Dressler D, Benecke R. Autonomic side effects of botulinum toxin type B treatment of cervical dystonia and hyperhidrosis. Eur Neurol 2003; 49(1): 34–8.
72. Dubow J, Kim A, Leikin J et al. Visual system side effects caused by parasympathetic dysfunction after botulinum toxin type B injections. Mov Disord 2005; 20(7): 877–80.
73. Tintner R, Gross R, Winzer UF, Smalky KA, Jankovic J. Autonomic function after botulinum toxin type A or B: a double-blind, randomized trial. Neurology 2005; 65(5): 765–7.
74. Comella CL, Jankovic J, Shannon KM et al. Comparison of botulinum toxin serotypes A and B for the treatment of cervical dystonia. Neurology 2005; 65(9): 1423–9.
75. Factor SA, Mohlo ES, Evans S, Feustel PJ. Efficacy and safety of repeated doses of botulinum toxin type B in type A resistant and responsive cervical dystonia. Mov Disord 2005; 20(9): 1152–60.

76. Jankovic J, Schwartz K, Donovan DT. Botulinum toxin treatment of cranial-cervical dystonia, spasmodic dysphonia, other focal dystonias and hemifacial spasm. J Neurol Neurosurg Psychiatry 1990; 53(8): 633–9.
77. Calace P, Cortese G, Piscopo R et al. Treatment of blepharospasm with botulinum neurotoxin type A: long-term results. Eur J Ophthalmol 2003; 13(4): 331–6.
78. Jankovic J, Schwartz KS. Longitudinal experience with botulinum toxin injections for treatment of blepharospasm and cervical dystonia. Neurology 1993; 43(4): 834–6.
79. Roggenkamper P, Jost WH, Bihari K et al. Efficacy and safety of a new Botulinum Toxin Type A free of complexing proteins in the treatment of blepharospasm. J Neural Transm 2006; 113(3): 303–12.
80. Costa J, Espirito-Santo C, Borges A et al. Botulinum toxin type A therapy for blepharospasm. Cochrane Database Syst Rev 2005; (1): CD004900.
81. Barnes MP, Best D, Kidd L et al. The use of botulinum toxin type-B in the treatment of patients who have become unresponsive to botulinum toxin type-A – initial experiences. Eur J Neurol 2005; 12(12): 947–55.
82. Price J, Farish S, Taylor H, O'Day J. Blepharospasm and hemifacial spasm. Randomized trial to determine the most appropriate location for botulinum toxin injections. Ophthalmology 1997; 104(5): 865–8.
83. Jankovic J. Apraxia of lid opening [letter; comment]. Mov Disord 1995; 10(5): 686–7.
84. Mackie IA. Riolan's muscle: action and indications for botulinum toxin injection. Eye 2000; 14(Pt 3a): 347–52.
85. Albanese A, Bentivoglio AR, Colosimo C et al. Pretarsal injections of botulinum toxin improve blepharospasm in previously unresponsive patients. J Neurol Neurosurg Psychiatry 1996; 60(6): 693–4.
86. Cakmur R, Ozturk V, Uzunel F, Donmez B, Idiman F. Comparison of preseptal and pretarsal injections of botulinum toxin in the treatment of blepharospasm and hemifacial spasm. J Neurol 2002; 249(1): 64–8.
87. Tintner R, Jankovic J. Botulinum toxin type A in the management of oromandibular dystonia and bruxism. In: Brin M, Hallett M, Jankovic J, eds. Philadelphia: Lippincott Williams and Wilkins; 2002: 343–50.
88. Tan EK, Jankovic J. Botulinum toxin A in patients with oromandibular dystonia: long-term follow-up. Neurology 1999; 53(9): 2102–7.
89. Brin M, Blitzer A, Herman S, Steward C. Oromandibular dystonia: treatment of 96 cases with botulinum A. In: Jankovic J, Hallett M, eds. Therapy with Botulinum Toxin. New York: Marcel Dekker; 1994: 429–35.
90. Watts MW, Tan EK, Jankovic J. Bruxism and cranial–cervical dystonia: is there a relationship? Cranio 1999; 17(3): 196–201.
91. Tan EK, Jankovic J. Treating severe bruxism with botulinum toxin. J Am Dent Assoc 2000; 131(2): 211–16.
92. Gibbs SR, Blitzer A. Botulinum toxin for the treatment of spasmodic dysphonia. Otolaryngol Clin North Am 2000; 33(4): 879–94.
93. Truong DD, Bhidayasiri R. Botulinum toxin therapy of laryngeal muscle hyperactivity syndromes: comparing different botulinum toxin preparations. Eur J Neurol 2006; 13 (Suppl 1): 36–41.
94. Blitzer A, Brin MF, Stewart CF. Botulinum toxin management of spasmodic dysphonia (laryngeal dystonia): a 12-year experience in more than 900 patients. Laryngoscope 1998; 108(10): 1435–41.
95. Langeveld TP, Drost HA, Baatenburg de Jong RJ. Unilateral versus bilateral botulinum toxin injections in adductor spasmodic dysphonia. Ann Otol Rhinol Laryngol 1998; 107(4): 280–4.
96. Tisch SH, Brake HM, Law M et al. Spasmodic dysphonia: clinical features and effects of botulinum toxin therapy in 169 patients – an Australian experience. J Clin Neurosci 2003; 10(4): 434–8.
97. Sataloff RT, Heman-Ackah YD, Simpson LL et al. Botulinum toxin type B for treatment of spasmodic dysphonia: a case report. J Voice 2002; 16(3): 422–4.
98. Warrick P, Dromey C, Irish JC et al. Botulinum toxin for essential tremor of the voice with multiple anatomical sites of tremor: a crossover design study of unilateral versus bilateral injection. Laryngoscope 2000; 110(8): 1366–74.
99. Bielamowicz S, Stager SV, Badillo A, Godlewski A. Unilateral versus bilateral injections of botulinum toxin in patients with adductor spasmodic dysphonia. J Voice 2002; 16(1): 117–23.
100. Bhattacharyya N, Tarsy D. Impact on quality of life of botulinum toxin treatments for spasmodic dysphonia and oromandibular dystonia. Arch Otolaryngol Head Neck Surg 2001; 127(4): 389–92.
101. Hogikyan ND, Wodchis WP, Spak C, Kileny PR. Longitudinal effects of botulinum toxin injections on voice-related quality of life (V-RQOL) for patients with adductory spasmodic dysphonia. J Voice 2001: 15(4): 576–86.
102. Chawda SJ, Munchau A, Johnson D et al. Pattern of premature degenerative changes of the cervical spine in patients with spasmodic torticollis and the impact on the outcome of selective peripheral denervation. J Neurol Neurosurg Psychiatry 2000: 68(4): 465–71.
103. Jankovic J. Botulinum toxin therapy for cervical dystonia. Neurotox Res 2006; 9(2–3): 145–8.
104. Comella CL, Thompson PD. Treatment of cervical dystonia with botulinum toxins. Eur J Neurol 2006; 13 (Suppl 1): 16–20.
105. Balash Y, Giladi N. Efficacy of pharmacological treatment of dystonia: evidence-based review including meta-analysis of the effect of botulinum toxin and other cure options. Eur J Neurol 2004; 11(6): 361–70.
106. Gelb DJ, Yoshimura DM, Olney RK, Lowenstein DM, Aminoff MJ. Change in pattern of muscle activity following botulinum toxin injections for torticollis [see comments]. Ann Neurol 1991; 29(4): 370–6.
107. Erdal J, Ostergaard L, Fuglsang-Frederiksen A et al. Long-term botulinum toxin treatment of cervical dystonia – EMG changes in injected and noninjected muscles. Clin Neurophysiol 1999; 110(9): 1650–4.
108. Buchman AS, Comella CL, Stebbins GT, Tanner CM, Goetz CG. Quantitative electromyographic analysis of changes in muscle activity following botulinum toxin therapy for cervical dystonia. Clin Neuropharmacol 1993; 16(3): 205–10.
109. Dressler D, Rothwell JC. Electromyographic quantification of the paralysing effect of botulinum toxin in the sternocleidomastoid muscle. Eur Neurol 2000 ; 43(1): 13–16.
110. Ostergaard L, Fuglsang-Frederiksen A, Sjo O, Werdelin L, Winkel H. Quantitative EMG in cervical dystonia. Electromyogr Clin Neurophysiol 1996; 36(3): 179–85.
111. Brans JW, Aramideh M, Koelman JH et al. Electromyography in cervical dystonia: changes after botulinum and trihexyphenidyl. Neurology 1998; 51(3): 815–19.
112. Van Gerpen JA, Matsumoto JY, Ahlskog JE, Maraganore DM, McManis PG. Utility of an EMG mapping study in treating cervical dystonia. Muscle Nerve 2000; 23(11): 1752–6.
113. Comella CL, Buchman AS, Tanner CM, Brown-Toms NC, Goetz CG. Botulinum toxin injection for spasmodic torticollis: increased magnitude of benefit with electromyographic assistance. Neurology 1992; 42(4): 878–82.
114. Barbano R, Wenqing F, Luergans S et al. Utility of electromyography in botulinum toxin injection for cervical dystonia. Mov Disord 2005; Suppl 10: S19.

115. Jankovic J. EMG-guided injections of botulinum toxin: an opposing viewpoint. Muscle Nerve 2001; 24: 1568–70.
116. Jordan SE, Ahn S, Freischlag JA et al. Selective botulinum chemodenervation of the scalene muscles for treatment of neurogenic thoracic outlet syndrome. Ann Vasc Surg 2000; 14(4): 365–9.
117. Herting B, Wunderlich S, Glockler T et al. Computed tomographically-controlled injection of botulinum toxin into the longus colli muscle in severe anterocollis. Mov Disord 2004; 19(5): 588–90.
118. Comella CL, Jankovic J, Brin MF. Use of botulinum toxin type A in the treatment of cervical dystonia. Neurology 2000; 55(Suppl 5): S15–S21.
119. Jankovic J. Treatment of cervical dystonia with botulinum toxin. Mov Disord 2004; 19 (Suppl 8): S109–15.
120. Ceballos-Baumann AO. Evidence-based medicine in botulinum toxin therapy for cervical dystonia. J Neurol 2001; 248 (Suppl 1): 14–20.
121. Jankovic J, Esquenazi A, Fehlings D et al. Evidence-based review of patient-reported outcomes with botulinum toxin type A. Clin Neuropharmacol 2004; 27(5): 234–44.
122. Greene P, Kang U, Fahn S et al. Double-blind, placebo-controlled trial of botulinum toxin injections for the treatment of spasmodic torticollis. Neurology 1990; 40(8): 1213–18.
123. Kessler KR, Skutta M, Benecke R. Long-term treatment of cervical dystonia with botulinum toxin A: efficacy, safety, and antibody frequency. German Dystonia Study Group. J Neurol 1999; 246(4): 265–74.
124. Lew MF, Brashear A, Factor S. The safety and efficacy of botulinum toxin type B in the treatment of patients with cervical dystonia: summary of three controlled clinical trials. Neurology 2000; 55(12 Suppl 5): S29–35.
125. Brashear A, Lew MF, Dykstra DD et al. Safety and efficacy of NeuroBloc (botulinum toxin type B) in type A-responsive cervical dystonia. Neurology 1999; 53(7): 1439–46.
126. Brin MF, Lew MF, Adler CA et al. Safety and efficacy of NeuroBloc (botulinum toxin type B) in type A-resistant cervical dystonia. Neurology 1999; 53(7): 1431–8.
127. Lew MF, Adornato BT, Duane DD et al. Botulinum toxin type B: a double-blind, placebo-controlled, safety and efficacy study in cervical dystonia. Neurology 1997; 49(3): 701–7.
128. Ondo WG, Gollomp S, Galvez-Jimenez N. A pilot study of botulinum toxin A for headache in cervical dystonia. Headache 2005; 45(8): 1073–7.
129. Anderson T, Rivest J, Stell R et al. Botulinum toxin treatment of spasmodic torticollis. J R Soc Med 1992; 85(9): 524–9.
130. Borodic GE, Pearce LB, Smith K, Joseph M. Botulinum A toxin for spasmodic torticollis: multiple vs single injection points per muscle. Head Neck 1992; 14(1): 33–7.
131. Brans JW, Lindeboom R, Snock JW et al. Botulinum toxin versus trihexyphenidyl in cervical dystonia: a prospective, randomized, double-blind controlled trial. Neurology 1996; 46(4): 1066–72.
132. Poewe W, Deuschl G, Nebe A et al. What is the optimal dose of botulinum toxin A in the treatment of cervical dystonia? Results of a double blind, placebo controlled, dose ranging study using Dysport. German Dystonia Study Group. J Neurol Neurosurg Psychiatry 1998; 64(1): 13–17.
133. Laubis-Herrmann U, Fries K, Topka H. Low-dose botulinum toxin-A treatment of cervical dystonia – a double-blind, randomized pilot study. Eur Neurol 2002; 47(4): 214–21.
134. Poewe W, Wissel J. Experience with botulinum toxin in cervical dystonia. In: Jankovic J, Hallet M, eds. Therapy with Botulinum Toxin. New York: Marcel Dekker; 1994: 267–78.
135. Skogseid IM, Kerty E. The course of cervical dystonia and patient satisfaction with long-term botulinum toxin A treatment. Eur J Neurol 2005; 12(3): 163–70.
136. Tarsy D. Comparison of acute- and delayed-onset posttraumatic cervical dystonia. Mov Disord 1998; 13(3): 481–5.
137. Jankovic J, Schwartz KS. Use of botulinum toxin in the treatment of hand dystonia. J Hand Surg (Am) 1993; 18(5): 883–7.
138. Jankovic J, Hunter C, Dolimbele BZ et al. Clinico-immunologic aspects of botulinum toxin type B treatment of cervical dystonia. Neurology 2006; 67(12): 2233–5.
139. Molloy FM, Shill HA, Kaelin-Lang A, Karp BI. Accuracy of muscle localization without EMG: implications for treatment of limb dystonia. Neurology 2002; 58(5): 805–7.
140. Pullman SL, Greene P, Fahn S, Pedersen SF. Approach to the treatment of limb disorders with botulinum toxin A. Experience with 187 patients. Arch Neurol 1996; 53(7): 617–24.
141. Ross MH, Charness ME, Sudarsky L, Logigian EL. Treatment of occupational cramp with botulinum toxin: diffusion of toxin to adjacent noninjected muscles. Muscle Nerve 1997; 20(5): 593–8.
142. Kruisdijk JJ, Koelman JH, Ongerboer de Visser BW, de Haan RJ, Speelman JD. Botulinum toxin for writer's cramp: a randomised, placebo-controlled trial and 1-year follow-up. J Neurol Neurosurg Psychiatry 2007; 78(3): 264–70.
143. Jankovic J, Schwartz K, Clemence W, Aswad A, Mordaunt J. A randomized, double-blind, placebo-controlled study to evaluate botulinum toxin type A in essential hand tremor. Mov Disord 1996; 11(3): 250–6.
144. Brin MF, Lyons KE, Doucette J et al. A randomized, double masked, controlled trial of botulinum toxin type A in essential hand tremor. Neurology 2001; 56(11): 1523–8.
145. Wissel J, Masuhr F, Schelosky L et al. Quantitative assessment of botulinum toxin treatment in 43 patients with head tremor. Mov Disord 1997; 12: 722–6.
146. Dressler D, Hallett M. Immunological aspects of Botox, Dysport and Myobloc/NeuroBloc. Eur J Neurol 2006; 13 (Suppl 1): 11–15.
147. Borodic G, Johnson E, Goodnough M, Schantz E. Botulinum toxin therapy, immunologic resistance, and problems with available materials. Neurology 1996; 46(1): 26–9.
148. Mejia NI, Vuong KD, Jankovic J. Long-term botulinum toxin efficacy, safety, and immunogenicity. Mov Disord 2005; 20(5): 592–7.
149. Dressler D, Bigalke H. Botulinum toxin type B de novo therapy of cervical dystonia: frequency of antibody induced therapy failure. J Neurol 2005; 252(8): 904–7.
150. Racette BA, McGee-Minnich L, Perlmutter JS. Efficacy and safety of a new bulk toxin of botulinum toxin in cervical dystonia: a blinded evaluation. Clin Neuropharmacol 1999; 22(6): 337–9.
151. Naumann M, Yakovleff A, Durif F. A randomized, double-masked, crossover comparison of the efficacy and safety of botulinum toxin type A produced from the original bulk toxin source and current bulk toxin source for the treatment of cervical dystonia. J Neurol 2002; 249(1): 57–63.
152. Jankovic J, Vuong KD, Ahsan J. Comparison of efficacy and immunogenicity of original versus current botulinum toxin in cervical dystonia. Neurology 2003; 60(7): 1186–8.
153. Racette BA, Stambuk M, Perlmutter JS. Secondary nonresponsiveness to new bulk botulinum toxin A (BCB2024). Mov Disord 2002; 17(5): 1098–100.
154. Hanna PA, Jankovic J. Mouse bioassay versus Western blot assay for botulinum toxin antibodies: correlation with clinical response. Neurology 1998; 50(6): 1624–9.
155. Gordon PH, Gooch CL, Greene PE. Extensor digitorum brevis test and resistance to botulinum toxin type A. Muscle Nerve 2002; 26(6): 828–31.
156. Dressler D, Bigalke H, Rothwell JC. The sternocleidomastoid test: an in vivo assay to investigate botulinum toxin antibody formation in humans. J Neurol 2000; 247(8): 630–2.

157. Birklein F, Walther D, Bigalke H, Winterholler M, Erbguth F. Sudomotor testing predicts the presence of neutralizing botulinum A toxin antibodies. Ann Neurol 2002; 52(1): 68–73.
158. Kessler KR, Benecke R. The EBD test – a clinical test for the detection of antibodies to botulinum toxin type A. Mov Disord 1997; 12(1): 95–9.
159. Cordivari C, Misra VP, Vincent A et al. Secondary nonresponsiveness to botulinum toxin A in cervical dystonia: the role of electromyogram-guided injections, botulinum toxin A antibody assay, and the extensor digitorum brevis test. Mov Disord 2006; 21(10): 1737–41.
160. Palace J, Nairne A, Hyman N, Doherty TV, Vincent A. A radioimmuno-precipitation assay for antibodies to botulinum A. Neurology 1998; 50(5): 1463–6.
161. Hanna PA, Jankovic J, Vincent A. Comparison of mouse bioassay and immunoprecipitation assay for botulinum toxin antibodies. J Neurol Neurosurg Psychiatry 1999; 66(5): 612–16.
162. Smith ME, Ford CN. Resistance to botulinum toxin injections for spasmodic dysphonia. Arch Otolaryngol Head Neck Surg 2000; 126(4): 533–5.
163. Park JB, Simpson LL, Anderson TD, Sataloff R. Immunologic characterization of spasmodic dysphonia patients who develop resistance to botulinum toxin. J Voice 2003; 17(2): 255–64.
164. Rollnik JD, Matzke M, Wohlfarth K, Dengler R, Bigalke H. Low-dose treatment of cervical dystonia, blepharospasm and facial hemispasm with albumin-diluted botulinum toxin type A under EMG guidance. An open label study. Eur Neurol 2000; 43(1): 9–12.
165. Sankhla C, Jankovic J, Duane D. Variability of the immunologic and clinical response in dystonic patients immunoresistant to botulinum toxin injections. Mov Disord 1998; 13(1): 150–4.
166. Dressler D, Bigalke H. Botulinum toxin antibody type A titres after cessation of botulinum toxin therapy. Mov Disord 2002; 17(1): 170–3.
167. Dressler D, Bigalke H, Benecke R. Botulinum toxin type B in antibody-induced botulinum toxin type A therapy failure. J Neurol 2003; 250(8): 967–9.
168. Atassi MZ. Basic immunological aspects of botulinum toxin therapy. Mov Disord 2004; 19 (Suppl 8): S68–84.
169. Dressler D. [Pharmacological aspects of therapeutic botulinum toxin preparations]. Nervenarzt 2006; 77(8): 912–21.
170. Tang X, Wan X. Comparison of Botox with a Chinese type A botulinum toxin. Chin Med J (Engl) 2000; 113(9): 794–8.
171. Dressler D. Electromyographic evaluation of cervical dystonia for planning of botulinum toxin therapy. Eur J Neurol 2000; 7(6): 713–18.

19

Surgery for dystonia

Joachim K Krauss and Thomas J Loher

INTRODUCTION

Surgical treatment options for patients with medically refractory dystonia are gaining increased attention and acceptance over the past few years.[1–3] Surgery can provide more permanent relief of disabling dystonic movement disorders, and it can effectively prevent secondary complications of dystonia. More recently, there has been considerable reinterest in functional stereotactic neurosurgery to treat dystonia, and deep brain stimulation (DBS) has become one of the most important therapeutic tools.[4,5] In the following sections, we provide a short overview on the history of surgical treatment of dystonia and discuss current treatment options.

HISTORY

The first operations for treatment of cervical dystonia (CD) were probably performed in ancient Greece. Early operative techniques consisted mainly of myotomies. Intradural denervation techniques were introduced in the late 19th century, and were popular throughout the 20th century.[6] In the 1970s, the concept of selective peripheral denervation using extradural approaches, including posterior ramisectomy and spinal accessory nerve sectioning, was developed and popularized by Bertrand.[7] Since side effects were clearly reduced with this technique, selective peripheral denervation has gained more and more popularity and has almost replaced intradural sectioning. In the 1970s, epidural dorsal column stimulation of the cervical spine was introduced to treat CD.[8] Although this method was attractive from a theoretical point of view, it has been largely abandoned since independent evaluation of outcome could not confirm its therapeutic benefit.[9]

Surgery of the basal ganglia circuitry for treatment of movement disorders was not performed until Meyers, in 1939, pioneered his innovative techniques.[10] After Spiegel and Wycis had introduced the method of functional stereotactic surgery in men in the late 1940s, ablative procedures targeting the thalamus and the pallidum were used in hundreds of patients with otherwise intractable dystonia.[11] Thalamotomies and pallidotomies were also used with success in patients with CD, and the results of more than 300 patients were reported in the literature.[12] In the late 1970s, functional stereotactic surgery for dystonia was almost abandoned for several reasons, including the general decline of movement disorders surgery at that time, the introduction of selective peripheral denervation, and the widespread and beneficial use of botulinum toxin (BTX) A soon thereafter. The reinterest in functional stereotactic surgery for dystonia followed the renaissance of movement disorders surgery for Parkinson's disease (PD). Finally, the introduction of DBS has facilated the performance of bilateral surgery in the same operative session without significant increase of side effects, and thus has replaced ablative surgery in many neurosurgical centers worldwide.

PERIPHERAL SURGERY FOR CERVICAL DYSTONIA

Peripheral surgery for CD, nowadays, is performed mainly in patients who do not achieve adequate benefit from BTX injections. The estimated frequency of primary non-responders to BTX injections is 6–14% of patients with CD, and BTX loses its efficacy with continued use because of the development of immunoresistance in about another 3–10% of patients.[13,14] Patients with secondary immunoresistance may benefit from newer types of BTX. Surgical treatment should be considered both in primary and in secondary non-responders to BTX. It may also be considered an alternative in selected patients after years of successful trials with BTX, because it can provide more permanent relief. Surgical treatment, in general, is indicated in those patients with functional disability caused by their dystonic movement disorder. Restriction of social activities because of embarrassment related to CD can be a major driving force, particularly in younger patients, to seek more invasive therapies. The operations most commonly used today aim at selectively weakening the dystonic muscles by nerve sectioning or myotomy. Nowadays, extradural procedures are performed most frequently, and, to a lesser extent, intradural nerve sectioning procedures. The denervation of muscles that are not involved in the production of dystonia should be avoided. The basic difference between intradural anterior cervical rhizotomy and extradural posterior ramisectomy is shown in Figure 19.1. In the past, operative procedures for treatment of CD were often performed as 'standard' procedures, not taking into account the specific pattern of dystonic activity in the individual patient. One of the crucial points of contemporary surgery for CD is tailoring the approach to the specific dystonic pattern of the individual patient, which may involve several successive operative steps, and the combined use of different surgical techniques.[15,16] Interestingly, it has been shown that dystonic activity in various combinations may result in a similar abnormal head posture, and that (actually) the pattern of activation of dystonic muscles may change in an individual patient.[17]

We have evaluated the symptomatic and functional outcome in a retrospective series of 46 consecutive patients who were operated on according to this algorithm, with independent assessment using the Toronto Western Spasmodic Torticollis Rating Scale (TWSTRS).[15] In this group, 76 surgical procedures were performed, including selective intradural and extradural denervation, and muscle sections. Global improvement at long-term follow-up at a mean of 6.5 years postoperatively was rated as excellent in 21% of patients, as marked in 27%, as moderate in 21%, as mild in another 21%, and as nil in 11%. Almost all mean TWSTRS subscores for severity of CD, functional disability, and pain were significantly improved. Mild transient side effects were present in 10% of the patients and included swallowing difficulties, severe neck pain or headaches, psychotic decompensation, and cellulitis at the site of the skin incision. Persistent side effects, however, occurred in only one patient. In this series, there were no significant differences in the distribution of outcome scores between patients with idiopathic and secondary dystonia, nor were there significant differences between patients who primarily did not respond to BTX injections and those who had developed secondary immunoresistance. There was a significant difference, however, with regard to the number of procedures performed. Patients with an excellent outcome had a higher number of surgical procedures on average than those patients who had achieved no benefit.

Selective peripheral denervation

Extradural sectioning of the posterior primary division of the cervical nerves is also known as ramisectomy. It was Bertrand who coined the term *selective peripheral denervation* for the combination of sectioning of the peripheral branch of the spinal accessory nerve to the sternocleidomastoid muscle combined with posterior ramisectomy from C1 to C6.[7,18] In contrast to anterior rhizotomy, there is no need for laminectomy and opening of the dura in posterior ramisectomy. The approach can be performed either unilaterally or bilaterally, depending on the pattern of dystonia.

Patients are operated on under general anesthesia.[19] There have been several modifications of the original Bertrand technique. With the patient in the sitting position, both the site for posterior ramisectomy and the site for sternocleidomastoid denervation can be draped. The disadvantage of this position is the danger of air embolism, which, however, occurs only rarely in daily practice.[20] A useful alternative is to perform the

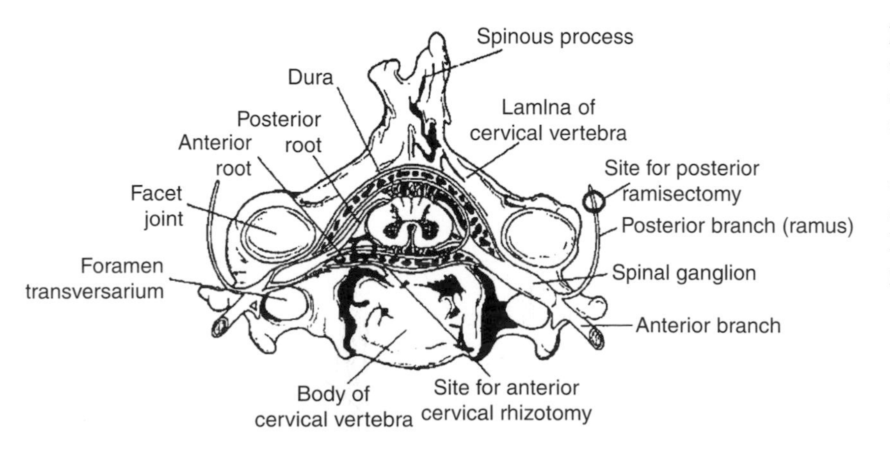

Figure 19.1 Schematic topographic anatomy of anterior cervical rhizotomy (intradural approach) and posterior ramisectomy (extradural approach). (Reproduced from Krauss et al,[6] with permission.)

ramisectomies in the prone position, and then the sternocleidomastoid denervation in the supine position. Using a 5 cm skin incision over the posterior margin of the sternocleidomastoid muscle, the trapezius branch of the spinal accessory nerve is first identified in the lateral neck triangle. Injury to the greater auricular nerve is carefully avoided. When the main trunk of the spinal accessory nerve is reached, branches to the sternocleidomastoid muscle are identified by electrical stimulation, and then sectioned and resected. Since the sternocleidomastoid may also be innervated by branches of the spinal nerves C1 and C2 or by recurrent nerves branching from the trapezius branch of the spinal accessory nerve, we have modified the original Bertrand technique and always complete the procedure with a myotomy and partial myectomy of the sternocleidomastoid.

Posterior ramisectomy is performed via a midline incision in the plane of the ligamentum nuchae until the posterior rim of the foramen magnum and the spinous processes of C2–C6 are reached. Then the cleavage plain between the more superficially located semispinalis capitis muscle and the more deeply located semispinalis cervicis and multifidus muscles on the involved side is entered (Figure 19.2). The inferior oblique capitis muscle is detached from its origin at the spinous process of C2. The posterior branches C3–C6 are found lateral to the facet joints, and are identified with the help of the surgical microscope and bipolar stimulation. After the main branches have been identified, they are sectioned and resected. Bipolar stimulation is then used to detect small residual branches. The C2 spinal ganglion is embedded in a rich venous plexus. With a unilateral approach, we usually perform a ganglionectomy at this site, including both the distal extradural portions of the roots and the rami. Since the greater occipital nerve is formed by the posterior C2 ramus, there is invariably a hypesthesia in the distribution of this nerve, which, however, in general, causes only little discomfort to the affected individual. It is more demanding to identify the suboccipital nerve, which is located between the arch of the atlas and the vertebral artery (Figure 19.3). It is also embedded in a venous plexus, which can result in brisk bleeding; this can be managed easily, however, by the application of Surgicel.

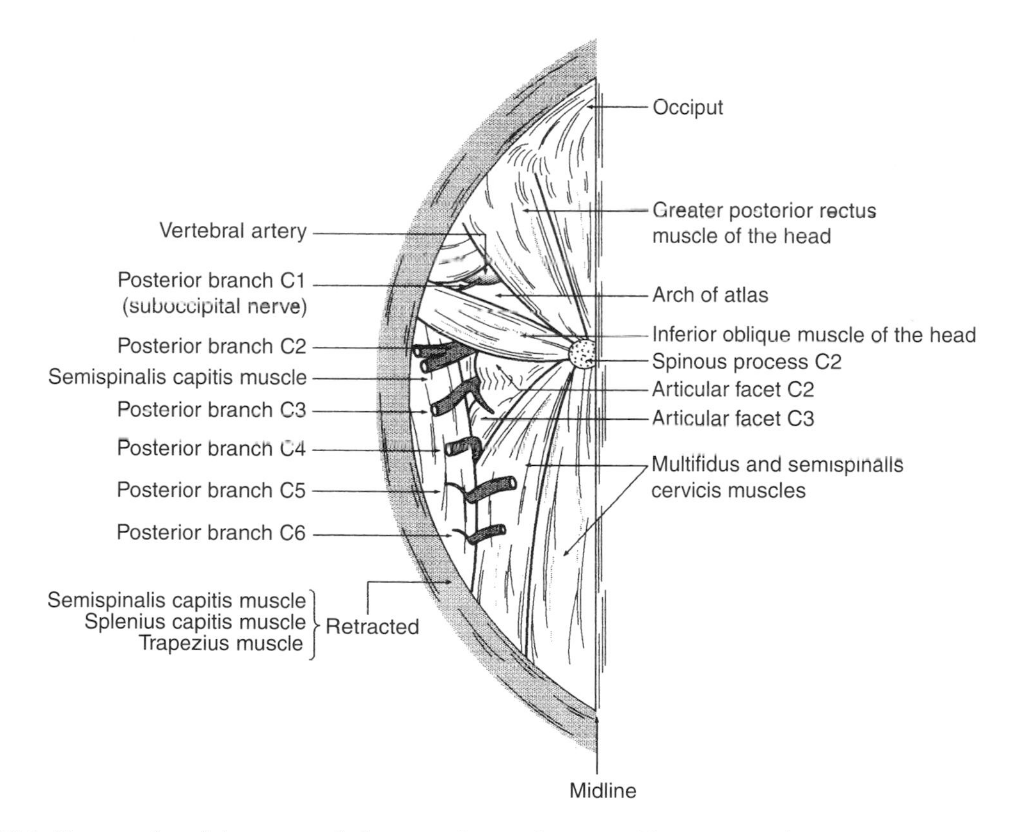

Figure 19.2 Topography of the approach for posterior ramisectomy. The posterior branches of C1–C6 can be reached within the natural cleavage plane between the more superficial semispinalis capitis muscle and the deeper multifidus and semispinalis cervicis muscles. (Reproduced from Braun and Richter,[19] with permission.)

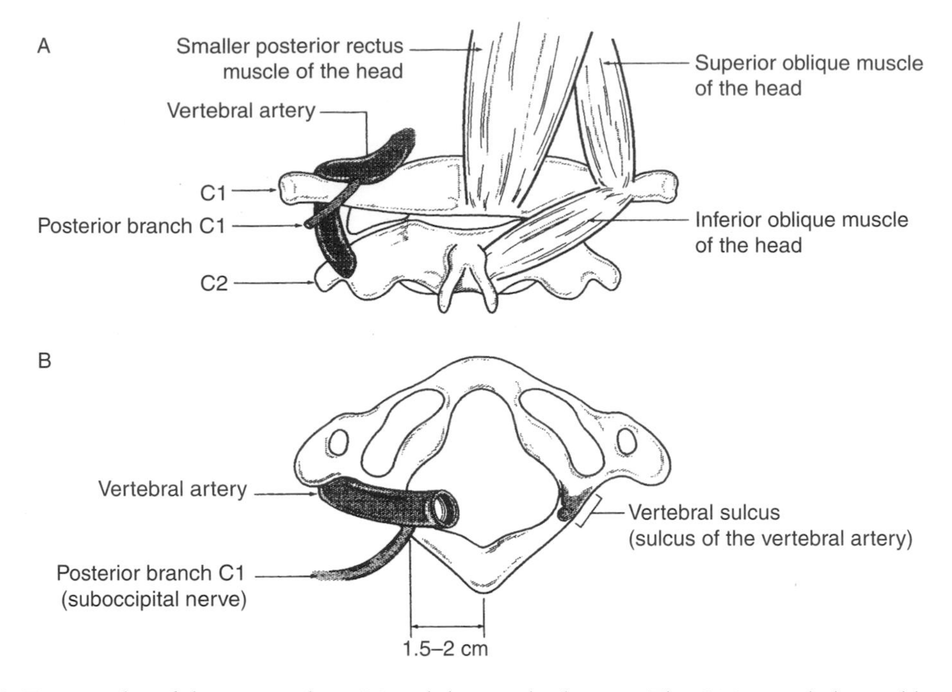

Figure 19.3 Topography of the approach to C1 and the vertebral artery. The C1 is mostly located between the vertebral artery and the arch of the atlas in the region of its vertebral sulcus about 1.5–2 cm from the midline. (A) Posterior (surgeon's) view. (B) View from above. (Reproduced from Braun and Richter,[19] with permission.)

Beneficial results have been reported in the range of 70–90% of patients in most series.[7,21,22] In a follow-up study on 140 patients at a mean of 33 months after surgery, 18 patients reported complete relief of their symptoms, 50 had marked relief, 34 moderate relief, and 19 had only minor relief, while another 19 patients had no improvement.[22] In this study, the result of surgery differed between primary and secondary non-responders to BTX injections. Whereas 80% of secondary non-responders were satisfied with their postoperative results, only 62% of the primary non-responders considered the operation had been helpful. Recurrence of CD was noted in 11% of patients. In a retrospective long-term study at a mean of 5 years after surgery, there was a reduction in dystonia by 30% in about one-third of patients.[23] In most studies, head tremor and phasic dystonic movements were improved to a lesser extent than dystonic postures. Since denervation of laryngeal and pharyngeal muscles is largely avoided, the frequency of side effects, in general, has been low. Side effects may include infection, paresthesias, and hypesthesia in the territory of the major occipital nerve, pain, and rarely transient dysphagia.[7,21–23] Chawda and colleagues demonstrated that patients with no or minimal degenerative changes of the cervical spine had significant improvement in pain and severity of CD after selective denervation, whereas no difference was found in those with more severe changes.[24] The authors concluded that effective early treatment of CD had a protective effect. Munchau and associates confirmed that reinervation is not infrequent after initially successful selective peripheral denervation.[22] In those cases, additional or repeat surgery can be useful. Occasionally, selective denervation can also be indicated in patients with fixed dystonic postures, with the goal not to correct the head position but to alleviate accompanying pain.[25]

Myotomy and myectomy

Myotomies and myectomies are rarely used as a first step in patients with CD, but these techniques can be helpful as an adjunct to selective denervation or for treatment of dystonic activities in muscles that cannot be denervated completely with ease.[26] Whereas the posterior neck muscles are denervated adequately by posterior ramisectomies, dystonic activity in the scalene muscles, the levator scapulae, and the omohyoid is not controlled by this approach. In such cases, selective myotomies/myectomies are useful. In patients who present with painful dystonic activity of the trapezius muscle that results in elevation and protraction of the shoulder or contributes to ipsilateral head tilt, partial myotomy and myectomy of the upper portion of the trapezius muscle can be performed with an asleep–awake–asleep operative technique.[26]

Chen has published the largest series on more extensive myotomies/myectomies for treatment of CD which were combined with selective peripheral denervations in certain patterns of CD.[27] Treatment algorithms included selective resections of dystonic muscles for various patterns of CD, such as rotational CD, tilt of the head, anterocollis, and retrocollis. In his series of 60 patients, excellent or marked improvement was described in 83% of patients. In a series of 15 patients with retrocollis, partial resections of the upper part of the trapezius muscles, the splenius, semispinalis capitis, and semispinalis cervicis muscles were performed bilaterally.[28] Outcome at follow-up at 3–10 years postoperatively was reported as excellent or marked improvement in 87% of patients without persistent side effects. The long-term results of non-selective sternocleidomastoid sectioning in another series of 11 patients, in contrast, were less favorable.[29]

Intradural rhizotomy and nerve sectioning

Intradural anterior cervical rhizotomy was the most common operation for CD before the advent of peripheral denervation.[30,31] Several variations of this procedure have been developed. The 'standard' procedure includes intradural sectioning of the C1–C3 anterior roots and those rootlets of the spinal accessory nerves which supply the sternocleidomastoid muscles. A small suboccipital craniotomy widening the posterior rim of the foramen magnum and laminectomies of the three upper cervical vertebrae are performed. After opening of the dura, the upper spinal cord, the medulla oblongata, the cerebellar tonsils, the upper cranial nerve roots, the spinal accessory nerves, and the blood vessels of the cervicomedullary junction and the upper cervical medulla are visualized with the operating microscope. The anterior roots are stimulated with a bipolar nerve stimulator and then divided. Any arterial blood vessels that accompany the nerve roots should be spared. Denervation with this approach, in general, is limited downward to the anterior root of C3 if it is performed bilaterally. The C4 root may be sectioned on one side but endangers functioning of the diaphragm. Thus, this intradural approach cannot control dystonic activity, which is mediated via the C4–C6 roots. Since the 'standard' approach was rather non-selective and resulted in high complication rates, modified techniques aimed to denervate the dystonic muscles and to preserve normal activity. Thus, for example in a patient with rotational CD, unilateral anterior rhizotomy would be combined with contralateral spinal accessory nerve section.

Both the reported results and the complication rates in different series were highly variable. Most studies claimed useful postoperative improvement in 60–90% of their patients.[30,31] It has been unclear, however, to what degree symptomatic amelioration of the abnormal postures or movements translated to improvement in functional disability with regard to the relatively high number of side effects. In the series of Friedman et al, the head was described to return to a neutral position in 59% of the patients postoperatively.[31] The likelihood of the head returning to a normal position postoperatively was inversely related to the duration of CD. Some studies have reported only very modest results after anterior intradural rhizotomy. Hernesniemi and Keränen, for example, reported no patient with an outcome considered as good based on their patients' self-assessments for the surgical result, disability, and working capacity.[29] Complications of the standard bilateral intradural denervation are frequent and may be persistent and disabling. Mortality with the standard procedure ranged between 0% and 1%, in general, but was as high as 12% in some series. Side effects include dysphagia, weakness of the neck, cerebrospinal fluid fistulas, and infection. Weak or unstable neck has been estimated to occur in about 40% of patients after bilateral rhizotomy, and transient dysphagia in about 30% of patients.[32] Radiologic swallowing abnormalities were described in as many as 95% of patients postoperatively, frequently representing aggravation of pre-existing pharyngeal dysfunction.[33] In rare cases, bilateral infarctions of the medulla oblongata with bilateral Wallenberg syndrome or ischemia of the upper spinal cord with tetraparesis were reported.[34] The procedure is much safer and accompanied by far less morbidity with selective approaches.

Microvascular decompression

Microvascular decompression (MVD) of the spinal accessory nerve for treatment of CD has been used in analogy to the therapeutic benefit of this procedure in other cranial neuropathies such as hemifacial spasm.[35] The existence of two pathogenetically different types of CD has been suggested by proponents of MVD. The first is CD of 'central' origin and the second is 'spasmodic torticollis of 11th nerve origin'.[36] However, it is difficult to understand how MVD of the spinal accessory nerve should work, both regarding the pathophysiologic concept of MVD and the fact that almost always other muscles than the sternocleidomastoid are involved in dystonic activity. Outcome data of MVD for treatment of CD are very limited. Often, nerve sectionings were performed in addition to MVD.[37] Jho and Jannetta claimed a cure of CD in 65% of their patients (13 of 20 patients), improvement considered as significant in 4 patients (20%), as moderate in 1 patient (5%), and as minimal in 2 patients on long-term follow-up between 5 and 10 years after MVD.[35] In some series high rates of surgical morbidity were described. Thus far, no prospective studies using appropriate assessment with standard rating scales have been published. With the present available data, microvascular decompression cannot be recommended as a treatment option for CD.

FUNCTIONAL STEREOTACTIC SURGERY

Current functional stereotactic surgical options include lesioning and DBS of the globus pallidus internus (GPi) and the thalamus. The pallidum was rediscovered in the mid 1990s as a target for dystonia, whereas DBS for treatment of dystonia was introduced only recently.[38–40] The indications for the different therapeutic options and the goals to be achieved depend on the distribution of dystonia, the severity, the etiology, the presence of other neurologic symptoms, and the patient's age. Hemidystonia, which is frequently secondary to contralateral caudatoputaminal lesions, may be stable after delayed onset and progression over several years, whereas idiopathic dystonia may still progressively spread to other body parts later on and then limit the benefit of surgery. Owing to the relatively small number of patient series, the variations in surgical methods, and the inconsistent outcome assessments, no definite recommendations about the best surgical options and ideal targets can be made for many dystonic disorders. In general, the GPi appears to be the preferred target for idiopathic genetic and other primary dystonias. The focus on the treatment of dystonia these days has shifted more and more to DBS because of the lower risk of performing bilateral surgery in one session.[4,5]

Thalamotomy

The target for thalamotomy for treatment of dystonia has been much more variable among different surgeons than thalamic targets for tremor. Thalamotomy has involved the nucleus ventralis oralis anterior and posterior, the nucleus ventralis oralis internus, the ventralis intermedius, the subthalamic region, the centrum medianum/nucleus parafascicularis complex, and the pulvinar thalami.[12] The comparison of the symptomatic and functional outcome of the reported series of thalamotomy is limited because of the heterogeneity of patients, variations of the target, differences in evaluation of outcome, and variable length of follow-up. Immediate postoperative improvement is less striking than in other movement disorders such as PD or essential tremor (ET). Often, further amelioration can be observed within months after the operation. Postoperative improvement has been reported, in general, in 25–80% of patients with generalized dystonia, and in 33–100% of patients with hemidystonia.[41–43] Andrew and colleagues found moderate or significant overall improvement in 25% of patients with generalized dystonia and in 100% of patients with hemidystonia; the benefit was more significant in secondary dystonia than in primary dystonia.[42] Tasker and associates described that 68% of patients with secondary dystonia had more than 25% clinical improvement, whereas this was the case in only 50% of patients with primary dystonia.[43] Patients with secondary dystonia also appeared to have more sustained improvement than patients with primary dystonia with thalamotomy. In the series of Tasker et al, 65% of patients with primary dystonia, but only 31% of patients with secondary dystonia, gradually lost the initial postoperative benefit. Immediate postoperative side effects were described in 7–47% of patients in different series. Transient side effects most commonly included confusion and contralateral weakness; similarly, as with PD, postoperative speech impairment has been observed more frequently after bilateral thalamotomies. Long-term follow-up has been rarely available. Cardoso et al reported moderate or significant improvement in 50% of patients with secondary dystonia at a mean follow-up of 41 months, and in 43% of patients with primary dystonia at a mean of 33 months.[44] Krauss et al observed sustained moderate improvement in 3 of 6 patients with post-traumatic hemidystonia at a mean follow-up of 18 years.[45]

Pallidotomy

The pallidal target for surgical treatment of dystonia is located in the posteroventral lateral GPi, basically at the same site as that used for pallidotomy in Parkinson's disease. Single-unit extracellular recording is helpful in our opinion to delineate the final target more precisely and to determine the external and internal borders of the pallidum. Most neurosurgeons place two radiofrequency lesions in the GPi, 2 mm apart, along the trajectory of the radiofrequency probe. Whereas improvement of phasic dystonic movements may be seen early after surgery, tonic dystonic postures improve over much longer time.

Pallidotomy has been reported to be effective in various dystonic disorders, including generalized dystonia, segmental dystonia, and hemidystonia, yielding about 50–80% improvement in most studies.[46–50] In the Baylor College of Medicine series, 14 out of 16 patients with generalized dystonia or hemidystonia benefited from meaningful improvement after pallidotomy.[41,48] Eleven patients had bilateral procedures, staged in 3 patients and concurrent in 8 patients. It was difficult to compare the efficacy of unilateral vs bilateral surgery, as the decision was clinically based upon the anatomic distribution of the dystonia. Patients with genetic dystonias (both DYT-1 positive and DYT-1 negative) consistently demonstrated marked improvement, whereas this was less dramatic and less consistent in secondary dystonia. At a mean of 1.5 years follow-up, improvement was sustained. Pallidotomy has been shown also to improve symptomatic dystonia resulting from other neurodegenerative diseases such as Hallervorden–Spatz disease and Huntington's disease in single cases.[51,52] In some studies, a partial recrudescence of dystonic symptoms over time has been noted. The response of dystonia to pallidotomy may depend on etiology, according to the experience made at different centers. It appears that patients with primary dystonia respond well to pallidotomy, whereas patients with secondary dystonia without structural lesions enjoy moderate improvement, and patients with secondary dystonia and structural brain lesions often have only minimal benefit.[53] Nevertheless, single patients with secondary dystonia may gain substantial benefit from pallidal surgery.[54] Overall, the response of secondary dystonia to pallidal surgery appears to be somewhat unpredictable, and many of these patients do not show much benefit.[55] Functional stereotactic surgery for choreoathetosis secondary to cerebral palsy (CP) is difficult to evaluate. Bilateral pallidotomies yielded limited benefit in such patients, with objective improvement of the movement disorder of up to 42%; however, this was at a high rate of persistent complications.[56,57]

Yoshor and colleagues recently compared the effectiveness of thalamotomy and pallidotomy in a retrospective series of 32 patients with primary and secondary dystonias.[50] Eighteen patients underwent thalamotomies, and 14 patients had pallidotomies. Although comparisons were limited according to various differences between the two surgical groups, patients with primary dystonia who underwent pallidotomy demonstrated significantly better long-term outcomes than did patients who underwent thalamotomy. In this series, patients with secondary dystonia experienced more modest improvement after either procedure, with little or no difference in outcomes between the two procedures.

Deep brain stimulation

Since its introduction a few years ago, pallidal DBS has become one of the mainstays in the treatment of medically refractory dystonia (for review see References 3–5). Pallidal DBS is performed with the quadripolar 3387 DBS electrode (Medtronic Minneapolis, MN, USA) which has 1.5 mm gaps between the single contacts. Patients with dystonia are stimulated continuously. For the initial programming we usually use bipolar settings with the deepest contact, most frequently contact 1 set to negative, and the next contact, usually contact 2 set to positive, while the other electrodes remain neutral. Initial stimulation settings include a frequency of 130 Hz, a pulse width of 210 μs, and amplitudes between 2.0 and 4.0 V as tolerated by the patient. During the next few months, the intensity of stimulation is gradually increased, staying below the threshold that elicits unwanted effects. The threshold for undesired effects such as perioral tightness, which also may involve some difficulty swallowing or speaking, dizziness, tingling, and capsular responses, tends to shift during progressive adjustment of stimulation amplitude. If no optimal benefit of the movement disorder is achieved upon chronic stimulation, alternative electrode contacts or combinations are activated. Some centers also start with monopolar stimulation, or use two contacts as cathodal with case or another contact anodal. DBS settings are adjusted within the first year after surgery. In general, only minimal adjustment, if any, is required later.

Sometimes it may take months before the full benefit of pallidal DBS is notable. In contrast, however, dystonia may reoccur within minutes or hours when the implantable pulse generators (IPGs) are switched off.[58] Since both pulse width and voltage are higher in dystonia patients than in Parkinson's disease, depletion of the IPG batteries may occur within 2 years. Amplitudes have ranged between 2.2 and 7.0 V in our dystonia patients. Most centers perform contemporaneous bilateral surgery to implant the electrodes. Failure of chronic GPi stimulation may result in a medical emergency, in particular in patients with the Kinetra, an IPG used for bilateral stimulation. Hardware failure caused by unilateral lead dysfunction results in a more gradual and progressive recurrence of symptoms, perhaps accounted for in part by the presence of the retained contralateral stimulation.

DBS has the advantages over lesional surgery of being reversible and adaptable. It avoids concern about the effects of lesioning on the developing brain in children and allows bilateral surgery to be undertaken more safely because of the reduced level of morbidity involved with DBS compared to lesions. However, DBS may include hardware failure, high costs, time-consuming follow-up as well as those related to the perioperative period, such as infection and possible intracranial hemorrhage. The overall rate of hardware-related problems has ranged from 8 to 65%.[59]

Several pilot studies have shown that DBS, in particular pallidal DBS, is reasonably safe and efficacious in a variety of dystonic disorders. DBS for treatment of dystonia has received FDA (Food and Drug Administration) approval in the form of an HDE (humanitarian device exemption) in the USA and CE (Conformité Europeene) certification in Europe. Larger studies are underway to validate the observations on DBS for dystonia being made in smaller studies that have been published. A French multicenter study investigated the effect of bilateral pallidal DBS in primary generalized dystonia, including blinded assessment of clinical outcome.[60] A German multicenter study is investigating the long-term outcome of GPi DBS for primary generalized and segmental dystonia by a randomized double-blind study design.[61] Furthermore, multicenter studies are being conducted to study the effect of pallidal DBS on tardive dystonia and cervical dystonia. Preliminary results of the Canadian study have become available.[62] It appears feasible now also to explore possible new indications for DBS, such as paroxysmal dystonia, blepharospasm-oromandibular dystonia, and other focal dystonias.

Cervical dystonia

Since CD is the most frequent dystonic movement disorder, DBS might be of special interest in this group of patients. In particular, pallidal DBS can be a very useful treatment option in those patients who do not respond satisfactorily to BTX injections and who are not good candidates for other less costly interventions. Serial selective peripheral surgery, as discussed above, is still considered the therapy of first choice in most of these patients. Peripheral surgery, however, is not indicated in a subset of CD patients, including those with head tremor and myoclonus, marked phasic dystonic movements, sagittal and lateral translation, anterocollis, and combined complex forms of CD. Although, at present DBS is limited mostly to such patients with more unusual manifestations of CD, it might be considered an alternative in other types of CD in the future.

Bilateral pallidal DBS is favored over unilateral DBS in CD for a variety of reasons. There is evidence from various studies that CD patients have bilateral basal ganglia dysfunction, regardless of the phenomenologic manifestation in the individual patient. Positron emission tomography (PET) investigations, for example, demonstrated higher glucose metabolism in the lentiform nucleus bilaterally in CD patients without significant differences regarding the laterality, the specific pattern, or the severity of CD.[63] Bilateral basal ganglia involvement was also shown in a single-photon emission computed tomography (SPECT) study investigating striatal D_2 receptor binding in CD patients.[64] Furthermore, transcranial magnetic stimulation studies revealed that there is considerable bihemispheric presentation of neck muscles.[65] Also, review of the early literature on ablative surgery for CD showed that patients who had bilateral surgery overall had better results than those who underwent unilateral surgery, although at a higher rate of side effects.[12] When a unilateral approach was chosen, there were quite different opinions on the side to be operated on. Cooper, for example, recommended thalamotomy contralateral to the dystonic sternocleidomastoid muscle, while Hassler and Dieckmann thought that an ipsilateral thalamotomy should be performed. This discussion has been revived recently, when opposing suggestions were made for unilateral DBS in CD patients based on the experience in single cases.[66]

Since the first patients with CD were treated by GPi DBS in the late 1990s, beneficial results have been reported by a number of centers.[38,62,67–73] Bilateral pallidal stimulation produces both symptomatic and functional improvement, including marked relief of pain in the long term in patients with complex CD.[38,67] In our series, the gradual amelioration of CD over months was reflected by improvement of a modified TWSTRS scale on subsequent follow-up examinations, and the mean scores were better at 1 year after surgery than at 3 months postoperatively. Formal follow-up evaluation, at 20 months after surgery, demonstrated a 63% improvement of the TWSTRS severity score, a 69% improvement of the disability score, and a 50% improvement of the pain score. These figures correspond well with those from the Oxford group, which showed similar amelioration for the subscores severity (64%), disability (60%), and pain (60%) at 19 months follow-up.[70] Our first patient has reached 9-year follow-up meanwhile. She still has marked benefit from continuous stimulation, but she underwent a total of three revisions over the years to replace fractured leads. Overall, 4 out of 5 patients with CD for whom we have long-term follow-up of 3 years or longer had sustained improvement comparable to 1 year postoperatively. In some patients, relief of pain preceded improvements observed in the other aspects of the TWSTRS scale. Single patients were reported in whom relief of pain was the most prominent feature.[69] Overall, there appears to be less interpatient variability in patients with CD than in patients with other dystonic disorders. We have used chronic pallidal stimulation also as an adjunct in patients with cervical dyskinesias and secondary cervical myelopathy prior to performing spinal surgery or spinal stabilization.[67,74]

The costs of chronic pallidal stimulation are relatively high for patients with CD. This is due to the relatively younger age of patients with CD as compared, for example, to those with Parkinson's disease, but also to the higher energy needed for chronic stimulation.

In particular, in this group of patients it would be desirable to develop new DBS strategies to reduce costs. Possible alternatives could include the development of rechargeable IPG batteries, the production of batteries that have a longer duration, or the exploration of other stimulation modes.

Generalized dystonia

The most beneficial results with pallidal DBS were reported in children with genetic DYT1-positive generalized dystonia. In their first publication on this subject, Coubes and colleagues described a mean improvement of 90% in the Burke–Fahn–Marsden Dystonia Movement Scale (BFMDMS) at a follow-up of at least 1 year after surgery in 7 patients (mean age of 14 years at operation).[75] Improvement was gradual within months after implantation of the electrodes. Six children managed to walk without assistance after surgery and became functionally normal. Drugs were reduced in all patients, resulting in improvement of alertness. All children returned to school. The Montpellier group recently reported follow-up data for a larger number of patients.[76] In this study, there was a mean improvement of 71% in the Burke–Fahn–Marsden (BFM) motor scores of 15 patients with primary DYT 1-positive dystonia 1 year after surgery, and a mean improvement of 74% in a group of 17 patients with primary dystonia of unknown etiology. Adverse effects have been minimal. Several other groups have reported similar results.[77–79] Nevertheless, single cases that did not achieve the expected dramatic postoperative benefit were also reported. Also, in adult patients with primary generalized dystonia, remarkable benefit is achieved with bilateral pallidal DBS. In two adult patients with a positive family history of dystonia, for example, BFM dystonia scores improved by 74% 3 months postoperatively, by 75% after 1 year, and by 74% after 2 years.[80] The improvement of the motor scores was accompanied by a 67% improvement of disability scores. In 12 patients with generalized dystonia from the Oxford group, there was a mean 48% improvement in the BFM severity scores, and a 38% improvement in the disability scores.[70] The lesser improvement in this group was most likely due to several issues such as greater variability in clinical background, the effect of treatment duration, and the duration of disease onset to treatment, which was more than 12 years. Overall, the response of generalized dystonia to pallidal DBS seems to depend on etiology, similar to the experience with pallidotomy.[53,81]

The recently published class III French multicenter study included blinded assessment of clinical outcome.[60] The mean improvement of the BFM rating scale in this study was 54% on average, and the mean improvement of disabilty was 44% at 1 year postoperatively. In addition, general health and physical functioning scores were significantly improved according to the SF-36. There was no permanent morbidity. It was also shown in this group of patients that no behavioral or mood changes were found. Also, there were no cognitive changes, except mild improvement in executive functions.[82] In the German randomized controlled multicenter study which included 40 patients, the range from baseline 3 months after randomization was significantly greater in the neurostimulation group (15.8 points on the BFM scale) than in the sham-stimulation group (1.4 points).[61] Substantial improvement in all movement symptoms except speech and swallowing was noted 6 months postoperatively.

Segmental and focal dystonia

Substantial benefit has also been described in patients with primary but more confined segmental dystonia.[70,83,84] Improvement with bilateral DBS in such cases ranged between 50% and 90% of dystonia scores. We reported on a 67-year-old man with risperidone-responsive segmental dystonia whose BFM motor scores improved by 86% at 9 months follow-up.[85] In this case, a more complex interaction with medication and stimulation was found, an issue that has been rather neglected thus far in DBS for dystonia. Although it has been claimed repeatedly that tardive dystonia, which often manifests as segmental or focal dystonia, is a good indication for pallidal DBS, little has been published on this subject. Nandi et al reported marked relief of tardive camptocormia with pallidal DBS in a patient whose movement disorder was otherwise refractory to medical treatment.[86]

Improvement of cranial dystonias was reported in patients who were operated on for segmental or generalized dystonia.[83,84,87] In a patient with Meige syndrome, BFM subscores had improved by 92% for eyes, by 75% for mouth, and by 33% for speech and swallowing at 2 years postoperatively.[88] Meige syndrome and other focal dystonias might be of interest to be further explored with pallidal DBS in the future.

In a recent study on a series of 14 patients with segmental dystonia who underwent pallidal or thalamic DBS, there were stable improvements of motor scores on follow-up at 17 months after surgery (preoperative BFM 53.8; at follow-up 15.5) which was paralleled by improved disability scores (preoperative BFM disability 6.0; at follow-up 3.9). In 3 patients stimulation-induced hypokinetic dysarthria occurred with higher voltages, which limited the therapeutical benefit in these patients.[89]

In the subgroup of 10 patients with pallidal DBS, there was a significant decrease of the total SF-36 scores by 40% at a mean of 7.5 months after surgery and by 51% at 17 months after surgery.[90]

Secondary dystonia

DBS for treatment of secondary dystonia is much more complex than that of primary dystonia. Although thought to be less effective in secondary dystonia, pallidal stimulation was reported to be successful in some individual cases.[81,83] Thalamic DBS has been suggested to be more useful in such cases, but data published thus far do not allow us to draw any conclusions. Before the routine use of GPi DBS for dystonia, patients with medically intractable dystonia underwent thalamic DBS in Grenoble.[83] Although there was little change in formal dystonia scores, about half of the patients achieved a good functional result. Thalamic stimulation was also efficient in patients with post-traumatic hemidystonia, postanoxic dystonia with basal ganglia necrosis, paroxysmal dystonia, and for the myoclonic component of myoclonic dystonia[91] (for review see References 4 and 5).

Promising results were described in 2 patients with choreoathetosis after bilateral GPi DBS.[92,93] Our experience with pallidal DBS in adult patients with cerebral palsy (CP) was more varied, and the benefit was minimal or irrelevant in some patients.[80] The mean improvement in BFM scores in 4 patients with choreoathetotic CP was 12% at 3 months postoperatively, 29% at 1 year, and 23% at 2 years, which was not significant as compared to preoperatively. Two of these patients thought they had achieved marked improvement at 2 years postoperatively, although results of objective evaluation were less impressive. In these 2 patients there was a minor but stable improvement in disability scores. This discrepancy between the objective and the subjective evaluation is remarkable, and is most likely due to the fact that even slight improvement may mean a lot for these severely disabled patients. Given the modest objective improvement, if any, in patients with choreoathetosis, however, it is difficult to recommend pallidal DBS for this indication, despite the positive self-rating of individual patients. Further studies are necessary before DBS is applied more widely for this indication.

Hemidystonia is a typical manifestation of secondary dystonia. As discussed above, the thalamus was the target of choice for ablative surgery in hemidystonia.[41,55] The results with pallidal DBS are rather heterogeneous. Whereas there was no or little improvement in some studies,[70] unilateral DBS contralateral to the hemidystonia resulted in sustained marked improvement of dystonia-associated pain, phasic dystonic movements, dystonic posture, and functional benefit at long-term follow-up in other patients.[54,83]

INTRATHECAL BACLOFEN

Intrathecal baclofen (ITB) has been used now for more than a decade to treat patients with dystonia.[94,95] In particular, patients with generalized secondary dystonia, and patients with both dystonia and spasticity are considered good candidates for this treatment option.[96,97] The mechanisms of action by which ITB treatment alters dystonia may involve both spinal and cranial levels. Intrathecal delivery of baclofen in dystonia patients results in reduction of dystonia and associated pain. In contrast to patients with spasticity, patients with dystonia require higher dosages of baclofen, they are more likely to become resistant to baclofen, and they are less likely to experience substantial improvement in function.

ITB is administered on a long-term basis through an implanted infusion pump. Pumps can be implanted in adults and in children weighing at least 20 lb (9 kg). Prior to pump implantation, patients may be screened with bolus injections of baclofen via lumbar puncture or by continuous infusion via an external micropump and an intrathecal catheter. Responses are expected within 6–12 hours. When the dystonia responds to the testing, a pump is implanted subcutaneously, usually in the right or left lower quadrant of the abdomen, and connected to an intrathecal catheter, which is inserted at approximately L2–3 and advanced cephalad to C7–T1. Regarding the need for numerous dose adjustments during chronic treatment, programmable pumps are clearly advantageous. Pumps are programmed postoperatively. Daily dosages for dystonia range from 200 to 2000 μg baclofen, usually between 500 and 1000 μg, which is higher than the dose needed to treat spasticity.

Sustained improvement of dystonia was reported in about 70% of published cases.[94] In a series of 86 patients with generalized dystonia ranging in age from 3 to 42 years (median age, 13 years), dystonia was associated with cerebral palsy in 71%.[98] Response to ITB was tested by continuous infusion in 72% of patients, and by bolus injections in 17%. Pumps were implanted in 77 patients. Dystonia scores were significantly decreased during follow-up up to 24 months. Patient questionnaires indicated that quality of life and ease of care improved in 86% of patients. Speech improved in 33% of patients, swallowing in 26%, upper limb function in 34%, and lower extremity function in 37%. Overall, surgical complications occurred in 38% of patients, including Cerebrospinal fluid (CSF) leaks, infections, and catheter problems, and ITB side effects in 26% of patients including constipation in 19%, decreased neck/trunk control in 8%, and drowsiness in 6%.

SURGERY FOR BLEPHAROSPASM

The mainstay in the treatment of blepharospasm is the local injection of BTX in the affected muscles. Surgical interventions are reserved for those patients who do not achieve adequate relief by the injections, or those who develop resistance with repeated injections.[99] It is important to note that patients with blepharospasm who do not benefit adequately from BTX injection may have a component of apraxia of eyelid opening. While Jordan and colleagues reported a 7% incidence of apraxia of eyelid opening in essential blepharospasm,[100] approximately 50% of patients with BTX failure who were referred for myectomy procedures were diagnosed with this condition.[101] Since patients in advanced stages of blepharospasm may become functionally blind and unable to care for themselves, contemporary surgery can be a valuable treatment option. Neurectomies and selective facial nerve avulsions directed at the denervation of the contracting muscles in blepharospasm have been largely abandoned because of their relatively high recurrence rates and frequent side effects.[102] Since Anderson and colleagues introduced and popularized selective myectomy procedures in the late 1970s,[103] these approaches have been adopted more widely. Currently, *extended limited myectomy* and *full myectomy* are the procedures of choice. *Full myectomy* is technically more demanding and complication rates are higher with this procedure.

The *extended limited myectomy* procedure has been suggested as the first step when considering myectomy operations.[101] The myectomy is performed through an eyelid crease incision, and involves the removal of the pretarsal orbicularis muscle, the preseptal orbicularis muscle, part of the orbital orbicularis muscle, and part of the corrugator superficialis muscle. In patients with apraxia of eyelid opening, the levator aponeurosis can be tightened to correct upper eyelid position, and also the lateral canthal tendon. This results in improvement of function and cosmesis while reducing squeezing in the upper eyelid. Few of these patients may require a frontalis suspension as a second procedure if the eyelids still do not open well enough. *Extended limited myectomy* has been described to result in less lymphedema, ecchymosis, and supraorbital hypersthesia, and patients recover much faster as compared with those after the *full myectomy* procedure. Also, this approach results in fewer corneal surface exposure problems and dry eyes. Often, patients in whom BTX injections had failed preoperatively respond to residual blepharospasm after *extended limited myectomy*.

Full myectomy is indicated in patients who did not achieve sufficient benefit with the more limited myectomy approach. It is performed through a brow incision above and a blepharoplasty incision in the lower eyelids. Then, the remaining orbicularis oculi muscles, and the procerus and corrugator muscles are removed as well, and the lateral canthal tendon is again tightened. Upper eyelid lymphedema is of utmost concern since it may last for weeks, months, and even years. Such patients may not be able to open their eyelids because of mechanical resistance, and the chronic swelling can be a difficult problem to resolve. The occurrence of chronic lymphedema is much rarer with the use of newer techniques. Other potential complications of the myectomy procedures include infection, hematoma, brow hair loss, eyelid retraction, trichiasis, and canthal deformity.

In a study from the Mayo Clinic, 94% of patients thought that myectomy procedures had provided both short-term and long-term benefits.[104] The long-term need for BTX injections was decreased in about 50% of patients, and increased efficacy or longer-lasting effects were noted, postoperatively. Patients with severe disability from blepharospasm benefited more from myectomies than did patients with relatively mild symptoms.

An alternative procedure, the so-called frontal sling operation, consists of frontalis suspension, which has been used earlier for treatment of ptosis.[105] In a series of 132 patients, improvement after surgery was achieved in 73% of patients. No serious corneal complications were observed. The beneficial effect of surgery, in general remained stable over the years. Most patients continued to have additional botulinum toxin injections. Frontalis suspension may be considered less-invasive surgery that is reversible upon removal of the silk or Gore-Tex sutures used in this procedure.

With regard to the recent development of pallidal DBS for treatment of dystonia, this new therapeutic modality might also be envisioned as an option in patients with severe and otherwise intractable blepharospasm. As outlined above, it has been used thus far successfuly in single patients with Meige syndrome, where it improved both orofacial dyskinesias and blepharospasm.[88,106]

REFERENCES

1. Jankovic J. Re-emergence of surgery for dystonia. J Neurol Neurosurg Psychiatry 1998; 65: 434.
2. Ondo WG, Krauss JK. Surgical therapies for dystonia. In: Brin MF, Comella C, Jankovic J, eds. Dystonia: Etiology, Clinical Features and Treatment. Philadelphia: Lippincott, Williams and Wilkins; 2004: 125–47.
3. Albanese A, Barnes MP, Bhatia KP et al. A systematic review on the diagnosis and treatment of primary (idiopathic) dystonia and

dystonia plus syndromes: report of an EFNS/MDS-ES Task Force. Eur J Neurol 2006; 13: 433–44.
4. Krauss JK. Deep brain stimulation for dystonia in adults: overview and developments. Stereotact Funct Neurosurg 2002; 78: 168–82.
5. Krauss JK, Yianni J, Loher TJ et al. Deep brain stimulation for dystonia. J Clin Neurophysiol 2004; 21: 18–30.
6. Krauss JK, Grossman RG, Jankovic J. Treatment options for surgery of cervical dystonia. In: Krauss JK, Jankovic J, Grossman RG, eds. Surgery for Parkinson's Disease and Movement Disorders. Philadelphia: Lippincott, Williams and Wilkins; 2001: 323–34.
7. Bertrand CM. Selective peripheral denervation for spasmodic torticollis: surgical technique, results, and observations in 260 cases. Surg Neurol 1993; 40: 96–103.
8. Gildenberg PL. Treatment of spasmodic torticollis by dorsal column stimulation. Appl Neurophysiol 1978; 41: 113–21.
9. Fahn S. Lack of benefit from cervical cord stimulation for dystonia. N Engl J Med 1985; 313: 1229.
10. Meyers R. The modification of alternating tremor, rigidity and festination by surgery of the basal ganglia. Res Publ Assoc Res Nerv Ment Dis 1942; 21: 602–65.
11. Spiegel EA, Wycis HT, Marks M et al. Stereotaxic apparatus for operations on the human brain. Science 1947; 106: 349–50.
12. Loher TJ, Pohle T, Krauss JK. Functional stereotactic neurosurgery for treatment of cervical dystonia: review of the experience from the lesional era. Stereotact Funct Neurosurg 2004; 82: 1–13.
13. Jankovic J, Schwartz K. Response and immunoresistance to botulinum toxin injections. Neurology 1995; 45: 1743–6.
14. Jankovic J. Treatment of cervical dystonia. In: Brin MF, Comella C, Jankovic J, eds. Dystonia: Etiology, Clinical Features and Treatment. Philadelphia: Lippincott, Williams and Wilkins, 2004: 159–66.
15. Krauss JK, Toups EG, Jankovic J et al. Symptomatic and functional outcome of surgical treatment of cervical dystonia. J Neurol Neurosurg Psychiatry 1997; 63: 642–8.
16. Taira T, Kobayashi T, Takahashi K et al. A new denervation procedure for idiopathic cervical dystonia. J Neurosurg 2002; 97(2 Suppl): 201–6.
17. Munchau A, Filipovic SR, Oester-Barkey A et al. Spontaneously changing muscular activation pattern in patients with cervical dystonia. Mov Disord 2001; 16: 1091–7.
18. Bertrand CM. Surgical management of spasmodic torticollis and adult-onset dystonia. In: Schmidek HH, Sweet WH, eds. Operative Neurosurgical Techniques, 3rd edn. Philadelphia: WB Saunders; 1995: 1649–59.
19. Braun V, Richter HP. Selective peripheral denervation and posterior ramisectomy in cervical dystonia. In: Krauss JK, Jankovic J, Grossman RG, eds. Surgery for Parkinson's Disease and Movement Disorders. Philadelphia: Lippincott Williams and Wilkins; 2001: 335–42.
20. Girard F, Ruel M, McKenty S et al. Incidences of venous air embolism and patent foramen ovale among patients undergoing selective peripheral denervation in the sitting position. Neurosurgery 2003; 53: 316–19.
21. Braun V, Richter HP. Selective peripheral denervation for spasmodic torticollis: 13-year experience with 155 patients. J Neurosurg 2002; 97(2 Suppl): 207–12.
22. Munchau A, Palmer JD, Dressler D et al. Prospective study of selective peripheral denervation for botulinum-toxin resistant patients with cervical dystonia. Brain 2001; 124: 769–83.
23. Ford B, Louis ED, Greene P et al. Outcome of selective ramisectomy for botulinum toxin resistant torticollis. J Neurol Neurosurg Psychiatry 1998; 65: 472–8.
24. Chawda SJ, Munchau A, Johnson D et al. Pattern of premature degenerative changes of the cervical spine in patients with spasmodic torticollis and the impact on the outcome of selective peripheral denervation. J Neurol Neurosurg Psychiatry 2000; 68: 465–71.
25. Weigel R, Rittmann M, Krauss JK. Spontaneous craniocervical osseous fusion resulting from cervical dystonia. J Neurosurg (Spine) 2001; 95: 115–18.
26. Krauss JK, Koller R, Burgunder JM. Partial myotomy/myectomy of the trapezius muscle with an asleep–awake–asleep anesthetic technique for treatment of cervical dystonia. J Neurosurg 1999; 91: 889–91.
27. Chen X. Selective resection and denervation of cervical muscles in the treatment of spasmodic torticollis: results in 60 cases. Neurosurgery 1981; 8: 680–8.
28. Chen XK, Ji SX, Zhu H et al. Operative treatment of bilateral retrocollis. Acta Neurochir 1991; 113: 180–3.
29. Hernesniemi J, Keränen T. Long-term outcome after surgery for spasmodic torticollis. Acta Neurochir 1990; 103: 128–30.
30. Hamby WB, Schiffer S. Spasmodic torticollis: results after cervical rhizotomy in 80 cases. Clin Neurosurg 1970; 17: 28–37.
31. Friedman AH, Nashold BS Jr, Sharp R et al. Treatment of spasmodic torticollis with intradural selective rhizotomies. J Neurosurg 1993; 78: 46–53.
32. Colbassani HJ Jr, Wood JH. Management of spasmodic torticollis. Surg Neurol 1986; 25: 153–8.
33. Horner J, Riski JE, Ovelmen-Levitt J et al. Swallowing in torticollis before and after rhizotomy. Dysphagia 1992; 7: 117–25.
34. Scoville WB. Motor tics of the head and neck: surgical approaches and their complications. Acta Neurochir 1978; 45: 338.
35. Jho HD, Jannetta PJ. Microvascular decompression for spasmodic torticollis. Acta Neurochir 1995; 134: 21–6.
36. Shima F, Fukui M, Kitamura K et al. Diagnosis and surgical treatment of spasmodic torticollis of 11th nerve origin. Neurosurgery 1988; 22: 358–63.
37. Freckmann N, Hagenah R, Herrmann HD et al. Bilateral microsurgical lysis of the spinal accessory nerve roots for treatment of spasmodic torticollis. Acta Neurochir 1986; 83: 47–53.
38. Krauss JK, Pohle T, Weber S et al. Bilateral stimulation of globus pallidus internus for treatment of cervical dystonia. Lancet 1999; 354: 837–8.
39. Coubes P, Echenne B, Roubertie A et al. [Treatment of early-onset generalized dystonia by chronic bilateral stimulation of the internal globus pallidus. Apropos of a case.] Neurochirurgie 1999; 45: 139–44. [in French]
40. Kumar R, Dagher A, Hutchison WD, Lang AE, Lozano AM. Globus pallidus deep brain stimulation for generalized dystonia: clinical and PET investigation. Neurology 1999; 53: 871–4.
41. Ondo WG, Desaloms M, Krauss JK et al. Pallidotomy and thalamotomy for dystonia. In: Krauss JK, Jankovic J, Grossman RG, eds. Surgery for Parkinson's Disease and Movement Disorders. Philadelphia: Lippincott, Williams and Wilkins; 2001: 299–306.
42. Andrew J, Fowler CJ, Harrison MJG. Stereotaxic thalamotomy in 55 cases of dystonia. Brain 1983; 106: 981–1000.
43. Tasker RR, Doorly T, Yamashiro K. Thalamotomy in generalized dystonia. Adv Neurol 1988; 50: 615–31.
44. Cardoso F, Jankovic J, Grossman RG et al. Outcome after stereotactic thalamotomy for dystonia and hemiballismus. Neurosurgery 1995; 36: 501–8.
45. Krauss JK, Mohadjer M, Braus DF et al. Dystonia following head trauma: a report of nine patients and review of the literature. Mov Disord 1992; 7: 263–72.
46. Bhatia KP. Posteroventral pallidotomy can ameliorate attacks of paroxysmal dystonia induced by exercise. J Neurol Neurosurg Psychiatry 1998; 65: 604–5.
47. Lozano AM, Kumar R, Gross RE et al. Globus pallidus internus pallidotomy for generalized dystonia. Mov Disord 1997; 12: 865–70.

48. Ondo WG, Desaloms JM, Jankovic J, Grossman RG. Pallidotomy for dystonia. Mov Disord 1998; 13: 693–8.
49. Vitek JL, Zhang J, Evatt M et al. GPi pallidotomy for dystonia: clinical outcome and neuronal activity. Adv Neurol 1998; 78: 211–19.
50. Yoshor D, Hamilton WJ, Ondo W et al. Comparison of thalamotomy and pallidotomy for the treatment of dystonia. Neurosurgery 2001; 48: 818–24.
51. Cubo E, Shannon KM, Penn RD et al. Internal globus pallidotomy in dystonia secondary to Huntington's disease. Mov Disord 2000; 15: 1248–51.
52. Justesen CR, Penn RD, Kroin JS et al. Stereotactic pallidotomy in a child with Hallervorden–Spatz disease. J Neurosurg 1999; 90: 551–4.
53. Alkhani A, Khan F, Lang AE et al. The response to pallidal surgery for dystonia is dependent on the etiology. Neurosurgery 2000; 47: 504.
54. Loher TJ, Hasdemir MG, Burgunder JM et al. Long-term follow-up study of chronic globus pallidus internus stimulation for posttraumatic hemidystonia. J Neurosurg 2000; 92: 457–60.
55. Krauss JK, Jankovic J. Head injury and posttraumatic movement disorders. Neurosurgery 2002; 50: 927–40.
56. Lin JJ, Lin SZ, Chang DC. Pallidotomy and generalized dystonia. Mov Disord 1999; 14: 1057–9.
57. Teo C. Functional stereotactic surgery of movement disorders in cerebral palsy. In: Krauss JK, Jankovic J, Grossman RG, eds. Surgery for Parkinson's Disease and Movement Disorders. Philadelphia: Lippincott, Williams and Wilkins; 2001: 410–15.
58. Grips E, Blahak C, Capelle HH et al. Patterns of reoccurrence of segmental dystonia after discontinuation of deep brain stimulation. Neurol Neurosurg Psychiatry 2007; 78: 318–20.
59. Rowe JG, Davies LE, Scott R et al. Surgical complications of functional neurosurgery treating movement disorders: results with anatomical localisation. J Clin Neurosci 1999; 6: 36–7.
60. Vidailhet M, Vercueil L, Houeto JL et al. French Stimulation du Pallidum Interne dans la Dystonie (SPIDY) Study Group. Bilateral deep-brain stimulation of the globus pallidus in primary generalized dystonia. N Engl J Med 2005; 352: 459–67.
61. Kupsch A, Benecke K, Muller J et al. Deep-Brain stimulation for Dystonia study group. Pallidal deep-brain stimulation in primary generalized or segmental dystonia. N Engl J Med 2006; 355: 1978–90.
62. Kiss ZH, Doig K, Eliasziw M et al. The Canadian multicenter trial of pallidal deep brain stimulation for cervical dystonia: preliminary results in three patients. Neurosurg Focus 2004; 17: E5.
63. Magyar-Lehmann S, Antonini A, Roelcke U et al. Cerebral glucose metabolism in patients with spasmodic torticollis. Mov Disord 1997; 12: 704–8.
64. Naumann M, Pirker W, Reiners K et al. Imaging the pre- and postsynaptic side of striatal dopaminergic synapses in idiopathic cervical dystonia: a SPECT study using (^{123}I) epidepride and (^{123}I) beta-CIT. Mov Disord 1998; 13: 319–23.
65. Thompson ML, Thickbroom GW, Mastaglia FL. Corticomotor representation of the sternocleidomastoid muscle. Brain 1997; 120: 245–55.
66. Krauss JK. Deep brain stimulation for cervical dystonia. J Neurol Neurosurg Psychiatry 2003; 74: 1598.
67. Krauss JK, Loher TJ, Pohle T et al. Pallidal deep brain stimulation in patients with cervical dystonia and severe cervical dyskinesias with cervical myelopathy. J Neurol Neurosurg Psychiatry 2002; 72: 249–56.
68. Parkin S, Aziz T, Gregory R et al. Bilateral internal globus pallidus stimulation for the treatment of spasmodic torticollis. Mov Disord 2001 16: 489–93.
69. Kulisevsky J, Lleo A, Gironell A et al. Bilateral pallidal stimulation for cervical dystonia: dissociated pain and motor improvement. Neurology 2000; 55: 1754–5.
70. Yianni J, Bain P, Giladi N et al. Globus pallidus internus deep brain stimulation for dystonic conditions: a prospective audit. Mov Disord 2003; 18: 436–42.
71. Bittar RG, Yianni J, Wang S et al. Deep brain stimulation for generalised dystonia and spasmodic torticollis. J Clin Neurosci 2005; 12: 12–16.
72. Botzel K, Steude U. [First experiences in deep brain stimulation for cervical dystonia]. Nervenarzt 2006; 77: 940–5. [in German]
73. Eltahawy HA, Saint-Cyr J, Poon YY et al. Pallidal deep brain stimulation in cervical dystonia: clinical outcome in four cases. Can J Neurol Sci 2004; 31: 328–32.
74. Loher TJ, Bärlocher CB, Krauss JK. Dystonic movement disorders and spinal degenerative disease. Stereotact Funct Neurosurg 2006; 84: 1–11.
75. Coubes P, Roubertie A, Vayssiere N et al. Treatment or DYT1-generalised dystonia by stimulation of the internal globus pallidus. Lancet 2000; 355: 2220–1.
76. Cif L, El Fertit H, Vayssiere N et al. Treatment of dystonic syndromes by chronic electrical stimulation of the internal globus pallidus. J Neurosurg Sci 2003; 47: 52–5.
77. Starr PA, Turner RS, Rau G et al. Microelectrode-guided implantation of deep brain stimulators into the globus pallidus internus for dystonia: techniques, electrode locations, and outcomes. J Neurosurg 2006; 104: 488–501.
77. Krause M, Fogel W, Kloss M et al. Pallidal stimulation for dystonia. Neurosurgery 2004; 55: 1361–70.
79. Katayama Y, Fukaya C, Kobayashi K et al. Chronic stimulation of the globus pallidus internus for control of primary generalized dystonia. Acta Neurochir Suppl 2003; 87: 125–8.
80. Krauss JK, Loher TJ, Weigel R et al. Chronic stimulation of the globus pallidus internus for treatment of non-DYT1 generalized dystonia and choreoathetosis: 2-year follow up. J Neurosurg 2003; 98: 785–92.
81. Eltahawy HA, Saint-Cyr J, Giladi N, Lang AE, Lozano AM. Primary dystonia is more responsive than secondary dystonia to pallidal interventions: outcome after pallidotomy or pallidal deep brain stimulation. Neurosurgery 2004; 54: 613–19.
82. Pillon B, Ardouin C, Dujardin K et al. French SPIDY Study Group. Preservation of cognitive function in dystonia treated by pallidal stimulation. Neurology 2006; 66: 1556–8.
83. Vercueil L, Pollak P, Fraix V et al. Deep brain stimulation in the treatment of severe dystonia. J Neurol 2001; 248: 695–700.
84. Bereznai B, Steude U, Seelos K et al. Chronic high frequency globus pallidus internus stimulation in different types of dystonia: a clinical, video, and MRI report of six patients presenting with segmental, cervical, and generalized dystonia. Mov Disord 2002, 17: 138–44
85. Wöhrle JC, Weigel R, Grips E et al. Risperidone-responsive segmental dystonia and pallidal deep brain stimulation. Neurology 2003; 61: 546–8.
86. Nandi D, Parkin S, Scott R et al. Camptocormia treated with bilateral pallidal stimulation. J Neurosurg 2002; 97: 461–6.
87. Muta D, Goto S, Nishikawa S et al. Bilateral pallidal stimulation for idiopathic segmental axial dystonia advanced from Meige syndrome refractory to bilateral thalamotomy. Mov Disord 2001; 16: 774–8.
88. Capelle HH, Weigel R, Krauss JK. Bilateral pallidal stimulation for blepharospasm-oromandibular dystonia (Meige syndrome). Neurology 2003; 60: 2017–8.
89. Krauss JK, Blahak C, Capelle HH et al. Prospective evaluation of deep brain stimulation in segmental dystonia: a series of 15 patients. Acta Neurochirurgica 2006; 148: 5.
90. Capelle HH, Blahak C, Kekelia K et al. Health-related quality of life in segmental dystonia is improved by bilateral pallidal chronic deep brain stimulation. Acta Neurochirurgica 2006; 148: 35.

91. Loher TJ, Krauss JK, Burgunder JM et al. Chronic stimulation of the ventrointermediate thalamus is effective for treatment of peripherally-induced dystonic paroxysmal nonkinesigenic dyskinesia. Neurology 2001; 56: 268–70.
92. Angelini L, Nardocci N, Estienne M et al. Life-threatening dystonia-dyskinesias in a child: successful treatment with bilateral pallidal stimulation. Mov Disord 2000; 15: 1010–12.
93. Gill S, Curran A, Tripp J et al. Hyperkinetic movement disorder in an 11-year-old child treated with bilateral stimulators. Dev Med Child Neurol 2001; 43: 350–3.
94. Albright AL. Intrathecal baclofen for treatment of dystonia. In: Krauss JK, Jankovic J, Grossman RG, eds. Surgery for Parkinson's Disease and Movement Disorders. Philadelphia: Lippincott Williams and Wilkins: 2001: 316–22.
95. Albright AL, Ferson SS. Intrathecal baclofen therapy in children. Neurosurg Focus 2006; 21: E3.
96. Narayan RK, Loubser PG, Jankovic J et al. Intrathecal baclofen for intractable axial dystonia. Neurology 1991; 41: 1141–2.
97. Penn RD, Gianino JM, York MM. Intrathecal baclofen for motor disorders. Mov Disord 1995; 10: 675–7.
98. Albright AL, Barry MJ, Shafton DH et al. Intrathecal baclofen for generalized dystonia. Dev Med Child Neurol 2001; 43: 652–7.
99. Patel BC. Surgical management of essential blepharospasm. Otolaryngol Clin North Am 2005; 38: 1075–98.
100. Jordan DR, Anderson RL, Digre KB. Apraxia of lid opening in blepharospasm. Ophthalmic Surg 1990; 21: 331–4.
101. Hwang IP, Anderson RL, Jordan DR. Surgical treatment of blepharospasm. In: Krauss JK, Jankovic J, Grossman RG, eds. Surgery for Parkinson's Disease and Movement Disorders. Philadelphia: Lippincott Williams and Wilkins; 2001: 382–92.
102. Bates AK, Halliday BL, Bailey CS, Collin JR, Bird AC. Surgical management of essential blepharospasm. Br J Ophthalmol 1991; 75: 487–90.
103. Anderson RL, Patel BC, Holds JB, Jordan DR. Blepharospasm: past, present, and future. Ophthal Plast Reconstr Surg 1998; 14: 305–17.
104. Chapman KL, Bartley GB, Waller RR et al. Follow-up of patients with essential blepharospasm who underwent eyelid protractor myectomy at the Mayo Clinic from 1980 through 1995. Ophthal Plast Reconstr Surg 1999; 15: 106–10.
105. Wabbels B, Roggenkamper P. Long-term follow-up of patients with frontalis sling operation in the treatment of essential blepharospasm unresponsive to botulinum toxin therapy. Graefes Arch Clin Exp Ophthalmol 2007; 245: 45–50.
106. Houser M, Waltz T. Meige syndrome and pallidal stimulation. Mov Disord 2005; 20: 1203–5.

20

Role of the physiotherapist

Jean-Pierre Bleton

INTRODUCTION

The usual treatment for pathologies affecting motor control involves motor rehabilitation, which explains the wide consensus of the medical profession regarding the use of rehabilitation to treat dystonia.[1] This therapy, which is now well developed and structured, aims to give patients as much independence as possible, in a palliative or curative way. Although physiotherapy seems to play an important role in the treatment of people suffering from dystonia, rehabilitation professionals have few reliable scientific studies upon which to build their approach, apart from the recent studies of Byl and McKenzie for writer's cramp[2] and an earlier study by Pierre Rondot on spasmodic torticollis.[3] Nevertheless, from the different approaches presented in the literature dealing with the rehabilitation of dystonia, it seems that rehabilitation focused on correcting the clinical abnormalities observed in dystonia reduces its severity.

Despite there being a great deal of similarity between the different forms of dystonia, each case is unique and requires its own rehabilitation program based on clinical evaluation.

REHABILITATION OF CERVICAL DYSTONIA OR SPASMODIC TORTICOLLIS

Many patients suffering from cervical dystonia (CD) or spasmodic torticollis (ST) are now referred to a physiotherapist by their neurologist to complement the effect of medical treatment and botulinum toxin injections. The specific rehabilitation of CD has long been a source of interest and comment, with the prescription of specialized exercises by such famous neurologists as Duchenne de Boulogne in 1862,[4] Brissaud in 1895,[5] and Meige and Feindel in 1901.[6] Today, rehabilitation is still recommended in association with medical treatment.

No one physiotherapy treatment has been found to be universally effective. Rather than one single method, there are several strategies, which deal with the various clinical presentations. The exercise program is selected in the light of the pathophysiology.

Elements of pathophysiology relevant to the development of rehabilitation programs

Muscular contraction is abnormal in dystonic patients. Dystonic movement reveals excessive co-contraction between agonistic and antagonistic muscles.[7,8] This pathologic muscular activity reduces the speed and force of the movement.[9] The rehabilitation strategy consists of rebalancing the activity between dystonic muscles and underperforming antagonistic muscles.

Continuing activity of the dystonic muscles leads to a deficit of the strength of their antagonists.[10] The rehabilitation program tries to focus selectively on the underperforming muscles and not to overflow on to other muscles.

Electromyographic (EMG) recording of passive neck movement shows a prominent paradoxical muscular activity of the dystonic muscles during their shortening. This pathologic localized postural reflex is called the 'shortening reaction' or Westphal's phenomenon.[11–13] Therefore, the objective of physiotherapy is to keep the head in the opposite direction, away from the torticollis side.

CD leads to abnormal reorganization of voluntary gestures. Instead of calling on synergistic muscles to carry out a movement, patients involve dystonic muscles that disturb the correct execution of the neck movements. This phenomenon is called overflow.[14]

The orientation, speed, localization, and intensity of the motor exercises are selected in order to obtain the specific intended contraction.

The intensity of dystonia varies according to the muscular effort, the degree of tension,[15–17] and the position of the body. CD is less important or even disappears when the body is relaxed. Thus, the physiotherapist chooses working positions (lying, sitting, or standing) adapted to the capabilities and tonic state of the patient.

Cutaneous stimulation of the dystonic muscles reinforces the pathologic activity.[18,19]

The close spatial relationship between the site of cutaneous stimulation and the contracting muscles explains why massage is not recommended in the treatment of dystonia. On the contrary, EMG recording shows reduction of myoelectric activity during an antagonistic gesture or sensory trick[20] (e.g. there is frequent reduction of myoelectric activity when the head is supported or leaning against a wall).[21]

Development of a specific rehabilitation program for cervical dystonia

Every CD case is unique, and therefore the physiotherapy approach must take into account the specific clinical presentation.[22] The physiotherapy management of the tonic forms aims to recover the balance between the actions of the different muscles that play a role in the position of the head.[23] On the other hand, the physiotherapy treatment of the myoclonic forms aims to remove involuntary and inappropriate head movements, by conscious and coordinated movements.

As the aim is to obtain stability of the head on midline, the physiotherapist develops an approach to treatment with realistic steps to be reached within a reasonable time frame. For some patients, treatment of pain is the priority, whereas for others it is stiffness of the neck or reawakening of specific muscles. Regular assessments allow the treatment to be constantly reshaped to fit the clinical evolution (Table 20.1).[24,25] When possible, physiotherapy assessment is performed before the botulinum toxin injections have modified the clinical presentation. The muscles identified as causing CD are a target for the botulinum toxin injections. This identification is also relevant to the physiotherapy treatment, which aims principally to relax the tension in the dystonic muscles and to reinforce the activity of the corrective muscles.

Pain management

Patients often complain of a sore neck or cervical discomfort. This seems to be due to the hyperactivity of the dystonic muscles.[26] The most common sites of pain are located on the sternoclavicular joint, acromioclavicular joint, spinous processes of lower cervical vertebrae, on the insertions of the sternocleidomastoid muscle (SCM) on the clavicle, and on the insertions of the trapezius muscle on the occipital bone. This kind of pain is often reduced by stretching the muscles concerned and by careful mobilization of the painful joints. Electrotherapy, in particular ultrasound therapy, is used for its thermic, vasomotor, and, fibrolytic properties.[27]

Orthopedic consequences

During the sessions, the physiotherapist should attempt to preserve the range of the different cervical and shoulder girdle movements and to decrease the tone of the involved muscles by using local or general relaxation techniques, gentle manual tractions of the cervical region, and deep breaths. Because the cervical region is a vulnerable area, mobilization must always be carried out with care.

Rehabilitation of the clonic form of cervical dystonia

Rehabilitation of the clonic form involves two stages of treatment.

The first stage consists of maintaining immobility for a gradually increasing length of time.[28] Initially, this immobility is sustained locally in the cervical region, then progressively during activities such as walking or moving the arms. The head can be kept immobile with the use of techniques such as a light touch on the cheek (equally effective whether performed by the patient or the physiotherapist), electrical or manual stimulation of the corrective muscles (often the SCM on the side of the pathologic rotation), or even rotation of the gaze to the side opposite to the CD (oculocephalogyric reflex), which induces contraction of the corrective cervical muscles. Patients train themselves to maintain immobility in front of a mirror or with the help of a myofeedback apparatus.[29,30] The supine position abolishes the spasms or noticeably moderates them. The support of the occipital bone against the horizontal plane of the table seems to play the principal role. The posture 'hands folded behind the head' decreases the intensity of the spasms and is taught as an exercise to repeat during the course of the day. Repetitions being a strong factor of improvement, patients are encouraged to constantly fight against the spasms and to organize their environment in order to facilitate corrective action.

The second stage of treatment is applied when patients are capable of maintaining their head immobile on their own. The aim is to suppress automatic and pathologic gestures and to develop conscious and natural movements. It relies on two basic principles: reinforcement of the weakened corrective muscular activity and

Surname:	**First name:**	Year of birth:
Starting date of spasmodic torticollis:		Duration of physiotherapy:

Clinical description: Observ. / modified-eyes closed

torticollis	right	left	
laterocollis	right	left	
	anterocollis	**retrocollis**	

displacement of the head	to the right	to the left	
displacement of the head	forwards	backwards	
pathologic position	fixed	spasmodic	
head tremor	yes	no	

participation of upper limbs	yes	no	
elevation of shoulder	right	left	no. of centimeters:
rotation of shoulder girdle	clockwise	counterclockwise	
participation of torso	yes	no	
participation of face	yes	no	

					Description
antagonistic movement	yes	no	antagonist	paradoxical	
factors which aggravate ST					
factors which improve ST					

Intensity of ST: !..................................!
Particular observations:

muscular tests	**right side**				**left side**			**Observations**
Sternocleidomast.	spasm	fibrosis	weakness		spasm	fibrosis	weakness	
splenius	spasm	fibrosis	weakness		spasm	fibrosis	weakness	
trapezius	spasm	fibrosis	weakness		spasm	fibrosis	weakness	
levator anguli	spasm	fibrosis	weakness		spasm	fibrosis	weakness	
Others:	spasm	fibrosis	weakness		spasm	fibrosis	weakness	
	spasm	fibrosis	weakness		spasm	fibrosis	weakness	

Botulinum toxin muscles injected:	Dates of injection:	
	1-	2-
	3-	4-

goniometric tests	**pathologic attitude**	**active cervical mobility**	**observ. / modif- eyes closed**
flexion			
extension			
right sided inclination			
left sided inclination			
right sided rotation			
left sided rotation			

PAIN Location: **Intensity:**
Particular difficulties reported by the patient:
Particular difficulties observed by therapist:
Comparison with previous assessment:

Table 20.1 ST Report Form. (Reproduced from Bleton,[24] with permission.)

recovery of normal synergy between the muscles involved. Myofeedback is a useful complement to the physiotherapy treatment, but, today, this approach has lost some of its appeal compared to current practice, which favors the development of the interaction between the patient and the physiotherapist.

Rehabilitation of the tonic form of cervical dystonia

In this presentation of CD, the rehabilitation strategy aims to reduce tension in the muscles responsible for the CD while reinforcing the action of the corrective muscles.[31] By acting upon both the hyperactive, dystonic muscles and their weakened antagonists, physiotherapy creates conditions which favor the maintenance of the head in a balanced position and prolongs the action of botulinum toxin injections carried out to weaken the muscles responsible for the CD.

The dystonic muscles relax in response to gentle but sustained traction of the neck. It then becomes possible to obtain a contraction of the corrective muscles, benefiting from the relaxation of their antagonists. The tractions are repeated as soon as the spasms reappear.

These mobilizations are carried out with the patient relaxed, lying on the back with the head resting on the plinth. In the rare situations where pressure on the occipital region triggers or increases spasms, the mobilizations can be carried out with the patient in prone position or on all fours.

The muscular approach consists of stretching each of the muscles responsible for the CD and controlling spasms by using 'favorable activities' – such as the direction of the gaze – that play a significant role in the correction of the cervical movement. The spasm intensity diminishes if the eyes are turned away from the spasm side. The positive effect of this oculocervical coordination is used in daily activities.[32] Other favorable activities are tactile inputs. Gentle friction on the jaw on the opposite side to the CD makes the head turn towards the stimulus as if pulled by a magnetic field.

Deficient muscles are reinforced by voluntary contraction (Figure 20.1). Static contractions in the inner range of movement are carried out in order to avoid muscular overflow and prevent the effect of the shortening reaction. The head is gradually shifted from the opposite side of the CD to the neutral position. Coordination of the action between deficient and dystonic muscles re-establishes localized postural balance. Patients learn how to immobilize the head in a lying position, then sitting, and finally upright. When patients have managed to control the head in the physiotherapy context, they then attempt to transfer this control to everyday life.

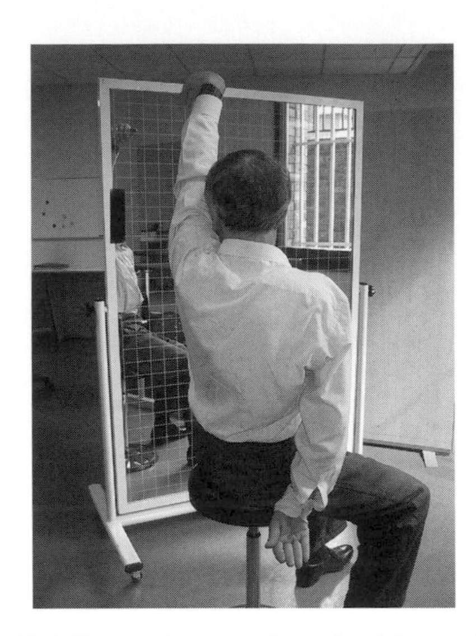

Figure 20.1 Dynamic correction of a right cervical dystonia.

Once the head is well positioned, one deals with the compensatory attitude of the upper body. The torso and shoulder girdle are frequently involved in the pathologic posture. Electrical muscle stimulation provides a boost to this muscular reinforcement.[33] The duration of the current, along with its onset and offset, are regulated so as to avoid sudden muscle jerks. The patient improves, not by remaining passive, but by accompanying the electrical stimulation with a voluntary corrective movement.

Patient involvement

As a matter of course, all sensory tricks and orthopedic appliances must be removed. Sensory tricks are a constant reminder of cervical dystonia and rigid cervical collars provoke nociceptive stimuli, which create spasms or increase their intensity. Patients must understand their condition and recognize the muscles involved in their particular case in order to correct their abnormal activity. Patients are advised about the organization of their environment in order to stimulate the contraction of the corrective muscles and to turn the gaze to the same side. Between treatment sessions, patients must respect the don't-make-it-worse rule by avoiding activities that increase the CD.[34] This is one way to facilitate control.

Physiotherapy and botulinum toxin

Even before the use of botulinum toxin, positive results had been observed after long months of treatment with myorelaxant drugs, intramuscular injections of alcohol, and rehabilitation. The use of botulinum toxin has changed the prognosis of CD; the short-term improvements are surprising, even if occasionally the long-term outcome is variable and sometimes inconsistent.[10] Pierre Rondot has shown in a review of 220 patients with isolated and idiopathic CD treated over a 14-year period that the best therapeutic results were obtained by combining anticholinergic drugs, local injections, and physiotherapy.[3] The weeks following the course of botulinum toxin injections are the ideal time to carry out physiotherapy treatment. Given the weakness of the dystonic muscles, the antagonistic muscles are more able to contract. At the end of the toxin's effective period, when muscular activity begins to interfere once more, rehabilitation continues unchanged. While awaiting the next injections, physiotherapy focuses on muscle relaxation.[35]

Although a prognosis cannot be reached during initial assessment, it can be suggested. Certain rules have been repeatedly confirmed through experience. Tonic form and simple CD in particular have a more positive outcome. Conversely, tremor forms and complex CD respond to a lesser degree to physiotherapy. Nevertheless, application of transcutaneous electrical nerve stimulation (TENS) can be an effective technique on dystonic tremor.[36]

Given that so few recent scientific studies have been published, it would be useful to investigate further the effectiveness of physiotherapy for CD.

TASK-SPECIFIC DYSTONIA: REHABILITATION OF WRITER'S CRAMP AND MUSICIAN'S CRAMP

Development of a specific rehabilitation program for writer's cramp

The treatment of writer's cramp is essentially very similar to that of CD. Botulinum toxin, combined with physiotherapy, is currently the best therapeutic approach.[37,38]

The effectiveness of rehabilitation depends on the capacity of patients suffering from writer's cramp to modify the sensorimotor program of writing through training.[39] In a preliminary study based on the publications of Byl et al,[40] EMG recording has shown disorganization of the representation of the fingers' somatotopia in the primary somatosensory cortex (S1) in patients suffering from a functional dystonia of the dominant upper limb.[41] The second study compared a cohort of patients who had been suffering from writer's cramp but were now clinically healed, and who had received only physiotherapy treatment, with a cohort of patients who also suffered from writer's cramp, but were not treated. This showed a reorganization of the somatotopic representation of the fingers at the level of S1 of the dominant upper limb in patients who had received physiotherapy treatment.[42]

The idea that rehabilitation is a legitimate treatment of writer's cramp has been gaining credibility since the middle of the 19th century, especially following the publications of Henry Meige, whose advice to write little, but slowly, in large, round, and straight movements still applies today.[43]

The aim of rehabilitation is not to enable patients with writer's cramp to write as they used to, but to help their dysgraphia evolve towards a more relaxed movement that is more fluid, legible, and better controlled. One of the foundations of rehabilitation relies on the principle of target muscles, the action of which is considered to be particularly pathogenic and the cause of the abnormality.[44] Once identified, these muscles undergo various relaxation techniques (stretching and corrective postures). The aim is to neutralize the muscles in order to break up the dystonic posture. Thus, rehabilitation adds its effects to those of botulinum toxin. Furthermore, the relaxation of the target muscles facilitates the corrective effect of the antagonists.

The lack of muscular coordination and of movement precision are not the only symptoms causing writer's cramp. The examination of some patients reveals signs of sensory impairment of the hand, which may be reversed with sensory training.[45,46] The inability to relax at will also plays an important part. de Ajuriaguerra has shown the benefits of relaxation for particularly anxious people, as well as when and how to use it.[47] Once patients are able to actively reach a state of muscular relaxation again (a feeling of heaviness in the arm), they are shown how to hold the writing instrument ergonomically. They then practice under supervision. Patients are given various exercises to develop the nimbleness of the fingers and, using a pencil, to regain fluidity and comfort in holding the writing instrument. It is then a matter of exercising the muscles in order to correct the dystonic posture by involving them in the drawing of curves, convex and concave lines, and complicated patterns.[48] The more the practice context is varied, the more the activity of writing becomes simple, precise, and comfortable. The picture-writing exercises and the materials used (long-bodied pencils, multisided pencils, large sheets of paper) are chosen to avoid reproducing the situation to which writer's cramp is initially linked.

Finally, the aim of the rehabilitation is not to improve one or more muscle actions, but instead to correct a gesture and modify a motor program (Figures 20.2 and 20.3). Hence, Kouindjy's suggestion, quoted by Macé de

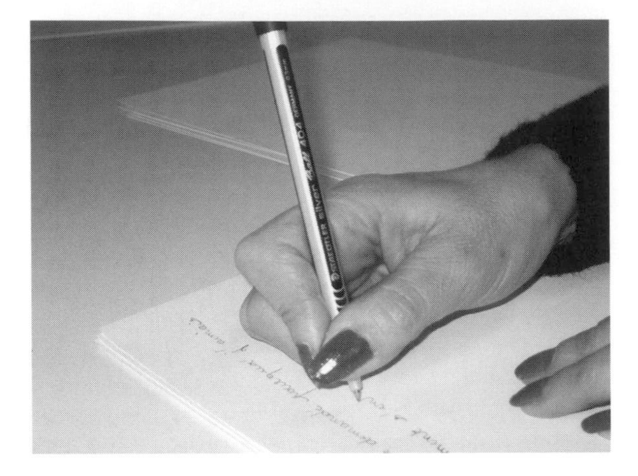

Figure 20.2 Abnormal holding of a pen.

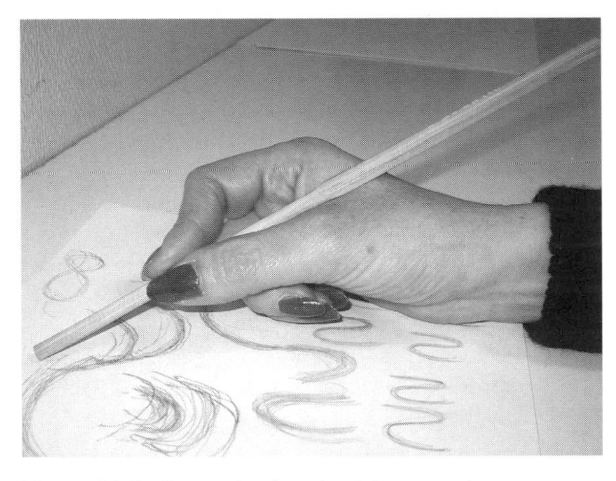

Figure 20.3 Corrective handwriting exercise.

Lépinay, to write with the wrist bent in flexion above the line of handwriting (*poignet renversé*) to overcome particularly persistent abnormalities in extension.[49]

Everyone's handwriting presents thoroughly individual characteristics. However, for the correction of writing dystonia, cursive handwriting is chosen, one of the essential characteristics being to encourage the linking of the letters with the effect of creating a synergy between the cursive movement of the shoulder and the writing movement of the hand.[50]

During the writing exercises, patients must take care to keep arms, shoulders, and chest relaxed, as well as to maintain calm and regular breathing. They must also try to avoid fragmenting words and separating letters. They must try to keep a balance between humps, ascending and descending loops, yet avoid too much pressure of the point of the writing instrument on the paper. The usual approach relies on a progressively more complex program. During this stage of the training, one must often exaggerate the size of the letters and slow the speed of the writing in order to enable patients to acquire control of the writing gesture. With practice, the handwriting returns to a normal size and speed. Given the very individualized nature of the exercises, sessions are on a one-to-one basis and require from patients a great deal of concentration. Therefore, exercises must be interrupted before signs of fatigue or discomfort appear. Sessions usually last between 30 and 45 minutes and end with relaxation techniques for the muscles. Patients are advised to practice the prescribed exercises regularly each day.

It takes 6–8 months to correct a writing dystonia. There is the risk of causing a relapse if rehabilitation is stopped too soon. A completed or successful rehabilitation is characterized by the disappearance of the abnormal posture, a more relaxed and faster movement, as well as an easier initiation of writing. The handwriting is rounder, more regular, and more legible. Patients can once again enjoy writing.

If the treatment fails, options are limited, apart from the use of information technology. Using the other hand may displace the problem, as the dystonia may in time affect that hand too. There are many special pens and devices offered to people suffering from writer's cramp. Few, however, have proved to be really effective.[51,52]

Development of a specific rehabilitation program for musician's cramp

This form of dystonia is a condition feared by musicians, as it leads to movement control problems that can interrupt their career, occasionally permanently. As in the case of writer's cramp, the dystonic posture is often one of rotation (e.g. hyper-pronation of the hand, excessive flexion of the wrist, arm internally rotated), and only appears during use of the musical instrument. Musicians lose mastery of the movement of their fingers and this is at the root of their distress. Examination frequently reveals musculoskeletal dysfunctions affecting not only the upper limbs but also the shoulder girdle and often the spine, as well as weakness of certain intrinsic muscles of the hand and an imbalance between the actions of agonistic and antagonistic muscles.[53]

The resemblance between writer's cramp and musician's cramp suggests a similar management, with rehabilitation being of primary importance.

Pain management

Although pain is not a predominant feature of musician's dystonia, some patients complain of pain related to muscular spasms. The treatment of these painful dystonias consists of resting the most affected part of the limb, often with the use of an orthosis. Prolonged immobilization is to be avoided, as it weakens the musculature and can be disheartening for the musician. One has often recourse to a rest, alternating the wearing of removable splints and gentle rehabilitation. In all cases, the resumption of playing the musical instrument occurs very gradually and is controlled by the physiotherapist, once pain is no longer present.

Correction of poor postures

It is important to watch patients playing their instruments in order to correct faulty postures. Rehabilitation is not limited to the hand, but addresses the whole of the upper limb and spine. Musicians must become conscious of the faulty postures that are at the origin of their dystonia. They must learn to relax the affected muscles, to deprogram the harmful movements, to correct the musculoskeletal dysfunctions, and eventually to relearn normal physiologic movements.[54] In front of a mirror, patients gain an awareness of their body and learn how to correct the abnormal postures. A muscular balance must be achieved, followed by relearning how to play the instrument with correct use of the body and of the adapted postures.

It takes at least 1 year to correct a musician's cramp. The quality and regularity of the treatment are important as is the active participation of patients in their own rehabilitation. With long and comprehensive rehabilitation programs, 'improvement of the symptoms is attained in most cases' of musician's cramp.[55] The satisfactory results obtained by correcting the pathologic postures and by teaching ergonomic positions highlight the importance of local factors in the appearance of task-specific dystonia, especially musician's cramp.[56]

GENERALIZED DYSTONIAS: REHABILITATION OF PRIMARY OR IDIOPATHIC TORSION DYSTONIA

The primary or idiopathic torsion dystonia (ITD) arise almost always in childhood. They begin very often with involuntary muscle contractions of the lower limbs, which spread progressively to the whole body. In general, they stabilize after adolescence, but having caused a significant motor handicap (loss of, or severe difficulties with walking, extension, or rotational spasms of the trunk and limbs, which greatly limit most functional activities).

The slightest movement provokes the dystonic muscle cramps, which may become permanent. Even if the cramp is continuous, its intensity is influenced by changes in position of the body, such as lying to sitting.[57] Emotion and stress are also aggravating factors. These clinical signs are diminished by sleep and by certain sensory tricks.

Children and adolescents with ITD pose a major therapeutic challenge, exceeding the limits of physiotherapy alone and requiring a multidisciplinary approach to deal with all of the psychological and educational issues and difficulties of daily life. Rehabilitation is an important part of the management of the dystonic child. Goals must be functional and the vision global. Treatment does not claim to make the symptoms disappear, but only to limit them to allow the child to lead as independent an existence as possible with the widest possible range of activities.

Development of a specific rehabilitation program for idiopathic torsion dystonia

The motor problems and the handicapping factors must be identified for each patient.[58] Solving these problems will involve not only the therapists but also the family and teachers. The rehabilitation of these children is different to that of children with cerebral palsy. Dystonic children have usually completed their neuromotor development before the appearance of the condition. Therefore it is not a question of facilitating a process of acquisition of motor skills, but one of reducing the involuntary muscular contractions that prevent children from using their motor potential. The activities of many of these children regress and reimprove due to variations in treatment efficacy or as a result of good and bad periods.

The search for physical comfort and painlessness

Pain only affects a small percentage of dystonic children. It occurs most with paravertebral muscle spasms, or with isolated intense cramps of certain muscles such as the hip adductors or biceps brachii. The asymmetrical distribution of cramps and of torsion postures leads to pain related to positioning. Traumatic lesions resulting from uncontrolled movements or falls may also cause pain. The treatment of pain is a priority as it disturbs rest, appetite, and schoolwork, and is the cause of anxiety and alterations in mood.

Muscular relaxation is obtained by:

- Placing the child in comfortable positions that require little effort and that maintain the body in flexion, as in sitting or lying on the side with knees against the chest. The spasms are sometimes less marked on all fours or in prone position, which can be considered as optimal rest positions for the patient.
- The use of relaxation techniques for the whole body, associated with deep breathing.

- The release of muscle tension in the 'starter muscles', the source of the spasms.

Rest and hydrotherapy in warm water favor muscular relaxation. The subject can then profit from this relaxation to attempt to produce voluntary muscle contractions that correct the worst deformities.

Prevention of orthopedic problems

Dystonic postures lead spontaneously to limb deformities and joint stiffness, which if not treated early may become irreversible. By acting upon the balance between the hyperactive dystonic muscles and their ineffective antagonists, it is possible to maintain and occasionally improve deformities. Orthopedic appliances such as corsets are poorly tolerated. The constraints they impose favor the appearance of muscular spasms or increase their intensity.

Physical activity

Physical activity includes localized exercises for the corrective muscles, dynamic in nature as well as exercises for the whole body, avoiding or limiting the onset of spasms. Placing the entire body in a flexed position diminishes the intensity of the spasms. It is then possible to benefit from this state of reduced pathologic tonic activity in order to obtain voluntary muscular contraction without triggering spasms.

Functional activity

Rehabilitation must help patients carry out activities essential to daily life, such as moving around independently, dressing, eating independently, and meeting basic hygiene requirements. This functional independence is necessary but not in itself sufficient, as the young patient must also go to school and have a social life and hobbies. Commonsense solutions can often overcome the difficulties associated with locations unadapted for persons with a handicap. Care must be taken to ensure that the time spent in rehabilitation does not disturb schooling.

Problems of written and verbal communication pose a major problem to the pursuit of studies:

- Verbal communication requires the advice and treatment of a speech therapist. Dysarthria is improved by general relaxation, control of breathing, and specific relaxation of the facial muscles. The dystonic child tries hard to communicate; therefore, attentive and benevolent listening on the part of the interlocutor is also essential.
- Writing is most commonly made possible through the use of school furniture adapted to the postural deficits of the child, and computer technology is overcoming the difficulties involved in holding a pen (digital recording, voice recognition software, or simplified keyboards).[59]

Although limited in what it can achieve, rehabilitation gives positive results in preventing joint deformity, in improving stability and comfort in different positions (lying, sitting, standing), and in allowing the patient, in many cases, to preserve or rediscover a certain degree of autonomy in walking. However, rehabilitation must not be considered merely as a treatment, but as a way of helping patients pursue their interests and passions and of allowing life to be lived to the full.

In the face of a condition with such a perplexing evolution, the slightest chance of improvement of any aspect of the handicap must be seized upon and made the object of a specific rehabilitation.[60] The contribution of family, friends, and teaching staff is of utmost importance for the successful integration of the child into everyday life.

CONCLUSION

The rehabilitation of dystonia is not restricted to the application of a few standard exercise programs. The objective is to correct the affected function through willful intervention. Such a rehabilitation program is as demanding for the patient as it is for the physiotherapist. Patients need information, stimulation, and motivation in order to find the inner resources to overcome their abnormality or handicap. In addition to correcting, or compensating for, the sensorimotor abnormalities, physiotherapy treatment must enable the reinsertion of patients with dystonia into family, social, and professional life as well as help them find within themselves a new dignity to their lives.

ACKNOWLEDGMENTS

I would like to thank Kari Hanet MEd BA and Laura Prendergast MSc BPhysio for their help in translating this text into English.

REFERENCES

1. Edwards S. Neurological Physiotherapy. London: Churchill Livingstone; 1996.
2. Byl NN, McKenzie A, Treatment effectiveness for patients with a history of repetitive hand use and focal hand dystonia: a planned, prospective follow-up study. J Hand Ther 2000; 13(4): 289–301.

3. Rondot P, Marchand MP, Dellatolas G. Spasmodic torticollis: review of 220 patients. Can J Neurol Sci 1991; 18: 143–51.
4. Duchenne (de Boulogne) GB. De l'Électrisation Localisée et Son Application à la Pathologie et à la Thérapeutique. Paris: Baillière et fils; 1862.
5. Brissaud E. Leçons sur Les Maladies. Nerveuses. Paris: Masson; 1895.
6. Meige H, Feindel E. Traitement des tics. Traitement par l'immobilisation des mouvements et les mouvements d'immobilisation. Méthode de Brissaud. Presse médicale 1901; 22: 125.
7. Rondot P. [Clinical and physiopathological study of contractures]. Rev Neurol (Paris) 1968; 118: 32–42. [in French]
8. Gelb DJ, Yoshimura DM, Olney RK, Lowenstein DH, Aminoff M. Changes in pattern of muscle activity following botulinum toxin injections for torticollis. Ann Neurol 1991; 29: 370–6.
9. Berardelli JC, Rothwell JC, Hallett M et al. The pathophysiology of primary dystonia. Brain 1998; 121: 1195–212.
10. Jedynak A, de Saint Victor JF. [Treatment of spasmodi torticollis by local injections of botulinum toxin]. Rev Neurol (Paris) 1990; 146: 440–3. [in French]
11. Westphal CFO. Uber eine dem Bilde der cerebrospinalen grauen Degeneration ähnliche Erkrankung des centrlen Nervensystems ohne anatomisschen Befund, nebst einigen Bemerkungen über paradoxe Contraction. Arch Psychiatr Nervenkr 1883; 14: 87–95.
12. Foix C, Thevenard A. Les réflexes de posture. Rev Neurol 1923; 30: 449–68.
13. Rondot P, Scherrer J. [Reflex contraction induced by passive shortening of the muscle in athetosis and position dystonias]. Rev Neurol 1966; 114: 329–37. [in French]
14. Feve A, Bathien N, Rondot P. Abnormal movements related potentials in patients with lesions of basal ganglia and anterior thalamus. J Neurol Neurosurg Psychiatry 1994; 57: 100–4.
15. Dykstra D, Ellingham C, Belfie A et al. Quantitative measurement of cervical range of motion in patients with torticollis treated with botulinum A toxin. Mov Disord 1993; 8: 38–42.
16. Van Zandijcke M. Cervical dystonia (spasmodic torticollis). Some aspects of the natural history. Acta Neurol Belg 1995; 95: 210–15.
17. Rondot P, Bleton JP. Syncinésies et mouvements involontaires spontanés. In: Chantraine A, ed. Rééducation Neurologique. Guide Pratique de Rééducation des Affections Neurologiques. Vélizy, Villacoublay: Arnette Initiatives santé; 1999: 269–80.
18. Ghika J, Regli F, Growdon JH. Sensory symptoms in cranial dystonia: a potentiel role in the etiology? J Neurol Sci 1993; 116: 142–7.
19. Hallet M. Is dystonia a sensory disorder? Ann Neurol 1995; 38: 139–40.
20. Stejskal L. Counterpressure in torticollis. J Neurol Sci 1980; 48: 9–19.
21. Monnier M. Le torticolis spasmodique; ses variations sous l'influence de diverses inductions motrices, sensitives, psychiques et végétatives. Schweizer Archiv für Neurologie und Psychiatrie 1937; 23: 345–61.
22. Cruchet R. Traité des Torticolis Spasmodiques, Spasmes, Tics, Rythmies du Cou, Torticolis Mental. Paris: Masson; 1907.
23. Deuschl G, Heinen F, Kleedorfer B et al. Clinical and polymyographic investigation of spasmodic torticollis. J Neurol 1992; 239: 9–15.
24. Bleton JP. Spasmodic Torticollis. Handbook of Rehabilitative Physiotherapy. Paris: Frison-Roche; 1994.
25. Tsui JK, Eisen A, Stoessi AJ, Calne S, Calne DB. Double-blind study of botulinum toxin in spasmodic torticollis. Lancet 1986; 2: 245–7.
26. Kutvonen O, Dastidar P, Nurmikko T. Pain in spasmodic torticollis. Pain 1997; 69: 279–86.
27. Patterson R, Little S. Spasmodic torticollis. Nerv Ment Dis 1943; 98: 571–99.
28. Zati A, Crémonini P. Le training autogène de Jacobson dans le traitement du torticolis psychogène. J Réadapt Méd 1993; 13: 3–6.
29. Korein J, Brudny J. Integrated EMG feedback in the management of spasmodic torticollis and focal dystonia: a prospective study of 80 patients. Res Publ Assoc Res Nerv Ment Dis 1976; 55: 385–426.
30. Bruce L, Bird BL, Catalo MF. Experimental analysis of E.M.G. feedback in treating dystonia. Ann Neurol 1978; 3: 310–15.
31. Cleeland CS. Behavioral techniques in the modification of spasmodic torticollis. Neurology 1973; 23: 1241–7.
32. Revel M, André-Deshays C, Minguet M. Cervicocephalic kinesthetic sensibility in patients with cervical pain. Arch Phys Med Rehabil 1991; 72: 288–91.
33. de Bisschop G, Corlobe P, Dumoulin J, Berthelin F. Musculation paravertébrale par stimulation électrique. Annales de Kinésithérapie 1994; 21: 245–50.
34. Jahanshahi M. Factors that ameliorate or aggravate spasmodic torticollis. J Neurol Neurosurg Psychiatry 2000; 68: 227–9.
35. Bleton JP. Physiotherapy for spasmodic torticollis. In: Bouvier G, de Soultrait F, Molina-Negro P, eds. Spasmodic Torticollis. Paris: Expressions Santé; 2006: 179–97.
36. Bending J, Cleeves L. Effect of electrical nerve stimulation on dystonic tremor. Lancet 1990; 336(8727): 1385–6.
37. Karp BI, Cole RA, Cohen LG et al. Long-term botulinum toxin treatment of focal hand dystonia. Neurology 1994; 44: 70–6.
38. Vidailhet M, Perkinden P, Gallouedec G, Vidal S, Sangla S. Les dystonies du membre supérieur: analyse sémiologique et prise en charge thérapeutique. In: Thoumie P, Pradat-Deihl P, eds. La Préhension. Paris: Springer-Verlag; 2000: 119–26.
39. Cottraux JA, Juenet C, Collet L. The treatment of writer's cramp with multimodal behaviour therapy and biofeedback: a study of 15 cases. Br J Psychiatry 1983; 142: 180–3.
40. Byl NN, Merzenich, MM, Jenkins WM. A primate genesis model of focal dystonia and repetitive strain injury: I. Learning-induced dedifferentiation of representation of the hand in the primary somatosensory cortex in adult monkeys. Neurology 1996; 47: 508–20.
41. Meunier S, Garnero L, Ducorps A et al. Human brain mapping in dystonia reveals both endophenotypic traits and adaptive reorganization. Ann Neurol 2001; 50: 521–7.
42. Meunier S, Bourdain F, Bleton JP et al. Cortical reorganization after behavioural training in writer's cramp. Poster P06.071, 55th Annual Meeting of the American Academy of Neurology, Honolulu, March 29 to April 5, 2003.
43. Meige H. Formule pour le Traitement de la Crampe des Écrivains. Paris: Masson; 1908.
44. Marion MH. Treatment of dystonias. Presse Med 1999; 28: 312–15. [in French]
45. Schenk T, Mai N. Is writer's cramp caused by a deficit of sensorimotor integration? Exp Brain Res 2001; 136: 321–30.
46. Zeuner KF, Bara-Jimenez W, Noguchi PS et al. Sensory training for patients with focal hand dystonia. Ann Neurol 2002; 51: 593–8.
47. de Ajuriaguerra J, Garcia Badaracco J, Trillat E, Soubiran G. [Treatment of writer's cramp by relaxation: the case process from the tonic experience]. Encéphale 1956; 2: 141–71. [in French]
48. Denner A. La psycho-motricité en thérapie par l'art. Psychologie Médicale 1992; 24: 1453–7.
49. Macé de Lépinay CE. Etude sur les Crampes Professionnelles (Spasmes Fonctionnels, Névroses Coordinatrices d'Occupation). Paris: Masson; 1909.
50. de Ajuriaguerra J, Auzias M, Denner A. L'Écriture de l'Enfant. 2 – La Rééducation de l'Écriture, 4th edn. Neuchâtel: Delachaux et Niestle; 1990.
51. Ranawaya R, Lang A. Usefulness of a writing device in writer's cramp. Neurology 1991; 41: 1136–8.
52. Tas N, Karatas GK, Sepici V. Hand orthosis as a writing aid in writer's cramp. Mov Disord 2001; 16: 1185–9.
53. Bejjani FJ, Glenn M, Kaye MD, Beham M. Musculoskeletal and neuromuscular conditions of instrumental musicians. Arch Phys Med Rehabil 1996; 77: 406–13.

54. Chamagne P. Functional dystonia in musicians: rehabilitation. Hand Clin 2003; 19: 309–16.
55. Tubiana R. Functional Disorders in Musicians. Paris: Elsevier; 2001.
56. Byl NN, Nagarajan SS, Merzenich MM, Roberts T, McKenzie A. Correlation of clinical neuromusculoskeletal and central somatosensory performance: variability in controls and patients with severe and mild focal hand dystonia. Neural Plast 2002; 9: 177–203.
57. Rondot P, Bathien N, Ziégler M. Les Mouvements Anormaux Paris: Masson; 1988.
58. Burke RE, Fahn S, Marsden CD et al. Validity and reliability of rating scale for the primary torsion dystonia. Neurology 1985; 35: 73–7.
59. Shahar E, Nowaczyk M, Tervo RC. Rehabilitation of communication impairment in dystonia musculorum deformans. Pediatr Neurol 1987; 3: 97–100.
60. McGuire TJ, Palaganas-Tosco A, Redford JB. Dystonia musculorum deformans: three cases treated on a rehabilitation unit. Arch Phys Med Rehabil 1988; 69: 373–6.

21

Role of the specialist dystonia nurse

Marianne King

INTRODUCTION

The development and implementation of the dystonia specialist nurse (DSN) role represents a valuable step forward in the creation of a more patient-focused service. The role includes one of educator, leader, researcher, resource manager, and clinician. It is suggested that a specialist nurse is able to see more patients in conjunction with the consultant, thereby reducing the consultant's work load, as well as decreasing the waiting list.[1,2] It enhances the service by reducing the number of complaints and waiting times for treatment, provides a more informal approach, and ensures up-to-date evidence-based practice. It also increases job satisfaction for the nurse, due to the dedicated nature of the role and ability to lead the service/practice development. This chapter highlights the advantages and disadvantages of a dystonia specialist nurse, as assessed within the UK healthcare system.

This chapter also provides a brief description of dystonia, the historical background to the treatment of dystonia, and the development of the DSN. It also looks at the reasons why the DSN role has developed and outlines the governmental influences on dystonia. Also discussed within the chapter are the reasons why patients with dystonia have had bad experiences and long waits for treatments. This all leads to why patients with dystonia need a service that is informal and predominantly patient-focused.

Clinical neuroscience is an expanding area of health care, and numerous specialist nurse posts are being developed. The expansion of these positions are part of the UK government's plans in bringing the health service into the 'twenty first century'.[3] According to the Code of Conduct for National Health Service (NHS) managers, the NHS plan will deliver services designed around the needs of the patients.[4,5] There is, however, the opportunity to be proactive in the development, implementation, and evaluation of specialist nurse posts, and the DSN is representative of this.

Dystonia is a movement disorder that has been poorly managed in the past. Many patients were (and are) misdiagnosed, and therefore receive inappropriate treatment.[6] Patients with chronic movement disorders, in whom no physical cause could be identified and therefore believed to be psychogenic in origin, were often referred to psychiatrists.[6] It was not until the latter part of the 19th century, with the development of neurology as a separate field of medicine, that patients were diagnosed as having a distinct neurologic conditions. The two World Wars, however, brought pharmacologic advances and, as a result, neurologic conditions such as epilepsy and Parkinson's disease were treated much more successfully.[6] With developments in neurologic medicine, there was also greater recognition of relatively rare neurologic disorders such as dystonia.[6–8]

Although dystonia is the third most prevalent neurologic movement disorder after essential tremor and Parkinson's disease,[7,8] many general practitioners (GPs) and other primary care physicians may never have seen anyone with dystonia. It is therefore not surprising that patients with dystonia have been misdiagnosed. Consequently, and also because many individuals with milder focal dystonia do not seek medical attention, the number of people with dystonia is probably higher than these estimates.[6,8–10] The need for people to acknowledge and understand dystonia is important: increased awareness leads to a more positive outlook for these patients.[11] As with any specialist nurse role, that of networking and communicating with other professionals is vital. A specialist dystonia nurse can be the link needed for better liaison between the primary care trusts (PCTs) and other healthcare professionals. This can be achieved by an increase in communication between primary and secondary care and by the development of various written leaflets and protocols. This is therefore a step in the right direction in increasing the awareness of the condition.

In this changing world of healthcare, the move towards more specialized areas of nursing is paramount due to the advances in technology education and extended nursing skills. Specialist nurses are the most suitable professional for raising awareness; they are best placed to take on the responsibilities of their patients, as they understand their needs and requirements.[1] Specialist nurses and nursing in general are concerned with health and the environment, which involves direct outcomes influencing patients, families, and communities.[3,11]

THE ROLE WITHIN NEUROSCIENCES

Within the UK, dystonia nurse specialists are relatively new roles which are evolving within neurosciences, ophthalmology, and ENT (ear, nose, and throat) departments. Specialist roles are developing in these areas due to the nature of the disease.[6–8] The development of DSNs in the UK began approximately 8 years ago, when one nurse had an overwhelming interest in dystonia. This nurse began his role funded as a university research nurse practitioner. The research was to test the theory that a fully qualified nurse could deliver botulinum toxin treatment and supportive care as effectively as the standard medical model. The project was successful; the nurse is now employed as a full-time outreach nurse for patients with dystonia and runs his own clinics. This nurse's work involved a more informal approach to dystonia.[11]

Dystonia services expanded within neurology, ophthalmology, and ENT approximately 20 years ago when botulinum toxin was more widely used for the treatment of dystonia.[6–8] These clinics ran for many years, treating patients with dystonia, strabismus, laryngeal dystonia, and hemifacial spasm, and seeing only about 10–15 patients per month. With the increasing number of cases of diagnosed dystonia, this inevitably led to an increase in number of patients in these clinics. Interestingly, however, dystonia services had never been formally audited until the late 1980s.

At this stage, purchasers of services did not realize that they were paying for expensive treatments. Treatment had been provided without specific allocation of resources to fund it. Increased number and throughput of botulinum toxin clinics further increased pressure on funding and led to increased follow-up intervals for patients receiving botulinum toxin.[6,9,12,13] A more recent review of the service identified the need for additional funding, and the possibility of involving private finance.[14] The number of dystonia referrals continues to increase, as a result of better recognition of the condition by GPs and awareness of the disease through access to the Internet. In addition, increased involvement of patient support groups and more active involvement of neurologists and specialist nurses with interest in dystonia has played a role. To deal with the greater numbers of patients with dystonia referred for assessment and treatment will require a proactive approach, and DSNs can play a key role in this.

STRUCTURED APPROACH TO DYSTONIA SERVICES

Dystonia presents differently in each individual and the degree of disability can fluctuate from person to person and from month to month.[15] The disease can cause profound deterioration in individual's health as well as severe social and financial difficulties. With the absence of cure or prevention, dystonia needs a well-coordinated case management. Figures 21.1–21.3 show the structured approach adopted in Neurosciences at Lancashire NHS Trust in the UK, where the key role for the nurse is assessment, counseling, and treatment of patients with botulinum toxin.

QUALITIES NEEDED FOR A DYSTONIA SPECIALIST NURSE

Patients' families and carers must be offered the widest possible range of support, treatment, and care.[16] This includes not only sensitivity to the needs of patients and others that may be involved in their care, but also an understanding of the roles of other interdisciplinary healthcare professionals who may need to be involved.

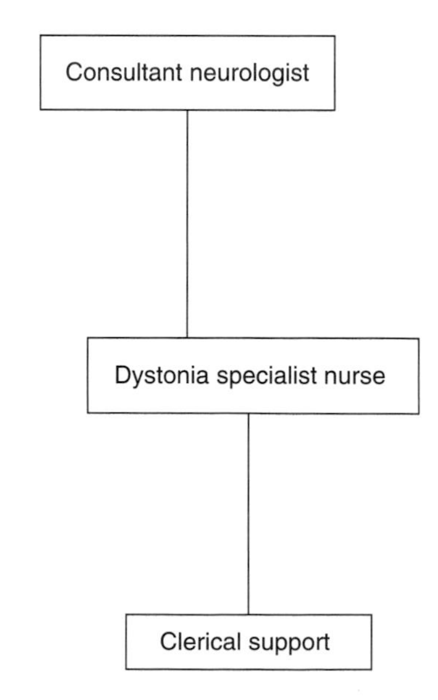

Figure 21.1 Organization of dystonia care team.

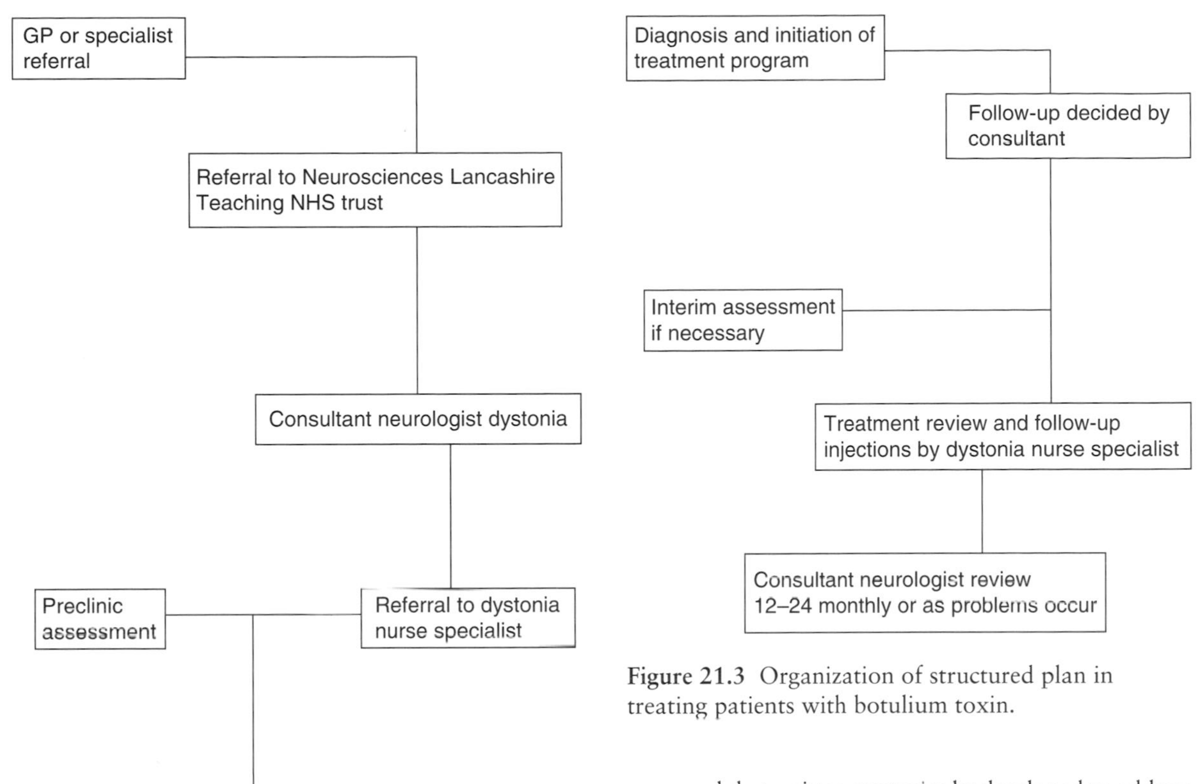

Figure 21.2 Organization of referral process.

Figure 21.3 Organization of structured plan in treating patients with botulium toxin.

With regular meetings and liaison with all these people, the DSN can provide a holistic approach to the care provided. The role of the DSN, therefore, would be to bring all these professionals together and provide a collaborative care pathway, continuity of care, and a high-quality service.

A specialist nurse needs extensive knowledge of his/her subject. Attending the Dystonia Society and support group meetings is an invaluable forum to meet patients and their carers who can keep up to date with new treatments. These meetings ensure a patient-led service by discussing patients' requirements. Therefore the role of the DSN is to listen to the patients and become their advocate. In doing so, the nurse also becomes an expert in dystonia, providing information, support, and guidance. Individuals with dystonia need alternative coping strategies: not only self-help but also involvement of other disciplines. The Commission for Health Improvements (CHI) recommends that hospitals need to improve patients' involvement in the care they receive and have proposed that written strategies be developed to address this.[16,17] The UK government policy 'The Expert Patient' states that 'patients with chronic illnesses know their needs best'.[18] These individuals need an advocate, and the DSN can do this, but they can only be patients' advocates by listening and working closely with them.

Part of the role is to educate others; therefore, presentations at conferences such as dystonia awareness days and neuroscience meetings, both locally and nationally, is a strategy to enhance this education role. The education of future dystonia nurses is very important to ensure quality services for all dystonia patients. According to the Royal College of Nursing (RCN) presentations are part of the specialist education strategy.[19] It is at these conferences that nurses often increase their knowledge and exchange and develop networks with nurses in the same and different specialities, sharing information and practice.[20] The DSN needs therefore to be able to educate others: not only patients but also other health professionals. They need to be able to liaise with all involved in providing a high-quality holistic approach.

Literature on nursing roles in dystonia is scarce. Literature about specialist nursing, in general, helps to define the role, looks at the qualities needed for the specialist role, and highlights the educational needs necessary. According to the UKCC (UK Central Council for Nursing and Midwifery) standards, there are no specific qualifications necessary; however, the document does highlight the need for nurses able to perform higher levels of judgment, discretion, and decision-making.[21] These higher levels lead to improved patient care by ensuring supervised practice, audit, research developments, and the teaching of others. This is achieved by having skilled leadership. These higher levels of judgment and decisions are based on:

- clinical practice
- care management
- clinical practice development
- clinical leadership.

As specialist nurses increase in numbers and evidence-based practice brings changes to patient care delivery, the role of the specialist nurse should be to sustain and spread knowledge so that those involved in healthcare delivery benefit:

> The need for the specialist practitioner to be expert in their field is essential, as the need to transform research into practice requires interest in the subject, organisation, intellectual vigour, clinical judgement skills and endurance.[19]

However, to ensure that the gap between theory and practice is closed, there must be closer links between knowledge generated and its implementation.[22] It is important, therefore, that specialist nurses are fully prepared for the roles and to ensure support, evaluation of the role, and further education. The right to claim such a status and all that it implies will only be given to those who are prepared to take up the heavy responsibilities for the continued development of both their knowledge and skills beyond that of initial qualifications and appointment to practice. Benner states that nursing develops in five stages from novice to expert.[21] Although Benner's ideas are correct, with each new situation we all become novices and one should never class oneself as a total expert since there are always new ways or ideas to explore. By involving others, the patient, is given the opportunities to have 'experts' in all fields. Therefore, the specialist nurse although never classed as a complete expert, will have the necessary expert knowledge and know where to find extended knowledge to teach others and be in touch with up-to-date advances in treatments.

Specialist nurses are involved with the delivery of direct and indirect patient care, becoming the coordinator of care between the primary and secondary delivery and ensuring continuity and providing emotional and psychological support.[10,12] Specialist roles were often developed because of local need, and, according to the RCN, they improved and increased information and developed a service that patients found acceptable.[19] This is, however, difficult to measure because of anecdotal and descriptive reviews.[24] There are few quantitative data available, although qualitative data show that specialist nurses are valuable in the care management of patients.[24,25] The reason for such poor quantitative data is that peoples' interpretations are difficult to quantify; often they find it difficult to explain why they think a service is good or bad. With the importance of audit and nursing governance, this quantitative data will become available and provide the evidence needed to demonstrate that the role is beneficial, cost-effective, and an improvement to services.[1,2]

Many individuals with dystonia have been treated unfairly in the past due to misdiagnosis and misreferral, and so there is a need for support and guidance. Providing information and listening may be all that is necessary for these patients to access and respond to treatment. One can argue then that this type of support could be offered by any nurse, although a nurse with extended knowledge and commitment to a service must be better equipped to deal with associated dystonia problems. One review states that the qualities needed to be a specialist nurse are 'adaptation to meet the challenging and changing needs of patients, families, nurses, physicians, trusts and to assist the government proposal'.[26] This commitment to a service brings added pressures to the post and the need for support from others is essential, and is best achieved by clinical supervision.[27] Thus, specialist nurses need the support of doctors, colleagues, and managers. Working with others is paramount, especially nurses within the same directorate and speciality, as this creates a learning environment as well as support and guidance.[27]

Education to practice has been debated extensively,[19,26,28,29] and many argue that education to degree level is essential, whereas others say experience and post basic education is all that is required. However, education improves knowledge, not only in the specialist subject but also in health politics, nursing research, and teaching methods.[30,31] For instance, education is invaluable when evaluating a business plan. This evaluation of the role provides evidence as a structured case/argument that the role is beneficial. Experience is also a critical requirement as it provides direct care delivery by teaching, assessing, and evaluating care given and also by providing consultation, change management, and providing advocacy for the patients.[24]

Many specialist nurses in the UK have, or are working towards, degree-level qualification, which brings them in line with other countries and will assist with consultant nurse posts in the future.[30–32] Without these skills, the role of the specialist nurse cannot be fulfilled. A clinical nurse specialist will assist in closing the theory practice gap, as the demand for evidence-based practice increases. Specialist nurse practitioners are often the contact between academia and practice, which can only be an advantage to nursing.[31–34]

According to many authors, nurse specialists deliver low-cost, high-quality care, providing medical intervention and alternative treatments for health care continually not only through illness but also during healthy periods.[1,32,35,36] Cost-effectiveness for specialist nurse service is a controversial area, as there may be an increase in cost through the initial setting up of a service, improved knowledge and uptake among patients and carers of possible services, and benefits for which they are entitled.[2] There will also be the extra patient referrals as the service improves and as dystonia becomes increasingly recognized. Many studies, however, have reported that specialist nurses are cost-effective by reducing hospital admissions and consultant-led outpatient appointments. This is achieved by working with set protocols, having nurse-led clinics, and managing their own patients.[1,24–26,34,37,38]

Although some studies have found no significant difference between medical and nursing treatment, the nurse's input appeared to be an effective innovation in care delivery.[1,2,24,38,39] Specialist nurses, in general, have more dedicated time with individual patients, compared with physicians, which may have a beneficial effect on the therapeutic experience and is felt to be an asset to any service.[40]

All nursing encourages patient-focused care, as nurses provide care based on the needs of patients after listening to them and involving them in decisions over care. However, this can have disadvantages, as patients seeing a specialist nurse can become focused only on their own illnesses and want treatments that they have seen on the Internet or have spoken with others about, which can sometimes be denied due to lack of evidence or lack of funding.

Figure 21.4 highlights the role and responsibilities of the specialist nurse practitioner and all are essential to ensure a smooth and successful dystonia clinic.

HOW THE SPECIALIST NURSE HELPS SERVICE DEVELOPMENT

Practice development, which is essential for the clinical nurse specialist role,[41] includes having some firm evidence-based criteria. Practice in the UK has been developing since nursing as a profession developed, but it has

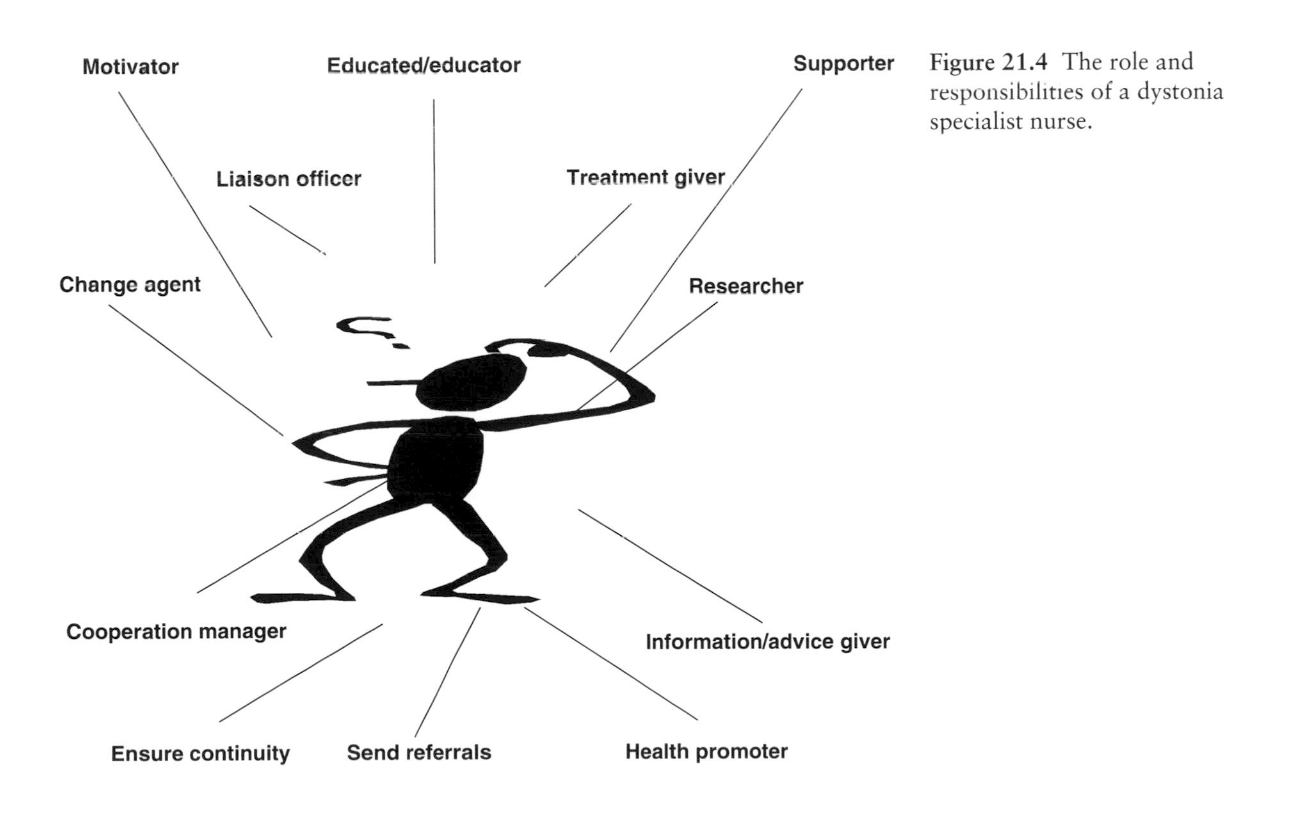

Figure 21.4 The role and responsibilities of a dystonia specialist nurse.

been accelerated since the introduction of the Post-Registration Education and Practice Project (PREPP).[42] PREPP guidelines also assist in the education and expert knowledge needed for such positions.[42] Nurses need to prove they are committed to lifelong learning by providing evidence that they ensure at least 5 study days within 3 years.[42]

With the development of dystonia specialist nurses came the introduction of nurse-led clinics. These provide better access to the service due to the specialist nurse taking on her own case load, which increases patient throughput and in turn leads to a decrease in the waiting times for patients with dystonia and an improvement in the services provided. The nurse-led clinics have smaller numbers, therefore creating more time for each patient instead of clinic appointments with a busy consultant. This can lead to fewer complaints.[37] One may question that if the patients seen are smaller in number, how does this improve service? The answer that a nurse's time is not restricted and therefore she is able to see more patients on extended days/hours and the patients have direct access to a telephone answering service. There is a minimal waiting list and patients referred to the dystonia clinic will not have to wait for months for treatment, as they have done in the past. Future developments could include the introduction of outreach clinics, meaning that patients will have access to the service near to their own homes and therefore minimize traveling times. Minimizing traveling time minimizes the stress of attending hospital,[11] which may involve travel of over 50 miles. Elderly patients without a mode of transport are reliant on hospital transport, which often cannot guarantee the requested time of pick up and return journeys. With all these advantages to the service, patient satisfaction should increase, with complaints conversely decreasing.

Research is another important aspect of clinical practice.[43,44] Nursing is said to have a poor track record in implementing research findings[43,44] and the development of specialist practitioners has improved this. Specialist nurses can be the innovators of research findings, liaising with other health professionals and ensuring evidence-based practice.[36] All specialist nurses are indirectly involved with the pharmaceutical companies who promote new treatments. Specialist nurses should have the skills to analyze trial data for new treatments and are often also directly involved with drug trials.[45] Nurses feel that when implementing research they come across barriers in the form of managers, doctors, and other nurses,[45] and have felt hampered by the medical profession in the area of research. Nurses cannot afford to be submissive, as they need to be looking at research and using best practice for their patients. This is highlighted with nurse governance, as nurses are now involved with decisions, therefore extending their authority in care giving.[46] Now that the basic nursing qualification is to diploma or degree level, nursing is working towards a professional status. Nurses are gaining a greater understanding of research and of the research process.[22] With this education, they are more likely to question procedures rather than just complete tasks.[44]

To ensure best practice, there must be good evidence-based protocols in place. With the introduction of standards, protocols, and competencies, and using audit to monitor the service, it can be ensured that what is said is being done is carried out. Design of protocols and standards for the dystonia specialist have been developed by a number of specialist nurses working together to achieve the best for patients.[45,47] Benchmarking and networking are strategies to ensure best practice is maintained. Benchmarking is a system developed to ensure that guidelines are written to enhance a better quality of care delivered to each patient.[46,47]

There are also national guidelines based on research evidence which are developed by a benchmarking group,[46–48] which should be multiprofessional and include patient representatives. Shared care protocols are key developments that involve the patients' GP to help with awareness of the disease and to involve others in the treatment and outcome of these patients.[49,50] Writing these protocols enables the service to be evaluated each year, and if the standards are not being achieved, the service must be amended. It also gives the specialist nurse evidence to support the notion that the service is an asset to directorates and trusts and other funding bodies.

The development of the dystonia service protocols has been paramount in the success of the service in other areas. These written guidelines provide a guidance for others who wish to develop such roles.[47] However, they should be considered as active documents, as there are always changes and innovations that must lead to the guidelines being reviewed and revised accordingly.[47,49] The implementation of any guidelines must be patient-centered, which means that one must recognize the patient's health problems and evaluate the outcomes and implement the evidence-based care within these guidelines. Guidelines for patients are best when patients have their say in what's best for them. This leads to guidelines that will be beneficial to nurses, patients, and doctors.[11,46,50]

The development of clinical competencies for a specialist nurse are vital and, with the guidance of others in the same field and the consultant in charge, these written competency statements act as legal documents to practice.[47] They also act as teaching material for others. It is essential that these protocols, standards, and competencies are written jointly with other dystonia nurses and with the patient's perspective in mind. Multiprofessional networking via the Internet offers opportunities for the development of competencies. In addition, it facilitates problem sharing and solving.[48,49] The Nursing and Midwifery Council (NMC) expects nurses to behave according to the standards and guidelines written.[4] It is therefore important that these developments are measured against NMC standards and good practice is upheld. These protocols will ensure that evidence-based practice in dystonia care is implemented, which, in turn, will improve patient satisfaction.

Specialist nurses also have a key role in assessing research developments to identify practice that may not only be beneficial to patients but may also be financially and clinically effective. After analyzing the research, specialist nurses need to instigate change. This change then needs to be part of an audit cycle to analyze the results and evaluate the effectiveness of change, with the ultimate goal of improving patient care.[51,52]

Dystonia specialist nurses need good leadership skills. These are enhanced by added education, experience, and commitment. Practice development tends to happen to nurses without thinking about it. The introduction of PREPP ensures all nurses are committed to lifelong learning, developing their skills so as not to be left behind. While working towards the specialist dystonia nurses position, leadership skills develop naturally as there is the need to be able to liaise with others and take peoples' opinions and experiences on board. Therefore, the specialist nurse needs to be an innovated change agent, researcher, teacher, counselor, and lifelong learner, so as to ensure quality care is given to each patient.

In the UK the government plays a large part in how the NHS develops. They have found that specialist nurses improve the quality of care delivered to patients economically. We can argue then that the government has pushed nurses into specialist roles by introducing targets, as one of the advantages with these roles is that they lower the waiting times to see a consultant.[32,53,54] However, specialist roles have not always been developed by medical influence;[47,55] nurses themselves have often been the instigation for these roles, by developing a particular interest within a specific field. Specialist roles may have been instigated from the extended roles developed within the NHS such as continence link nurses, infection control nurses, and pain management nurses.

Specialist nurses, as highlighted in many reviews, are an asset to the service, providing holistic care to patients. Owing to the lack of quantitative evidence, the reason for this is hard to establish. However, a patient who has a personal nurse giving information and support, who sees them every visit and is at the end of a phone, appears to have enhanced outcome compared with one who does not have access to a specialist nurse. Information has been highlighted as an improvement seen by the majority of patients,[11,24,40] although not by all.[56]

To summarize, a specialist nurse's role is one of direct and indirect caregiver with experience in a specific field, performing higher levels of judgment and decisions with discretion. These nurses should be capable of degree-level education and have the responsibility to supervise evidence-based practice, oversee audit, develop research strategies, and be seen as an educator. The specialist nurse's role will also enhance the service development by ensuring government targets are met and being economically viable and that patients are given the treatment when and how they deserve.[57]

REFERENCES

1. Fitzpatrick ER. Analysis and synthesis of the role of the advanced practice nurse. Clin Nurse Spec 1998; 123: 106–7.
2. McGrath D. The cost effectiveness of nurse practitioner. Nurse Pract 1990; 15: 40–2.
3. DOH Guidelines to Developing a New Career Framework for Nurses. London: HMSO; 2002.
4. Allergan. Cervical Dystonia Botulinum, Toxin A. Burlington: Adelphi Communications Ltd; 1996.
5. Dressler D. Botulinum Toxin Therapy. Properties of Botulinum Toxin. Stuttgart: Thieme: 2000.
6. Lees AJ. In: Moore P, ed. Botulinum Toxin Treatment. London: Blackwell Science; 1999.
7. Marsden CD. The Dystonias. BMJ 1990; 300: 139–44.
8. Athena. Living With Dystonia. Élan Pharmaceuticals Ltd. London: Packer Forbes Communications; 2000.
9. Davis S. Disabled people in hospital: evaluating the CNS role. Nurs Stand 2001; 15(21): 33–7.
10. Fulton T. It all depends on your point of view. Clin Nurse Spec 2002; 16(5): 229–50.
11. Élan. Practical considerations for the clinical use of Botulinum Toxin. Élan Pharma Ltd. 2002.
12. Department of Health. The New NHS. Modern Dependable. London: HMSO; 1997.
13. Ipsen. Selected In Effectiveness Proven In Us. 2000.
14. Department of Health. The NHS Plan For Investment: A Plan For Reform. London: HMSO; 2000
15. Commission for Health Improvements. Clinical Governance Review Chorley and South Ribble NHS Trust and Preston Acute NHS Trust. Commission For Health Improvements; 2001.
16. Department of Health. The Expert Patient Government Guidelines. London: HMSO; 2002.
17. Royal College of Nursing. Specialities In Nursing. London: RCN; 1999.
18. Ashworth P. Writing And Submitting Abstracts For Conference Presentations. Nurse Researcher.
19. Nursing and Midwifery Council. Scope of Professional Practice. London: UKCC; 2001.
20. Kitson A, Ahmed LB, Harvey G, Seers K, Thompson DR. From research to practice: one organizational model for promoting research-based practice. J Adv Nurs 1996; 23(3): 430–40.
21. Benner P. From Novice To Expert. California: Addison Wesley; 1984.
22. De Broe S, Christopher F, Waugh N. The role of specialist nurses in multiple sclerosis: a rapid and systematic review. Health Technol Assess 2001; 5(17): 1–47.

23. Adams SR. A description of the role, activities and skills of the clinical nurse specialist in the United States. Clin Nurse Spec 1999; 13(4):
24. Redkopp MA. Clinical nurse specialist role confusion: the need for identity. Clin Nurse Spec 1997; 11:
25. Wright PB. Clinical supervision and primary nursing. Br J Nurs 1994; 3(1): 23–9.
26. Gibson F, Bamford O. Focus group interviews to examine the role and development of the clinical nurse specialist. J Nurs Manage 2001; 9(6): 331–42.
27. Department of Health. The NHS Plan Changes For Nurses Midwives Therapists and Other NHS Staff. London: HMSO; 2001.
28. Castledine G. Can we standardize titles and levels in nursing? Br J Nurs 2001; 10(13): 891.
29. Castledine G. The qualities needed to become an expert nurse. Br J Nurs 1999; 8(9): 626.
30. Beecroft PC, Papenhausen JL. What is a specialist? Clin Nurse Spec 1988; 2(3): 109–12.
31. Walsh M. Nurses and nurse practitioners. Part 2: Perspectives on care. Nurs Stand 1999; 13(25): 36–40.
32. Scott RA. A description of the roles, activities and skills of clinical nurse specialist in the United States. Clin Nurse Spec 1999; 13(4): 183–90.
33. Chase LK, Johnson KS, Laffoon TA, Jacobs RS, Johnson ME. CNS role: an experience in retitling and role classification. Clin Nurse Spec 1996; 10(1): 41–5.
34. Hamric AB, Spross JA, Hanson CM. The Clinical Nurse Specialist in Theory and Practice. 1993: 20–7.
35. Tang P. Evaluation of nurse specialist pilot scheme. In: A Systematic Review 20001 Debroe Et Al
36. Tucker S, Gretchen S, Clark J, Sikkink V, Stears R. Enhancing psychiatric nursing practice role of an advanced practice nurse. Clin Nurse Spec 1999; 13(3): 133–9.
37. Armstrong P. The role of the clinical nurse specialist. Nurs Stand 1999: 13(16): 40–2.
38. Tijuis GJ, Zwiderman AH, Hazes JW, Breedveld FC, Vieland PM. Two-year follow-up of a randomized controlled trial of a clinical nurse specialist intervention, inpatient and day patient team care in rheumatoid arthritis. J Adv Nurs 2003; 41(1): 34–43.
39. Clarke CL, Wilcockson J. Professional and organisational learning: analysing the relationship with the development of practice. J Adv Nurs 2001; 34(2): 264–72.
40. UKCC. PREP and You. London: HMSO; 1995.
41. ADDER. Action For Dystonia. Diagnosis, Education and Research. Durham, UK: ADDER; Charity No 1077578, 2000.
42. Foundation of Nursing Studies. Reflection for Action. London: Foundation Of Nursing Studies; 1996.
43. Nolan M, Morgan L, Curran M et al. Evidence-based care: can we overcome the barriers? Br J Nurs 1998; 7(20): 1273–8.
44. Hess R. Measuring nursing governance. Nurs Res 1998; 47(1): 35–42.
45. Duff LA, Kitson AL, Seers K, Humphries D. Clinical guidelines: an introduction to their development and implementation. J Adv Nurs 1996; 23(5): 887–95.
46. Humphris D (ed.) The Basis of Role Specialism in Nursing. In: The Clinical Nurse Specialist. London: Macmillan; 1994: 1–15.
47. Nursing and Midwifery Council. Standards for Specialist Education and Practice. UKCC. London: HMSO. Following Registration Transitional Arrangements Specialist Practitioner Registrars Letter London
48. McDonough KJ. A shared governance system more structured than substance. J Nurs Admin 1996; 26(2): 14–19.
49. Nursing and Midwifery Council. Code of Professional Conduct for NHS Managers. United Kingdom Central Council For Nursing Midwifery and Health Visiting, 3rd edn. London: NMC; 2002.
50. Department of Health. A First Class Service Quality in The New NHS. London: HMSO; 1998.
51. Antai-Otoung D. Team building in a health care setting. Am J Nurs 1997; 9(7): 48–51.
52. Davidzhar R. Leading with charisma. J Adv Nurs 1993; 18: 675–9.
53. Head S. Nurse practitioners: the new pioneers. Nurs Times 1988; 84(20): 27–8.
54. Ibbotson K. The role of the clinical nurse specialist: a study. Nurs Stand 1999; 14(9): 35–8.
55. Kerrison P. A Diploma In The Job: The Clinical Nurse Specialist. London: Macmillan; 1990: 1–15.
56. Mills M, Sullivan K. The importance of information giving for patients newly diagnosed with cancer: a review of the literature. J Clin Nurse 1999; 8: 631–42.
57. Department of Health. National Service Framework for Long Term Conditions. London: HMSO; 2001.

22

Dystonia and quality of life

Stefan J Cano and Thomas T Warner

Outcomes of dystonia have been traditionally evaluated using objective clinical indices measuring disease markers such as head movement, shoulder elevation, and tremor. Although such indices provide important data, they are limited as they do not give valuable information regarding patients' perceptions of their condition. Therefore, patient-reported rating scales are used to measure broader health outcomes such as quality of life (QL). This chapter provides information on dystonia and QL. It has three aims:

1. To provide an introduction to QL.
2. To describe QL research in dystonia.
3. To critically appraise current research with the view to recommendations for future studies.

AN INTRODUCTION TO QUALITY OF LIFE

Background

During the past two decades, there has been a transition from solely measuring traditional clinical outcomes to the inclusion of a wider range of health variables, including QL. This shift has occurred for a number of reasons. The narrow definition of health in terms of morbidity and mortality has been replaced by the broader definition: a 'complete state of physical, mental and social well-being and not merely the absence of disease or infirmity'.[1] In addition, rising standards of living, aging populations, and the development of health technology have led to a shift in attention from curing acute diseases to the management of more complex, chronic conditions, including many neurologic disorders such as dystonia. Additionally, healthcare providers increasingly demand that clinicians demonstrate evidence of cost-effectiveness, in which the benefits of treatment are weighed against the costs of that intervention.[2]

What is quality of life?

Health cannot be measured directly. The complex and abstract nature of health has led to a continuing debate on how best to measure it.[3] Health measurement relies on the use of health indicators to represent various dimensions of health, and so researchers have developed measures to elicit patients' opinion about various aspects of health such as QL. Health measurement, therefore, can be described as the field of study concerned with the development of methods for measuring patient-reported outcomes.

The terms QL, health-related QL, health status, and functional status are often used interchangeably in the health measurement literature. Although there is a lack of conceptual clarity regarding these terms,[4] there is broad agreement on the core minimum set of health concepts[5] that should be measured. These include physical and mental health, social functioning, and general health perceptions.

Why measure quality of life?

Despite the recent acceptance of QL data, some clinicians have regarded these as 'soft science'[6] preferring 'hard data' such as tangible variables measured with mechanical instruments (e.g. blood counts) or clinician judgment. However, it can be argued that many of the so-called 'hard outcomes' reported in the literature are actually 'softer' than first supposed.[7] For example, data obtained from medical records contain information about subjective states that have been collected using non-standardized methods.[8] Also, traditional disease-staging techniques are observer-dependent and subject to considerable variation.[9] In contrast, it has been shown that patient-based data are good predictors of long-term outcome.[10] For example, QL data are accurate predictors of outcome in hypertension, diabetes, chronic obstructive pulmonary disorder, and ischemic heart disease,[11] and mortality in the general population.[12] Thus, patients' views and perceptions of their own health are an essential part of healthcare evaluation.[13]

How is quality of life measured?

Two main conceptual approaches to health measurement have been identified.[14,15] The standard needs approach describes measuring QL as the extent to which certain universal needs are met. This approach advocates that there are a standard set of life circumstances that are required for optimal functioning. Although a subjective phenomenon, QL is viewed as an objective characteristic of an individual. In contrast, the psychological processes approach views QL as constructed from individual evaluations of personally salient aspects of life. This approach sees QL as being made up of perception of life circumstances, dependent on the psychological make-up of an individual, rather than on their life circumstances alone. The central assumption of this approach is that each person is the best source of judgments about QL and one cannot assume that all people will value different circumstances in the same way.

Many types of patient-reported rating scale can be classed as following the standard needs approach, including generic (e.g. Medical Outcomes Study Short Form-36[16]), disease-specific (e.g. the Cervical Dystonia Impact Profile[17]), and site-specific measures (e.g. Oxford Hip Score[18]). For more details on different types of measure see Chapter 23 on dystonia rating scales.

In contrast to using generic or specific measures using predetermined content, proponents of the psychological processes approach argue that listing items in measurement scales does not capture the subjectivity of human beings and the individual structure of values. In short, prescribing items using a preordained definition of QL and matching the person to the definition (i.e. 'goodness of fit'), does not let us know whether all the domains, pertinent and meaningful to each respondent, are included. This viewpoint has influenced the development of 'individualized' measures such as the Schedule for the Evaluation of Individual Quality Of Life (SEIQoL).[19] This measure allows individuals to nominate important domains of QL and weight those domains in order of importance. Another measure, the Patient Generated Index (PGI), asks individuals to identify those aspects of life that are personally affected by health.[20] The advantage of these measures includes a claim for validity, as the areas of importance are selected by the individuals involved in completing the measures. The main disadvantages are that some of these measures require trained interviewers, which translates into a need for greater resources, and lower practicality. Also, it is not easy to produce population-based comparative or normative data given the variation in each individual completed measure.[21]

The majority of existing patient-reported rating scales follow the standard needs approach. Research into individualized measures is still in its infancy and more work is required before the relative advantages and disadvantages of the two approaches can be discerned.[21] There is no existing dystonia research using individualized measures and, as such, the studies presented in this chapter follow the standard needs approach.

QUALITY OF LIFE RESEARCH IN DYSTONIA

This section focuses on generic patient-rated scales used to measure QL or aspects of QL in dystonia research. Dystonia and QL study descriptives are presented, followed by measures and QL domains, and a summary of main findings. Chapter 23 on dystonia rating scales describes disease-specific measures in greater detail.

Study descriptives

Twenty-six studies have investigated aspects of QL in generalized dystonia, cervical dystonia (CD), and blepharospasm using generic patient-reported rating scales. The majority of studies have analyzed cohorts of CD patients. Sample sizes ranged from 6 to 289, with a median sample size of 64 (85% of the studies included less than 100 patients). In general, response rates were not reported, but when they were, they were generally high (>84%). Mean age ranged from 41 to 57 years. The percentage of women in the samples ranged from 48% to 81%, which reflects the preponderance of females with focal dystonias.[22,23]

Domains and measures

Eighteen generic rating scales have been used: the most commonly used were the Beck Depression Inventory, Medical Outcomes Study Short-Form-36, and the Rosenberg Self-Esteem Scale. Table 22.1 shows the type of measures and domains measured. Studies have predominantly focused on psychological outcomes such as depression, anxiety, and self-esteem. Table 22.2 shows domains measured.

Findings

As described above, QL measures should include a number of physical, psychological, and social dimensions. Dystonia research has included aspects of all of the following areas.

Table 22.1 Types of generic measures categorized by domain with associated studies

Domain	Measure	Study references
Depression	Beck Depression Inventory	27–29, 31, 32, 40, 50, 53, 54
Health-related QL	Medical Outcomes Study Short Form-36	28, 30, 32, 34, 47, 53
Self-esteem	Rosenberg Self-Esteem Scale	31, 32, 40, 50
Psychological functioning	Sickness Impact Profile	42–44, 51
Health-related QL	Medical Outcomes Study Short Form-20	35, 39
	Euroqol-5D	34, 36, 46
	Nottingham Health Profile	37, 38
Disease acceptance	Acceptance of Illness Scale	32, 50
Anxiety	Spielberger Trait Anxiety Scale	25, 50
	Beck Anxiety Inventory	32, 46
Negative expectancy	Hopelessness Scale	26
Locus of control	Multi-Dimensional Health Locus of Control Scale	31
Psychological functioning	Bradburn's Present Feelings Scale	50
Psychological distress	Symptom Checklist-90R	33
Pain descriptors	Finnish Pain Questionnaire	24
	McGill Pain Questionnaire	46
Health State	Euroqol-5D	34
QL	Nottingham Health Profile	37

Physical health

Pain is described as an important symptom, with CD patients using descriptors such as 'tiring', 'continuous', and 'tugging'.[24]

Mental health

The majority of studies using generic measures have evaluated the psychological impact of dystonia. Studies have described CD patients as similar to cervical spondylosis patients on anxiety[25] and negative expectancies,[26] but experiencing more depression.[26–28] Long-term follow-up has revealed that levels of depression do not change over time.[29] Levels of self-esteem and self-deprecation are similar to patients with Parkinson's disease,[30] but CD patients believe in internal locus of control (i.e. they feel personal control over their own lives and health as opposed to being controlled by others or outside forces).[31] However, there is some contradiction in the literature. For example, whereas one study emphasizes the need to consider psychological well-being in the treatment of CD patients,[32] another argues that CD patients experience low psychological distress,[33] although the last study included patients with dystonia as part of a complex regional pain syndrome and therefore is not a form of primary torsion dystonia.

General health-related quality of life

The most common health-related QL measure used to assess the impact of dystonia has been the Medical Outcomes Study Short Form-36 (SF-36). The SF-36 contains questions on general health and well-being in 8 multi-item scales. Each scale is scored from 0 (indicating worst possible health) to 100 (indicating best

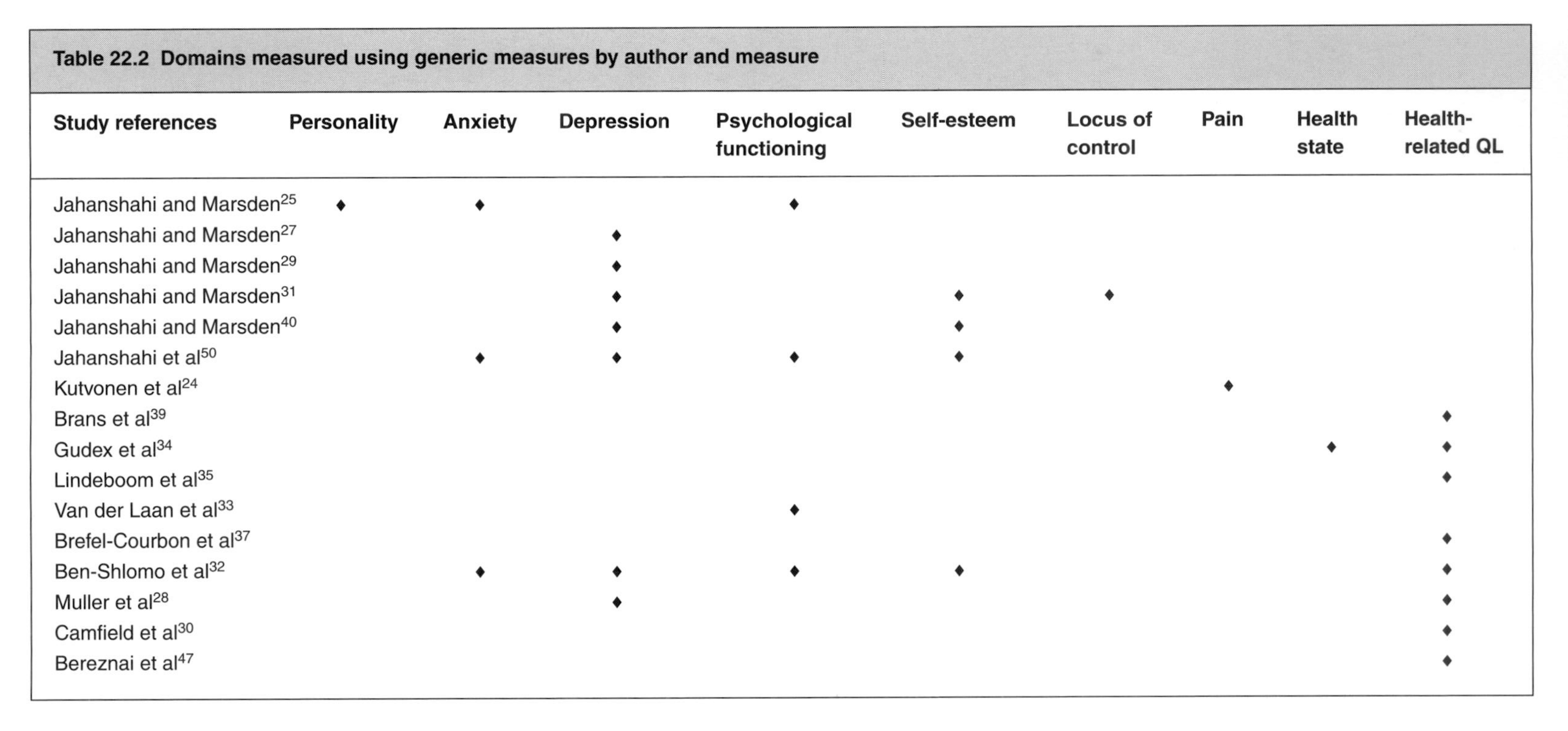

Table 22.2 Domains measured using generic measures by author and measure

Study references	Personality	Anxiety	Depression	Psychological functioning	Self-esteem	Locus of control	Pain	Health state	Health-related QL
Jahanshahi and Marsden[25]	♦	♦		♦					
Jahanshahi and Marsden[27]			♦						
Jahanshahi and Marsden[29]			♦						
Jahanshahi and Marsden[31]			♦		♦	♦			
Jahanshahi and Marsden[40]			♦		♦				
Jahanshahi et al[50]		♦	♦	♦	♦				
Kutvonen et al[24]							♦		
Brans et al[39]									♦
Gudex et al[34]								♦	♦
Lindeboom et al[35]									♦
Van der Laan et al[33]				♦					
Brefel-Courbon et al[37]									♦
Ben-Shlomo et al[32]		♦	♦	♦	♦				♦
Muller et al[28]			♦						♦
Camfield et al[30]									♦
Bereznai et al[47]									♦

possible health). Two component scores make up overall physical and mental dimensions. In a study of blepharospasm, women were found to score lower (i.e. poorer health-related QL) in all SF-36 domains than male patients.[28,34] In addition, 37% of patients were found to be depressed. Patients with CD have been found to have poorer health-related QL than UK controls, particularly in the areas of SF-36 physical role limitation (42 vs 86), pain (55 vs 82), and health perception (46 vs 74).[30] This trend has been supported in other studies.[28,34] Dimension scores are comparable to data from patients with mild to moderate multiple sclerosis (EDSS 3-6), moderate Parkinson's disease, and moderate epilepsy.[30]

One study has attempted to model QL variables in CD patients.[32] Patients with CD (n = 289) were recruited from seven European countries. Data on QL were collected using the SF-36. It was found that SF-36 physical and mental component scores were predicted by self-esteem and self-deprecation, educational level, employment status, social support, response to botulinum toxin, disease severity, social participation, stigma, acceptance of illness, anxiety, and depression. The strongest predictors of QL were found to be anxiety and depression. The authors also present a conceptual scheme in which QL is associated with a number of explanatory and intermediary variables (Figure 22.1).

Finally, a recent study has provided evidence-based guidelines for using the SF-36 in CD research.[52] To do this, the hypothesized relationships between items, scales, and summary measures of the SF-36 were tested using psychometric analyses in data from a postal survey of 235 people with CD. Although the majority of subscales performed adequately, the Role Physical and Role Emotional subscales had substantial floor and/or ceiling effects. Evidence did not support computing SF-36 Physical and Mental Component summary scores. Guidelines were proposed that include the recommendation that these subscale and summary scores should be reported with caution.

Treatment effects

The majority of studies investigating treatment have focused on the use of botulinum toxin type A (BTX-A) in CD,[28,34–41] with a few studies investigating the impact of type B (BTX-B).[42–44] These studies have used generic measures to focus on the impact of treatment on aspects of psychological functioning and general health-related QL. Fewer studies have investigated surgery, including muscle sections,[45] denervation,[46] or deep brain stimulation.[47,53,54] Surgical studies have focused on aspects of psychological functioning, pain, and general health-related QL, although one study used

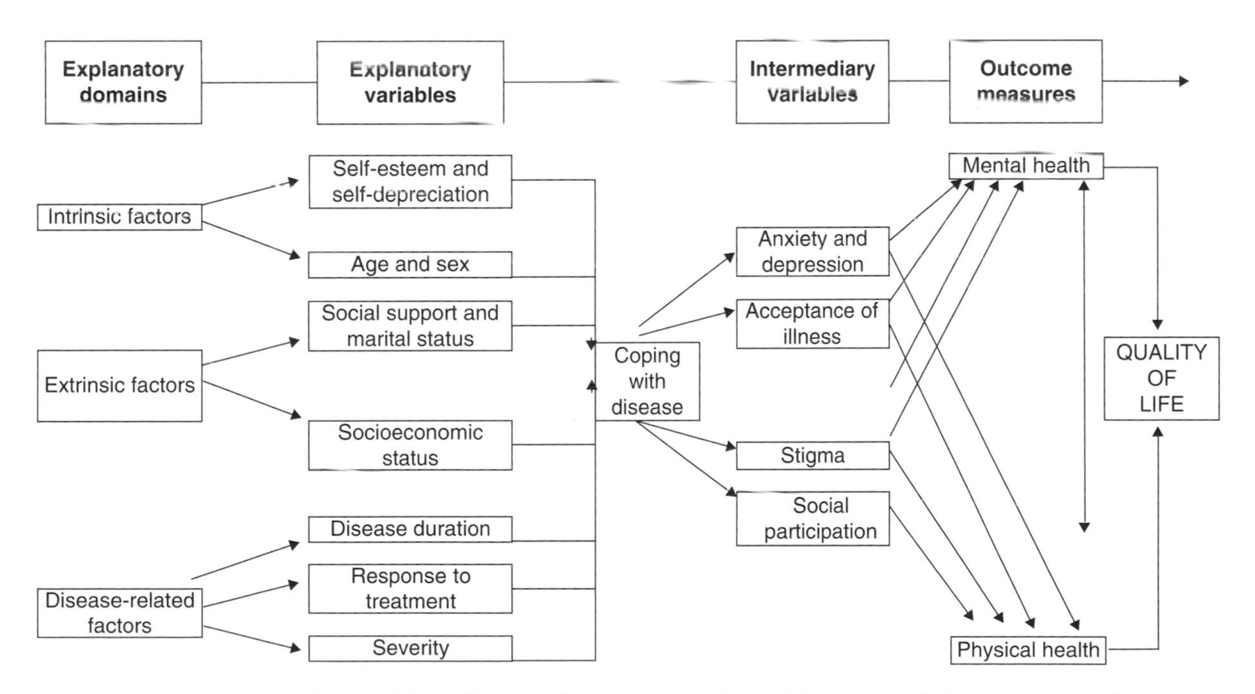

Figure 22.1 Conceptual scheme of the influence of factors on quality of life in cervical dystonia. (Reproduced from Ben-Shlomo et al,[32] with permission.)

a Parkinson's disease self-report scale (PDQ39) as there was no specific dystonia measure available.[54] Interpretation of data from this measure should be treated with caution.

Most studies report improvement, but have either been unable to discriminate between patients[35] or have described small changes post-treatment.[34,36] For example, whereas one study[35] found that the Medical Outcomes Study-Short Form-20 detected improvement in CD patients following BTX-A, a study assessing the efficacy of BTX-B[42–44] showed no significant improvement as measured by the Sickness Impact Profile. A large French study of deep brain stimulation in primary generalized dystonia showed improvements in global health as determined by the SF-36.[53] Table 22.3 shows a summary of the findings of treatment effects by measure.

CRITICAL APPRAISAL OF QUALITY OF LIFE RESEARCH

QL research in dystonia is a growing field and many widely accepted generic measures have been used to assess aspects of QL. However, sample sizes have been low, and much of the research into patient reported outcomes of dystonia is limited, focusing primarily on psychological dimensions of patient well-being. Also, none of the generic measures have been psychometrically tested for suitability with dystonia patients. There is little conformity in the number and types of measures used in each of the studies, reducing the extent to which findings can be compared. The vast majority of research focuses on CD, with few or no studies on other types of dystonia.

Table 22.3 Treatment effects

Treatment	Measure	*n*	Assessment period (range)	Percentage of studies reporting significant improvement ($p < 0.05$)
BTX-A (type A)	Beck Depression Inventory[28,40]	26 to 131	B, 30 weeks P	100
	Euroqol-5D[34,36]	196	4, 6 weeks P	100
	MOS-20[39]	54 to 64	3, 12 months P	100
	NHP[37,38]	20 to 21	B, 7 months P	50
	Rosenberg Self-Esteem Scale[40]	26	B, 30 weeks P	0
	SF-36[28,34,36]	131 to 196	4, 6 weeks P	50
BTX-B (type B)				
Surgery (denervation)	Sickness Impact Profile[42–44,51]	122	B, 4 weeks P	0
	Beck Anxiety Index[46]	62	B, 3, 18 months P	0
	Beck Depression Inventory[46]	62	B, 3, 18 months P	100
	Euroqol-5D[46]	62	B, 3, 18 months P	100
	McGill Pain Questionnaire[46]	62	B, 3, 18 months P	100
	Rosenberg Self-Esteem Scale[46]	62	B, 3, 18 months P	0

B = baseline; P = post-treatment.

Regarding measuring the impact of treatment, generic measures may be limited, as they may be unable to address important aspects of outcome that are affected by a particular disease, and are generally not sensitive enough to detect changes in outcome which occur in response to treatment or over time.[48] This is highlighted by significant floor and ceiling effects found on a number of SF-36 dimensions.[30,52] Thus, measures used in these studies appear, in general, not to address the pertinent areas of health impact of dystonia. In addition, the majority of studies report the statistical significance of findings but not effect sizes, which may misrepresent the true changes experienced by patients.[49] Disease-specific measures should be more appropriate to assess therapies but at present the vast majority of existing disease-specific measures have not been comprehensively evaluated from a scientific point of view. Therefore, the full impact of treatment has yet to be addressed.

CONCLUSIONS AND RECOMMENDATIONS

Dystonia has far-reaching effects on QL. Research in QL is growing but has thus far focused largely on CD patients and is largely limited to psychological outcomes. There is little consistency or comparability in the rating scales used, making meta-analysis difficult. We suggest the following areas for future research:

- Large studies are required to assess the impact of all types of dystonia on a broad range of QL measures.
- Studies should present the psychometric properties of generic scales used to show appropriateness of measures in dystonia patient groups.
- We recommend that there is conformity in the types of measures used in each of the studies, allowing for comparison. Comprehensive measurement would include generic measures used in conjunction with an appropriately validated disease-specific measure (e.g. CDIP-58).

REFERENCES

1. World Health Organisation. Constitution of the World Health Organisation. Geneva: WHO Basic Documents; 1948.
2. Robinson R. The policy context. Br Med J 1993; 307: 994–6.
3. McDowell I, Newell C. Measuring Health: A Guide to Rating Scales and Questionnaires. New York: Oxford University Press; 1987.
4. Hunt S. The problem of quality of life. Qual Life Res 1997; 6: 205–12.
5. Scientific Advisory Committee of the Medical Outcomes Trust. Assessing health status and quality of life instruments: attributes and review criteria. Qual Life Res 2002; 11: 193–205.
6. Feinstein A. Clinical biostatistics XLI. Hard science, soft data, and the challenge of choosing clinical variables in research. Clin Pharmacol Ther 1977; 22: 485–98.
7. Guyatt GH, Feeny D, Patrick D. Issues in quality-of-life measurement in clinical trials. Control Clin Trials 1991; 12(Suppl 4): 81S–90S.
8. Cleary PD, Greenfield S, McNeil BJ. Assessing quality of life after surgery. Control Clin Trials 1991; 12(4 Suppl): 189S–203S.
9. Bowling A. Measuring disease. Buckingham: Open University Press; 1995.
10. Cleary P. Subjective and objective measures of health: which is better when? J Health Serv Res Policy 1997; 2(1): 3–4.
11. Parkerson GR Jr, Broadhead WE, Tse CK. Health status and severity of illness as predictors of outcomes in primary care. Med Care 1995; 33(1): 53–66.
12. Miilunpalo S, Vuori I, Oja P et al. Self-rated health status as a health measure: the predictive value of self-reported health status on the use of physician services and on mortality in the working-age population. Clin Epidemiol 1997; 50(5): 517–28.
13. Lohr KN. Applications of health status assessment measures in clinical practice. Overview of the third conference on advances in health status assessment. Med Care 1992; 30(5 Suppl): Ms1–14.
14. Browne J, McGee H, O'Boyle C. Conceptual approaches to the assessment of quality of life. Psychol Health 1997; 12: 737–51.
15. Bowling A. Measuring Health: A Review of Quality of Life Measurement Scales, 2nd edn. Buckingham: Open University Press; 1997.
16. Ware JJ, Sherbourne C. The MOS 36-item Short-Form Health Survey (SF-36): 1. Conceptual framework and item selection. Med Care 1992; 30(6): 473–83.
17. Cano S, Warner T, Linacre M et al. Development and validation of a new patient-based rating scale for cervical dystonia – the Cervical Dystonia Impact Profile (CDIP-58). Neurology 2004; 63: 1629–33.
18. Dawson J, Fitzpatrick R, Murray D et al. The problem of 'noise' in monitoring patient-based outcomes: generic, disease-specific and site-specific instruments for total hip replacement. Health Serv Res Policy 1996; 1(4): 224–31.
19. Browne JP, O'Boyle CA, McGee HM et al. Development of a direct weighting procedure for quality of life domains. Qual Life Res 1997; 6: 301–9.
20. Ruta DA, Garratt AM, Leng M et al. A new approach to the measurement of quality of life. The Patient-Generated Index. Med Care 1994; 32(11): 1109–26.
21. Fitzpatrick R, Davey C, Buxton M et al. Evaluating Patient-Based Outcome Measures for Use in Clinical Trials. Southampton: National Co-ordinating Centre for Health Technology Assessment; 1998: 1–73.
22. Nutt J, Muenter M, Aaronson A et al. Epidemiology of focal and generalised dystonia in Rochester, Minnesota. Mov Disord 1988; 3(3): 188–94.
23. Duffey P, Butler A, Hawthorne M et al. The epidemiology of the primary dystonias in the North of England. Dystonia 3. Adv Neurol 1998; 78: 121–5.
24. Kutvonen O, Dastidar P, Nurmikko T. Pain in spasmodic torticollis. Pain 1997; 69: 279–86.
25. Jahanshahi M, Marsden C. Personality in torticollis: a controlled study. Psychol Med 1988; 18: 375–87.
26. Jahanshahi M, Marsden C. Depression in torticollis: a controlled study. Psychol Med 1988; 18: 925–33.
27. Jahanshahi M, Marsden C. Body concept, disability, and depression in patients with spasmodic torticollis. Behav Neurol 1990; 3: 117–31.
28. Muller J, Kemmler G, Wissel J et al. The impact of blepharospasm and cervical dystonia on health-related quality of life and depression. J Neurol 2002; 249(7): 842–6.

29. Jahanshahi M, Marsden C. A longitudinal follow-up study of depression, disability, and body concept in torticollis. Behav Neurol 1990; 3: 233–46.
30. Camfield L, Ben-Shlomo Y, Warner T. Impact of cervical dystonia on quality of life. Mov Disord 2002; 17(4): 838–41.
31. Jahanshahi M. Psychosocial factors and depression in torticollis. J Psychosom Res 1991; 35(4/5): 493–507.
32. Ben-Shlomoy, Camfield L, Warner T; ESDE Collaborative group. What are the determinants of quality of life in people with cervical dystonia? J Neurol Neuosurg Psychiatry 2002; 2(5): 608–14.
33. van der Laan L, van Spaendonck K, Horstink M, Goris R. The Symptom Checklist-90 Revised questionnaire: no psychological profiles in complex regional pain syndrome-dystonia. J Pain Symptom Manager 1999; 17(5): 357–62.
34. Gudex C, Hawthorne M, Butler A et al. Effect of dystonia and botulinum toxin treatment on health-related quality of life. Mov Disord 1998; 13(6): 941–6.
35. Lindeboom R, Brans J, Aramideh M et al. Treatment of cervical dystonia: a comparison of measures for outcome assessment. Mov Disord 1998; 13(4): 706–12.
36. Gudex C, Hawthorne M, Butler A et al. Measuring patient benefit from botulinum toxin in the treatment of dystonia. Pharmacoeconomics 1997; 12(6): 675–84.
37. Brefel-Courbon C, Simonetta-Moreau M, More C et al. A pharmacoeconomic evaluation of botulinum toxin in the treatment of spasmodic torticollis. Clin Neuropharmacol 2000; 23(4): 203–7.
38. Odergren T, Tollback R, Borg J. Efficacy of botulinum toxin for cervical dystonia. A comparison of methods for evaluation. Scand J Rehabil Med 1994; 26: 191–5.
39. Brans J, Lindeboon R, Aramideh M et al. Long-term effect of botulinum toxin on impairment and functional health in cervical dystonia. Neurology 1998; 50: 1461–3.
40. Jahanshahi M, Marsden C. Psychological functioning before and after treatment of torticollis with botulinum toxin. J Neurol Neurosurg Psychiatry 1992; 55: 229–31.
41. Brans J, Lindeboom R, Snoek J et al. Botulinum toxin versus trihexyphenidyl in cervical dystonia: a prospective, randomised, double-blind controlled trial. Neurology 1996; 46: 1066–72.
42. Lew M, Adornato B, Duane D et al. Botulinum toxin type B: a double-blind placebo-controlled, safety and efficacy study in cervical dystonia. Neurology 1997; 49: 701–7.
43. Lew M, Brashear A, Factor S. The safety and efficacy of botulinum toxin type-B in the treatment of patients with cervical dystonia; summary of the three controlled clinical trials. Neurology 2000; 55(Suppl 5): S229–35.
44. Brashear A, Lew M, Dyskstra D et al. Safety and efficacy of NeuroBloc (botulinum toxin type B) in type A-responsive cervical dystonia. Neurology 1999; 53: 1439–46.
45. Krauss J, Toups E, Jankovic J et al. Symptomatic and functional outcome of surgical treatment of cervical dystonia. J Neurol Neurosurg Psychiatry 1997; 63: 642–8.
46. Munchau A, Palmer J, Dressler D et al. Prospective study of selective peripheral denervation for botulinum-toxin resistant patients with cervical dystonia. Brain 2001; 124: 769–83.
47. Bereznai B, Steude U, Seelos K et al. Chronic high-frequency globus pallidus internus stimulation in different types of dystonia: a clinical, video, and MRI report of six patients presenting with segmental, cervical and generalised dystonia. Mov Disord 2002; 17(1): 138–44.
48. Guyatt GH, Feeny DH, Patrick DL. Measuring health-related quality of life. Ann Intern Med 1993; 118(8): 622–9.
49. Beaton D, Bombardier C, Katz J et al. A taxonomy for responsiveness. J Clin Epidemiol 2001; 54: 1204–17.
50. Jahanshahi M, Brown R, Whitehouse C et al. Contact with a nurse practitioner: a short-term evaluation study in Parkinson's disease and dystonia. Behav Neurol 1994; 7: 189–96.
51. Lew M. Botulinum Type B: an effective treatment of alleviating pain associated with cervical dystonia. J Back Musculoskeletal Rehabil 2002; 16(1): 3–9.
52. Cano SJ, Thomas AJ, Bhatia K et al. Evidence-based guidelines for using the Short Form 36 in cervical dystonia. Mov Disord 2007; 22: 122–6.
53. Vidailhet M, Vercueil L, Houeto J-L et al. Bilateral deep brain stimulation of globus pallidus in primary generalised dystonia. N Engl J Med 2005; 352: 459–67.
54. Halbig T, Gruber D, Kopp U et al. Pallidal stimulation in dystonia: effects on cognitive function and quality of life. J Neurol Neurosurg Psychiatry 2005; 76: 1713–16.

23

Dystonia rating scales

Stefan J Cano and Thomas T Warner

In recent years the importance of evaluating the impact of disease and treatments on health has become clear. However, health cannot be measured directly and, instead, indicators should be used to represent clinical outcomes. Increasingly, rating scales are used to score aspects of disease (e.g. symptoms) or elicit patients' opinion about aspects of health (e.g. psychological well-being).[1] This chapter provides information on dystonia rating scales. It has three aims:

1. To provide an introduction to the use and development of rating scales.
2. To describe existing dystonia rating scales.
3. To critically evaluate scales with the view to recommendations for future directions of research.

AN INTRODUCTION TO RATING SCALES

Background

The origins of scale development can be traced back to psychophysics in the 1800s, which claimed that people are able to make subjective judgments about physical stimuli, such as the brightness of lights of varying intensity and the loudness of different sounds, in an accurate and internally consistent manner. The next three-quarters of a century revealed that the logarithmic relationship did not fit all types of stimuli, and in the mid-1950s, the logarithmic approach was replaced by Stevens' Power Law. This new approach recognized that the relationship between stimulus and subjective responses was not linear.[2] This law has been since tested and has been used to argue that people can make subjective judgments in a consistent manner, even when asked to make abstract comparisons. This is particularly relevant to the health measurement field in which many rating scales incorporate such comparisons.[1]

The use of rating scales in health research began at the beginning of the 20th century.[3] However, it was not until the end of the 1940s that rating scales were used in neurology.[4] At the same time, psychometricians extended the basic principles of rating scale development, and the essential scientific properties of rating scales (e.g. reliability and validity)[5–7] became well established. In the 1970s, broader aspects of health began to be included in clinical research (e.g. activities of daily living[8]) and the last two decades have witnessed increasing recognition of the importance of rating scales for all aspects of health measurement.[9,10]

Science

Although scale evaluation methods (i.e. psychometrics) have been used in the social sciences for the best part of the last century, they have been slow to transfer to health research.[11] However, it is clear that for scales to be useful they need to be rigorously evaluated.[12] At a minimum, this should include psychometric evaluations of reliability, validity, and, when assessing treatment effects, responsiveness. Table 23.1 shows a summary of the main traditional psychometric properties.

In brief, the reliability of a measure is the degree to which it is free from random error. Reliability is an important property of a rating scale, because it is essential to establish that any changes observed in patient groups, due to a treatment, are due to the treatment and not to problems in the scale.[13] There are two general approaches to evaluate reliability: internal consistency (a function of the number of items and their covariation within a scale) and test–retest reproducibility (whether a measure yields the same results on repeated applications). Validity is the extent to which a scale measures what it intends to measure.[14] There are two main types of validity: content validity (how well a

Table 23.1 Summary of reliability, validity, and responsiveness – definitions and types

Psychometric property	Definition	Main types	Statistic/method of assessment
Reliability	The degree to which a measure is free from random error	1. Internal consistency 2. Test–retest reproducibility	1. Cronbach's coefficient α 2. Intraclass correlation coefficient
Validity	The extent to which an instrument measures what it intends to measure	1. Content validity 2. Construct validity	1. Qualitative methods 2. Pearson product–moment correlation
Responsiveness	The ability of a measure to detect significant change over time	Magnitude of detected change	Effect size

measure covers important parts of the target health components) and construct validity (testing the expected relations of health dimensions to each other, both internally and externally). Finally, if a new scale is to be used in evaluating the effects of a given intervention (e.g. botulinum toxin injections), responsiveness needs to be evaluated. Responsiveness is the ability of a measure to detect significant change over time, such as a meaningful reduction in symptoms from the patient's perspective.[15]

Types of rating scale

Scales can be considered either generic (i.e. applicable across patient groups or diseases) or specific (i.e. developed for a specific patient group or condition). Table 23.2 summarizes the main types of rating scale. Generic measures are useful, as they permit direct comparisons of different patient populations.[16] However, they may be unable to address important aspects of outcome that are affected by a particular disease, and are generally not as sensitive as specific measures to detect clinical change.[17] There are two main types of specific measure: disease-specific measures are developed for a specific disease or condition (e.g. dystonia), whereas site-specific measures assess health problems in a specific part of the body (e.g. Oxford Hip Score[18]). Specific measures ensure more comprehensive assessment of important outcome domains, and are generally more sensitive in detecting the effects of treatment on outcome and changes in outcome over time.[19] However, they do not allow comparisons between different patient groups.[13]

What makes a good rating scale?

The features that determine high-quality rating scales have been widely published.[12,13,20] Central to these guidelines is the tenet that as scales represent various dimensions of health, they should incorporate patients' opinions and be tested to ensure scientific rigour. In short, current guidelines for good practice state that measures should be developed from an item pool formed from patient interviews, expert opinion, and literature review. This should be followed by field testing involving large numbers of the target patient group: first, to carry out item reduction to select the best indicators of outcome; second, to comprehensively evaluate the measurement properties of the final instrument in an independent sample.

A full evaluation of rating scales extends beyond the basic components of reliability, validity, and responsiveness.[12] Scale developers also need to consider conceptual issues (e.g. conceptual and empirical bases for content) as well as practical concerns (e.g. time taken to complete the scale). The current gold standard for evaluating rating scales has been set out by the Scientific Advisory Committee of the Medical Outcomes Trust (SAC).[12] These criteria form a defined set of eight key attributes for rating scales: conceptual and measurement model; reliability; validity; responsiveness; interpretability; respondent and administrative burden; alternate forms; and cultural and language adaptations. Each criterion has a number of requirements (e.g. validity is divided into content-, construct-, and criterion-related). A general rule of thumb is that the more

Table 23.2 Summary of the main types of rating scale

Type	Description	Use	Example
Generic	Applicable for use across diseases	Permits direct comparisons of different patient populations Enhance the generalizability of a study	Medical Outcome Study Short Form-36
Disease-specific	Developed for use in a specific condition (e.g. dystonia)	Ensure comprehensive assessment of important outcome domains Sensitive to detecting effects of treatment	The Cervical Dystonia Impact Scale (CDIP-58)
Site-specific	Assess health problems in a specific part of the body (e.g. hip)	Ensure comprehensive assessment of important outcome domains Sensitive in detecting the effects of treatment	Oxford Hip Score

criteria evaluated and fulfilled, the better the quality of scales. The next section describes dystonia rating scales. This is followed by a critical appraisal of these scales using the SAC guidelines.

DISEASE-SPECIFIC RATING SCALES FOR DYSTONIA

This chapter focuses on disease-specific ratings developed for patients with dystonia. The preceding chapter in this book (Dystonia and Quality of Life) describes further types of measure used in dystonia research. Ten rating scales have been developed for generalized dystonia, cervical dystonia (CD), and craniocervical dystonia. In this section, each scale is presented, including its purpose, a description of its content, and psychometric evaluation described in the associated development/validation paper(s). Table 23.3 summarizes the content and evaluation of each of the scales and Table 23.4 summarizes psychometric data where reported. First, clinician-rated scales are presented, followed by patient-rated scales.

Clinician-rated scales

Four clinical rating scales have been developed to assess the impact of dystonia.

Toronto Western Spasmodic Torticollis Rating Scale (TWSTRS)[21,22]

Purpose The TWSTRS measures symptom severity, disability, and pain in patients with CD. It has mainly been used in treatment trials.

Content Three main scales: clinician-rated symptom severity, patient-rated disability (including activities of daily living), and pain scales. The symptom scale rates severity of head movements on 2-, 4-, and 5-point scales. In addition, duration of symptoms, sensory tricks, shoulder elevation, and range of motion are rated on 3-, 4-, 5-, and 6-point scales. The disability scale (on 6-point scales) comprises six areas, including daily activities, work, reading, and driving. The pain scale rates severity, duration, and degree on 6-point scales.

Psychometric data Reliability and validity have been presented: the TWSTRS scales have been shown to have acceptable inter-rater reliability (ICC $>0.71–0.85$); evidence for validity is shown by moderate within-scale correlations ($r >0.61–0.68$).

Unified Dystonia Rating Scale (UDRS) and Global Dystonia Rating Scale (GDS)[23]

Purpose The UDRS and GDS measure the severity of the symptoms of dystonia. These measures focus on individual body areas.

Table 23.3 Dystonia rating scales – description and psychometric data

Measure	Description	Reported psychometrics
Clinician-rated scales		
Toronto Western Spasmodic Torticollis Rating Scale (TWSTRS)[22]	Three main scales: • symptom severity scale – neurologist-rated • disability scale – patient-rated (including work, daily activities) • pain scale – patient-rated (presence, severity)	*Reliability* Inter-rater reliability (α): • 0.71–0.85 (range) *Validity (r)* • 0.61–0.68 (range)
Unified Dystonia Rating Scale (UDRS) and Global Dystonia Rating Scale (GDS)[23]	Two main scales: • Two symptom scales – neurologist-rated	*Reliability* Internal consistency: • $\alpha > 0.91$ • inter-rater reliability ICC >0.71 • weighted $\kappa = 0.52$–0.90
Burke–Fahn–Marsden Scale[24]	Two main scales: • movement scale – neurologist-rated • disability scale – patient-rated (includes speech, hygiene, daily activities)	*Reliability* Movement scale: • inter-rater (>0.85) • intra-rater (>0.98) *Construct validity (r)* Movement scale: • with global severity (>0.69) • with disability scale (0.70)
Tsui Scale[25,40]	Three scores: • Movement (clinician-rated) • Tremor (clinician-rated)	*Reliability* Inter-rater ($r > 0.85$)
Patient-rated scales		
Cervical Dystonia Impact Scale (CDIP-58)[26–28]	Eight 5-point scales made up of: three symptom scales (i.e. head and neck, pain and discomfort, sleep); two activity scales (i.e. upper limb activities, walking); three psychosocial scales (i.e. annoyance, mood, psychosocial functioning)	*Rasch* • MNSQ infit <1.5 • even spread of item calibrations • hierarchical structure *Reliability* • $\alpha > 0.92$ • item-total correlation >0.64 • test–retest >0.83 *Validity* • within-scale analyses and comparisons with external measures (e.g. SF-36 ($r = 0.48$–0.66), GHQ ($r = 0.30$–0.66) and HADS ($r = 0.31$–0.80)) • Responsiveness effect sizes (0.23–0.66)

(*Continued*)

Table 23.3 (Continued)

Measure	Description	Reported psychometrics
Body Concept Scale (BCS)[30]	One scale (four factors) Body concept scale – patient-rated (22 items)	*Reliability* • $\alpha = 0.95$ • test–retest (1 month) = 0.87 *Construct validity* • BCS and total = 0.44 • BCS and Beck Depression Inventory = 0.41 • PCA produce four-factor structure
Functional Questionnaire for disability[30]	One scale (four factors) Functional disability scale – patient-rated (27 items)	*Reliability* • $\alpha = 0.92$ (27 items) • Test–retest (1 month) = 0.93 *Validity* • PCA produce four-factor structure
Ways of Coping Checklist[31]	Patient-rated 64 items (six factors: wish-fulfilling fantasy; threat-minimization; negative reappraisal/coping; cognitive restructuring; religious faith; instrumental coping)	*Reliability* $\alpha > 0.70$ (64 items)
Freiberg Questionnaire for dystonia (torticollis version)[34]	Patient-rated (including medical history, course of disease, previous treatment, current neurologic, and psychosocial changes) Psychosocial changes section includes 23 items covering five areas (profession, everyday life, social life, family, psychological well-being)	*Reliability* $\alpha > 0.87$ (two factors) *Validity* Two-factor model 'psychological distress': • (loadings 0.56–0.83) and 'functional disability' • (loadings 0.55–0.81), explaining 59.4% of the variance
Craniocervical Dystonia Questionnaire-24[29]	Patient-rated 24 items (five scales: stigma; emotional well-being; pain; ADL; social/family life)	*Reliability* $\alpha > 0.77$ (all scales) *Validity* CDQ-24 correlated with SF-36 subscales measuring similar aspects (Pearson's correlation $r = 0.50$–0.73; $p < 0.001$) *Responsiveness* Statistical significant change ($p < 0.001$)

For abbreviations, please see text.

Table 23.4 Dystonia rating scales – description and psychometric data

Scale	MOT criteria							
	Conceptual and measurement model	Reliability	Validity	Responsiveness	Interpretability	Burden	Alternative modes of administration	Cultural and language adaptations or translations
TWSTRS[22]		✓	✓					
Burke–Fahn–Marsden Scale[24]		✓	✓					
UDRS and GDS[23]		✓						
Tsui Score[25,40]		✓						
CDIP-58[26–29]	✓	✓	✓	✓	✓	✓		
Body Concept Scale[30]		✓	✓					
Functional Disability Questionnaire[30]		✓	✓					
Ways of Coping Checklist[31]		✓						
Freiberg questionnaire for dystonia[34]		✓	✓					
Craniocervical Dystonia Questionnaire-24[29]		✓	✓	✓				

✓ = evaluation reported.
No tick = no evaluation reported.
For abbreviations, please see text.

Content There are two clinician-rated symptom scales. The UDRS has ratings for 14 body areas, including head, trunk, and limbs. For each area, there is a 5-point severity scale (ranging from no dystonia to extreme) and a 5-point duration rating (ranging from at rest to with action). The GDS provides a global severity rating in each body area on a 0–10 scale (ranging from 0 = no dystonia to 10 = severe dystonia). The total score is the sum of the scores for all body areas.

Psychometric data Only reliability has been presented. The UDRS and GDS scales have been shown to have acceptable internal consistency (α >0.91), and acceptable inter-rater reliability for total scores (ICC >0.71). However, more variable inter-rater reliability was found when examining body area scores (weighted κ = 0.52–0.90).

Burke–Fahn–Marsden Dystonia Scale[24]

Purpose The Burke–Fahn–Marsden Dystonia Scale[24] measures movement and disability for primary torsion dystonias. It has mainly been used in treatment trials.

Content There are two main scales: a clinician rated movement scale and a patient-rated disability scale. The movement scale rates severity of movement affecting different body parts on a 5-point scale. Body areas include the head, trunk, and limbs. Trunk and limb movements are assigned a weight of 1, and scores from eyes, mouth, and neck are 'down-weighted' (0.5) on the premise that they cause less disability. The disability scale (also on 5 points) comprises seven areas of daily activities, including writing, dressing, and walking.

Psychometric data Reliability and validity have been presented. The movement scale has been shown to have acceptable inter- and intra-rater reliability (r >0.85, r >0.98, respectively). Evidence for construct validity has been found in the form of correlations with global severity and disability scale (r >0.69).

Tsui Scale[25]

Purpose The Tsui Scale measures movement and tremor in CD. It has mainly been used in botulinum toxin trials.

Content There are three main scores: clinician-rated movement and tremor scales. Amplitude of head movement and position are scored on 4-point scales: these scores are added (maximum score = 9) and multiplied by a value that is assigned on the basis of the type of head movement (1 = intermittent or 2 = constant movements). Tremor is rated on a 3-point scale, ranging from absent to severe and multiplied by 1 (intermittent movement) or 2 (constant movement). Thirdly, shoulder elevation is rated on a 4-point scale.

Psychometric data Only reliability has been presented. The scale has been shown to have acceptable inter-rater reliability (r >0.85).

Patient-report scales

Six patient-reported rating scales have been developed to assess the impact of dystonia.

Cervical Dystonia Impact Scale (CDIP-58)[26–28]

Purpose The CDIP-58 measures eight areas of health impacted upon by CD and was developed for use in clinical research, audit, and treatment trials.

Content Fifty-eight items made up of eight 5-point scales, ranging from 4 to 10 items in length: three symptom scales (i.e. head and neck, pain and discomfort, sleep); two activity scales (i.e. upper limb activities, walking); and three psychosocial scales (i.e. annoyance, mood, psychosocial functioning). Eight summary scale scores are generated by summing items and then transformed to a 0–100 scale. High scores indicate worse health.

Psychometric data Development strategy and traditional and new psychometric data techniques are presented. CDIP-58 was developed in three phases following standard guidelines.[12] New psychometric techniques (Rasch analyses) revealed that the CDIP-58 performed well (e.g. good mean square infit (MNSQ) <1.5, even spread of item calibrations and hierarchical structure). In addition, traditional psychometric properties have been supported (e.g. Cronbach's α = 0.92–0.97, item-total correlation = 0.64–0.91, test–retest = 0.83–0.96). Within scale analyses and comparisons with external measures (e.g. Medical Outcomes Study Short Form-36 (SF-36) (r = 0.48–0.66), General Health Questionnaire (GHD) (r = 0.30–0.66), and Hospital Anxiety and Depression Scale (HAD) (r = 0.31–0.80)). Moderate to high effect sizes reveal the CDIP-58 is good at detecting the impact of botulinum toxin on all eight health dimensions.[28]

Craniocervical Dystonia Questionnaire-24 (CDQ-24)[29]

Purpose The CDQ-24 measures the impact of craniocervical dystonia on five health-related quality of life domains. It was developed for use in clinical research.

Content Twenty-four items, forming five scales: stigma, emotional well-being, pain, activities of daily living, and social/family life. Items are rated on a 5-point scale (18 items based on frequency – never to always; 6 items based on severity – not at all to very severely). High scores indicate worse health.

Psychometric data A 29-item pool was developed based on semi-structured interviews of patients with cervical dystonia (CD) and blepharospasm (BSP). This questionnaire was sent to 203 patients with CD and BSP, resulting in the 24-item version (CDQ-24). Validity and reliability data were assessed in 231 patients with CD and BSP. Internal consistency and reliability: Cronbach's α value range from 0.77 to 0.89. CDQ-24 subscales showed moderate to high correlations with those SF-36 subscales measuring similar aspects (Pearson's correlation $r = 0.50–0.73$; $p < 0.001$, each). Statistical sensitivity to change supported significant improvements of all CDQ-24 subscores in the de-novo patients from baseline to 4-week follow-up.

Functional Disability Questionnaire[30]

Purpose The Functional Disability Questionnaire measures disability due to CD. Four areas are included: social, physical activity, self-care, and leisure activities.

Content There are 27 items, forming four factors: social disability, physical activity, self-care, and leisure activities. Each item is rated on a 4-point scale, ranging from 1 (not affected) to 4 (severely affected). Subscores for each factor are derived by summation of raw scores. High scores indicate worse health.

Psychometric data Reliability and validity have been presented. The scale has been shown to have acceptable internal consistency (Cronbach's $\alpha = 0.92$) and test–retest reliability (ICC = 0.93). Construct validity is supported by principal components analysis (PCA).

Body Concept Scale[30]

Purpose The Body Concept Scale measures the impact of CD on body concept.

Content There are 22 semantic differential scales, forming four factors: speed/strength, postural/movement-related, evaluative/esthetic, and tension. Each item is rated on a 7-interval semantic scale. Subscores for each factor are derived by summation of raw scores. High scores indicate a more negative body concept.

Psychometric data Reliability and validity have been presented. The scale has been shown to have acceptable internal consistency (Cronbach's $\alpha = 0.95$), and test–retest reliability (ICC = 0.87). Construct validity is supported by moderate correlations of the scale and disfigurement ratings and the Beck Depression Inventory (0.44 and 0.41, respectively).

Ways of Coping Checklist[31]

Purpose The Ways of Coping Checklist measures coping in CD and was adapted from an original scale devised by Folkman and Lazarus[32] and revised by Felton et al.[33]

Content There are 64 items, forming six factors: wish-fulfilling fantasy, threat-minimization, negative reappraisal/coping, cognitive restructuring, religious faith, and instrumental coping. Subscores for each factor are derived by summation of raw scores. High scores indicate poorer coping.

Psychometric evaluation Reliability and validity have been presented. The scale has been shown to have acceptable internal consistency (Cronbach's $\alpha = 0.70$). Construct validity supported by principal components analysis.

Freiberg Questionnaire for dystonia (torticollis version)[34]

Purpose The Freiberg Questionnaire measures behavioral aspects of CD.

Content This multi-item questionnaire consists of open-ended, dichotomous, and 5-point response options. Items include medical history, course of disease, previous treatment, current neurologic, and psychosocial changes. The psychosocial changes section includes 23 items, covering five areas (profession, everyday life, social life, family, and psychological well-being).

Psychometric data Reliability and validity have been presented on the psychosocial changes subscale. This scale is shown to have acceptable internal consistency (Cronbach's $\alpha = 0.87$). Construct validity was supported by principal components analysis.

CRITICAL EVALUATION OF DYSTONIA RATING SCALES

Researchers have a number of options when selecting a measure for outcome studies. In order to make recommendations for dystonia scale selection for future studies, current measures were examined to determine how they have been developed and evaluated.

Strengths

Existing dystonia scales cover a wide range of important outcomes, including symptoms, activities of daily living, and aspects of psychosocial functioning, which provide researchers with a good range of alternative measures for different research aims. Measures are either clinician-rated, patient-rated, or a combination of both, which also provides choice in the mode of administration and allows the combination and comparison of clinician and patient ratings. Finally, some psychometric data are presented for each of the scales, providing further useful information for instrument selection.

Weaknesses

There are a number of drawbacks to the majority of existing scales. The main limitations of clinician-rated scales are that they are predominantly observer-dependent and do not incorporate the patient's perspective of physical, psychological, and social health impact of the disorder.[35,36] Therefore, additional patient-report rating scales must be used to overcome this. However, the majority of the patient scales focus on a narrow range of outcomes, primarily on psychological dimensions. Only one disease-specific scale (CDIP-58) has been developed following standard guidelines (i.e. patient-generated item pool, item reduction, and psychometric evaluation)[12,13,20] and fulfils many of the SAC scale evaluation criteria.[12] For the remainder of the measures, the psychometric properties were limited. For example, reliability and validity analyses of the Burke–Fahn–Marsden Scale[24] and TWSTRS[22] were confined to inter-rater reliability and some construct validity.

The lack of appropriately evaluated scales has implications for clinical research. For example, in CD research a number of studies have investigated the treatment effects of botulinum toxin type A (BTX-A),[36–50] botulinum toxin type B (BTX-B),[51–56] drug treatment,[57] and surgery.[58,59] Most studies report improvement, but have either been unable to discriminate between patients,[36] or have described small changes post-treatment.[42,45] However, as none of the CD scales used in these studies had been developed appropriately or been evaluated for responsiveness, it is difficult to disentangle treatment and measurement effects. This poses serious questions about the validity of the findings.

New developments in rating scale assessment

Rating scale use and development in dystonia research is still in its infancy, and only recently have studies been carried out using rigorous methodologies. Despite this, the health measurement field is moving quickly, and techniques applicable to dystonia studies are being developed and advanced. The methods described in this chapter are termed *traditional* psychometric methods and are currently the most commonly used methods of rating scale development and validation.[12,60] It is important that neurologists be familiar with these methods of rating scale evaluation but also be aware of their limitations which restrict the impact of their use in research and routine clinical practice.

From a research perspective, the first limitation of these traditional methods is that raw scores are non-linear counts and not interval measures. This potentially biases the interpretation of scores and score changes, and may result in treatment effectiveness being underestimated.[61,62] A second limitation is that raw scores are scale-dependent. Therefore, different scales purporting to measure the same health construct cannot be accurately equated, or their results combined for systematic reviews and meta-analyses.[63] A third limitation is that the traditional psychometric properties of scales are sample-dependent and, therefore, not necessarily stable across different samples.[64] This means that before using a rating scale in different patient populations, new validation data must first be collected and analyzed. A fourth limitation is that rating scales tend to cover a limited spectrum of quality of life. Samples in clinical studies often extend outside of the range of the scale, resulting in floor and ceiling effects. These represent subsamples of patients for whom health changes will not be detected, or be underestimated by scales.

From a clinical perspective, rating scales developed using traditional psychometric techniques provide raw scores that are not precise enough for individual patient clinical decision-making. Importantly for neurologists, this means that scales developed using such methods are valid for population-based research, but are not necessarily valid as clinical measurement tools for individual patients. Such rating scales cannot be used in routine clinical practice.[65]

These limitations of summed rating scales were recognized some time ago in education and psychology. Research led to the development of Rasch item analysis[66] and Item Response Theory (IRT)[67] models. These new psychometric methods convert raw scores into interval measures using a log odds-ratio transformation.[68] Recently, Rasch methodology has been used in questionnaire development as a means of increasing the clinical utility of new questionnaires for individual patients. There are two clinically relevant issues. First, as a consequence of the mathematics of the model, it is legitimate to sum items to produce total scores and, in turn, the total scores produce interval-level measures from ordinal level rating scale data.[68] Thus, when items (data) fit the model, we can be confident that items can be summed to produce valid total scores, and that we are able to measure consistently across the whole range of disease impact. This improves the accuracy with which clinical change can be measured. Secondly, Rasch analysis provides estimates for patients (and items) that are independent of the sampling distribution of items (and patients). Among other benefits, this allows for accurate estimates suitable for individual person measurement. This can help directly inform upon patient monitoring, management, and treatment.

The latent advantages of this new approach to rating scale development are significant. If neurologists perceive that a 'research questionnaire' also provides useful clinical information regarding an individual patient's outcome, they may be more likely to offer the questionnaire to their patients in the context of prospective studies and clinical trials. Patients, as well, may be more likely to complete questionnaires if they perceive that they are deriving some direct benefit by providing the information. This can improve communication with the patient, allowing the physician to be more effective in addressing the specific issues of a patient. Thus, the clinical utility of a questionnaire that is able to measure health-related quality of life in clinical settings is the potential to improve clinical outcomes for individual patients with dystonia.

Another exciting prospect of these new methods is that by providing information about item performance, not available using traditional psychometric methods, these new techniques can be used to create banks of items with known characteristics.[69] These calibrated item banks lay the foundation for rapid and efficient individual patient measurement using computer algorithms,[70] which in turn opens the door to computer-adaptive testing.[71] In this technique, rather than giving the same set of items to each individual, the items are selected based on the ability level or other characteristics.[72]

CONCLUSIONS AND RECOMMENDATIONS

There is little consistency or comparability in dystonia rating scales used in current research, making meta-analysis difficult. Much of the emphasis is on observer (clinician)-rated scales, which do not often take account of the patient's perspective of the health impact of dystonia. Much of the research into patient-reported outcomes of dystonia is limited, focusing primarily on psychological dimensions of patient well-being. The majority of the dystonia rating scales do not meet the rigorous scientific standards required (i.e. reliability, validity, and responsiveness). Therefore, for future research, the following recommendations can be made:

- Clinician-rated scales: the TWSTRS and the Burke–Fahn–Marsden Dystonia Scale are the most popular measures for dystonia studies, the UDRS and GDS are new scales for general dystonia, but there is a need for new measures to be developed and evaluated following standard guidelines.
- Patient-rated scales: for CD research, the CDIP-58 should be used, as it is the only existing measure to have followed recommended guidelines and have extensive testing using both traditional and new psychometric methods.
- There is a need for more dystonia-specific validated measures to assess the health impact beyond CD, including the effectiveness of treatment.

It is appropriate when designing trials to use both clinician-rated and patient-rated scales to assess new treatments. In the long term, the use of appropriate dystonia rating scales is vital as policy and patient decisions based on outcome studies depend on scientific quality.

REFERENCES

1. McDowell I, Newell C. Measuring Health: A Guide to Rating Scales and Questionnaires. New York: Oxford University Press; 1987.
2. Stevens S. Mathematics, measurement and psychophysics. In: Stevens S, ed. Handbook of Experimental Psychology. New York: Wiley; 1951.
3. Kaska S, Weinstein J. Historical perspective. Ernest Amory Codman, 1869–1940. A pioneer of evidence-based medicine: the end result idea. Spine 1998; 23(5): 629–33.
4. Herndon R. Handbook of Neurologic Rating Scales. New York: Demos Vermande; 1997.
5. Cronbach LJ. Coefficient alpha and the internal structure of tests. Psychometrika 1951; 16: 297–334.
6. Cronbach L, Meehl P. Construct validity in psychol tests. Psychol Bull 1955; 52: 281–301.
7. Campbell D, Fiske D. Convergent and discriminant validation by the multi trait-multimethod matrix. Psychol Bull 1959; 56: 81–105.
8. Katz S, Downs T, Cash H, Grotz R. Progress in development of the index of activities of daily living (ADL). Gerontologist 1976; 10: 20–30.
9. Cleary P. Subjective and objective measures of health: which is better when? J Health Serv Res Policy 1997; 2(7): 3–4.
10. Hobart J. Measuring disease impact in disabling neurological conditions: are patients' perspectives and scientific rigor compatible? Curr Opin Neurol 2002; 15: 721–4.
11. Hobart JC, Lamping DL, Thompson AJ. Evaluating neurological outcome measures: the bare essentials [editorial]. J Neurol Neurosurg Psychiatry 1996; 60(2): 127–30.
12. Scientific Advisory Committee of the Medical Outcomes Trust. Assessing health status and quality of life instruments: attributes and review criteria. Qual Life Res 2002; 11: 193–205.

13. Fitzpatrick R, Davey C, Buxton M, Jones D. Evaluating Patient-Based Outcome Measures for Use in Clinical Trials. Southampton: National Coordinating Centre for Health Technology Assessment; 1998: 1–73.
14. Messick S. Validation of inferences from persons' responses and performances as scientific enquiry into score meaning. Am Psychol 1995; 50(9): 741–9.
15. Deyo RA, Diehr P, Patrick DL. Reproducibility and responsiveness of health status measures. Statistics and strategies for evaluation. Control Clin Trials 1991; 12(4 Suppl): 142S–58s.
16. Bergner M, Rothman ML. Health status measures: an overview and guide for selection. Amu Rev Public Health 1987; 8: 191–210.
17. Wiebe S, Guyatt G, Weaver B, Matijevic S, Sidwell C. Comparative responsiveness of generic and specific quality-of-life instruments. J Clin Epidemiol 2003; 56: 52–60.
18. Dawson J, Fitzpatrick R, Murray D, Carr A. The problem of 'noise' in monitoring patient-based outcomes: generic and disease-specific instruments for total hip replacement. J Health Serv Res Policy 1996; 1: 224–31.
19. Patrick DL, Deyo RA. Generic and disease-specific measures in assessing health status and quality of life. Med Case 1989; 27: S217–32.
20. McDowell I, Jenkinson C. Development standards for health measures. J Health Serv Res Policy 1996; 1(4): 238–46.
21. Consky E, Basinski A, Belle L, Ranawaya R, Lang A. The Toronto Western Spasmodic Torticollis Rating Scale (TWSTRS): assessment of validity and inter-rater reliability. Neurology 1990; 40(Suppl 1): 445.
22. Consky E, Lang A. Clinical assessment of patients with cervical dystonia. In: Jankovic J, Hallett M, eds. Therapy with Botulinum Toxin. New York: Marcel Dekker; 1994: 211–37.
23. Comella C, Leurgans S, Wuu J et al. Rating scales for dystonia: a multicentre assessment. Mov Disord 2003; 18(3): 303–12.
24. Burke R, Fahn S, Marsden C et al. Validity and reliability of a rating scale for the primary torsion dystonias. Neurology 1985; 35: 73–7.
25. Tsui JK, Eisen A, Stoessl AJ, Calne S, Calne DB. Double-blind study of botulinum toxin in spasmodic torticollis. Lancet 1986: 2: 245–6.
26. Cano SJ, Warner TT, Linacre JM et al. Capturing the true burden of dystonia on patients: the Cervical Dystonia Impact Profile (CDIP-58). Neurology 2004: 63(9): 1629–33.
27. Cano SJ, Hobart J, Fitzpatrick R et al. Patient-based outcomes of cervical dystonia: a review of rating scales. Mov Disord 2005; 19: 1054–9.
28. Cano SJ, Hobart JC, Edwards M et al. CDIP-58 can measure the impact of botulinum toxin treatment in cervical dystonia. Neurology 2006; 67: 2230–2.
29. Muller J, Wissel J, Kemmler G et al. Craniocervical dystonia questionnaire (CDQ-24): development and validation of a disease-specific quality of life instrument. J Neurol Neurosurg Psychiatry 2004; 75(5): 749–53.
30. Jahanshahi M, Marsden C. Body concept, disability, and depression in patients with spasmodic torticollis. Behav Neurol 1990; 3: 117–31.
31. Jahanshahi M. Psychosocial factors and depression in torticollis. J Psychosom Res 1991; 35(4–5): 493–507.
32. Folkman S, Lazarus R. An analysis of coping in a middle-aged community sample. J Health Soc Behav 1980; 21: 219–39.
33. Felton B, Revenson T, Hinrichsen G. Stress and coping in the explanation of psychological adjustment among chronically ill adults. Soc Sci Med 1984; 18: 889–98.
34. Scheidt C, Rayki O, Nickel T et al. Spasmodic torticollis – a multicenter study on behavioural aspects I: introduction and methods. Behav Neurol 1996; 9: 25–31.
35. Lindeboom R, de Haan R, Aramideh M, Brans J, Speelman J. Treatment outcomes in cervical dystonia. Mov Disord 1996; 11: 371–6.
36. Lindeboom R, Brans J, Aramideh M, Speelman H, De Haan R. Treatment of cervical dystonia: a comparison of measures for outcome assessment. Mov Disord 1998; 13(4): 706–12.
37. Jahanshahi M, Marsden C. Psychological functioning before and after treatment of torticollis with botulinum toxin. J Neurol Neurosurg Psychiatry 1992; 55: 229–31.
38. Brans J, Lindeboom R, Snoek J et al. Botulinum toxin versus trihexyphenidyl in cervical dystonia: a prospective, randomised, double-blind controlled trial. Neurology 1996; 46: 1066–72.
39. Odergren T, Tollback R, Borg J. Efficacy of botulinum toxin for cervical dystonia. A comparison of methods for evaluation. Scand J Rehabil Med 1994; 26: 191–5.
40. Wissel J, Maguhr F, Schelosky L, Ebersbach G, Poewe W. Quantitative assessment of botulinum toxin treatment in 43 patients with head tremor. Mov Disord 1997; 12: 722–6.
41. Tarsy D. Comparison of clinical rating scales in treatment of cervical dystonia with botulinum toxin. Mov Disord 1997; 12(1): 100–2.
42. Gudex C, Hawthorne M, Butler A, Duffey P. Measuring patient benefit from botulinum toxin in the treatment of dystonia. Pharmacoeconomics 1997; 12(6): 675–84.
43. Brans J, Lindeboon R, Aramideh M, Speelman J. Long-term effect of botulinum toxin on impairment and functional health in cervical dystonia. Neurology 1998; 50: 1461–3.
44. Odergren T, Hjaltason H, Kaakkola S et al. A double blind, randomised, parallel group study to investigate the dose equivalence of Dysport and Botox in the treatment of cervical dystonia. J Neurol Neurolsurg Psychiatry 1998; 64(1): 6–12.
45. Gudex C, Hawthorne M, Butler A, Duffey P. Effect of dystonia and botulinum toxin treatment on health related quality of life. Mov Disord 1998; 13(6): 941–6.
46. Brefel-Courbon C, Simonetta-Moreau M, More C et al. A pharmacoeconomic evaluation of botulinum toxin in the treatment of spasmodic torticollis. Clin Neuropharmacol 2000; 23(4): 203-7.
47. Wissel J, Kanovsky P, Ruzicka E et al. Efficacy and safety of a standardised 500 unit dose of Dysport (Clostridium botulinum toxin type A haemaglutinin complex) in a heterogeneous cervical dystonia population: results of a prospective, multicentre, randomised, double-blind, placebo-controlled, parallel group study. J Neurol 2001; 248: 1073–8.
48. Muller J, Kemmler G, Wissel J et al. The impact of blepharospasm and cervical dystonia on health-related quality of life and depression. J Neurol 2002; 249(7): 842–6.
49. Naumann M, Yakovleff A, Durif F. A randomized, double-masked, crossover comparison of the efficacy and safety of botulinum toxin type A produced from the original bulk toxin source and current bulk toxin source for the treatment of cervical dystonia. J Neurol 2002; 249(1): 57–63.
50. Ranoux D, Gury C, Fondarai J, Mas J, Zuber M. Respective potencies of Botox and Dysport: a double blind, randomised, crossover study in cervical dystonia. J Neurol Neurosurg Psychiatry 2002; 72(4): 459–62.
51. Truong D, Cullis P, O'Brien C et al. BotB (Botulinum toxin type B): evaluation of safety and tolerability in botulinum toxin type A-resistant dystonia patients (preliminary study). Mov Disord 1997; 12(5): 772–5.
52. Lew M, Adornato B, Duane D et al. Botulinum toxin type B: a double-blind placebo-controlled, safety and efficacy study in cervical dystonia. Neurology 1997; 49: 701–7.
53. Brashear A, Lew M, Dyskstra D et al. Safety and efficacy of NeuroBloc (botulinum toxin type B) in type A-responsive cervical dystonia. Neurology 1999; 53: 1439–46.
54. Brin M, Lew M, Adler C et al. Safety and efficacy and NeuroBloc (botulinum toxin type B) in type A-resistant cervical dystonia. Neurology 1999; 53: 1431–8.
55. Lew M, Brashear A, Factor S. The safety and efficacy of botulinum toxin type B in the treatment of patients with cervical

dystonia: summary of the three controlled clinical trials. Neurology 2000; 55(12-Suppl 5): S29–35.

56. Lew M. Botulinum type B: an effective treatment of alleviating pain associated with cervical dystonia. J Back Musculoskeletal Rehabil 2002; 16(1): 3–9.
57. Muller J, Wenning G, Wissel J et al. Riluzole therapy in cervical dystonia. Mov Disord 2002; 17(1): 198–200.
58. Krauss J, Toups E, Jankovic J, Grossman R. Symptomatic and functional outcome of surgical treatment of cervical dystonia. J Neurol Neurosurg Psychiatry 1997; 63: 642–8.
59. Ford B, Louis E, Greene P, Fahn S. Outcome of selective ramisectomy for botulinum toxin resistant torticollis. J Neurol Neurosurg Psychiatry 1998; 65(4): 472–8.
60. Hobart J, Lamping D, Freeman J et al. Evidence-based measurement – which disability scale for neurologic rehabilitation? Neurology 2001; 57: 639–44.
61. Wright BD, Linacre JM. Observations are always ordinal; measurements, however, must be interval. Arch Phys Med Rehabil 1989; 70: 857–60.
62. Wright BD. Fundamental measurement for outcome evaluation. In: Smith RM, ed. Physical Medicine and Rehabilitation: State of the Art Reviews. Philadelphia: Hanley & Belfus; 1997: 261–88.
63. Bjorner JB, Ware JEJ. Using modern psychometric methods to measure health outcomes. Med Outcomes Trust Monitor 1998; 3(2): 1–5.
64. McHorney CA, Ware JEJ, Lu JFR, Sherbourne CD. The MOS 36-Item Short-Form Health Survey (SF-36): III. Tests of data quality, scaling assumptions and reliability across diverse patient groups. Med Care 1994; 32(1): 40–66.
65. McHorney CA, Tarlov AR. Individual-patient monitoring in clinical practice: are available health status surveys adequate? Qual Life Res 1995; 4: 293–307.
66. Rasch G. Probabilistic Models for Some Intelligence and Attainment Tests. Copenhagen: Danish Institute for Educational Research; 1960.
67. Lord FM, Novick MR. Statistical Theories of Mental Test Scores. Reading, MA: Addison-Wesley; 1968.
68. Wright B, Stone M. Best Test Design: Rasch Measurement. Chicago: MESA Press; 1979.
69. Wright B. Solving measurement problems with the Rasch model. J Educ Measure 1977; 14(2): 97–116.
70. Wainer H, Dorans NJ, Flaugher R et al, eds. Computerized Adaptive Testing: A Primer. Hillsdale, New Jersey: Lawrence Erlbaum Associates; 1990.
71. Revicki DA, Cella DF. Health status assessment for the twenty-first century: item response theory, item banking and computer adaptive testing. Qual Life Res 1997; 6(6): 595–600.
72. Linacre J. Computer-adaptive testing: a methodology whose time has come. In: Chae S, Kang U, Jeon E, Linacre J, eds. Development of Computerised Middle School Achievement Tests. Seoul: Komesa Press; 2000.

Index

Page references to *figures, tables and boxes* are shown in *italics*. Genes and genetic loci have been grouped in the index.